Comprehensive Review in Clinical Neurology

A Multiple Choice Question Book for the Wards and Boards

ESTEBAN CHENG-CHING, M.D.
Clinical Associate
Cleveland Clinic Neurological Institute
Department of Neurology
Cleveland, Ohio

LAMA CHAHINE, M.D.
Fellow
Parkinson's Disease and Movement
Disorders Center
University of Pennsylvania
Philadelphia, Pennsylvania

ERIC P. BARON, D.O.
Staff
Cleveland Clinic Neurological
Institute
Center for Headache and Pain
Center for Regional Neurology
Cleveland, Ohio

ALEXANDER RAE-GRANT, M.D.
Staff
Cleveland Clinic Neurological
Institute
Mellen Center for Multiple Sclerosis
Treatment and Research
Cleveland Clinic Lou Ruvo Center for
Brain Health
Cleveland, Ohio

Wolters Kluwer | Lippincott Williams & Wilkins
Health
Philadelphia · Baltimore · New York · London
Buenos Aires · Hong Kong · Sydney · Tokyo

Acquisitions Editor: Frances Destefano
Product Manager: Tom Gibbons
Vendor Manager: Alicia Jackson
Senior Manufacturing Manager: Benjamin Rivera
Marketing Manager: Brian Freiland
Creative Director: Doug Smock
Production Service: Aptara, Inc.

© 2011 by LIPPINCOTT WILLIAMS & WILKINS, a WOLTERS KLUWER business
Two Commerce Square
2001 Market Street
Philadelphia, PA 19103 USA
LWW.com

Printed in China

Library of Congress Cataloging-in-Publication Data
Cheng-Ching, Esteban, author.
Comprehensive review in clinical neurology : a multiple choice question book for the wards and boards / Esteban Cheng-Ching, M.D., Department of Neurology, Cleveland Clinic, Cleveland, Ohio, Lama Chahine, M.D., Eric Baron, D.O., Alexander Rae-Grant, M.D.
    p. ; cm.
Includes bibliographical references and index.
    ISBN 978-1-60913-348-1 (pbk. : alk. paper)   1. Nervous system–Diseases–Examinations, questions, etc.   2. Neurology–Examinations, questions, etc.   I. Chahine, Lama, author. II. Baron, Eric (Eric P.), author.   III. Rae-Grant, Alexander, author.   IV. Title.
    [DNLM: 1. Nervous System Diseases–Examination Questions.   2. Clinical Medicine–methods–Examination Questions. WL 18.2]
RC356.C44 2011
616.80076—dc22
                                                                                    2010054296

Care has been taken to confirm the accuracy of the information presented and to describe generally accepted practices. However, the authors, editors, and publisher are not responsible for errors or omissions or for any consequences from application of the information in this book and make no warranty, expressed or implied, with respect to the currency, completeness, or accuracy of the contents of the publication. Application of the information in a particular situation remains the professional responsibility of the practitioner.

The authors, editors, and publisher have exerted every effort to ensure that drug selection and dosage set forth in this text are in accordance with current recommendations and practice at the time of publication. However, in view of ongoing research, changes in government regulations, and the constant flow of information relating to drug therapy and drug reactions, the reader is urged to check the package insert for each drug for any change in indications and dosage and for added warnings and precautions. This is particularly important when the recommended agent is a new or infrequently employed drug.

Some drugs and medical devices presented in the publication have Food and Drug Administration (FDA) clearance for limited use in restricted research settings. It is the responsibility of the health care providers to ascertain the FDA status of each drug or device planned for use in their clinical practice.

To purchase additional copies of this book, call our customer service department at (800) 638-3030 or fax orders to (301) 223-2320. International customers should call (301) 223-2300.

Visit Lippincott Williams & Wilkins on the Internet: at LWW.com. Lippincott Williams & Wilkins customer service representatives are available from 8:30 am to 6 pm, EST.

10 9 8 7 6 5 4 3 2

Preface

Anyone who studies neurology immediately recognizes not only its fascinating complexities but also the many different types of learning skills that one calls upon to understand it and commit it to memory. As medical students rotating in neurology, and later as neurology residents and fellows, it was clear to us that while there were great and grand neurology textbooks written by giants in the field, a study guide that offered clear explanations, simplifying complex concepts, and presenting information in an easily understandable format, while allowing for study of large amounts of information in a timely manner, was not available. As our board examinations neared, we were unable to identify a board review book that satisfied the minimum criteria for what we felt was the ideal study guide: comprehensive yet concise, case-based, with an abundance of images and diagrams, and perhaps most importantly, a question-and-answer (Q&A) multiple-choice type format. As chief residents organizing board review sessions for our neurology resident colleagues, we found this format to be the most effective and enjoyable way to learn neurology. With these criteria in mind, we envisioned and set out to write *Comprehensive Review in Clinical Neurology*.

In neurology perhaps more than any other specialty, clinical vignettes increase learning efficiency by illustrating examples and placing sometimes challenging neuroscience concepts into clinical practice. With this in mind, the majority of questions in this book are case-based. A multitude of radiographic and pathologic images are carefully selected to supplement information in the cases while also contributing to knowledge of these respective areas. The anatomic diagrams and other graphics provide visual aids to consolidate information presented in the discussions. The book is organized so that the reader can review chapters in their entirety or select individual questions from each chapter for review. Despite the Q&A format, topical review is possible with this book as well: the chapters are organized by topics, the index is comprehensive, and most importantly, reference is made in the discussion to different questions related to a specific concept. This book is strengthened by the renowned specialists who painstakingly reviewed the chapters and contributed valuable suggestions and images.

We feel that *Comprehensive Review in Clinical Neurology* will be useful to the whole spectrum of those learning neurology, from medical students and junior residents beginning their neurology education to senior neurology residents and fellows studying for the neurology board examination, and even to staff physicians reviewing for maintenance-of-certification examinations. Because neurology is a key component of all specialties related to neuroscience, psychiatrists, neurosurgeons, geriatricians, and psychologists will benefit from this book as well. We hope that readers of this book will enjoy it and learn from it.

Esteban Cheng-Ching
Lama Chahine
Eric Baron
Alexander Rae-Grant

Acknowledgments

We thank our colleagues in neurology, for whom this book is written; our patients, who make this book necessary; and our families, who have made this book possible.

To my parents and brothers, for showing me the path to follow.
To my wife Catalina, for your love and support ... always ...

Esteban

To my parents, for everything you have done for me, and to my sisters, family members, and friends. Thank you for all the support over the years.

Lama

Thanks to my wife Jen for continuous support and patience during the writing of this book. Thanks also to my mom, dad, brother and family for molding me into who I am today.

Eric

Personal thanks to Drs. Cheng-Ching, Chahine, and Baron, who goaded this book into existence, and to my family, Mary Bruce, Michael, Tucker, George, and Sasha.

Alex

Many thanks to the experts who contributed their time and efforts to the review of this book:

Cranial Nerves and Neuro-ophthalmology—Dr. Gregory Kosmorsky, Dr. Neil Cherian, and Dr. Richard Drake

Vascular Neurology—Dr. Ken Uchino

Neurocritical Care—Dr. Edward Manno

Headache—Dr. Stewart Tepper and Dr. Jennifer Kriegler

Adult and Pediatric Epilepsy and Sleep—Dr. Andreas Alexopoulos and Dr. Charles Bae

Movement Disorders – Dr. Krishe Menezes

Neuro-oncology—Dr. Glen Stevens

Neuromuscular I (Neurophysiology, Plexopathy, and Neuropathy)—Dr. Robert Shields, Dr. Jinny Tavee, Dr. David Polston, and Dr. Steven Shook

Neuromuscular II (Adult and Pediatric Muscle, Autonomic Nervous System, and Neuromuscular Junction Disorders)—Dr. Lan Zhou and Dr. Robert Shields

Neuromuscular III (Disorders of the Spinal Cord and Motor Neurons)—Dr. Richard Lederman and Dr. Erik Pioro

Cognitive and Behavioral Neurology—Dr. Michael Parsons

Psychiatry—Dr. Mayur Pandya

Child Neurology—Dr. David Rothner, Dr. Gary Hsich, and Dr. Sumit Parikh

Infectious Diseases of the Nervous System—Dr. Carlos Isada

Neurologic Complications of Systemic Diseases and Pregnancy—Dr. Rami Khoriaty

Nutritional and Toxic Disorders of the Nervous System—Dr. Edward Covington

Abbreviations

ACA	Anterior cerebral artery
ACTH	Adrenocorticotropic hormone
AED	Antiepileptic drug
AIDS	Acquired immunodeficiency syndrome
AMPA	Alpha-amino-3-hydroxyl-5-methyl-4-isoxazole-propionate
ANA	Anti-nuclear antibodies
ATP	Adenosine triphosphate
BPM	Beats per minute
CJD	Creutzfeld-Jakob disease
cm	Centimeter
CMAP	Compound motor action potential
CNS	Central nervous system
CSF	Cerebrospinal fluid
CT	Computed tomography
DLB	Dementia with Lewy bodies
DNA	Deoxyribonucleic acid
DWI	Diffusion weighted imaging
ECA	External carotid artery
EEG	Electroencephalogram
EMG	Electromyography
ESR	Erythrocyte sedimentation rate
FDA	Food and drug administration
FDG	Fluoro-deoxy-glucose
FLAIR	Fluid attenuated inversion recovery
FTD	Frontotemporal dementia
GABA	Gamma-aminobutyric acid
GTP	Guanosine triphosphate
HIV	Human immunodeficiency virus
HSV	Herpes simplex virus
HTLV	Human lymphotrophic virus
Hz	Hertz
ICA	Internal carotid artery
ICP	Intracranial pressure
ICU	Intensive care unit
INR	International normalized ratio
L	Liter
MCA	Middle cerebral artery
μL	Microliter
mEq	Milliequivalents
mL	Milliliter
MLF	Medial longitudinal fasciculus
mm Hg	Millimiter of mercury
mm	Millimiter
MR	Magnetic resonance
MRA	Magnetic resonance angiogram
MRI	Magnetic resonance image
MRV	Magnetic resonance venogram
ms	Milliseconds
NCS	Nerve conduction studies
NMDA	N-methyl-D-aspartic acid
NSAID	Non-steroidal anti-inflammatory drugs
PCA	Posterior cerebral artery
PCR	Polymerase chain reaction
PET	Positive emission tomography
PPRF	Paramedian pontine reticular formation
RBC	Red blood cell count
REM	Rapid eye movements
RNA	Ribonucleic acid
SAH	Subarachnoid hemorrhage
SNAP	Sensory nerve action potential
STIR	Short TI inversion recovery
TIA	Transient ischemic attack
VDRL	Venereal disease research laboratory
WBC	White blood cell count
WHO	World Health Organization

Contents

Chapter 1

Cranial Nerves and Neuro-ophthalmology

Questions

Questions 1–3

1. Which of the following represents the actions of the superior oblique muscle?
    a. The primary action is eye elevation and secondary action is intorsion
    b. The primary action is eye depression and secondary action is extorsion
    c. The primary action is eye elevation and secondary action is extorsion
    d. The primary action is eye depression and secondary action is intorsion
    e. The primary action is eye depression and secondary action is adduction

2. Which of the following represents the actions of the inferior rectus muscle?
    a. The primary action is eye elevation and secondary action is extorsion
    b. The primary action is eye depression and secondary action is extorsion
    c. The primary action is eye elevation and secondary action is intorsion
    d. The primary action is eye depression and secondary action is adduction
    e. The primary action is eye depression and secondary action is intorsion

3. Which of the following muscles is not innervated by the oculomotor nerve?
    a. Superior rectus
    b. Inferior oblique
    c. Lateral rectus
    d. Inferior rectus
    e. Medial rectus

Questions 4–6

4. A 58-year-old man presents with a left-sided headache and neck pain that occurred during weight lifting. He was concerned because he felt like his left eye was "droopy." On examination, you confirm that he has slight ptosis of the left eye. What is the cause of this finding?
    a. Overactivity of the parasympathetics
    b. Impairment in oculomotor nerve function

    c. Underactivity of the sympathetics
    d. Underactivity of the parasympathetics
    e. Overactivity of the sympathetics

5. Which of the following is not a known association with this disorder?
    a. Depression of the left lower eyelid
    b. Miosis of the left pupil
    c. Depression of the left upper eyelid
    d. Left-sided facial anhidrosis
    e. Enophthalmos of the left eye

6. During your examination, you attempt to better localize the extent of the lesion. Which of the following findings would suggest that the lesion is proximal to the carotid bifurcation?
    a. Depression of the left upper eyelid
    b. Left-sided facial anhidrosis
    c. Miosis of the left pupil
    d. Elevation of the left lower eyelid
    e. Enophthalmos of the left eye

Questions 7–10

7. You are consulted on a 76-year-old man who is referred for right eyelid ptosis and right pupillary constriction. He also mentions that when he exerts himself, he notices that the right side of his face does not seem to sweat like the left side. Using this information, which of the following would not be a probable cause for these symptoms?
    a. A tumor affecting C8-T2 spinal levels
    b. A lesion between hypothalamus and ciliospinal center of Budge
    c. Tumor in the right lung apex
    d. Large hematoma formation under the subclavian artery following attempted central line placement
    e. Internal carotid dissection involving the midcervical region

8. Which of the following is false regarding the sympathetic pathway to the orbit and face?
    a. The oculosympathetic fibers travel with the ophthalmic division of the trigeminal nerve (V1) to the orbit
    b. The sympathetic fibers arise from the posterior thalamus
    c. The ciliospinal center of Budge is located at spinal levels C8 to T2
    d. The vasomotor and sweat fibers travel to the face along the ECA
    e. The superior cervical ganglion is located near the level of the carotid bifurcation

9. You are determined to further try to localize the lesion. After placing 4% cocaine eye drops in his eyes, you notice that the left eye dilates further, whereas the right eye remains unchanged. Which of the following can be definitively concluded on the basis of this finding?
    a. The lesion lies between the second- and third-order sympathetic neurons of the right eye
    b. There is sympathetic denervation to the right eye
    c. The lesion lies between the first- and second-order sympathetic neurons of the right eye
    d. The lesion lies between the first- and second-order sympathetic neurons, and third order sympathetic neurons of the right eye
    e. This finding is nonconfirmatory of a Horner's syndrome

10. You next use 1% hydroxyamphetamine eye drops to help you localize the lesion further. After instillation, both pupils dilate. Which of the following can be definitively concluded on the basis of this finding?
    a. The lesion involves the third-order sympathetic neurons of the right eye
    b. This finding disproves the presence of a true Horner's syndrome
    c. The lesion lies between the second- and third-order sympathetic neurons of the right eye
    d. The lesion lies between the first- and third-order sympathetic neurons of the right eye
    e. The lesion is proximal and does not involve the third-order sympathetic neurons of the right eye

Questions 11–14

11. A 61-year-old woman with a history of diabetes, hyperlipidemia, and hypertension presents to the emergency department with double vision that she woke up with this morning. On examination, you find that she has a complete left oculomotor nerve palsy with intact pupillary function. Which of the following is the most likely cause of her examination findings?
    a. Myasthenia gravis
    b. Brainstem infarction involving the midbrain
    c. Diabetic oculomotor nerve palsy
    d. Aneurysmal compression of the oculomotor nerve
    e. Neoplastic infiltration of the oculomotor nerve

12. Which of the following is false regarding the oculomotor nuclear complex?
    a. The inferior rectus subnucleus innervates the ipsilateral inferior rectus muscle
    b. The superior rectus subnucleus innervates the contralateral superior rectus muscle
    c. The inferior oblique subnucleus innervates the contralateral inferior oblique muscle
    d. A single lesion to the levator palpebrae superioris nucleus will result in bilateral ptosis
    e. The medial rectus subnucleus innervates the ipsilateral medial rectus muscle

13. Which of the following is true regarding the course of the oculoparasympathetic innervation of the eye?
    a. The parasympathetic fibers travel on the peripheral aspect of the ophthalmic division of the trigeminal nerve (V1)
    b. The parasympathetic fibers travel on the peripheral aspect of the oculomotor nerve
    c. The parasympathetic fibers travel together with the sympathetic fibers along the oculomotor nerve
    d. The parasympathetic fibers travel on the central aspect of the ophthalmic division of the trigeminal nerve (V1)
    e. The parasympathetic fibers travel on the central aspect of the oculomotor nerve

14. Which of the following is false regarding the pupillary light response and oculoparasympathetic pathways?
    a. The lateral geniculate body is not involved in the afferent pathway of the pupillary light response
    b. The efferent pathway of the pupillary light response begins in the Edinger–Westphal nucleus
    c. Each pretectal nucleus receives light input from the contralateral visual hemifield
    d. The preganglionic parasympathetic fibers originate from the pretectal nuclei
    e. The ciliary muscle is activated for accommodation, resulting from increased curvature of the lens

4 Chapter 1

Questions 15–17

15. A 9-year-old girl presented to your office with complaints of diplopia. This began after she had a bad fall off her bicycle, hitting her head. On the basis of the directions of gaze noted on your examination, and shown in Figure 1.1, what nerve is involved?

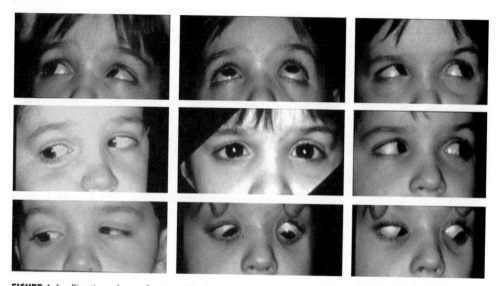

FIGURE 1.1   Directions of gaze. Courtesy of Dr. Gregory Kosmorsky. Shown also in color plates

    a. Right trochlear nerve
    b. Left trochlear nerve
    c. Right abducens nerve
    d. Left abducens nerve
    e. Left oculomotor nerve

16. In this type of nerve lesion, which of the following corrective head positions would be expected to lessen the severity of diplopia?
    a. Head tilted left
    b. Head tilted forward (flexion)
    c. Head rotated left
    d. Head tilted right
    e. Head rotated right

17. Which of the following is true regarding the course and innervation of this nerve?
    a. The motor neurons that this nerve originates from innervate the ipsilateral superior oblique muscle
    b. The motor neurons that this nerve originates from innervate the contralateral inferior oblique muscle
    c. This nerve passes between the posterior cerebral and superior cerebellar arteries
    d. This nerve has the shortest intracranial course
    e. The axons from this nerve decussate prior to exiting ventrally at the level of the midbrain

Questions 18–19

18. A 68-year-old woman with diabetes, hypertension, and hyperlipidemia presents to your office for diplopia. Her extraocular motor examination is seen in Figure 1.2. On pupillary examination, you note that her right pupil is dilated and nonreactive. Which of the following nerves is affected?

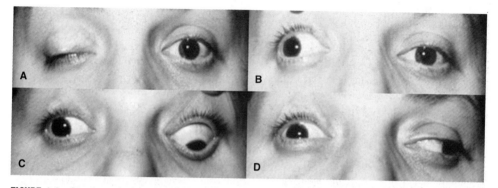

FIGURE 1.2 Directions of gaze. Courtesy of Dr. Gregory Kosmorsky. Shown also in color plates. **A,** looking forward in primary gaze; **B,** looking forward in primary gaze with right eyelid lifted; **C,** looking down; **D,** looking left

    a. Right oculomotor nerve
    b. Left oculomotor nerve
    c. Right abducens nerve
    d. Left abducens nerve
    e. Right trochlear nerve

19. Which of the following would be the least likely cause of this patient's findings?
    a. Aneurysm of the basilar tip
    b. Aneurysm of the PCA
    c. Aneurysm of the SCA
    d. Aneurysm of the PICA
    e. Aneurysm of the Pcomm

Questions 20–22

20. A 42-year-old woman with a history of multiple sclerosis presents for a complaint of recent onset of diplopia, especially when she looks to the right. On examination, you find that on right lateral gaze she has impaired adduction of the left eye and nystagmus of the abducted right eye. Where do you suspect this lesion is localized?
    a. Left PPRF
    b. Left MLF
    c. Left MLF and left PPRF
    d. Right MLF
    e. Right PPRF

21. Your patient returns 2 weeks later with complaints of diplopia in all directions of gaze. On examination, you find that she now has exotropia of both eyes on primary gaze and no voluntary horizontal adduction. Where do you localize her findings to?

a. Left MLF and right PPRF
b. Bilateral PPRFs
c. Right MLF and right PPRF
d. Bilateral abducens nucleus
e. Right and left MLF

22. Three months after treatment with pulse corticosteroid therapy and return of normal extraocular function, your patient presents to you again with new ocular complaints. On examination, you find that she has no horizontal movements of the right eye and only has abduction of the left eye associated with nystagmus. Where do you localize her current findings to?
a. Right abducens nucleus and left MLF
b. Right PPRF
c. Left PPRF and right MLF
d. Right abducens nucleus and right MLF
e. Bilateral MLF

23. Which of the following cranial nerves would most likely be affected in a patient presenting to your office with papilledema, headache, and significant obstructive hydrocephalus?
a. Facial nerve
b. Trochlear nerve
c. Abducens nerve
d. Trigeminal nerve
e. Oculomotor nerve

Questions 24–25

24. A 34-year-old woman with diabetes presents to your office complaining of mild left eye ache and an increased left pupil size that she noticed in the mirror yesterday. On examination, you find that her right pupil reacts normally to light, but her left pupil is nonreactive to direct and consensual light, or to accommodation. What do you suspect as the likely cause?
a. Argyll–Robertson pupil from neurosyphilis
b. Optic neuritis
c. Aneurysmal compression of oculomotor nerve
d. Tonic (Adie's) pupil
e. Diabetic cranial neuropathy

25. In the chronic stage of this disease process, which of the following pupillary findings are most often seen?
a. Miotic with intact pupillary light response, but minimal-to-absent accommodation
b. Miotic with minimal-to-absent pupillary light response and minimal-to-absent accommodation
c. Mydriatic with minimal-to-absent pupillary light response, but intact accommodation
d. Mydriatic with minimal-to-absent pupillary light response and minimal-to-absent accommodation
e. Miotic with minimal-to-absent pupillary light response, but intact accommodation

Questions 26–28

26. A 29-year-old woman with a history of hypertension presents with complaints of right eye pain on eye movement, impaired and blurry vision, and the feeling that some colors "don't look right." On examination, you notice that her right pupil is poorly responsive to direct light, but responds briskly on consensual response light stimulation of the left eye. Her visual acuity is significantly impaired in the right eye, as is red color perception. Which of the following is not a possible cause of this finding?

a. Bilateral asymmetric optic nerve disease
b. Severe macular disease
c. Optic chiasm involvement
d. Right optic nerve disease
e. Right lateral geniculate body lesion

27. Her fundoscopic examination of the right eye is shown in Figure 1.3. What diagnosis do you suspect?

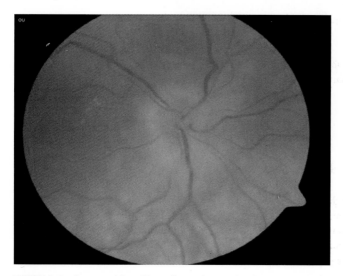

FIGURE 1.3   Courtesy of Anne Pinter. Shown also in color plates

a. Papilledema
b. Giant cell arteritis
c. Posterior ischemic optic neuropathy
d. Acute optic neuritis
e. Anterior ischemic optic neuropathy

28. A brain MRI with contrast confirms your suspicion. Which of the following would be the most appropriate next course of treatment?

a. Oral prednisone taper
b. Intravenous methylprednisolone followed by an oral prednisone taper
c. Observation, initiate treatment at the next episode
d. Begin interferon therapy
e. Begin plasma exchange

29. A 52-year-old man with diabetes, hypertension, and hyperlipidemia presents with severe painless visual blurring and "cloudiness" in the left eye which he woke with this morning. The fundoscopic examination findings of the left eye are shown in Figure 1.4. What diagnosis do you suspect?

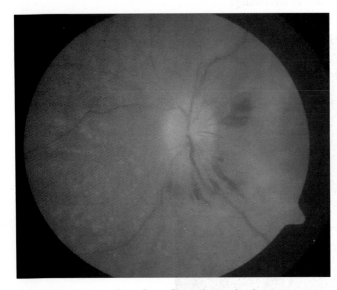

FIGURE 1.4   Courtesy of Anne Pinter. Shown also in color plates

a. Acute optic neuritis
b. Giant cell arteritis
c. Posterior ischemic optic neuropathy
d. Papilledema
e. Anterior ischemic optic neuropathy

Questions 30–31

30. A 64-year-old man presents with a right homonymous hemianopia. Which of the following is the most likely localization for this finding?
a. Left upper lip of the calcarine cortex
b. Right optic tract
c. Left parietal lobe
d. Left lateral geniculate body
e. A temporal lobe infarct

31. A 57-year-old woman presents with a left upper quadrantanopsia. Which of the following would be the most likely localization?
a. Right lower bank of the calcarine cortex
b. Right upper bank of the visual cortex
c. Right parietal lobe
d. Left upper bank of the calcarine cortex
e. Left lower bank of the visual cortex

32. A 67-year-old female with a chronic neurologic disease describes a long progressive loss of vision in the left eye greater than the right eye over the past 15 years. Her fundoscopic examination of the left eye is seen in Figure 1.5, and she has a relative afferent pupillary defect in the same eye. What do you suspect as the cause of this finding?

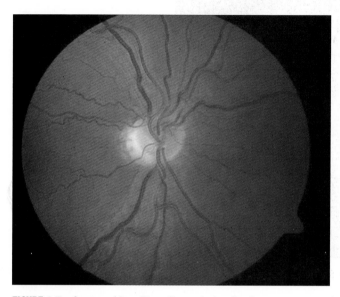

FIGURE 1.5   Courtesy of Anne Pinter. Shown also in color plates

    a. Acute optic neuritis
    b. Papilledema
    c. Posterior ischemic optic neuropathy
    d. Optic atrophy
    e. Anterior ischemic optic neuropathy

33. A 56-year-old male with diabetes presents with 1 week of fever, double vision, and visual blurring. He has proptosis bilaterally, bilateral abduction weakness, visual acuity 20/50 in the right eye and 20/100 in the left, and facial numbness in V2 on the right eye. You suspect the following diagnosis:
    a. Midbrain infarction with hypothalamic hyperthermia
    b. Chronic meningitis with cranial nerve palsies
    c. Cavernous sinus involvement with *mucormycosis*
    d. Diabetic third nerve palsy
    e. Idiopathic cranial polyneuropathy

Questions 34–36

34. A 58-year-old female with a history of hypertension, diabetes, and hyperlipidemia presents to the emergency department for left "facial droop." She woke this morning and noticed unilateral facial paralysis on the left, which was not present the prior night. She also reports hyperacusis in the left ear and says food tastes different. There have been no other new symptoms over the last year of any kind. On examination, you notice left facial droop and inability to close the left eye. She is unable to wrinkle the left side of her forehead. What is the most likely diagnosis?

a. Acute pontine stroke
b. Cholesteatoma
c. Lyme disease
d. Bell's palsy
e. Multiple sclerosis

35. What is the most appropriate diagnostic and/or management strategy at this time?

a. Brain MRI and MRA of circle of Willis
b. Brain CT angiogram
c. Lumbar puncture
d. MRI of the internal auditory canals
e. Observation

36. What initial treatment do you recommend at this time for this patient?

a. Prednisone
b. Doxycycline
c. Otolaryngology consult
d. Referral to a neurosurgeon for peripheral nerve decompression
e. Electric nerve stimulation

37. Which of the following cranial nerves does not have a synapse in the thalamus before terminating in the cortex?

a. Trigeminal nerve
b. Optic nerve
c. Olfactory nerve
d. Vestibulocochlear nerve
e. Facial nerve

38. A 43-year-old man with a history of right-sided Bell's palsy the prior year, who made a good recovery, comes to you complaining of excessive tearing of the right eye, mainly when he is eating. What do you attribute this to?

a. Early recurrence of Bell's palsy
b. Absence of normal facial nerve inhibition of overactivity due to prior damage from Bell's palsy
c. Reinnervation of lacrimal glands by glossopharyngeal nerve axons after facial nerve injury
d. Reinnervation of lacrimal glands by trigeminal nerve axons after facial nerve injury
e. Reinnervation of lacrimal glands by misdirected facial nerve axons

Questions 39–43

39. A 56-year-old woman with hypertension, diabetes, and hyperlipidemia presents to the emergency department with complaints of severe vertigo, unsteadiness, nausea, and vomiting. These symptoms began this morning and she has had several exacerbations since then, each lasting about a minute or so, especially on neck extension. Her examination is normal with exception of nystagmus and nausea brought on by certain head movements. You are trying to decide if her vertigo is central or peripheral in origin. What would be the next step in evaluation of this patient?

a. Brain MRI to evaluate for stroke
b. Brain MRI to evaluate for acoustic schwannoma
c. Dix–Hallpike maneuver
d. Avoiding neck rotation and Dix–Hallpike maneuver until vertebral dissection is ruled out by neck MRI with fat saturation
e. Epley maneuver

40. Which of the following is most suggestive of central vertigo?
a. Suppression of nystagmus by visual fixation
b. Absent nystagmus latency
c. Preserved walking with mild unsteadiness toward one direction
d. Horizontal nystagmus with a torsional component
e. Unilateral decrease in hearing

41. Which of the following is incorrect regarding nystagmus from a peripheral etiology?
a. The fast phase of nystagmus is directed toward the affected side
b. Nystagmus is suppressed by visual fixation
c. Amplitude of nystagmus increases with gaze directed toward the fast phase
d. The slow phase of nystagmus is directed toward the affected side
e. Amplitude of nystagmus increases with gaze directed toward the unaffected side

42. What is the pathophysiology for the disease process you suspect in this patient?
a. Vertebral dissection
b. Acute pontine stroke
c. Acute infarct of vestibular nuclei
d. Canalithiasis
e. Acoustic schwannoma

43. What would be the best initial treatment at this time for this patient?
a. Begin anticoagulation with heparin
b. Referral to neurosurgery for schwannoma resection options
c. Nasogastric tube placement to prevent aspiration until further evaluation is complete
d. Decrease blood pressure to prevent dissection extension
e. Epley maneuver

Questions 44–46

44. Regarding the vestibular sensory organs, which of the following is correct?
a. The ampulla is located within the saccule
b. The otolithic organs are more sensitive to vertical motion of the head
c. The semicircular canals contain otoconia that are involved in detecting motion
d. The ampulla is located within the utricle
e. The semicircular canals are considered otolithic organs

45. Which of the following is correct regarding the vestibuloocular reflex (VOR) when the head is turned to the right side in a purely horizontal plane, while the eyes are focused directly ahead on an object?
a. The right medial rectus would be inhibited
b. The left lateral rectus would be activated
c. The right superior rectus would be inhibited

    d. The left superior oblique would be activated

    e. The right inferior oblique would be activated

46. You are consulted on a comatose 79-year-old man who was found down at home for an unknown amount of time. On the basis of cold calorics, you suspect that he is not brain dead. If the ice water is infused into the left ear canal, which of the following responses would not be expected in a patient with an intact brainstem?

    a. The left lateral rectus is activated

    b. There will be tonic deviation of the eyes to the left

    c. The right lateral rectus is inhibited

    d. The right medial rectus is activated

    e. There will be a slow conjugate movement directed to the right

Questions 47–49

47. Which of the following muscles is not innervated by the trigeminal nerve?

    a. Mylohyoid

    b. Lateral pterygoid

    c. Posterior belly of the digastric

    d. Tensor veli palatini

    e. Tensor tympani

48. Which of the following muscles is not innervated by the facial nerve?

    a. Stapedius

    b. Tensor tympani

    c. Stylohyoid

    d. Posterior belly of the digastric

    e. Buccinator

49. Which of the following muscles is innervated by the glossopharyngeal nerve?

    a. Mylohyoid

    b. Stylopharyngeus

    c. Stylohyoid

    d. Posterior belly of the digastric

    e. Tensor veli palatini

Questions 50–54

50. A 39-year-old woman presents to your office with left-sided facial weakness involving the entire left half of the face. Taste is impaired and sound is excessively loud in her left ear. She denies problems with dry or runny eyes. A lesion in which of the following facial nerve locations could explain these symptoms?

    a. The left facial nerve nucleus

    b. Between the geniculate ganglion and the stapedius nerve

    c. Between the chorda tympani and the stylomastoid foramen

    d. Between the stapedius nerve and the chorda tympani

    e. Between the facial nerve nucleus and the geniculate ganglion

51. If this patient presented with the same symptoms, except that she only had the left facial weakness and taste impairment, without the hearing complaints mentioned above, where would you expect the lesion to be?

a. Between the geniculate ganglia and the stapedius nerve
b. The left facial nerve nucleus
c. Between the facial nerve nucleus and the geniculate ganglia
d. Between the chorda tympani and the stylomastoid foramen
e. Between the stapedius nerve and the chorda tympani

52. Which of the following is true regarding the facial nerve and its branches?
a. The chorda tympani provides parasympathetic innervation to the nasal glands
b. The greater petrosal nerve provides parasympathetic innervation to the lacrimal glands
c. Parasympathetic innervation to the lacrimal glands travels in the ophthalmic (V1) branch of the trigeminal nerve
d. The chorda tympani provides innervation for taste sensation to the posterior one-third of the tongue
e. The pterygopalatine ganglion contains the nerve cell bodies of taste axons for the tongue

53. Which of the following cranial nerve nuclei supplies the parasympathetics to the head and neck?
a. Superior salivatory nucleus
b. Nucleus ambiguus
c. Inferior salivatory nucleus
d. Nucleus solitarius
e. Dorsal motor nucleus of vagus

54. Which of the following glands are not innervated by the facial nerve?
a. Lacrimal glands
b. Nasal mucosal glands
c. Sublingual glands
d. Parotid glands
e. Submandibular glands

Questions 55–57

55. Which of the following cranial nerve nuclei is involved in the sensation of taste?
a. Superior salivatory nucleus
b. Nucleus ambiguus
c. Inferior salivatory nucleus
d. Nucleus tractus solitarius
e. Dorsal motor nucleus of vagus

NTS – both taste & baro reflexes.
(rostral NTS).

56. Which of the following cranial nerve nuclei receives the initial afferent signals in the baroreceptor reflex?
a. Superior salivatory nucleus
b. Nucleus ambiguus
c. Inferior salivatory nucleus
d. Nucleus tractus solitarius   (caudal NTS).
e. Dorsal motor nucleus of vagus

57. Which of the following cranial nerve nuclei innervates the muscles of the pharynx and larynx?
a. Superior salivatory nucleus
b. Nucleus ambiguus

c. Inferior salivatory nucleus
d. Nucleus tractus solitarius
e. Dorsal motor nucleus of vagus

Questions 58–60

58. A 67-year-old male presents with symptoms suspicious for cavernous sinus thrombosis. Which of the following nerves is not located in the cavernous sinus?
a. Mandibular branch of the trigeminal nerve
b. Trochlear nerve
c. Abducens nerve
d. Oculomotor nerve
e. Maxillary branch of the trigeminal nerve

59. Regarding the trigeminal nerve, which of the following is correct?
a. The maxillary division supplies the skin of the lower lip
b. The ophthalmic division innervates the entire cornea
c. The mandibular division provides sensory innervation to the upper teeth
d. The mandibular division provides tactile sensation to the anterior two-thirds of the tongue
e. The trigeminal nerve provides the afferent and efferent limbs of the corneal reflex

60. Regarding the course of the trigeminal nerve from the cranium, which of the following is incorrect?
a. The maxillary division exits through the foramen rotundum
b. The ophthalmic division exits through the superior orbital fissure
c. The ophthalmic and maxillary divisions are the only trigeminal divisions that travel through the cavernous sinus
d. The three divisions of the trigeminal nerve arise from the sphenopalatine ganglion
e. The mandibular division exits through the foramen ovale

61. Which of the following is true regarding the hypoglossal nerve (cranial nerve XII)?
a. A lesion to the hypoglossal nerve causes contralateral tongue deviation on tongue protrusion
b. Corticobulbar input to the hypoglossal nucleus is by crossed innervation only
c. Each genioglossus muscle pulls the tongue anterior and lateral
d. The genioglossus and palatoglossus are the largest hypoglossal-innervated muscles
e. If tongue deviation was due to an upper motor neuron lesion, the deviation would be contralateral to the lesion

62. Which of the following is incorrect regarding the accessory nerve?
a. A lesion in the corticobulbar fibers affects the ipsilateral sternocleidomastoid (SCM)
b. Activation of the accessory nerve causes ipsilateral head rotation
c. A lesion in the corticobulbar fibers affects the contralateral trapezius
d. Activation of the accessory nerve causes ipsilateral head tilt
e. An accessory nerve lesion will cause ipsilateral shoulder drop

63. A 68-year-old man with an extensive history of smoking is hospitalized for aspiration pneumonia. You are consulted for generalized weakness. Besides generalized weakness, you notice that he has a poor gag reflex as well as a slightly lowered left soft palate with mild deviation of the uvula to the right. Which of the following is correct?

a. The afferent limb of the gag reflex is mediated by the vagus nerve
b. This patient has clinical findings of a left glossopharyngeal nerve lesion
c. This patient has clinical findings of a right-sided vagus nerve lesion
d. The efferent limb of the gag reflex is mediated by the glossopharyngeal nerve
e. The gag reflex is mediated by the nucleus ambiguus

Answer Key

1. d	**12.** c	**23.** c	**34.** d	**45.** b	**56.** d
2. b	**13.** b	**24.** d	**35.** e	**46.** e	**57.** b
3. c	**14.** d	**25.** e	**36.** a	**47.** c	**58.** a
4. c	**15.** b	**26.** e	**37.** c	**48.** b	**59.** d
5. a	**16.** d	**27.** d	**38.** e	**49.** b	**60.** d
6. b	**17.** c	**28.** b	**39.** c	**50.** b	**61.** e
7. e	**18.** a	**29.** e	**40.** b	**51.** e	**62.** b
8. b	**19.** d	**30.** d	**41.** a	**52.** b	**63.** e
9. b	**20.** b	**31.** a	**42.** d	**53.** a	
10. e	**21.** e	**32.** d	**43.** e	**54.** d	
11. c	**22.** d	**33.** c	**44.** b	**55.** d	

Answers

1. d, 2. b, 3. c

There are six muscles for each eye: superior oblique, inferior oblique, superior rectus, inferior rectus, medial rectus, and lateral rectus. Each muscle has a primary action and a secondary action (except the medial rectus and lateral rectus, which work only in the horizontal plane). The secondary action of the "superior" muscles is intorsion, whereas that of the "inferior" muscles is extorsion. The primary and secondary actions, respectively, of each muscle are described below:

Superior oblique: Depression/intorsion
Inferior oblique: Elevation/extorsion
Superior rectus: Elevation/intorsion
Inferior rectus: Depression/extorsion
Medial rectus: Adduction
Lateral rectus: Abduction

All extraocular muscles are innervated by the oculomotor nerve except for two: the superior oblique (innervated by the trochlear nerve) and the lateral rectus (innervated by the abducens nerve).

Wilson-Pauwels L, Akesson EJ, Stewart PA, et al. Cranial Nerves in Health and Disease, 2nd ed. Ontario: B.C. Decker Inc., 2002.

4. c, 5. a, 6. b

There are several muscles with varied innervation involved in the resting state of the eyelids, and lesion location will cause different severities of clinical signs. The upper and lower eyelids open and close due to facial nerve innervation of the orbicularis oculi. The levator palpebrae superioris helps with opening of the upper eyelid and is innervated by the oculomotor nerve. Müller's muscle arises from the undersurface of the levator palpebrae superioris, and has sympathetic innervation, contributing to 1 to 2 mm of upper eyelid elevation. The sympathetics also innervate the superior and inferior tarsal muscles that contribute to slight upper eyelid elevation and lower eyelid depression, respectively. Due to the sympathetic innervation of the eyelid muscles, slight over-elevation of the eyelid may be seen in high sympathetic states (such as fear), and subtle ptosis may be seen in low sympathetic states (such as fatigue). In normal patients, the upper eyelid should cover the superior 1 to 1.5 mm of the limbus (junction of the sclera with the cornea), and the lower eyelid should lie at the inferior limbus.

This patient has a left-sided Horner's syndrome due to reduced sympathetic innervation to the left eye. This patient likely has a left internal carotid dissection that has affected the sympathetic fibers running along it. Horner's syndrome is characterized by ptosis of the upper eyelid (due to impaired superior tarsal and Müller's muscles, which normally contribute to upper eyelid elevation and unopposed orbicularis oculi action), slight elevation of the lower eyelid (due to impaired inferior tarsal function, which normally contributes to lower eyelid depression), pupillary miosis (impaired pupillodilator function) and facial anhidrosis (if dissection (or other lesion) extends proximal to the region of the carotid bifurcation, because sweating fibers travel primarily with ECA), and enophthalmos (appearance of enophthalmos from decrease in palpebral fissure).

Beard C. Müller's superior tarsal muscle: Anatomy, physiology, and clinical significance. Ann Plast Surg. 1985; 14:324–333.

Biousse V, Touboul PJ, D'Anglejan-Chatillon J, et al. Ophthalmologic manifestations of internal carotid artery dissection. Am J Ophthalmol. 1998; 126(4):565–577.

7. e, 8. b, 9. b, 10. e

This patient has a classic Horner's syndrome. The sympathetic pathway to the eye is a three-neuron pathway. Horner's syndrome can result from a lesion anywhere along this pathway. The first-order neurons (central neurons) originate in the posterior hypothalamus (not thalamus) and descend through the brainstem to the first synapse, located in the lower cervical and upper thoracic spinal cord (levels C8 to T2). This spinal segment is called the ciliospinal center of Budge. The second-order neurons (preganglionic neurons) exit the spinal cord, travel across the apex of the lung, under the subclavian artery, and ascend the neck and synapse in the superior cervical ganglion, near the bifurcation of the carotid artery at the level of the angle of the mandible. The third-order neurons (postganglionic neurons) travel with the branches of the carotid artery. The vasomotor and sweat fibers branch off at the superior cervical ganglion near the level of the carotid bifurcation and travel to the face with the ECA. The oculosympathetic fibers continue with the ICA, through the cavernous sinus to the orbit, where they then travel with the ophthalmic (V1) division of the trigeminal nerve to their destinations. These pathways are illustrated in Figure 1.6.

Differentiation between causes of Horner's syndrome can be difficult and depends on location along the pathway. In general, a lesion to the first-order neurons (central neurons) will be associated to brainstem or other focal neurologic findings from a central lesion. A second-order (preganglionic) lesion is often associated with lesions of the neck, mediastinum, or lung apex. A third-order (postganglionic) lesion is often associated with pain or headache, caused by conditions such as a skull base tumor, or carotid dissection. Cocaine 4% or 10% eye drops are sometimes used for confirmation of a Horner's syndrome. Cocaine blocks the reuptake of norepinephrine released at the neuromuscular junction of the iris dilator muscle, allowing more local availability of norepinephrine. Following instillation of cocaine, the sympathetically denervated eye will not respond and the anisocoria will become more pronounced. (The Horner's pupil will not change, but the unaffected pupil will become more dilated.) Therefore, in this patient, this test will only confirm the sympathetic denervation and the presence of a Horner's syndrome,

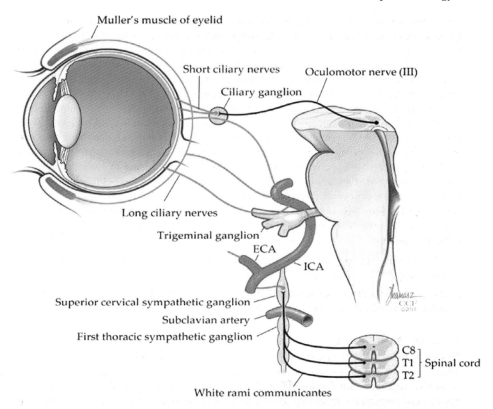

Muller's muscle of eyelid

Short ciliary nerves

Ciliary ganglion

Oculomotor nerve (III)

Long ciliary nerves

Trigeminal ganglion

ECA

ICA

Superior cervical sympathetic ganglion

Subclavian artery

First thoracic sympathetic ganglion

C8
T1 }- Spinal cord
T2

White rami communicantes

FIGURE 1.6 Sympathetic innervation to the eye. ECA; ICA. Illustration by Joseph Kanasz, BFA. Reprinted with permission of the Cleveland Clinic Center for Medical Art and Photography. © 2010. All rights reserved. Shown also in color plates

but will not further localize it. Hydroxyamphetamine 1% eye drops will differentiate between a lesion affecting the first- or second-order neurons from a third-order neuron. There is no pharmacologic test to distinguish between a first- and second-order lesion. Hydroxyamphetamine causes release of stored norepinephrine in the third-order neurons. Following instillation, if the Horner's pupil dilates, the lesion is either first- *or* second order. If the Horner's pupil does not dilate, there is a third-order lesion. This correlates with the finding of anhidrosis on the right face in this patient, consistent with a first- or second-order neuron lesion.

Kardon R. Anatomy and physiology of the autonomic nervous system. In: Walsh and Hoyt Clinical Neuro-ophthalmology, 6th ed, Miller NR, Newman NJ, Biousse V, Kerrison JB (Eds), Baltimore, MD: Williams & Wilkins; 2005; 649–712.

Kardon RH, Denison CE, Brown CK, Thompson HS. Critical evaluation of the cocaine test in the diagnosis of Horner's syndrome. Arch Ophthalmol. 1990; 108:384–387.

Maloney WF, Younge BR, Moyer NJ. Evaluation of the causes and accuracy of pharmacologic localization in Horner's syndrome. Am J Ophthalmol. 1980; 90:394–402.

11. c, 12. c, 13. b, 14. d

Using the findings, this patient most likely has a diabetic cranial nerve palsy involving the oculomotor nerve. A complete pupil-sparing oculomotor nerve palsy without other neurologic findings is most often caused by ischemia to the oculomotor nerve. This is frequently associated with diabetes, especially in the setting of other vascular risk factors. The pupil sparing in diabetic oculomotor nerve palsies is explained on the basis of the anatomy of the nerve itself. The pupillomotor fibers travel along the peripheral aspects of the oculomotor nerve, whereas the somatic fibers to the muscles innervated by the oculomotor nerve travel centrally. The terminal branches of the arterial supply to the nerve are most affected by microvascular changes from diabetes and other risk factors as the vessels decrease in diameter from the periphery of the nerve to the central regions. Therefore, the supply to the periphery of the nerve (where the pupillomotor fibers reside) is spared, whereas the central fibers are affected. Compressive lesions (such as PCA aneurysms) typically affect the peripheral pupillomotor fibers, leading to pupil dilatation with poor response to light (although rarely there may be some pupil sparing).

At the level of the superior colliculus in the dorsal midbrain, there are paired and separate oculomotor subnuclei for the inferior rectus, medial rectus, and inferior oblique—all providing ipsilateral innervation. It is rare for these muscles to be affected in isolation from central lesions without nearby subnuclei also being affected. There is a paired superior rectus subnucleus that provides contralateral innervation. There are paired midline Edinger–Westphal subnuclei providing parasympathetic innervation to the iris sphincters and ciliary muscles. There is also a midline subnucleus providing innervation to both levator palpebrae superioris muscles. Therefore, a lesion to this single midline nucleus can cause bilateral ptosis; it would be rare to affect only this nucleus without affecting nearby structures, so other clinical findings are expected to be present.

The optic pathways are illustrated in Figure 1.7. Afferent neurons beginning in retinal ganglion cells (carrying signals from light stimulation) travel through the optic nerve to the optic chiasm where decussation occurs. Nasal retinal fibers (carrying information from temporal fields) decussate at the chiasm and travel in the contralateral optic tract. Temporal retinal fibers

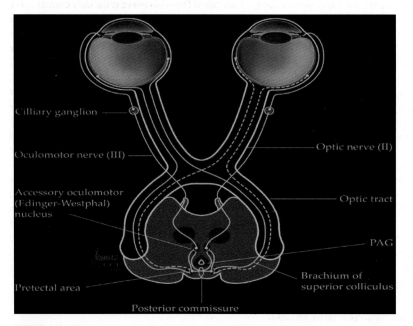

FIGURE 1.7 Pupillary light reflex. Periaqueductal gray (PAG). Illustration by Joseph Kanasz, BFA. Reprinted with permission of the Cleveland Clinic Center for Medical Art and Photography. © 2010. All rights reserved. Shown also in color plates

(carrying information from nasal fields) travel ipsilaterally in the optic tract. In the optic tracts, some neurons project to the ipsilateral lateral geniculate body (for vision) and a few leave the optic tract, ipsilaterally enter the brachium of the superior colliculus, and synapse in the ipsilateral pretectal nuclei (for pupillary response). Therefore, each pretectal nucleus receives light input from the contralateral visual hemifield. From each pretectal nucleus, the afferent fibers travel via interneurons and synapse ipsilaterally and contralaterally in the Edinger–Westphal nuclei, respectively, completing the afferent arm. From the Edinger–Westphal nucleus, efferent preganglionic parasympathetic fibers travel concurrently through the bilateral oculomotor nerves to the ciliary ganglia, which innervate the iris sphincter muscles and the ciliary muscles, resulting in pupillary constriction and ciliary muscle activation that leads to accommodation (for near vision) from increased curvature of the lens.

Myasthenia gravis would present more often with bilateral fatigable ptosis. Neoplastic infiltration would be a slower process. Brainstem infarct would have additional neurologic features.

Brazis PW, Masdeu JC, Biller J. Localization in Clinical Neurology, 5th ed. Philadelphia, PA: Lippincott Williams & Wilkins; 2007.

Leigh RJ, Zee DS. The Neurology of Eye Movements, 3rd ed. New York, NY: Oxford University Press; 2006.

Sanders S, Kawasaki A, Purvin VA. Patterns of extra-ocular muscle weakness in vasculopathic pupil-sparing, incomplete, third nerve palsies. J Neuroophthalmol. 2001; 21:256–259.

Wilson-Pauwels L, Akesson EJ, Stewart PA, et al. Cranial Nerves in Health and Disease, 2nd ed. Ontario: BC Decker Inc; 2002.

15. b, 16. d, 17. c

This patient has a left trochlear nerve palsy (cranial nerve IV). This nerve is the only cranial nerve that exits dorsally from the brainstem. Of note, the trochlear nerves decussate just before they exit dorsally at the level of the inferior colliculi of the midbrain. Therefore, motor neurons from each trochlear nucleus innervate the contralateral superior oblique muscle. After exiting, the trochlear nerve curves ventrally around the cerebral peduncle and passes between the posterior cerebral and superior cerebellar arteries, lateral to the oculomotor nerve. Although it is the smallest nerve, the trochlear nerve has the longest intracranial course due to this dorsal exit, making it more prone to injury, as seen in this patient. The trochlear nerve innervates the superior oblique muscle, which allows for depression and intorsion of the eye, especially when the eye is adducted.

Patients with trochlear nerve palsies may complain of vertical diplopia and/or tilting of objects (torsional diplopia). Because of loss of intorsion and depression from the superior oblique muscle, the affected eye is usually extorted and elevated due to unopposed action of its antagonist, the inferior oblique. Objects viewed in primary position or downgaze may appear double (classically, when going down a flight of stairs). Symptoms of diplopia often improve with head tilting to the contralateral side of the lesion, and the patient adapts to this primary head position to avoid the diplopia. In this patient, vertical and torsional diplopia due to her left trochlear nerve palsy improve with the head tilted toward the right and with the head slightly flexed (chin downward). This occurs because the left eye is in a slightly extorted and elevated position in primary gaze due to the lesion. On tilting right, the right eye must intort, and when it matches the same degree that the left eye is extorted, the diplopia improves.

Brazis PW, Masdeu JC, Biller J. Localization in Clinical Neurology, 5th ed. Philadelphia, PA: Lippincott Williams & Wilkins; 2007.

Wilson-Pauwels L, Akesson EJ, Stewart PA, et al. Cranial Nerves in Health and Disease, 2nd ed. Ontario: BC Decker Inc; 2002.

18. a, 19. d

This patient has a right oculomotor nerve palsy (cranial nerve III) in the classic "down and out" position. Aneurysms involving all the choices except the posteroinferior cerebellar artery (PICA) are the most likely to cause a complete oculomotor nerve palsy with pupillary involvement. The oculomotor nerve and nucleus are discussed in questions 11 to 14. Briefly to review, the oculomotor nerve supplies the levator palpebrae superioris muscles of the eyelid (single central nucleus controls both sides) and four extraocular muscles: medial rectus (ipsilateral nucleus), superior rectus (contralateral nucleus), inferior rectus (ipsilateral nucleus), and inferior oblique (ipsilateral nucleus). The actions of these muscles are discussed in questions 1 to 3, and paresis of the levator palpebrae leads to ptosis. In the setting of an oculomotor palsy, the unopposed actions of the nonparetic muscles innervated by the trochlear and abducens nerve lead to the "down and out" position in primary gaze (as shown in Figure 1.2). The oculomotor nerve also carries the parasympathetic fibers from the Edinger–Westfall nucleus that supply the ciliary muscle and the iris sphincter as detailed in questions 11 to 14. After exiting the brainstem and entering the subarachnoid space, the oculomotor nerve passes between the posterior cerebral and superior cerebellar arteries (near the basilar tip), in proximity to the posterior communicating artery, as well as the uncus of the temporal lobe. Therefore, aneurysms in any of these arteries could potentially cause a compressive lesion of the oculomotor nerve. Uncal herniation also is a classic cause of third nerve palsy, although the patient is often comatose by the time this would occur. As compression occurs, the parasympathetics are often first involved given their peripheral distribution in the nerve, as discussed in question 11.

Brazis PW, Masdeu JC, Biller J. Localization in Clinical Neurology, 5th ed. Philadelphia, PA: Lippincott Williams & Wilkins; 2007.

Wilson-Pauwels L, Akesson EJ, Stewart PA, et al. Cranial Nerves in Health and Disease, 2nd ed. Ontario: BC Decker Inc; 2002.

20. b, 21. e, 22. d

In question 20, this patient has a left internuclear ophthalmoplegia (INO) resulting from a left MLF lesion. INO is characterized by impaired adduction of the affected side and nystagmus of the abducting contralateral eye (the normal side).

The pathways mediating horizontal eye movements are illustrated in Figure 1.8. The PPRF is also known as the conjugate gaze center for horizontal eye movements. The PPRF receives contralateral cortical input. Normally, on horizontal eye movement initiated by the contralateral premotor frontal cortex, the PPRF activates the ipsilateral abducens nerve and, thus, the ipsilateral lateral rectus muscle. From the activated ipsilateral abducens nerve, fibers cross the midline, enter into the contralateral MLF, and activate the contralateral medial rectus subnucleus of the oculomotor complex and, thus, the contralateral medial rectus muscle. The end result is a finely coordinated gaze deviation to one side, with abduction of one eye and adduction of the other.

An INO results from a lesion in the MLF, ipsilateral to the impaired adducting eye, as it runs through the pons or midbrain tegmentum. Patients may complain of horizontal diplopia on lateral gaze, which is not usually present in primary gaze. The classic findings include impaired adduction on lateral gaze (the side of the affected MLF), with nystagmus in the contralateral abducting eye. Slowing of the adducting eye may be a sign of a partial INO, as can be detected on optokinetic nystagmus testing.

There are some important variations of INO. A bilateral INO, due to bilateral MLF lesions, will cause exotropia of both eyes and is known as "wall-eyed bilateral INO" (WEBINO), as

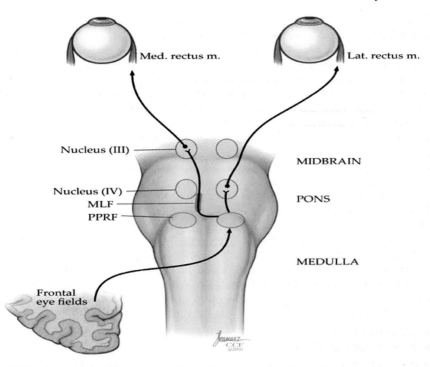

FIGURE 1.8   Pathways of horizontal gaze. MLF, medial longitudinal fasciculus; PPRF, paramedian pontine reticular formation. Illustration by Joseph Kanasz, BFA. Reprinted with permission of the Cleveland Clinic Center for Medical Art and Photography. © 2010. All rights reserved. Shown also in color plates

depicted in question 21. A lesion to both the ipsilateral abducens nucleus or PPRF and ipsilateral MLF results in loss of all horizontal eye movements on that side, and abduction of the contralateral eye is the only lateral eye movement retained (which is also typically associated with abduction nystagmus). This finding is known as the "one-and-a-half syndrome" and is described in question 22.

Brazis PW, Masdeu JC, Biller J. Localization in Clinical Neurology, 5th ed. Philadelphia, PA: Lippincott Williams & Wilkins; 2007.

Frohman EM, Frohman TC, Zee DS, et al. The neuro-ophthalmology of multiple sclerosis. Lancet Neurol. 2005; 4:111–121.

23. C

The abducens nerve (cranial nerve VI) is prone to a stretching injury, especially as it passes over the petrous ridge, and is the most likely nerve to be involved with elevated intracranial pressure. An abducens nerve palsy due to elevated intracranial pressure is often bilateral and is termed a "false localizing sign" because this long cranial nerve could be affected anywhere along its path, and does not necessarily reflect a specific central lesion. The action of the abducens nerve is purely abduction of the eye due to its innervation of the lateral rectus muscle.

Patel SV, Mutyala S, Leske DA, et al. Incidence, associations, and evaluation of sixth nerve palsy using a population-based method. Ophthalmology. 2004; 111(2):369–375.

24. d, 25. e

This patient has an idiopathic tonic (Adie's) pupil. It is thought to result from a lesion in the post-ganglionic parasympathetic pathway to either the ciliary ganglion or the short ciliary nerves and is most often attributed to viral etiology, although evidence is lacking. Acutely, there is unilateral mydriasis and the pupil does not constrict to light or accommodation because the iris sphincter and ciliary muscle are paralyzed. Sectoral palsy of part of the iris sphincter may be involved, and is considered the earliest and most specific feature. Patients often complain of photophobia, visual blurring, and ache in the orbit. Within a few days to weeks, denervation supersensitivity to cholinergic agonists develops and this is most often tested with low-concentration pilocarpine 0.125%, in which the tonic pupil will constrict but the normal pupil is unaffected by the low concentration. Eventually, slow, sustained constriction to accommodation and slow redilation after near constriction occur, and the baseline pupil decreases slightly in size (in ambient light), whereas the other features remain. In general, the chronic stage is characterized by the pupillary light reflex rarely improving, whereas the accommodation reflex does improve, although it often remains slower (tonic). This is termed "light-near dissociation." It is sometimes associated with diminished or absent deep tendon reflexes and this is referred to as "Holmes–Adie syndrome," or Adie's syndrome.

Argyll–Robertson pupils are classically associated with neurosyphilis. They are characterized by bilateral irregular miosis with little to no constriction to light, but constriction to accommodation without a tonic response as opposed to Addie's pupil. Optic neuritis would be associated with a relative afferent pupil defect. An aneurysm would likely have more oculomotor involvement (although not necessarily). Diabetic oculomotor neuropathy is classically associated with pupil sparing, although the appearance of Argyll–Robertson pupils can occur as well.

Brazis PW, Masdeu JC, Biller J. Localization in Clinical Neurology, 5th ed. Philadelphia, PA: Lippincott Williams & Wilkins; 2007.

Loewenfeld IE, Thompson HS. Mechanism of tonic pupil. Ann Neurol. 1981; 10(3):275–276.

Thompson HS, Kardon RH. The Argyll Roberson pupil. J Neuroophthalmol. 2006; 26(2):134–138.

26. e, 27. d, 28. b

This finding is called a relative afferent pupillary defect (RAPD), also known as a Marcus Gunn pupil, and is most commonly caused by a lesion anywhere from the optic nerve to the optic chiasm. In general, retrochiasmal lesions do not cause a pure RAPD. However, a RAPD combined with contralateral hemianopia secondary to an optic tract lesion may occur infrequently. Retinal lesions, refractive errors, amblyopia, and disease of the lens, cornea, and retina do not cause RAPD, although rarely, severe macular disease has been associated with RAPD. The pathway of the pupillary light reflex is discussed in detail in questions 11 to 14. RAPD is frequently seen in optic neuritis. A lesion to the lateral geniculate body would cause a homonymous hemianopia. This structure is involved in vision and not in pupillary responses.

This patient's fundoscopic examination reveals optic nerve edema consistent with optic neuritis. Optic neuritis develops over hours to days and is associated with symptoms of reduced color perception (especially red, called red desaturation), reduced visual acuity (especially central vision), visual loss, eye pain, and photopsias. Only one-third of patients have papillitis with hyperemia and swelling of the disc, blurring of disc margins, and distended veins. The rest of cases have only retrobulbar involvement, and therefore, have a normal fundoscopic examination.

The Optic Neuritis Treatment Trial (ONTT) randomized patients to one of three groups: oral prednisone for 14 days with a 4-day taper versus intravenous methylprednisolone followed by oral prednisone for 11 days with a 4-day taper versus oral placebo for 14 days. The intravenous methylprednisolone group showed faster visual recovery, but at 1 year, visual outcomes were similar. The intravenous methylprednisolone group also had a reduced risk of conversion to multiple sclerosis (MS) within the first 2 years compared with the other groups. At 5 years, there were no differences in the rates of multiple sclerosis between treatment groups though. Interestingly, only the oral prednisone group was found to have a higher 2-year risk of recurrent optic neuritis compared to both the intravenous methylprednisolone and placebo groups. At 10 years, the risk of recurrent optic neuritis was still higher in the oral prednisone group when compared with the intravenous methylprednisolone group, but not the placebo groups.

Papilledema is not present in this fundoscopic examination. An early finding in papilledema is loss of spontaneous venous pulsations, although the absence of spontaneous venous pulsations can also be a normal variant. Disc margin splinter hemorrhages may be seen early also. Eventually, the disc becomes elevated, the cup is lost, and disc margins become indistinct. Blood vessels appear buried as they course the disc. Engorgement of retinal veins lead to a hyperemic disc. As the edema progresses, the optic nerve head appears enlarged and may be associated with flame hemorrhages and cotton wool spots, as a result of nerve fiber infarction. Anterior ischemic optic neuropathy (AION) is discussed in later questions. In giant cell arteritis (GCA), the optic disc is more often pallid, rather than hyperemic.

Beck RW, Cleary PA, Anderson MM Jr, et al. A randomized, controlled trial of corticosteroids in the treatment of acute optic neuritis. The Optic Neuritis Study Group. N Engl J Med. 1992; 326:581–588.

The Optic Neuritis Study Group. The 5-year risk of MS after optic neuritis. Experience of the Optic Neuritis Treatment Trial. Optic Neuritis Study Group. Neurology. 1997; 49:1404–1413.

29. e

This patient has anterior ischemic optic neuropathy (AION). AION is considered to be the most common optic nerve disorder in patients older than age 50. It can also affect the retrobulbar optic nerve in isolation, in which case it is termed posterior ischemic optic neuropathy (diagnosis of exclusion). Patients often have risk factors for cardiovascular and cerebrovascular diseases, such as diabetes and hypertension. AION is a result of ischemic insult to the optic nerve head. Clinically, it presents with acute, unilateral, usually painless visual loss, although 10% of patients may have pain that can be confused with optic neuritis. Fundoscopic examination shows optic disc edema (unless retrobulbar), hyperemia with splinter hemorrhages, and crowded and cupless disc.

The painless vision loss is one key feature in differentiating AION from optic neuritis, which is often associated with painful eye movements. Optic neuritis is discussed in question 26. In addition, optic neuritis presents more often in younger (especially female) patients and may be associated with disc edema (but not always), but without splinter hemorrhages. In contrast to giant cell arteritis (GCA), the optic disc edema in AION is more often hyperemic rather than pallid, as would be more common in GCA. Papilledema is not present in this fundoscopic examination and is discussed in question 26.

Hayreh SS, Zimmerman MB. Nonarteritic anterior ischemic optic neuropathy: Natural history of visual outcome. Ophthalmology. 2008; 115:298–305.

Rucker JC, Biousse V, Newman NJ. Ischemic optic neuropathies. Curr Opin Neurol. 2004; 17:27–35.

30. d, 31. a

The visual pathways are illustrated in Figure 1.9. A right homonymous hemianopia could be caused by a left lateral geniculate body lesion, and a left upper quadrantanopia could be caused by a lesion to the right lower bank of the calcarine cortex. A homonymous hemianopia is caused by lesions of the retrochiasmal visual pathways that consist of the optic tract, lateral geniculate nucleus, optic radiations, and the cerebral visual (calcarine, occipital) cortex. At the optic chiasm, the retinal ganglion afferents from the temporal retina (nasal visual field) continue in the ipsilateral lateral optic chiasm and pass into the ipsilateral optic tract, whereas the retinal ganglion afferents from the nasal retina (temporal visual field) decussate in the optic chiasm and continue into the contralateral optic tract. Therefore, beyond the optic chiasm, each optic tract contains crossed and uncrossed nerve fibers relaying visual information from the contralateral visual field. The optic tracts continue to the lateral geniculate body. Beyond the lateral geniculate body, the optic radiations continue carrying the visual information from the contralateral visual field to the primary visual cortex in the occipital lobe. The superior fibers of the optic radiations carry information from the inferior visual field as they pass through the parietal lobe. The inferior fibers of the optic radiations carry information from the superior visual field as they pass through the temporal lobe, forming Meyer's loop. When this visual information reaches the visual cortex, the upper bank of the calcarine cortex receives projections representing the inferior visual field, whereas the lower bank of the calcarine cortex receives information representing the superior visual field.

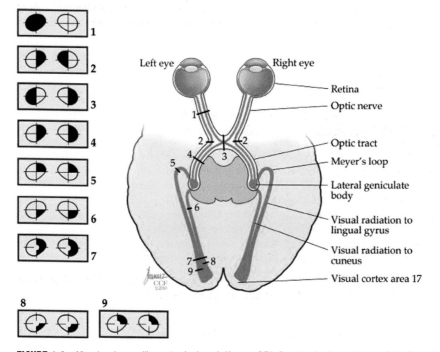

FIGURE 1.9   Visual pathways. Illustration by Joseph Kanasz, BFA. Reprinted with permission of the Cleveland Clinic Center for Medical Art and Photography. © 2010. All rights reserved. Shown also in color plates

Brazis PW, Masdeu JC, Biller J. Localization in Clinical Neurology, 5th ed. Philadelphia, PA: Lippincott Williams & Wilkins; 2007.

32. d

The fundoscopic examination reveals optic nerve atrophy, consistent with a long-standing history of multiple sclerosis. The other choices are described in questions 26 and 29. Signs of chronic optic neuritis include persistent visual loss, color desaturation (especially red), and possibly a persistent relative afferent pupillary defect. Optic atrophy occurs and the disc appears shrunken and pale, especially in the temporal half, and this pallor extends beyond the margins of the disc.

Bradley WG, Daroff RB, Fenichel GM, Jankovic J. Neurology in Clinical Practice, 5th ed. Philadelphia, PA: Elsevier; 2008.

Ropper AH, Samuels MA. Adams and Victor's Principles of Neurology, 9th ed. New York, NY: McGraw-Hill; 2009.

33. c

This patient has mucormycosis involving the cavernous sinus and posterior orbits. This can occur in poorly controlled diabetes. It causes proptosis, visual blurring, and unilateral or bilateral cavernous sinus syndrome (combination of III, IV, VI, V2 and VI cranial nerve involvement), and visual acuity may also be impaired. The contents of the cavernous sinus are illustrated in Figure 1.10. A chronic meningitis would not cause proptosis. A midbrain infarction could cause third and fourth nerve palsies, but would not cause facial numbness or visual blurring. A third nerve palsy would not present in this fashion. Idiopathic cranial polyneuropathy is a diagnosis of exclusion and would not cause proptosis.

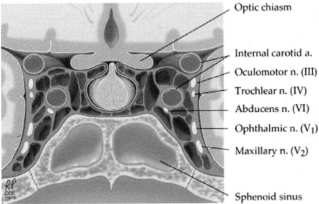

Optic chiasm

Internal carotid a.

Oculomotor n. (III)

Trochlear n. (IV)

Abducens n. (VI)

Ophthalmic n. (V₁)

Maxillary n. (V₂)

Sphenoid sinus

FIGURE 1.10   Cavernous sinus. Illustration by Ross Papalardo, BFA. Reprinted with permission of the Cleveland Clinic Center for Medical Art and Photography. © 2010. All rights reserved. Shown also in color plates

Bradley WG, Daroff RB, Fenichel GM, Jankovic J. Neurology in Clinical Practice, 5th ed. Philadelphia, PA: Elsevier; 2008.

Ropper AH, Samuels MA. Adams and Victor's Principles of Neurology, 9th ed. New York, NY: McGraw-Hill; 2009.

34. d, 35. e, 36. a

This patient most likely has Bell's palsy. No testing is necessary at this time and steroids should be initiated. "Bell's palsy" is the term often used for an acute peripheral facial nerve palsy of unknown cause. It is frequently seen in the third trimester of pregnancy or in the first postpartum week and is also seen in patients with diabetes. A herpes simplex–mediated viral inflammatory mechanism has been proposed as a controversial etiology. Other common viruses have also been associated with Bell's palsy, including varicella-zoster virus as in Ramsay–Hunt syndrome. Ischemia of the facial nerve has also been suggested, especially in patients with diabetes.

Patients with Bell's palsy typically present with relatively abrupt onset of unilateral facial paralysis, which often includes difficulty closing the eye, drooping eyebrow, mouth droop with loss of nasolabial fold, loss of taste sensation on the anterior two-thirds of the tongue (in distribution of facial nerve), decreased tearing, and hyperacusis. Patients may complain of discomfort behind or around the ear prior to symptom onset. There may also be a history of recent upper respiratory infection. It is important to differentiate between a peripheral and central (upper motor neuron) lesion. Sparing of the forehead muscles suggests a central lesion because of bilateral innervation to the facial subnuclei innervating the forehead, as opposed to unilateral facial subnucleus innervation of the ipsilateral lower face (below the eye). However, a lesion to the facial nerve nucleus itself in the pons can lead to complete facial paralysis (of both the upper and lower face). Bell's palsy should classically involve only the facial nerve, although additional cranial nerve involvement has been infrequently reported, including the trigeminal, glossopharyngeal, and hypoglossal nerves. Some studies have reported ipsilateral facial sensory impairment suggesting trigeminal neuropathy, although this sensation has often been attributed to abnormal perception on the basis of "droopy" facial muscles.

Diagnostic studies are not necessary in all patients. Those with a typical history and examination consistent with Bell's palsy do not need further studies initially. Imaging should be considered if there is slow progression beyond 3 weeks, if the physical signs are atypical, or if there is no improvement at 6 months. If imaging is pursued, an MRI with and without gadolinium is optimal. Electrodiagnostic studies may be considered in patients with clinically complete lesions for prognostic purposes if they do not improve. If the history suggests an alternate etiology, evaluation should be targeted as such. A pontine stroke would be unlikely to affect only the facial nerve nucleus without affecting surrounding structures; hemiparesis contralateral to the facial nerve palsy would suggest involvement of corticospinal structures, as in Millard–Gubler syndrome (see Chapter 2), and ipsilateral impairment of eye abduction would suggest involvement of the ipsilateral cranial nerve VI nucleus, as in Foville's syndrome (see Chapter 2). These additional focal symptoms should prompt investigation for pontine infarct. This patient did not have a history or symptoms consistent with Lyme disease or multiple sclerosis. Multiple sclerosis would be highly suspected in a young patient with bilateral Bell's palsy, although Lyme disease and sarcoidosis would also be in the differential. A cholesteatoma would present with a much slower onset.

Treatment of Bell's palsy has been controversial. In general, early treatment with oral glucocorticoids for all patients with Bell's palsy is recommended and optimal treatment should begin within 3 days of symptom onset. There have been two large clinical trials showing no significant benefit for antiviral therapy, so its use is controversial. Some feel that the addition of antivirals to glucocorticoids is beneficial anecdotally, especially in those with severe facial palsy and suggest early combined prednisone (60 to 80 mg per day) plus valacyclovir (1000 mg three times daily) for 1 week in these patients. Artificial tears and eye patches should also be used for eye protection when needed. Nerve stimulation and surgical decompression are not routinely recommended on the basis of current evidence.

Prognosis of Bell's palsy depends on severity of the lesion, and in general, clinically incomplete lesions tend to recover better than complete lesions. In addition, the prognosis is favorable if some recovery is seen within the first 21 days of onset.

Bradley WG, Daroff RB, Fenichel GM, Jankovic J. Neurology in Clinical Practice, 5th ed. Philadelphia, PA: Elsevier; 2008.

Engstrom M, Berg T, Stjernquist-Desatnik A, et al. Prednisolone and valaciclovir in Bell's palsy: A randomised, double-blind, placebo-controlled, multicentre trial. Lancet Neurol. 2008; 7:993–1000.

Grogan PM, Gronseth GS. Practice parameter: Steroids, acyclovir, and surgery for Bell's palsy (an evidence-based review): Report of the Quality Standards Subcommittee of the American Academy of Neurology. Neurology. 2001; 10;56(7):830–836.

Sullivan FM, Swan IR, Donnan PT, et al. Early treatment with prednisolone or acyclovir in Bell's palsy. N Engl J Med. 2007; 357:1598–1607.

37. c

The olfactory nerve is the only nerve listed that does not have a synapse in the thalamus prior to traveling to the cortex. Afferents for all sensory modalities, except for the olfactory nerve, have a synapse in the thalamus prior to terminating in the cortex. From the olfactory bulb, secondary neurons project directly to the olfactory cortex and then have direct connections to the limbic area. The limbic area plays a role in memory formation and this explains why some smells provoke specific emotions and memories. The olfactory cortex has connections with autonomic and visceral centers, including the hypothalamus, thalamus, and amygdala. This may explain why some smells can cause changes in gut motility, nausea, and vomiting. The facial nerve has autonomic fibers descending from the thalamus to the superior salivatory nucleus. It also has sensory afferents for taste that travel to the ventral postero-medial (VPM) nucleus of the thalamus and subsequently to the cortex.

Wilson-Pauwels L, Akesson EJ, Stewart PA, et al. Cranial Nerves in Health and Disease, 2nd ed. Ontario: BC Decker Inc; 2002.

38. e

This phenomenon is called "crocodile tears", and results when misdirected regenerating facial nerve axons originally supplying the submandibular and sublingual salivary glands innervate the lacrimal gland through the greater petrosal nerve. This results in abnormal unilateral lacrimation when eating. In addition, some axons from the motor neurons to the labial muscles involved in smiling may regenerate and misdirect to the orbicularis oculi, which results in closure of the eye on smiling. This phenomenon is termed synkinesis. The reverse may also occur and result in twitching of the mouth on blinking.

Wilson-Pauwels L, Akesson EJ, Stewart PA, et al. Cranial Nerves in Health and Disease, 2nd ed. Ontario: BC Decker Inc; 2002.

39. c, 40. b, 41. a, 42. d, 43. e

A provoking maneuver should be done to evaluate for benign paroxysmal positional vertigo (BPPV) in patients such as this with a typical history. History and examination are less consistent for acute stroke, vertebral dissection or a slow-growing acoustic schwannoma. BPPV is most commonly attributed to calcium debris in a semicircular canal (canalithiasis) and most commonly occurs in the posterior canal. This debris likely represents loose otoconia made up of calcium carbonate crystals within the utricular sac that have migrated into the semicircular canal. The Dix–Hallpike maneuver is most commonly done for this reason and is performed as follows. With the patient sitting, the neck is extended and turned to one side. The patient is then rapidly brought back to a supine position, so that the head hangs over the edge of the bed. This position is kept until 30 seconds have passed if no nystagmus occurs. The patient is then returned to a sitting position and observed for another 30 seconds for nystagmus. Then the maneuver is repeated with the head turned to the other side. This maneuver is most useful for diagnosing posterior canal BPPV (the most common form), and the nystagmus is usually characterized by beating upward and torsionally. After it stops and the patient is sitting again, the nystagmus may occur in the opposite direction (reversal). Besides posterior BPPV, there are three other types of BPPV, including anterior canal, horizontal canal, and pure torsional BPPV. Anterior canal BPPV (superior canal BPPV) has similar provoking factors as posterior canal BPPV, but the nystagmus is downbeat and torsional. Horizontal canal BPPV is provoked by turning the head while lying down and sometimes by turning it in the upright position, but not by getting in or out of bed or extending the neck. Therefore, the nystagmus is elicited by a lateral head turn in the supine position, rather than with the head extended over the edge of the bed, and is characterized by horizontal nystagmus beating toward the floor after turning the affected ear down. The nystagmus lasts less than 1 minute, pauses for a few seconds, and then a reversal of the nystagmus is seen. Pure torsional nystagmus may mimic a central lesion, and results from canalithiasis, simultaneously involving both the anterior and posterior canals, though is less common. This form of BPPV tends to persist longer than other forms of BPPV.

Absence of nystagmus latency would be suggestive of a central lesion. Central nystagmus has the following characteristics: nonfatiguing, absent latency (onset of nystagmus immediately after provocative maneuver), not suppressed by visual fixation, duration of nystagmus is greater than 1 minute, and may occur in any direction. Although purely torsional or vertical nystagmus is classically central in origin, pure torsional BPPV may mimic central nystagmus. Central vertigo is usually subjectively less severe than peripheral vertigo, but gait impairment, falls, and unsteadiness are much more pronounced and other neurologic signs often coexist. Hearing changes and tinnitus are usually absent. Peripheral nystagmus is characterized by fatigability with repetition, latency typically of 2 to 20 seconds, suppression by visual fixation, duration of nystagmus less than 1 minute, unidirectional, and usually horizontal, occasionally with a torsional component. Walking is typically preserved, although unilateral instability may exist. Hearing changes and tinnitus are more common with peripheral lesions.

A unilateral peripheral vestibular lesion, such as in BPPV, leads to an asymmetry in vestibular activity. This results in a slow drift of the eyes away from the target in one direction (toward the affected side and away from the unaffected side), followed by a fast cortical corrective movement to the opposite side (toward the unaffected side, away from the affected side). The amplitude of nystagmus increases with gaze toward the side of the fast phase (toward the unaffected ear and away from the affected ear), and this is known as Alexander's law. As above, peripheral nystagmus is suppressed by visual fixation and this helps differentiate it from central nystagmus.

Initial treatment of BPPV is symptomatic and should begin with a particle-repositioning maneuver, consisting of a sequence of head and body repositioning with the goal of moving the debris from the semicircular canal back into the utricular cavity. The most commonly used is the Epley maneuver, or modified Epley maneuver, although other variations exist. These specific sequences are beyond the scope of this discussion. The Epley maneuver is most efficacious for posterior canal repositioning, whereas anterior and horizontal canal repositioning often require different maneuvers. Self-treatment exercises should be given for the patient to use at home.

Postmaneuver activity restrictions, such as use of a cervical collar and maintenance of an upright head position for 2 days after treatment, had previously been recommended to prevent return of particles into the semicircular canal. Recent studies have shown no significant benefit from postmaneuver activity restrictions, or the use of meclizine.

Bradley WG, Daroff RB, Fenichel GM, Jankovic J. Neurology in Clinical Practice, 5th ed. Philadelphia, PA: Elsevier; 2008.

De la Meilleure G, Dehaene I, Depondt M, et al. Benign paroxysmal positional vertigo of the horizontal canal. J Neurol Neurosurg Psychiatry. 1996; 60:68–71.

Imai T, Takeda N, Uno A, et al. Three-dimensional eye rotation axis analysis of benign paroxysmal positioning nystagmus. ORL J Otorhinolaryngol Relat Spec. 2002; 64:417–423.

Korres S, Riga M, Balatsouras D, Sandris V. Benign paroxysmal positional vertigo of the anterior semicircular canal: Atypical clinical findings and possible underlying mechanisms. Int J Audiol. 2008; 47:276–282.

Oas JG. Benign paroxysmal positional vertigo: A clinician's perspective. Ann NY Acad Sci. 2001; 942:201–209.

44. b, 45. b, 46. e

The vestibular sensory organs consist of the otolithic organs and semicircular canals. The otolithic organs are the saccule and utricle, and these two organs are expansions of the membranous labyrinth. Within each of these organs there is a macula, which is a layer of hair cells overlain by a heavy gelatinous otolithic membrane covered by calcium carbonate particles (the otoconia). During linear acceleration of the head, the head moves relative to the otoconia. This results in bending of the hair cells and a subsequent change in neuronal activation. The otolithic organs detect linear and vertical motions of the head relative to gravity.

There are three semicircular canals within each vestibular apparatus on each side, oriented at right angles to each other. These are tubes of membranous labyrinth extending from each utricle. Therefore, there are two horizontal canals, two vertically directed anterior canals, and two vertically directed posterior canals. The semicircular canals contain endolymph and an ampulla. Each ampulla contains sensory hair cells, which are embedded in a gelatinous cap termed the cupula, and does not contain otoconia. During head rotation, inertia causes the endolymph to lag behind and push on the cupula. Similar to the otolithic organs, this bends the hair cells and causes neuronal activation. The semicircular canals are more sensitive to angular motions of the head.

Information regarding head movement is transmitted to the ocular motor nuclei, resulting in eye movement in an equal and opposite amount to the head turn, allowing the eyes to remain stationary in space despite head movement. This phenomenon is termed the vestibuloocular reflex (VOR). Head movement in the direction of a semicircular canal will excite that respective semicircular canal and the correlative extraocular muscles. The VOR keeps the line of sight stable in space while the head is moving (e.g., keeping your eyes focused on one object while shaking your head back and forth). This occurs because each semicircular canal has excitatory and inhibitory projections to agonist and antagonist extraocular muscles (one per eye; the agonistic muscle is activated, whereas the antagonistic muscle is inhibited). Each semicircular canal has excitatory projections to a pair of agonistic extraocular muscles (one in each eye) and inhibitory projections to a pair of antagonistic extraocular muscles (one in each eye). The medial and lateral recti adduct and abduct the eye, respectively, in a purely horizontal plane. When the head turns right, the right horizontal canal is stimulated. This leads to excitation of the right medial rectus and left lateral rectus, along with inhibition of the right lateral rectus and left medial rectus.

Cold caloric testing is done to assess brainstem integrity (which helps define whether brain death is present or not) and this is a passive way to evaluate the VOR. It should be done using cold water at 30°C and by bringing the head of the bed to 30° from horizontal in order to bring the horizontal canals into a more vertical plane for optimal testing. The temperature difference between the body and the infused water creates a convective current in the endolymph of the nearby horizontal semicircular canal. Hot and cold water produce currents in opposite directions and therefore a horizontal nystagmus in opposite directions. With cold water infusion, the endolymph falls within the semicircular canal, decreasing the rate of vestibular afferent firing and both eyes then slowly deviate toward the ipsilateral ear. Therefore, if cold water is infused into the left ear, the following will occur; excitatory signals are sent to the left lateral rectus and right medial rectus, as well as inhibitory signals to the left medial rectus and right lateral rectus. This results in tonic deviation of the eyes to the left. In a healthy person with normal functioning cortex, following a latency of about 20 seconds, nystagmus appears and may persist up to 2 minutes. The fast phase of nystagmus reflects the cortical correcting response and is directed away from the side of the ice water stimulus. If the cortical circuits are impaired (e.g., comatose state, as in this patient), the nystagmus will be suppressed and not present, and only the tonic deviation will be evident (with intact brainstem). The opposite of these findings should occur with warm water. Nystagmus is named in the direction of the fast phase and thus the well-known mnemonic COWS (cold opposite warm same) for caloric testing.

Purves D, Augustine GA, Fitzpatrick D, et al. Neuroscience, 4th ed. Sunderland, MA: Sinauer Associates Inc; 2008.

Wilson-Pauwels L, Akesson EJ, Stewart PA, et al. Cranial Nerves in Health and Disease, 2nd ed. Ontario: BC Decker Inc; 2002.

47. c, **48.** b, **49.** b

The trigeminal nerve innervates the anterior belly of the digastric, whereas the posterior belly is innervated by the facial nerve. The tensor tympani is innervated by the trigeminal nerve and not the facial nerve. The only muscle innervated by the glossopharyngeal nerve is the stylopharyngeus muscle.

The muscles innervated by the trigeminal nerve are medial and lateral pterygoids, masseter, deep temporal, anterior belly of the digastric, mylohyoid, tensor veli palatini, and tensor tympani.

The muscles innervated by the facial nerve are stapedius, posterior belly of the digastric, stylohyoid, frontalis, occipitalis, orbicularis oculi, corrugator supercilii, procerus, buccinator, orbicularis oris, nasalis, levator labii superioris, alaeque nasi, zygomaticus major and minor, levator anguli oris, mentalis, depressor anguli oris, depressor labii inferioris, risorius, and platysma.

Wilson-Pauwels L, Akesson EJ, Stewart PA, et al. Cranial Nerves in Health and Disease, 2nd ed. Ontario: BC Decker Inc; 2002.

50. b, **51.** e, **52.** b, **53.** a, **54.** d

The facial nerve (cranial nerve VII) is a mixed nerve, containing motor fibers to the facial muscles, parasympathetic fibers to the lacrimal, submandibular, and sublingual salivary glands, special sensory afferent fibers for taste from the anterior two-thirds of the tongue, and somatic sensory afferents from the external auditory canal and pinna. Lesions of the facial nerve can easily be localized by remembering the course of the facial nerve and where the branches arise, keeping in mind that everything before the lesion would be unaffected and everything after the lesion would be affected. A lesion anywhere from the facial nerve nucleus to the distal branches can cause facial weakness in a peripheral distribution. Determining which other facial nerve functions are involved is what helps localize the lesion.

Two roots arise from the pontomedullary junction and merge to form the facial nerve. One of these roots provides motor innervation to the facial muscles. The second root is a mixed visceral nerve carrying parasympathetic fibers and is called the nervus intermedius. The preganglionic cell bodies of the parasympathetics are scattered in the pontine tegmentum, which are called the superior salivatory nuclei (SSN), and their fibers travel in the nervus intermedius. The facial nerve courses laterally through the cerebellopontine angle with the vestibulocochlear nerve to the internal auditory meatus leading to the facial, or fallopian, canal. The facial canal is located in the petrous part of the temporal bone and consists of labyrinthine, tympanic, and mastoid segments. Within the labyrinthine segment, the facial nerve bends sharply backward. At this genu, there is a swelling that forms the geniculate ganglion. This ganglion contains nerve cell bodies of taste axons from the tongue and somatic sensory axons from the external ear, auditory meatus, and external surface of the tympanic membrane.

The parasympathetic greater petrosal nerve arises from the geniculate ganglion and is the first branch of the facial nerve. The greater petrosal nerve leaves the geniculate ganglion anteriorly, enters the middle cranial fossa extradurally, and enters the foramen lacerum en route to the pterygopalatine (sphenopalatine) ganglion. From the pterygopalatine ganglion, postganglionic fibers travel with branches of the maxillary portion of the trigeminal nerve (V2) to supply the lacrimal and mucosal glands of the nasal and oral cavities.

After the geniculate ganglion region and the branch of the greater petrosal nerve, the facial nerve axons then pass backward and downward toward the stylomastoid foramen. The next branch as the facial nerve passes downward is the nerve to the stapedius, prior to exit from the stylomastoid foramen. The stapedius muscle dampens the oscillations of the ossicles of the middle ear. Impairment of the stapedius nerve and muscle will cause hyperacusis, in which sounds are much louder. Question 50 refers to a lesion between the geniculate ganglion/greater petrosal nerve (normal lacrimation) and nerve to the stapedius (hyperacusis).

After the branch of the stapedius nerve and just before the exit from the stylomastoid foramen, the facial nerve gives off the third branch, the chorda tympani nerve. The chorda tympani nerve passes near the tympanic membrane, where it is separated from the middle ear cavity by a mucus membrane. It continues anteriorly and joins the lingual nerve of V3 where it carries general sensory afferents for the anterior two-thirds of the tongue. The chorda tympani contains secretomotor fibers to sublingual and submandibular glands, as well as visceral afferent fibers for taste. The cell bodies of the gustatory neurons lie in the geniculate ganglion and travel via the nervus intermedius back to the nucleus tractus solitarius (gustatory nucleus). Therefore, the nervus intermedius carries efferents from the superior salivatory nucleus and taste afferents to the nucleus tractus solitarius. It is important to remember that the parotid glands are innervated by the glossopharyngeal nerve, whereas all other glands in the head and face are innervated by the facial nerve. Question 51 refers to a lesion between the nerve to the stapedius (absent hyperacusis) and the chorda tympani (impaired taste).

The facial nerve then exits at the stylomastoid foramen, turns anterolaterally, and travels through the parotid gland. After the facial nerve exits the stylomastoid foramen, it gives off different branches to the various facial muscles.

Monkhouse WS. The anatomy of the facial nerve. Ear Nose Throat J. 1990; 69(10):677–683.

Wilson-Pauwels L, Akesson EJ, Stewart PA, et al. Cranial Nerves in Health and Disease, 2nd ed. Ontario: BC Decker Inc; 2002.

55. d, 56. d, 57. b

The nucleus tractus solitarius is involved with both taste and baroreceptor reflexes. The rostral part of this nucleus is involved with taste and receives taste afferents from the facial nerve (anterior two-thirds of the tongue), glossopharyngeal nerve (posterior one-third of the tongue), and the vagus nerve (base of tongue, epiglottis, and pharynx). The caudal part of this nucleus is involved in the baroreceptor reflexes. Baroreceptors in the wall of the carotid sinus are stimulated by increased blood pressure and the glossopharyngeal afferents travel to the caudal nucleus tractus solitarius. As a result, interneurons stimulate the dorsal motor nucleus of the vagus nerve, leading to activation of parasympathetic vagal efferents projecting to the heart and causing slowing of the heart rate. The nucleus ambiguus is the central nucleus responsible for innervation of the muscles of the larynx and pharynx, innervated by the glossopharyngeal and vagus nerves (with some laryngeal muscle innervation contributed by the spinal accessory nerve).

The superior salivatory nucleus is the source of parasympathetic innervation to the head and neck. The inferior salivatory nucleus innervates the parotid gland via the glossopharyngeal nerve.

Crossman AR, Neary D. Neuroanatomy; An Illustrated Colour Text, 2nd ed. London, UK: Churchill-Livingstone; 2000.

Wilson-Pauwels L, Akesson EJ, Stewart PA, et al. Cranial Nerves in Health and Disease, 2nd ed. Ontario: BC Decker Inc; 2002.

58. a, 59. d, 60. d

The trigeminal nerve carries sensory information from the face, and supplies the sensory and motor innervation to the muscles of mastication. The nerve emerges from the midlateral surface of the pons. Its sensory ganglion (trigeminal or gasserian or semilunar ganglion) sits in a depression (Meckel's or trigeminal cave) in the floor of the middle cranial fossa. Three primary divisions emerge from the gasserian ganglion (not the sphenopalatine ganglion, which is discussed below): the ophthalmic (V1), maxillary (V2), and mandibular (V3).

The ophthalmic division (V1) leaves the gasserian ganglion and exits the cranium through the cavernous sinus and the superior orbital fissure en route to the orbit. It branches into the tentorial, frontal, lacrimal, and nasociliary nerves. It mediates the afferent limb of the corneal reflex while the efferent limb is provided by the facial nerve. The V1 division supplies sensation to the skin of the nose, upper eyelid, forehead, and scalp (as far back as lambdoidal suture); upper half of cornea, conjunctiva, and iris, mucus membranes of frontal, sphenoidal, and ethmoidal sinuses, upper nasal cavity and septum, and lacrimal canals; and dura mater of the anterior cranial fossa, falx cerebri, and tentorium cerebelli.

The maxillary division (V2) leaves the gasserian ganglion, travels through the cavernous sinus, exits the cranium through the foramen rotundum, enters the sphenopalatine fossa, and then enters the orbit through the inferior orbital fissure. Branches include the zygomatic, infraorbital, superior alveolar, and palatine nerves. The V2 division supplies sensation to the lower eyelid, lateral nose, upper lip and cheek, lower half of cornea, conjunctiva, and iris; mucus membranes of maxillary sinus, lower nasal cavity, hard and soft palates, and upper gum; teeth of the upper jaw; and dura mater of the middle cranial fossa.

The mandibular division (V3) leaves the gasserian ganglion, exits the cranium through the foramen ovale, travels in the infratemporal fossa, and branches into the buccal, lingual, inferior alveolar, and auriculotemporal nerves. The V3 division does not travel through the cavernous sinus and is therefore spared in cavernous sinus thrombosis. Besides the muscles of mastication, V3 supplies sensation to skin of the lower lip, lower jaw, chin, tympanic membrane, auditory meatus, upper ear; mucus membranes of floor of the mouth, lower gums, anterior two-thirds of the tongue (not taste, which is facial nerve), and teeth of lower jaw; and dura mater of the posterior cranial fossa (although most of posterior fossa innervation arises from upper cervical nerves).

The cavernous sinus contains the ICA (siphon), postganglionic sympathetic fibers, and cranial nerve VI on the medial wall (adjacent to the sphenoid sinus), whereas cranial nerves III, IV, V1, and V2 are found along the lateral wall. The cavernous sinus receives blood from the middle cerebral vein and drains into the jugular vein (via the inferior petrosal sinus) and into the transverse sinus (via the superior petrosal sinus). The two cavernous sinuses are connected by intercavernous sinuses that lie anterior and posterior to the hypophysis forming a venous circle around it.

The sphenopalatine ganglion (pterygopalatine ganglion) is a parasympathetic ganglion found in the pterygopalatine fossa. It is the largest of four parasympathetic ganglia of the head and neck, along with the submandibular ganglion, otic ganglion, and ciliary ganglion. The sphenopalatine ganglion is associated with the branches of the trigeminal nerve. It supplies the lacrimal glands, paranasal sinuses, glands of the mucosa of the nasal cavity and pharynx, the gingiva, and the mucus membrane and glands of the hard palate.

Brazis PW, Masdeu JC, Biller J. Localization in Clinical Neurology, 5th ed. Philadelphia, PA: Lippincott Williams & Wilkins; 2007.

Crossman AR, Neary D. Neuroanatomy; An Illustrated Colour Text, 2nd ed. London, UK: Churchill-Livingstone; 2000.

Wilson-Pauwels L, Akesson EJ, Stewart PA, et al. Cranial Nerves in Health and Disease, 2nd ed. Ontario: BC Decker Inc; 2002.

61. e

Most of the corticobulbar projections to the hypoglossal nuclei are bilateral, although there is one exception. The cortical neurons that drive the genioglossus muscles project only to the contralateral hypoglossal nucleus. There is one genioglossus muscle on each side of the tongue and they pull the tongue anterior and medial. Therefore, if tongue deviation is due to an upper motor neuron lesion affecting the genioglossus projections, tongue deviation will be contralateral. A lower motor neuron lesion causes ipsilateral tongue deviation.

The hypoglossal nerve provides innervation to all intrinsic tongue muscles and three (genioglossus, styloglossus, and hypoglossus) of the four extrinsic tongue muscles, with the fourth (palatoglossus) being innervated by the vagus nerve.

Wilson-Pauwels L, Akesson EJ, Stewart PA, et al. Cranial Nerves in Health and Disease, 2nd ed. Ontario: BC Decker Inc; 2002.

62. b

Activation of the accessory nerve causes ipsilateral head tilt and contralateral head rotation. The accessory nerve innervates the sternocleidomastoid and the trapezius muscle on each side. The action of each sternocleidomastoid (SCM) is to pull the mastoid process toward the clavicle, resulting in contralateral head rotation and turning of chin to the contralateral side (ipsilateral head tilt). Each SCM is innervated by the ipsilateral motor cortex, whereas each trapezius is innervated by the contralateral motor cortex.

Wilson-Pauwels L, Akesson EJ, Stewart PA, et al. Cranial Nerves in Health and Disease, 2nd ed. Ontario: BC Decker Inc; 2002.

63. e

The gag reflex is mediated by the nucleus ambiguus. The afferent limb is by the glossopharyngeal nerve and the efferent limb is by the vagus nerve. The vagus nerve exits the cranium through the jugular foramen with the glossopharyngeal and spinal accessory nerves. It innervates the palatal, pharyngeal, and laryngeal muscles via the nucleus ambiguus. A vagus nerve lesion will cause impaired swallowing (likely the cause of this patient's aspiration pneumonia), hoarse voice, and flattening and lowering of the palate, which causes the uvula to point toward the contralateral side. The dorsal motor nucleus of the vagus supplies parasympathetic innervation to the heart, lungs, gastrointestinal (GI) tract, and trachea. The vagus nerve also supplies sensation to the base of the tongue, epiglottis, and pharynx.

Wilson-Pauwels L, Akesson EJ, Stewart PA, et al. Cranial Nerves in Health and Disease, 2nd ed. Ontario: BC Decker Inc; 2002.

Buzz Phrases	Key Points
Central nystagmus	Nonfatiguing, absent latency, not suppressed by visual fixation, duration of nystagmus greater than 1 minute, any direction, but purely torsional or vertical direction is classically central in origin (although pure torsional BPPV may mimic)
Central vertigo	Subjectively less severe vertigo than peripheral, more prominent gait impairment, other neurologic signs coexist, absent hearing changes and tinnitus
Peripheral nystagmus	Fatigable, latency present, suppression by visual fixation, duration of nystagmus is less than 1 minute, direction is unidirectional and usually horizontal with a torsional component
Peripheral vertigo	Subjectively more severe, walking typically preserved, hearing changes and tinnitus common
Taste anterior two-thirds of tongue	Facial nerve
Tactile sensation anterior two-thirds of tongue	Trigeminal nerve
Taste posterior one-third of tongue	Glossopharyngeal nerve
Parasympathetic source to head and neck	Superior salivatory nucleus
Motor nuclei to pharyngeal and laryngeal muscles	Nucleus ambiguus
Provides innervation to the parotid gland by glossopharyngeal nerve	Inferior salivatory nucleus
Nuclei for taste sensation	Rostral nucleus solitarius
Nuclei for baroreceptor reflex	Caudal nucleus solitarius
Nuclei for parasympathetic output to chest, thorax, and GI tract	Dorsal motor nucleus of vagus
Corneal reflex	Afferent: trigeminal nerve Efferent: facial nerve
Gag reflex	Afferent: glossopharyngeal nerve Efferent: vagus nerve
Pupil-sparing third nerve palsy	Diabetic pupil/diabetic cranial nerve palsy
Ptosis, miosis, anhidrosis (when proximal to carotid bifurcation)	Horner's syndrome
Fourth nerve palsy	Contralateral head tilt

(*continued*)

Buzz Phrases	Key Points
Argyll–Robertson pupil	Neurosyphilis; accommodation reflex present, pupillary reflex absent
Marcus Gunn pupil	Afferent pupillary defect: no response to direct light, but response to consensual light in contralateral eye present
"Down and out pupil"	Third nerve palsy
Painful vision loss	Optic neuritis
Painless vision loss	Anterior ischemic optic neuropathy
Cocaine 4% or 10% eye drops	Confirmation of Horner's pupil (no change in size of Horner's pupil; unaffected side dilates)
Hydroxyamphetamine 1% eye drops: Horner's pupil dilates	First- *or* second-order Horner's pupil
Hydroxyamphetamine 1% eye drops: Horner's pupil does not dilate	Third-order Horner's pupil

Chapter 2

Vascular Neurology

Questions

1. A 65-year-old patient with diabetes presents with a TIA. According to the ABCD2 score that assesses stroke risk in someone with TIA, which of the following is not a predictor of occurrence of a stroke?
    a. Diabetes
    b. Age of 60 years or more
    c. Hypertension
    d. Duration of neurologic symptoms
    e. Hyperlipidemia

2. A 42-year-old woman with diabetes, hypertension, and hyperlipidemia is brought to the emergency department for unresponsiveness. An MRI is shown in Figure 2.1. Which of the following will most likely be encountered in this patient?
    a. Vertical gaze impairment
    b. Hemisensory symptoms
    c. Hemiparesis
    d. Quadriplegia with impaired horizontal gaze
    e. Aphasia

3. A 49-year-old man with history of hypertension presents to the emergency department with acute onset of right hemiparesis and aphasia about 45 minutes ago. The National Institutes of Health Stroke Scale (NIHSS) score is 14. Which of the following is the best next step?
    a. Start intravenous tissue plasminogen activator (tPA)
    b. Get a brain CT scan
    c. Give aspirin 325 mg once
    d. Start intravenous heparin
    e. Get a brain MRI

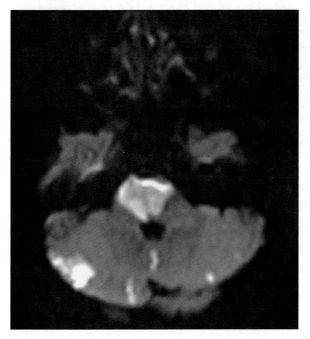

FIGURE 2.1 Axial diffusion-weighted MRI

4. A 49-year-old woman presents with acute onset of hemiplegia, progressing to quadriplegia over the next 2 hours. On examination she seems awake; however, she is unable to verbalize. She cannot move her eyes horizontally but is able to move them vertically and blink. Which of the following is the most likely cause?
   a. Bilateral thalamic infarcts
   b. Lateral medullary infarct
   c. Top of the basilar occlusion
   d. Infarct affecting the base of the pons bilaterally
   e. Infarct affecting the dorsal midbrain

5. Which of the following is correct regarding thrombosis of the venous sinuses?
   a. Diplopia with a sixth cranial nerve palsy is specific for cavernous sinus thrombosis
   b. Headache is present in less than 50% of cases ~ 90%
   c. Increased intracranial pressure is uncommon — com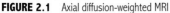
   d. Superior sagittal sinus thrombosis may produce bilateral thalamic venous infarcts — ✓
   e. Seizures are more common in venous infarcts as compared to arterial infarcts

6. A 51-year-old man presents with ataxia. An MRI is obtained and is shown in Figure 2.2. Which of the following will most likely result from this injury?
   a. Vertigo, nystagmus, and right sided ptosis and miosis
   b. Vertical gaze impairment
   c. Right third and sixth nerve palsies
   d. Hemisensory loss to pain and temperature on the left side of the face
   e. Hemisensory loss to pain and temperature on the right side of the body

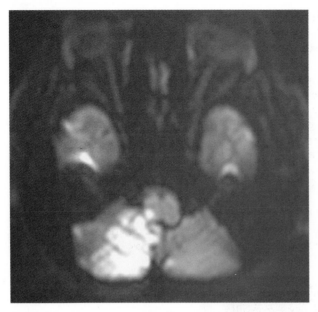

FIGURE 2.2 Axial diffusion-weighted MRI

7. A 34-year-old man presents with vertigo and neck pain after riding a "very wild" roller coaster. The examination demonstrates anisocoria with mild ptosis on the left side, nystagmus, and left side ataxia. Which of the following is the best diagnostic test?
    a. Carotid ultrasound
    b. Transcranial doppler ultrasonography
    c. Transthoracic echocardiogram with bubble study
    d. Cerebral angiogram
    e. Time-of-flight MRA

8. A 69-year-old woman presents to the emergency department at 2 hours and 35 minutes from the onset of left hemiparesis and hemineglect. Her National Institutes of Health Stroke Scale (NIHSS) score is 16. A brain CT scan shows no hemorrhage. Which of the following statements is correct regarding tissue plasminogen activator (tPA)?
    a. The risk of hemorrhage with tPA is similar to placebo.
    b. Earlier administration carries a better prognosis and a lower risk of hemorrhage.
    c. There is no maximum dose.
    d. The use of tPA improves short-term but not long-term clinical outcomes.
    e. tPA should not be administered beyond 2 hours from the onset of symptoms.

9. A 72-year-old woman with a history of diabetes presents with a transient visual disturbance on the right side. On further questioning, she reports that she experienced a transient dimness of the vision of the right eye, progressing from the upper visual field to the lower visual field like a "shade" falling. This lasted for about 10 minutes and resolved on its own. Which of the following is correct?
    a. This patient is having transient ischemia of the left occipital cortex
    b. A transcranial doppler will demonstrate increased velocities in the basilar artery

, c. The right ICA is stenotic with an atherosclerotic plaque
   d. The left ICA is stenotic with an atherosclerotic plaque
   e. Fundoscopic examination will demonstrate papilledema

10. A 40-year-old man presents with tinnitus, unilateral hearing loss, nausea, vomiting, and vertigo. On examination, he has nystagmus, ipsilateral ataxia, ipsilateral Horner's syndrome, and contralateral sensory deficits to pain and temperature of the arm, trunk, and leg. Which of the following is the most likely diagnosis?   *very similar to PICA*
,   a. Anterior inferior cerebellar artery (AICA) stroke - *but w/ ~~~ Ipsilateral Hearing loss.*
    b. Posterior inferior cerebellar artery (PICA) stroke
    c. Midbrain infarct
    d. Occipital lobe infarct
    e. Superior cerebellar infarct

11. A 59-year-old woman presents with altered mental status. There is restricted diffusion on the MRI which is shown in Figure 2.3. Which of the following is the most likely diagnosis?

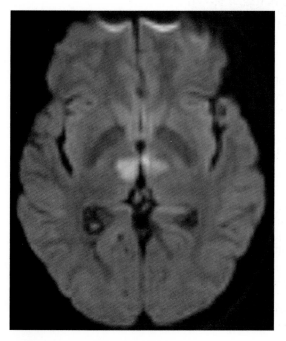

FIGURE 2.3   Axial diffusion-weighted MRI

   a. Bilateral anterior choroidal artery stroke
   b. Stroke from occlusion of the recurrent artery of Heubner
, c. Stroke from occlusion of the artery of Percheron
   d. Stroke from occlusion of the pericallosal artery
   e. Superior sagittal sinus thrombosis

12. A 49-year-old woman with anxiety, depression, hypertension, and diabetes presents to the emergency department with a sensory deficit affecting her right face, arm, trunk, and leg, which started yesterday in the evening. The symptoms reached their peak on the morning of presentation. There are no motor deficits on examination. Which of the following is correct?

   a. No further work up is needed, and the patient can be discharged from the emergency department
   b. Given the lack of motor deficits, her symptoms are most likely related to anxiety
   c. The most likely location of the lesion is in the cortex
   d. Cardioembolism is the most likely etiology
   e. Small vessel disease is the most likely etiology

13. A 52-year-old man with history of smoking, diabetes mellitus, and hypertension presents with acute onset of left hemiparesis affecting the face, arm, and leg. He recognizes the left side of his body and acknowledges the deficits. His gaze is not deviated. Which is the most likely location of the vascular occlusion?

   a. Trunk of the right MCA before the bifurcation
   b. Right lenticulostriate branches of the MCA
   c. Superior division of the right MCA
   d. Right PCA
   e. Inferior division of the right MCA

14. A 59-year-old woman with a history of atrial fibrillation and hypertension presents with right hemiparesis affecting mainly the face and arm. Her eyes are deviated toward the left. She seems to be able to understand and follow commands, however, cannot verbalize, and appears frustrated when asked questions because she cannot answer. Where is the location of the vascular occlusion?

   a. Trunk of the MCA before the bifurcation
   b. Lenticulostriate branches of the left MCA
   c. Superior division of the left MCA
   d. Inferior division of the left MCA
   e. Penetrating branches at the level of the pons

15. A 51-year-old man with hypertension and diabetes presents with left leg weakness associated with urinary incontinence. This patient was known to have a normal circle of Willis based on a previous MRA performed for other reasons. Where is the most likely vascular occlusion?

   a. Right ACA proximal to the origin of anterior communicating artery
   b. Right ACA distal to the origin of the anterior communicating artery
   c. Anterior communicating artery
   d. Superior division of the right MCA
   e. Inferior division of the right MCA

16. Which of the following is correct regarding the recurrent artery of Heubner?

   a. It is a penetrating branch of the ACA
   b. It is a penetrating branch of the PCA
   c. It provides bilateral perfusion to the thalamus

d. Provides perfusion to the posterior limb of the internal capsule

e. Originates from the main trunk of the MCA

17. The lenticulostriate branches provide perfusion to all of the following structures except:
    a. Part of the head and body of the caudate
    b. Posterior limb of the internal capsule
    c. The putamen
    d. External part of the globus pallidus
    e. Anterior limb of the internal capsule

18. A 31-year-old man presents with dizziness, vertigo, and hoarseness after having chiropractic neck manipulation by an unexperienced practitioner. On examination, the patient has nystagmus, findings of Horner's syndrome on the right side, paralysis of the right palate, decreased sensation to pinprick on the right side of the face and left hemibody, and right-sided ataxia. Which of the following is the most likely diagnosis?
    a. Right medial medullary syndrome
    b. Right lateral medullary syndrome
    c. Left medial medullary syndrome
    d. Left lateral medullary syndrome
    e. Right pontine infarct

19. Which of the following options is correct regarding the vascular supply of the thalamus?
    a. It is primarily provided by the anterior circulation
    b. The anterior choroidal artery supplies the ventral posteromedial nucleus
    c. The posterior choroidal artery supplies the ventral anterior nucleus
    d. The paramedian branches supply the dorsomedial nucleus
    e. The posterior choroidal artery arises from the posterior communicating artery and supplies the pulvinar

20. A 49-year-old man presents with ataxia. His brain CT scan is shown in Figure 2.4. Which of the following is the most likely artery involved? × Superior Cerebellar stroke
    a. Anterior inferior cerebellar artery (AICA)
    b. Superior cerebellar artery (SCA)
    c. Posterior inferior cerebellar artery (PICA)
    d. PCA
    e. Vertebral artery

21. You are asked to see a 42-year-old right-handed woman with diabetes and dilated cardiomyopathy who developed acute "confusion." On examination, she does not follow commands and is speaking fluently and saying multiple phrases that do not make sense. She seems to have a visual defect in the right hemifield. An MRI is obtained and shows evidence of a stroke. Where is the most likely vascular occlusion?
    a. Trunk of the left MCA prior to the bifurcation
    b. Lenticulostriate branches of the left MCA
    c. Superior division of the left MCA
    d. Inferior division of the left MCA
    e. Penetrating branches at the level of the pons

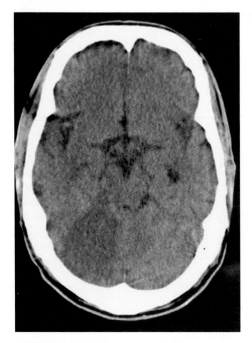

FIGURE 2.4   Axial CT

22. What syndrome can you expect in a patient with the MRA shown in Figure 2.5?
    a. Wallenberg's syndrome
    b. Parinaud's syndrome
    c. A left MCA syndrome
    d. Locked-in syndrome
    e. Dejerine-Roussy syndrome

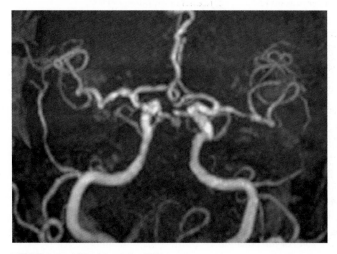

FIGURE 2.5   MRA of the circle of Willis

23. An MRI is shown in Figure 2.6. Which of the following is correct regarding this condition?

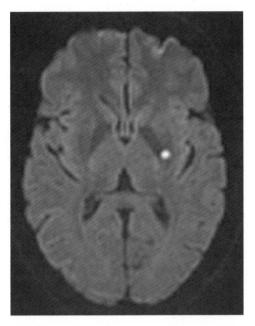

FIGURE 2.6 Axial diffusion-weighted MRI

    a. Aphasia and neglect are common neurologic manifestations
    b. Echocardiogram with bubble study and Holter monitor are indicated
    c. Pathologic analysis of this lesion would demonstrate microhemorrhages in the affected area
    d. It is caused by occlusion of a penetrating vessel and intimately related to hypertension
    e. The most common presentation in this case is pure sensory deficits

24. Which is the abnormality in the MRA shown in Figure 2.7?

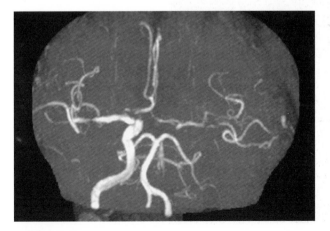

FIGURE 2.7 MRA

a. Absence of the left vertebral artery
b. Basilar occlusion
c. Left MCA occlusion
d. Left ICA occlusion
e. Fetal posterior cerebral arteries

25. Which of the following is incorrect regarding the anterior choroidal artery?
    a. It is a branch of the ICA
    b. It supplies the posterior limb of the internal capsule
    c. It supplies the anterior limb of the internal capsule
    d. It supplies a part of the geniculocalcarine tract
    e. It supplies the choroid plexus in the lateral ventricles

26. A 49-year-old patient presents with acute onset of neurologic symptoms. A cerebral angiogram is shown in Figure 2.8. Which is the abnormality in this angiogram?

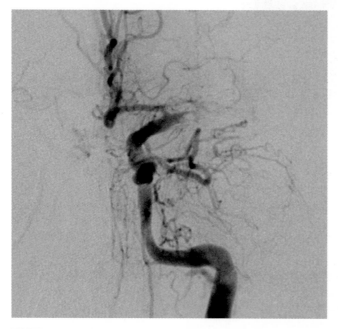

FIGURE 2.8 Angiogram

    a. Left MCA occlusion
    b. Left vertebral artery occlusion
    c. ACA occlusion
    d. ICA occlusion
    e. This is a normal angiogram

27. Which of the following is the most likely mechanism of the stroke shown in Figure 2.9?
    a. Cardioembolic
    b. Lacunar strokes

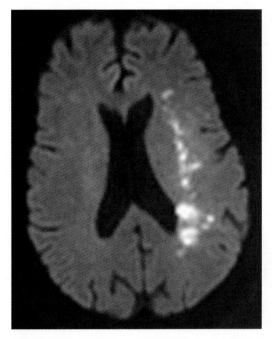

FIGURE 2.9 Axial diffusion-weighted MRI

   c. Embolic from large artery atherosclerosis
   d. Hypotension in the setting of carotid stenosis
   e. Venous infarction

28. A 39-year-old woman presents with Horner's syndrome on the left side, with vertigo, ataxia, and sensory changes on the left side of the face and right side of the body. Which of the following is the most likely cause?
   a. Left carotid artery dissection
   b. Right carotid artery dissection
   c. Left vertebral artery dissection
   d. Right vertebral artery dissection
   e. Right MCA stroke

29. A 52-year-old woman presents to the emergency department with acute onset of right hemiparesis. A CT scan is obtained and is shown in Figure 2.10. Which of the following is correct?
   a. This patient is at risk of vasospasm
   b. The cause of the symptoms is a lacunar stroke
   c. The patient may need suboccipital craniectomy for decompression
   d. The patient has a hypertensive hemorrhage
   e. The patient has an MCA occlusion

30. A 59-year-old man with a history of diabetes, hypertension, and hyperlipidemia presents with a blood pressure of 60/30 mm Hg and confusion. His creatine kinase is very elevated with an MB

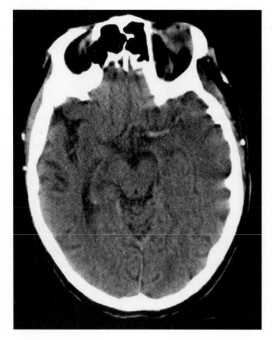

FIGURE 2.10 Axial CT

fraction of 12%. His troponin is elevated, and the electrocardiogram shows ST depressions in the inferior leads. After stabilization he is noticed to have left side weakness, more prominent in the shoulder abductors and hip flexors. Which of the following is the most likely underlying mechanism of his weakness?

a. Weakness from a myopathy
b. Internal capsule lacunar infarction
c. Hypotension in the setting of a left internal carotid stenosis
d. Hypotension in the setting of a right internal carotid stenosis
e. Cardioembolic event associated with arrhythmia

31. A 57-year-old man presents with acute onset of paralysis of the right arm and leg sparing the face, loss of position and vibration sensation on the right side of the body, and dysarthria. On examination, it is also noticed that the tongue deviates to the left. Which of the following is the most likely diagnosis?

a. Right lateral medullary syndrome
b. Left medial medullary syndrome
c. Right medial medullary syndrome
d. Right pontine infarct
e. Left lateral medullary syndrome

32. A 65-year-old woman went on a roller coaster ride. About 3 weeks later, she had an episode of what sounds like amaurosis fugax in the left eye. She complains of headaches, feels weak "all over," and states that her shoulders have been aching for at least 6 months. She also reports that when eating, she gets tired of chewing and her jaw hurts. Initial noninvasive imaging studies of

the brain and intracranial and extracranial circulation are unremarkable. Besides checking an ESR, which of the following is the best next step?

a. Cerebral angiogram
b. CT angiogram of the neck
c. Start heparin and bridge to warfarin
d. Schedule a temporal artery biopsy
e. Start steroids

33. A 49-year-old woman presents with acute onset of right side facial weakness, involving both the upper and lower face, and left hemiplegia. Which of the following is the most likely diagnosis?

a. Right pontine infarct   *Millard - Gubler syndrome.*
b. Left pontine infarct
c. Right midbrain infarct
d. Left midbrain infarct
e. Right MCA infarct

34. A 42-year-old woman presents for evaluation of headaches and is found to have a left MCA bifurcation aneurysm. The patient asks about risks. Which of the following is not correct?

a. Patients with previous aneurysmal rupture have a higher risk of SAH
b. Smoking is a risk factor for aneurysmal rupture
c. Anterior circulation aneurysms have a higher risk of rupture when compared with posterior circulation aneurysms
d. Patient age should be taken into consideration when formulating the management strategy
e. Uncontrolled hypertension may be a risk for aneurysmal rupture

35. A 59-year-old right-handed man presents with neurologic deficits. A brain CT scan is obtained and is shown in Figure 2.11. Which of the following manifestations would <u>not</u> be seen in this patient as a result of this lesion?

a. Right homonymous hemianopia
b. Anomia
c. Alexia
d. Visual agnosia
e. Expressive aphasia

36. A 52-year-old woman with diabetes comes to the clinic with a sudden onset of vertical diplopia with limited adduction and vertical movements of the right eye. She also has tremor and choreoa-thetotic movements on the left side of her body. Which of the following is the most likely diagnosis?

a. Right ventral mesencephalic tegmentum infarct
b. Left ventral mesencephalic tegmentum infarct
c. Right pontine infarct
d. Left pontine infarct
e. Quadrigeminal plate infarct

37. A right-handed patient presents with acute onset of neurologic deficits, and an MRI of the brain is obtained and is shown in Figure 2.12. Which of the following manifestations may be seen in this patient?

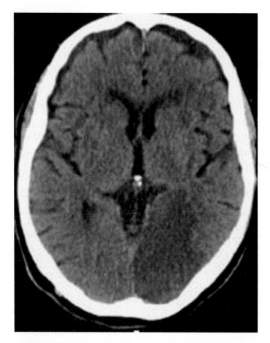

FIGURE 2.11 Axial CT

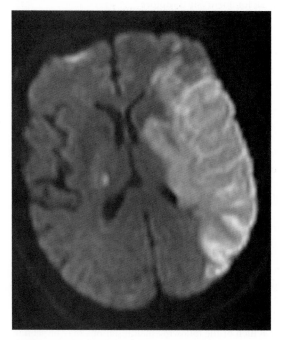

FIGURE 2.12 Axial diffusion-weighted MRI

    a. Neglect of the left side of the body
    b. Gaze deviation toward the right
    c. Global aphasia
    d. Paresis of the right leg more than face and arm
    e. Left homonymous hemianopsia

38. Which of the following patients should be managed with antiplatelet agents for stroke prevention?
    a. A 50-year-old man who suffered an ST-elevation myocardial infarction last week and has an ejection fraction of 30% with anterior wall akinesis and a left ventricular thrombus
    b. A 49-year-old woman with a mechanical heart valve
    c. A 52-year-old man with hyperthyroidism and intracranial atherosclerotic stenosis
    d. A 76-year-old man with atrial fibrillation, diabetes, hypertension, and congestive heart failure
    e. A 70-year-old man with an intracardiac thrombus

39. A 49-year-old right-handed man with a history of atrial fibrillation and hypertension presents with acute onset of right hemiparesis affecting the face, arm, and leg. His gaze is deviated toward the left, and he seems to have a right homonymous hemianopsia. He is globally aphasic. What is the location of vascular occlusion?
    a. Trunk of the MCA before the bifurcation
    b. Left lenticulostriate branches of the MCA
    c. Inferior division of the left MCA
    d. Penetrating branches at the level of the pons
    e. Superior division of the left MCA

40. Which of the following is incorrect regarding the intracranial circulation?
    a. The ACA and MCA are branches of the ICA
    b. The PCAs are branches of the basilar artery
    c. The pericallosal artery arises from the anterior circulation
    d. Lenticulostriate branches arise from the PCA
    e. The recurrent artery of Heubner arises from the ACA

41. A 50-year-old woman with hypertension presents to the clinic with a history of TIA about a month ago. Aspirin 81 mg was started at that time. Cardioembolic work up was negative, carotid ultrasound demonstrated nonsignificant stenosis, and low-density lipoprotein (LDL) was 110 mg/dL. Which of the following agents has been shown to prevent recurrent cerebrovascular events and should be used in this patient?
    a. Statins
    b. Warfarin
    c. Tissue plasminogen activator (tPA)
    d. Heparin
    e. Hormone replacement therapy

42. A patient presents with limited upward gaze bilaterally, nystagmus on attempted convergence, and skew deviation. The pupils are fixed with abnormal accommodation and light-near dissociation. Where is the lesion?
    a. Ventral midbrain
    b. Pons
    c. Medulla

  d. Bilateral thalami
  e. Quadrigeminal plate

43. A 53-year-old woman who underwent coronary artery bypass surgery 5 days ago develops acute onset of right hemiparesis and aphasia. As per the nurse, the patient had shaking of her right arm just prior to the onset of the neurologic deficits. A brain CT scan obtained 30 minutes from the onset of symptoms shows no hemorrhage and no evidence of acute stroke. The patient's blood pressure is 170/100 mm Hg, and her blood glucose is 48 mg/dL. The National Institutes of Health Stroke Scale (NIHSS) score is initially 16 prior to the CT scan, but at a second evaluation after the scan the NIHSS score is 6. A decision is made not to give her intravenous tPA. Which of the following is not a contraindication to give this therapy?
  a. Major surgery within the last 14 days
  b. Seizure at the onset
  c. Rapidly improving or minor symptoms
  d. Glucose less than 50 mg/dL or more than 400 mg/dL
  e. CT scan of the brain showing no evidence of acute infarct

44. A 50-year-old man has a history of stroke in the right MCA distribution. The MRA shows a severe stenosis of the right MCA. As initial therapy, which of the following treatment options has evidence to support its use?
  a. Surgical bypass
  b. Angioplasty
  c. Stent placement
  d. Warfarin
  e. Aspirin

45. A 59-year-old man presents with sudden onset of right hemiparesis and aphasia. The National Institutes of Health Stroke Scale (NIHSS) score is 18. A brain CT scan is obtained and you calculate the Alberta Stroke Program Early CT Score (ASPECTS). Which of the following is correct?
  a. A score of 4 supports the use of intravenous tissue plasminogen activator (tPA)
  b. Three CT scan cuts are required to calculate this score (two)
  c. The maximum score is 20 (0)
  d. A score of 7 or less is associated with increased dependence and death
  e. The minimum score is 3

46. Which of the following is incorrect regarding the ICA?
  a. The cervical segment extends from the bifurcation to the carotid canal at the skull base and has no branches
  b. The petrous segment is located in the petrous region of temporal bone
  c. The ophthalmic artery arises from the ophthalmic segment
  d. The cavernous segment runs within the cavernous sinus
  e. The anterior choroidal artery arises from the petrous segment

47. A 69-year-old woman with history of a right MCA territory stroke, hypertension, hyperlipidemia, and diabetes comes with recurrent symptoms of left side numbness. A carotid artery ultrasound is obtained to determine if an endarterectomy is indicated. Which of the following is incorrect?
  a. A right carotid stenosis of more than 70% is an indication for endarterectomy in this patient
  b. A left carotid stenosis of less than 50% is not treated surgically

c. A right carotid occlusion is not treated surgically
d. A right carotid stenosis of 60% will benefit from surgical treatment
e. If the left carotid stenosis is more than 70%, medical treatment is superior to surgery

48. A 61-year-old man with a history of diabetes on insulin, hyperlipidemia, and hypertension presents with transient left hemiparesis without speech problems, lasting for 20 minutes and resolving. Which of the following is incorrect?
a. The patient should be evaluated as soon as possible
b. Stroke work up should be initiated, including noninvasive imaging of the extracranial arteries
c. The risk of stroke is highest in the period immediately following and soon after a TIA
d. A brain MRI will be helpful to rule out brain infarction
e. A period of observation is indicated before thrombolysis, to determine if the patient has a TIA rather than a stroke

49. A 69-year-old man presents with acute neurologic deficits. His brain CT scan is shown in Figure 2.13. Which of the following is the most likely etiology?

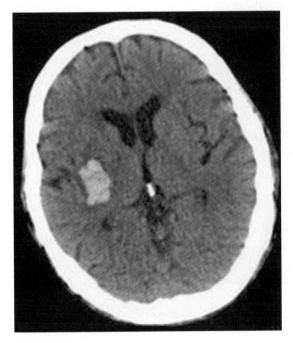

FIGURE 2.13 Axial CT

a. Amyloid angiopathy
b. Intracranial aneurysm
c. Anticoagulation
d. Hypertension
e. Sinus venous thrombosis

50. A 14-year-old girl comes for evaluation with a presumptive diagnosis of Moyamoya. Which of the following is incorrect regarding this condition?
   a. There is bilateral stenosis of the intracranial internal carotid arteries and other arteries of the circle of Willis
   b. There is extensive collateral circulation seen on angiography as a "puff of smoke."
   c. Affects predominately children and adolescents
   d. Cerebral ischemia and hemorrhage may occur
   e. Anticoagulation has proven to be of benefit in these patients

51. An 82-year-old man presents with an intracranial hemorrhage (ICH) affecting the entire left temporal lobe. He has a history of three ICHs in the past. An MRI obtained a few years ago for evaluation of dementia and prior to his current hemorrhage is shown in Figure 2.14. Which of the following is the most likely diagnosis?

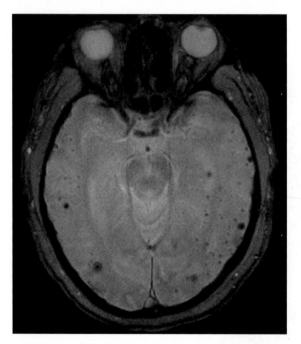

FIGURE 2.14 Axial gradient echo sequence MRI

   a. Amyloid angiopathy
   b. Intracranial aneurysm
   c. Anticoagulation
   d. Hypertension
   e. Sinus venous thrombosis

52. A 49-year-old woman suffers an acute stroke producing significant sensory loss on the left hemibody. About 3 weeks later, the patient comes back to the clinic and complains of severe painful sensation when touched superficially, as well as deep burning pain in the same region. Which of the following is the most likely diagnosis?

    a. Medullary infarct
    b. Midbrain infarct
    c. Caudate infarct
    d. Pontine infarct
    e. Thalamic infarct

53. Which of the following is incorrect regarding the posterior circulation?

    a. The posterior choroidal arteries arise from the posterior circulation
    b. The anterior choroidal arteries arise from the posterior circulation
    c. The anterior spinal artery arises from the intracranial vertebral arteries
    d. The posterior inferior cerebellar artery (PICA) arises from the vertebral arteries
    e. A segment of the vertebral artery runs through the transverse foramina of C5-C6 to C2

54. A 29-year-old woman, smoker, on oral contraceptives, with a history of antiphospholipid antibodies and a recent untreated left middle ear infection, developed right hemiparesis and later became comatose. An MRI is obtained and is shown in Figure 2.15. Which of the following is most likely diagnosis?

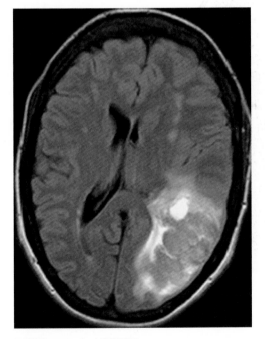

FIGURE 2.15 Axial FLAIR MRI

    a. Hypertensive hemorrhage
    b. PCA stroke with hemorrhagic transformation
    c. Hemorrhage associated with amyloid angiopathy

     d. Venous infarct with hemorrhage
     e. SAH

55. A 49-year-old woman with hypertension presents with a TIA suggestive of ischemia in the territory of the right MCA. Imaging studies suggest a 60% stenosis of the right MCA. Based on available evidence, which of the following treatment plans is least warranted in this patient?
     a. Start warfarin
     b. Start aspirin
     c. Start clopidogrel
     d. Start a statin in addition to an antiplatelet agent
     e. Start aspirin with dipyridamole.

56. A 61-year-old man presents with acute onset of diplopia and difficulty using his right hand. On examination, he has a left third nerve palsy, right-sided tremors, and ataxia, but no choreoathetotic movements. Which of the following is the most likely diagnosis?
     a. Left hemispheric infarct
     b. Left pontine infarct
     c. Left midbrain infarct
     d. Right pontine infarct
     e. Right midbrain infarct

57. A 40-year-old woman with history of diabetes and hypertension presents with a severe headache. An MRV is obtained and is shown in Figure 2.16. Which of the following is correct regarding this condition?

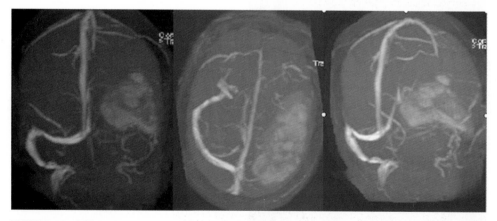

FIGURE 2.16 MRV

     a. Echocardiogram with bubble study and Holter monitor should be obtained to look for the embolic source
     b. Given the history of hypertension and diabetes, further investigation for other prothrombotic causes is not needed
     c. A middle ear infection may be the etiological factor
     d. Anticoagulation is contraindicated
     e. Endovascular therapy plays no role in this disease group

58. A 67-year-old man with history of atrial fibrillation and a recent TIA comes for evaluation. A decision is made to put him on warfarin. Which of the following factors is not routinely taken into account to assess the stroke risk in patients with atrial fibrillation?

   a. Age
   b. History of congestive heart failure
   c. History of hypertension
   d. History of a prior stroke
   e. History of renal disease

59. Which of the following is incorrect regarding the venous system?

   a. Veins of the scalp communicate with the dural venous sinuses via emissary veins
   b. Ophthalmic veins drain into the cavernous sinus
   c. Cavernous sinus drains to the superior and inferior petrosal sinuses
   d. The vein of Labbe is the superior anastomotic vein
   e. The vein of Rosenthal is a deep vein

60. A 52-year-old patient with a history of migraines and multiple "mini strokes," is being treated with aspirin. He presents with a new pure motor stroke, and the MRI shows multiple subcortical lacunes and diffuse white matter changes. Routine stroke work up is negative, and he does not have history of diabetes, hypertension, or hyperlipidemia. He is discharged and gets lost to follow up, coming back about 3 years later for evaluation of dementia. His wife reported that the patient has three siblings who had strokes at young ages, and his father also had strokes and developed dementia early in life. The patient subsequently dies, and an autopsy is performed, with a histopathologic specimen of his brain shown in Figure 2.17. Which of the following is correct regarding this condition?

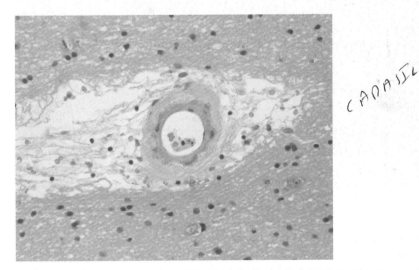

FIGURE 2.17 Brain specimen. (Courtesy of Dr. Richard A. Prayson.) Shown also in color plates

   a. It is autosomal recessive
   b. Parkinsonism is a classic feature

Central Autosomal dominant arteriopath SIC

c. It is associated with *NOTCH3* mutation *(Chromosome 19)*

d. It is an X-linked disorder

e. Migraine headaches are not associated with this condition

61. A 45-year-old man suffers an ST-elevation myocardial infarction requiring percutaneous trans-luminal coronary angiography with stent placement in the left anterior descending artery. Subsequently, the patient develops right hemiplegia and diplopia, worse when looking upwards and to the right. The patient has limited adduction and upgaze of the left eye. Which is the most likely diagnosis?

a. Right pontine infarct

b. Left midbrain infarct

c. Left pontine infarct

d. Right midbrain infarct

e. Left internal capsule infarct

62. A brain MRI is shown in Figure 2.18. Which of the following is the most likely diagnosis?

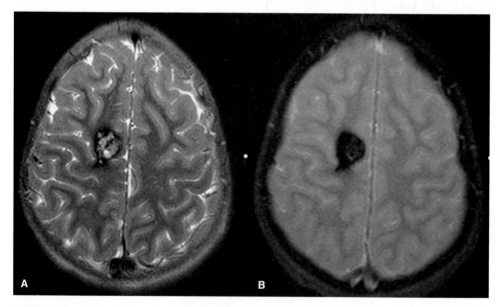

FIGURE 2.18   A: Axial T2-weighted MRI; **B:** Axial gradient echo sequence MRI

a. Arteriovenous malformation (AVM)

b. Cavernous malformation

c. Dural arteriovenous fistula (DAVF)

d. Venous angioma

e. Capillary telangiectasias

63. Which of the following is incorrect regarding cerebral arterial circulation?

a. The left common carotid artery most commonly arises from the aortic arch

b. The left vertebral artery arises from the left subclavian artery

c. The right common carotid artery arises from the innominate artery
d. The left common carotid artery may arise from the innominate artery in some cases
e. The common carotid artery divides into external and internal carotid arteries at the level of C7 (c4)

64. A 52-year-old man presents with progressive lower extremity weakness over the past 6 months. He reports that last week he woke up one day and his legs could not move at all. His MRI is shown in Figure 2.19. A vascular anomaly is suspected. Which of the following is the most likely diagnosis?

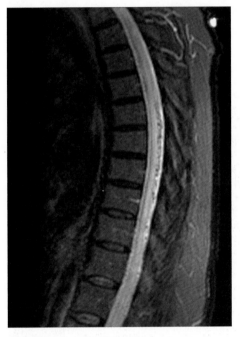

FIGURE 2.19 Sagittal STIR MRI

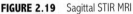

a. Epidural hematoma
b. Cavernous malformation
c. DAVF
d. Venous angioma
e. Spinal cord infarct

65. Based on imaging studies shown in Figure 2.20, which of the following is correct?
a. This is a hyperacute bleed
b. This is not a hemorrhage
c. This is an old hemorrhage, probably more than 1 month old
d. This hemorrhage is about 1 week old
e. This hemorrhage occurred within the last 24 hours

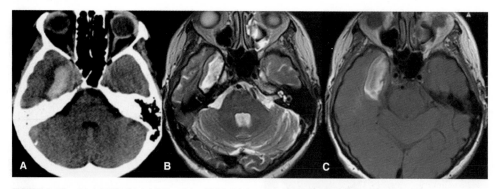

FIGURE 2.20   (a) Axial CT; (b) Axial T2-weighted MRI; (c) Axial T1-weighted precontrast MRI

Answer key

1. e	12. e	23. d	34. c	45. d	56. c
2. d	13. b	24. d	35. e	46. e	57. c
3. b	14. c	25. c	36. a	47. e	58. e
4. d	15. b	26. a	37. c	48. e	59. d
5. e	16. a	27. d	38. c	49. d	60. c
6. a	17. e	28. c	39. a	50. e	61. b
7. d	18. b	29. e	40. d	51. a	62. b
8. b	19. d	30. d	41. a	52. e	63. e
9. c	20. b	31. b	42. e	53. b	64. c
10. a	21. d	32. e	43. e	54. d	65. d
11. c	22. d	33. a	44. e	55. a	

Answers

1. **e**

Hyperlipidemia is not a part of the ABCD2 scoring system.

Identification of risk factors that predict stroke after TIA is important in the assessment of patients presenting with a TIA. The ABCD2 score provides an evaluation of this risk. Points are given for the following risk factors:

– Age of 60 years or more: 1 point
– Blood pressure of 140/90 mm Hg or greater: 1 point
– Clinical symptoms: 1 point for speech impairment without weakness and 2 points for focal weakness
– Symptom Duration: 1 point for 10 to 59 minutes and 2 points for 60 minutes or more
– Diabetes: 1 point

The 2-day risk of stroke is 0% for scores of 0 to 1, 1.3% for scores of 2 to 3, 4.1% for scores of 4 to 5, and 8.1% for scores of 6 to 7.

Easton JD, Saver JL, Albers GW, et al. Definition and evaluation of transient ischemic attack. Stroke. 2009; 40:2276–2293.

2. d

The MRI shown in Figure 2.1 demonstrates restriction on DWI of the pons bilaterally, as well as in the cerebellum. Most likely this patient will have quadriplegia and impaired horizontal gaze, findings consistent with locked-in syndrome. Other neurologic manifestations may be present given the extensive stroke in this important structure. However, the other manifestations listed in the options would not be present in this patient.

Goetz CG. Textbook of Clinical Neurology, 3rd ed. Philadelphia, PA: Saunders Elsevier; 2007.

Ropper AH, Samuels MA. Adams and Victor's Principles of Neurology, 9th ed. New York, NY: McGraw-Hill, 2009.

3. b

A brain CT scan should be obtained before any therapy is started.

This patient's clinical presentation is consistent with an acute stroke. If this is an acute ischemic stroke, and there are no contraindications, intravenous tissue plasminogen activator (tPA) should be given since the patient presented within the time window for this therapy.

When a patient presents to the emergency department with acute onset of focal neurologic symptoms suggestive of a stroke, and if stable from the hemodynamic and respiratory standpoint, steps should be taken to ensure appropriate treatment in a timely manner. The National Institutes of Health Stroke Scale (NIHSS) is a point system utilized to assess patients presenting with a stroke in which different neurologic functions are examined, including consciousness; vision and eye movement; movement of the face, arm, and leg; sensation; coordination; speech; and language. Points are given for impairments of these functions. The maximum score is 42, with higher scores representing worse neurologic deficits.

The first thing to do is to obtain a brain CT scan to rule out an intracranial hemorrhage (ICH). A brain CT scan will also help to determine if there are other structural lesions and/or already established ischemic changes. If there is no evidence of hemorrhage, an exclusion criteria checklist should be assessed, and if there are no contraindications and if the patient is within the time window, intravenous tPA should be given. The dose is 0.9 mg/kg, with a 10% bolus and the rest over 1 hour, with a maximum dose of 90 mg.

The time window approved on the basis of the National Institute of Neurological Disorders and Stroke (NINDS) tPA trial is 3 hours. However, a recent study (European Cooperative Acute Stroke Study 3 or ECASS3), showed that this medication, when given between 3 and 4.5 hours after the onset of symptoms, can improve clinical outcomes in patients with acute ischemic stroke, with NIHSS score of less than 25 on admission, without exclusion criteria as per the NINDS tPA trial, and with no history of prior clinical stroke or diabetes.

Aspirin may be needed, but a CT scan is a priority to rule out ICH. Intravenous heparin should not be used in the treatment of acute ischemic stroke. A brain MRI is sensitive to detect infarcted tissue, however, is not practical, since it takes time to obtain, and is not widely available in an emergency setting.

Hacke W, Kaste M, Bluhmki E, et al. Thrombolysis with alteplase 3 to 4.5 hours after acute ischemic stroke. N Engl J Med. 2008; 359:1317–1329.

The National Institute of Neurological Disorders and Stroke rt-PA Stroke Study Group. Tissue plasminogen activator for acute ischemic stroke. N Engl J Med. 1995; 335:1581–1587.

4. d

This patient has a locked-in syndrome, which is caused by a basilar occlusion leading to bilateral lesions at the base of the pons, affecting the long tracts but preserving the reticular activating system. These patients are awake, consciousness is preserved, and they can blink and move their eyes vertically; however, they are quadriplegic, unable to speak, and with impairment of horizontal eye movements.

Top of the basilar syndrome results from occlusion at the top of the basilar artery causing infarcts of various structures including the midbrain, thalamus, and temporal and occipital lobes. The manifestations are complex and varied, including combinations of behavioral abnormalities, alteration of consciousness, pupillary manifestations, disorders of ocular movements, visual field defects, and motor and/or sensory deficits.

Infarcts in the other locations will not produce the clinical manifestations that this patient has.

Goetz CG. Textbook of Clinical Neurology, 3rd ed. Philadelphia, PA: Saunders Elsevier; 2007.

Ropper AH, Samuels MA. Adams and Victor's Principles of Neurology, 9th ed. New York, NY: McGraw-Hill; 2009.

5. e

Seizures occur in 40% of the patients with venous sinus thrombosis, which is a higher percentage than that in patients with arterial strokes. In patients with venous sinus thrombosis, headache is the most frequent symptom, seen in about 90% of cases in adults. Given the occlusion of venous drainage along with hemorrhagic infarct and edema, patients may develop increased intracranial pressure. Diplopia caused by a sixth cranial nerve palsy has nonlocalizing value and may be a manifestation of increased intracranial pressure.

In patients with venous infarcts, focal neurologic findings will be present depending on the area affected along the thrombosed venous sinus. Thrombosis of the deep venous system may lead to deep venous infarcts, including bilateral thalamic infarcts. This is not seen with superior sagittal sinus thrombosis, which instead can lead to infarcts in the parasagittal cortex bilaterally along the sinus.

Ropper AH, Samuels MA. Adams and Victor's Principles of Neurology, 9th ed. New York, NY: McGraw-Hill; 2009.

Stam J. Thrombosis of the cerebral veins and sinuses. N Engl J Med. 2005; 352:1791–1798.

6. a

This MRI demonstrates restricted diffusion in the lateral medulla and cerebellum, which manifests with Wallenberg's syndrome. A lateral medullary infarct is caused by occlusion of the posterior inferior cerebellar artery (PICA), and often from occlusion of the vertebral artery.

Wallenberg's syndrome, or lateral medullary syndrome, involves the following structures:

– Vestibular nuclei, causing vertigo, nystagmus, nausea, and vomiting.
– Descending tract and nucleus of the fifth cranial nerve, producing impaired sensation on the ipsilateral hemiface.
– Spinothalamic tract, producing loss of sensation to pain and temperature in the contralateral hemibody.
– Sympathetic tract, manifesting with ipsilateral Horner's syndrome with ptosis, miosis, and anhidrosis.
– Fibers of the ninth and tenth cranial nerves, presenting with hoarseness, dysphagia, ipsilateral paralysis of the palate and vocal cord, and decreased gag reflex.
– Cerebellum and cerebellar tracts, causing ipsilateral ataxia and lateropulsion.
– Nucleus of the tractus solitarius, causing loss of taste.

Patients may present with combinations of these manifestations and not always with a complete syndrome. Other clinical manifestations, such as hiccups, are typically seen in this syndrome, but may not be explained by a lesion to a specific structure in the brainstem.

The other manifestations are unlikely to result from the anatomic localization of this infarct.

Goetz CG. Textbook of Clinical Neurology, 3rd ed. Philadelphia, PA: Saunders Elsevier; 2007.

Park MH, Kim BJ, Koh SB, et al. Lesional location of lateral medullary infarction presenting hiccups (singultus). J Neurol Neurosurg Psychiatry. 2005; 76:95–98.

Ropper AH, Samuels MA. Adams and Victor's Principles of Neurology, 9th ed. New York, NY: McGraw-Hill; 2009.

7. d

This patient likely has a left vertebral artery dissection causing a lateral medullary syndrome. The gold standard diagnostic test for an arterial dissection is a conventional angiogram, demonstrating the narrowing of the vessel, the extension of the dissection with an intimal flap, or double lumen.

Ultrasonography is noninvasive and is useful in the initial assessment; however, the dissection may not be visualized, and ultrasound may not be able to determine the extent of the dissection.

Transcranial Doppler ultrasonography is less useful and does not provide direct visualization of the dissection.

An echocardiogram with bubble study is not indicated.

MRA with a time-of-flight sequence may also be helpful to assess the flow at the site of the dissection; however, it does not provide information about the vessel wall. An MRI with fat-suppression techniques is helpful to assess the vessel wall and surrounding tissues, and very useful in nonocclusive dissections, when conventional angiogram will not give information about the vessel wall.

Patients with arterial dissections will have strokes either from vessel occlusion or from embolism originating in the dissected vessel wall. Treatment ranges from antiplatelet agents to anticoagulation, and in some cases endovascular techniques to open the vessel. However, there is no evidence to dictate which treatment is the best option.

Ropper AH, Samuels MA. Adams and Victor's Principles of Neurology, 9th ed. New York, NY: McGraw-Hill; 2009.

Schievink WI. Spontaneous dissection of the carotid and vertebral arteries. N Engl J Med. 2001; 344:898–906.

8. b

Tissue plasminogen activator (tPA) is a thrombolytic agent that is used intravenously for the treatment of acute ischemic stroke. Earlier administration correlates with better prognosis and lower risk of hemorrhage when compared with later administration of the medication.

The tPA for acute ischemic stroke trial was published in 1995 and performed by the National Institute of Neurological Disorders and Stroke (NINDS) Study Group. In this trial, intravenous t-PA was given to eligible patients with acute ischemic stroke within 3 hours from onset of symptoms. These patients were given 0.9 mg/kg of the drug, 10% as a bolus and the rest over 1 hour. The maximum dose is 90 mg.

Symptomatic intracranial hemorrhage (ICH) occurred in 6.4% of the patients who received intravenous tPA, compared with 0.6% in those who received placebo. The time window from symptom onset to allowable time for tPA administration was 3 hours; however, it was determined that the earlier the administration, the better the prognosis and the lower the risk of hemorrhage.

Patients who received intravenous tPA had improved clinical outcomes and were at least 30% more likely to have minimal or no disability at 3 months. The mortality at 3 months was 17% in the tPA group and 21% in the placebo group.

Administration of intravenous tPA is indicated in patients with an acute ischemic stroke presenting within 3 hours from symptom onset when no contraindications are identified.

Based on the European Cooperative Acute Stroke Study 3 (ECASS3), the use of intravenous tPA between 3 and 4.5 hours from the onset of symptoms has been shown to be beneficial in select patients. However, 4 additional exclusion criteria exist: National Institutes of Health Stroke Scale (NIHSS) 25 or greater, age >80, history of both stroke and diabetes, and any anticoagulant use, regardless of prothrombin time or INR.

Hacke W, Kaste M, Bluhmki E, et al. Thrombolysis with alteplase 3 to 4.5 hours after acute ischemic stroke. N Engl J Med. 2008; 359:1317–1329.

The National Institute of Neurological Disorders and Stroke rt-PA Stroke Study Group. Tissue plasminogen activator for acute ischemic stroke. N Engl J Med. 1995; 335:1581–1587.

9. c

This patient had transient monocular blindness or amaurosis fugax, which may represent atherosclerotic stenosis of the ipsilateral ICA, in this case the right side.

The retinal artery originates from the ophthalmic artery, which is a branch of the ICA. Transient occlusion of the retinal or ophthalmic arteries may manifest as amaurosis fugax.

Amaurosis fugax is often described as a painless visual loss: a "shade" or "curtain" moving in the vertical plane, with a rapid onset and brief duration of few minutes. Vision is most commonly recovered completely; however, the presentation of amaurosis fugax in a patient with an underlying ICA stenosis, may herald the occurrence of a stroke. For this reason, when a patient complains of amaurosis fugax, investigations should be obtained to rule out ICA stenosis. Other more rare but potential causes include giant cell arteritis, and embolism.

The other options listed do not correlate with the presentation of amaurosis fugax.

Goetz CG. Textbook of Clinical Neurology, 3rd ed. Philadelphia, PA: Saunders Elsevier; 2007.

Ropper AH, Samuels MA. Adams and Victor's Principles of Neurology, 9th ed. New York, NY: McGraw-Hill; 2009.

10. a

This patient has an infarct in the distribution of the anterior inferior cerebellar artery (AICA). The clinical presentation is very similar to that of a posterior inferior cerebellar artery (PICA) stroke or Wallenberg's syndrome; however, the difference is the ipsilateral deafness that occurs with AICA infarcts, as a consequence of involvement of the lateral pontomedullary tegmentum. By imaging, AICA infarcts affect the cerebellum more ventrally as compared with PICA infarcts.

Infarcts in the other locations will not produce the clinical manifestations depicted in this case.

Goetz CG. Textbook of Clinical Neurology, 3rd ed. Philadelphia, PA: Saunders Elsevier; 2007.

Ropper AH, Samuels MA. Adams and Victor's Principles of Neurology, 9th ed. New York, NY: McGraw-Hill; 2009.

11. c

Figure 2.3 shows bilateral thalamic infarction, which can be seen with occlusion of the artery of Percheron.

The P1 segment of the PCA gives rise to interpeduncular branches that will provide vascularization to the medial thalamus. Most frequently, these branches arise from each PCA separately and will give perfusion to the thalamus on its respective side. In some cases, a single artery called the artery of Percheron will arise from the P1 segment on one side and will supply the medial thalami bilaterally. This is a normal variant. If an occlusion of the artery of Percheron occurs, the result will be an infarct in the medial thalamic structures bilaterally.

The anterior choroidal arteries do not supply the medial thalamus. The recurrent artery of Heubner is a branch of the ACA that supplies the anterior limb of the internal capsule, the inferior part of the head of the caudate and the anterior part of the globus pallidus.

The pericallosal artery is one of the subdivisions of the ACA, running along the corpus callosum, and does not supply the thalamus.

Thrombosis of the deep venous structures may produce venous infarcts in the thalamus, but this is not seen with superior sagittal sinus thrombosis.

Goetz CG. Textbook of Clinical Neurology, 3rd ed. Philadelphia, PA: Saunders Elsevier; 2007.

Ropper AH, Samuels MA. Adams and Victor's Principles of Neurology, 9th ed. New York, NY: McGraw-Hill; 2009.

12. e

This patient presents with pure sensory symptoms, which can be seen in a pure sensory lacunar infarct. A lacunar stroke occurs from occlusion of small penetrating arteries, as a consequence of chronic hypertension. Diabetes and hyperlipidemia also play a role but to a lesser degree. These small vessels develop lipohyalinosis with vessel wall degeneration and luminal occlusion. Atherosclerosis of the parent vessel may occlude the opening of these small penetrating branches, or predispose to the entry of embolic material that will occlude them.

These lacunes occur in the putamen, caudate nuclei, thalamus, basis pontis, internal capsule, and deep hemispheric white matter. Symptoms will depend on the location, and several syndromes have been reported including the following:

– Pure motor, usually involving face, arm, and leg equally, and the most frequent location is in the territory of the lenticulostriate branches, affecting the posterior limb of the internal capsule, but has also been described with lacunes in the ventral pons.
– Pure sensory, with hemisensory deficit involving the contralateral face, arm, trunk, and leg from a lacune in the thalamus.
– Clumsy-hand dysarthria occurs more frequently from a lacune in the paramedian pons contralateral to the clumsy hand, but it may also occur from a lacune in the posterior limb of the internal capsule.
– Ataxic-hemiparesis, in which the ataxia is on the same side of the weakness, but out of proportion to the weakness, and this occurs from lacunes in the pons, midbrain, internal capsule, or parietal white matter.

The clinical manifestations of these lacunar infarcts may have a sudden onset; however, it is not infrequent to see a stepwise "stuttering" progression of the neurologic deficits over minutes, and sometimes over hours to even days.

This patient should undergo evaluation, and MRI with diffusion-weighted sequences should be obtained. Even though diabetes control is important, hypertension plays a major role in the pathogenesis of lacunar strokes, and strict blood pressure control may prevent further events.

Ropper AH, Samuels MA. Adams and Victor's Principles of Neurology, 9th ed. New York, NY: McGraw-Hill; 2009.

13. b

This patient has a lacunar pure motor stroke syndrome. The infarct is most likely in the posterior limb of the internal capsule on the right side, from occlusion of one or many of the lenticulostriate branches of the MCA. These lenticulostriate branches provide vascular supply to the putamen, part of the head and body of the caudate nucleus, the outer globus pallidus, the posterior limb of the internal capsule, and the corona radiata.

Occlusion of the trunk of the MCA will, in addition to weakness, cause other sensory deficits and cortical findings, such as hemineglect, particularly with nondominant strokes. Strokes in the territory of the divisions of the MCA will not present with a pure motor syndrome, and the motor findings will affect the face and arm more than the leg.

A PCA stroke will present with visual and sensory deficits.

Blumenfeld H. Neuroanatomy through Clinical Cases, 1st ed. Sunderland, MA: Sinauer Associates; 2002.

Goetz CG. Textbook of Clinical Neurology, 3rd ed. Philadelphia, PA: Saunders Elsevier; 2007.

Ropper AH, Samuels MA. Adams and Victor's Principles of Neurology, 9th ed. New York, NY: McGraw-Hill; 2009.

14. c

This patient has an infarct in the distribution of the superior division of the left MCA. There is hemiparesis affecting mainly arm and face, probably from ischemia to the lateral hemispheric surface. Eye deviation toward the left occurs from unopposed action originating from the right frontal eye fields, given that the left frontal eye fields are dysfunctional. This patient has a Broca's or motor aphasia, in which she is able to understand and follow commands but cannot verbalize. It is common for these patients to seem frustrated since they can understand and know what they want to say but cannot speak. Broca's aphasia occurs from ischemia in the territory of the superior division of the MCA affecting the dominant inferior frontal gyrus. On the other hand, ischemia in the territory of the inferior division of the MCA in the dominant hemisphere will cause a Wernicke's rather than a Broca's aphasia.

A left MCA trunk occlusion will likely produce a global aphasia, and will also produce ischemia in the lenticulostriate arteries territory, therefore presenting with hemiparesis or hemiplegia affecting face, arm, and leg.

An infarct in the territory of the lenticulostriate branches will not present with cortical findings such as aphasia. A pontine stroke will not produce a brachiofacial hemiparesis with motor aphasia.

Blumenfeld H. Neuroanatomy through Clinical Cases, 1st ed. Sunderland, MA: Sinauer Associates; 2002.

Goetz CG. Textbook of Clinical Neurology, 3rd ed. Philadelphia, PA: Saunders Elsevier; 2007.

Ropper AH, Samuels MA. Adams and Victor's Principles of Neurology, 9th ed. New York, NY: McGraw-Hill; 2009.

15. b

This patient has ischemia in the territory of the right ACA. Given that both ACAs communicate via the anterior communicating artery, an occlusion proximal to the anterior communicating artery may not produce significant clinical manifestations. Therefore, to produce symptoms, the occlusion must occur in the segment distal to the anterior communicating artery.

An infarction occurring from an ACA occlusion distal to the anterior communicating artery presents with contralateral sensorimotor deficits of the lower extremity, sparing the arm and face. There may be urinary incontinence due to involvement of the medial micturition center in the paracentral lobule; sometimes deviation of the eyes to side of the lesion and paratonic rigidity occur.

An anterior communicating artery occlusion does not produce clinical manifestations in patients with otherwise normal perfusion dynamics.

An MCA distribution infarct would produce manifestations in the arm and face rather than in the lower extremity.

Blumenfeld H. Neuroanatomy Through Clinical Cases, 1st ed. Sunderland, MA: Sinauer Associates; 2002.

Goetz CG. Textbook of Clinical Neurology, 3rd ed. Philadelphia, PA: Saunders Elsevier; 2007.

Ropper AH, Samuels MA. Adams and Victor's Principles of Neurology, 9th ed. New York, NY: McGraw-Hill; 2009.

16. a

The ACA supplies the anterior three quarters of the medial surface of the frontal lobe. Proximal to the circle of Willis and prior to the anterior communicating artery, deep penetrating branches come off the ACA segment of the anterior communicating artery, the recurrent artery of Heubner being the largest of these deep branches. These branches supply the anterior limb of the internal capsule, the inferior part of the head of the caudate nucleus, and the anterior part of the globus pallidus.

Ropper AH, Samuels MA. Adams and Victor's Principles of Neurology, 9th ed. New York, NY: McGraw-Hill; 2009.

17. e

The MCA has superficial and deep branches. The deep penetrating or lenticulostriate branches supply the putamen, part of the head and body of the caudate nucleus, the external part of the globus pallidus, the posterior limb of the internal capsule, and the corona radiata. The anterior limb of the internal capsule is supplied by the recurrent artery of Heubner and deep branches coming from the ACA.

The superficial branches of the MCA supply the lateral convexity, including the lateral and inferior parts of the frontal lobe, parietal lobe, superior parts of the temporal lobe, and insula.

Ropper AH, Samuels MA. Adams and Victor's Principles of Neurology, 9th ed. New York, NY: McGraw-Hill; 2009.

18. b

This patient has Wallenberg's syndrome, or a lateral medullary syndrome, in this case caused by an infarct on the right side. Based on the history, the etiology is likely secondary to vertebral artery dissection. In this patient, the structures affected are the vestibular nuclei, the descending sympathetic tract on the right side, the right fifth, ninth, and tenth cranial nerve nuclei, right cerebellum and/or its connections, and right spinothalamic tract affecting the sensation on the contralateral side. These findings are consistent with an infarct in the lateral medulla on the right side.

Wallenberg's syndrome, or lateral medullary syndrome, involves the following structures:

- Vestibular nuclei, causing vertigo, nystagmus, nausea, and vomiting.
- Descending tract and nucleus of the fifth cranial nerve, producing impaired sensation on the ipsilateral hemiface.
- Spinothalamic tract, producing loss of sensation to pain and temperature in the contralateral hemibody.
- Sympathetic tract, manifesting with ipsilateral Horner's syndrome with ptosis, miosis, and anhidrosis.
- Fibers of the ninth and tenth cranial nerves, presenting with hoarseness, dysphagia, ipsilateral paralysis of the palate and vocal cord, and decreased gag reflex.
- Cerebellum and cerebellar tracts, causing ipsilateral ataxia and lateropulsion.
- Nucleus of the tractus solitarious, causing loss of taste.

Patients may present with combinations of these manifestations and not always with a complete syndrome. Other clinical manifestations, such as hiccups, are typically seen in this syndrome but may not be explained by a lesion to a specific structure in the brainstem.

Goetz CG. Textbook of Clinical Neurology, 3rd ed. Philadelphia, PA: Saunders Elsevier; 2007.

Ropper AH, Samuels MA. Adams and Victor's Principles of Neurology, 9th ed. New York, NY: McGraw-Hill; 2009.

19. d

The vascular supply of the thalamus originates mainly from the posterior circulation.
There are four major arteries supplying four regions of the thalamus:

1. The tuberothalamic artery, also known as polar artery, originates from the posterior communicating artery and supplies the anterior portion of the thalamus, especially the ventral anterior nucleus.
2. The thalamoperforating or paramedian artery originates from the P1 segment of the PCA and supplies the medial aspect of the thalamus, especially the dorsomedial nucleus.
3. The thalamogeniculate artery originates from the P2 segment of the PCA and supplies the lateral aspect of the thalamus, including the ventral lateral group of nuclei.
4. The posterior choroidal artery arises from the P2 segment of the PCA and provides vascularization to the posterior aspect of the thalamus, where the pulvinar is located.

The anterior choroidal artery does not supply the thalamus.

Carrera E, Bogousslavsky J. The thalamus and behavior. Effects of anatomically distinct strokes. Neurology. 2006; 66:1817–1823.

20. b

Figure 2.4 shows an infarct that involves mainly the right cerebellar hemisphere superiorly, consistent with a superior cerebellar artery (SCA) stroke. The CT scan shows a slice at the level of the midbrain; therefore, it is certain that this is the superior cerebellum.
The SCA supplies most of the superior half of the cerebellar hemisphere, including the superior vermis, the superior cerebellar peduncle, and part of the upper lateral pons.
The anterior inferior cerebellar artery (AICA) supplies the inferolateral pons, middle cerebellar peduncle, and a strip of the ventral cerebellum between the posterior inferior cerebellar and superior cerebellar territories.
The posterior inferior cerebellar artery (PICA) supplies the lateral medulla, most of the inferior half of the cerebellum and the inferior vermis.
A PCA lesion will not produce cerebellar strokes.

A vertebral artery lesion may account for PICA strokes but not strokes in SCA territory.

Blumenfeld H. Neuroanatomy through Clinical Cases, 1st ed. Sunderland, MA: Sinauer Associates; 2002.

21. d

This patient has an infarct in the inferior division of the MCA, which supplies the superior parietal and posterior temporal regions. The patient has clinical findings suggestive of a Wernicke's (receptive) aphasia, in which the patient speaks fluently but what she says does not make sense, and she is not able to understand spoken language or follow commands. This occurs from ischemia to the posterior aspect of the superior temporal gyrus. Patients with ischemia in the territory of the inferior division of the MCA will also present with agitation and confusion, cortical sensory deficits in the face and arm, as well as visual defects in the contralateral hemifield.

An MCA trunk occlusion will affect not only the cortex but also the deep subcortical structures provided by lenticulostriate branches, therefore presenting with cortical findings as well as a dense hemiparesis.

A stroke in the territory of the superior division of the MCA will manifest with an expressive rather than a receptive aphasia.

Stroke in the territory of the lenticulostriate branches will not present with cortical findings. A pontine stroke will not produce an aphasia.

Blumenfeld H. Neuroanatomy Through Clinical Cases, 1st ed. Sunderland, MA: Sinauer Associates; 2002.

Goetz CG. Textbook of Clinical Neurology, 3rd ed. Philadelphia, PA: Saunders Elsevier; 2007.

Ropper AH, Samuels MA. Adams and Victor's Principles of Neurology, 9th ed. New York, NY: McGraw-Hill; 2009.

22. d

The most prominent finding in the MRA shown in Figure 2.5 is the absence of a basilar artery, probably from an occlusion. A pontine stroke from the basilar occlusion will likely result in a locked-in syndrome. Basilar occlusion may occur from local thrombosis of the basilar artery itself, thrombosis of both vertebral arteries, or thrombosis of a single vertebral artery when it is the dominant vessel. Embolism can occur as well, frequently lodging distally in the vessel.

Wallenberg's syndrome occurs from an infarct of the lateral medulla, and is usually caused by involvement of the posterior inferior cerebellar artery (PICA), or the parent vertebral artery.

Parinaud's syndrome is characterized by supranuclear paralysis of eye elevation, defect in convergence, convergence-retraction nystagmus, light-near dissociation, lid retraction, and skew deviation of the eyes. The lesion is localized in the dorsal midbrain and is classically seen with pineal tumors compressing the quadrigeminal plate; however, it can occur from midbrain infarcts.

This patient does not have significant disease of the left MCA.

Dejerine-Roussy syndrome is caused by thalamic infarct, and even though this patient may have lesions in the thalamus, other manifestations are more likely to predominate.

Goetz CG. Textbook of Clinical Neurology, 3rd ed. Philadelphia, PA: Saunders Elsevier; 2007.

Ropper AH, Samuels MA. Adams and Victor's Principles of Neurology, 9th ed. New York, NY: McGraw-Hill; 2009.

23. d

The MRI shown in Figure 2.6 demonstrates a very small area of restricted diffusion consistent with a lacunar stroke, which is caused by the occlusion of a small penetrating vessel. This condition is intimately related to hypertension.

The pathologic basis of lacunes is lipohyalinosis of small penetrating branches but not microhemorrhages.

Given that this is a disease of small vessels, studies to look for a cardioembolic source are not required.

Given the location of the lacune in this case, it is unlikely for this patient to present with a pure sensory syndrome, which will be seen more frequently with thalamic lacunes.

Aphasia and neglect are manifestations of infarcts affecting the cortex and are not seen with subcortical strokes.

Ropper AH, Samuels MA. Adams and Victor's Principles of Neurology, 9th ed. New York, NY: McGraw-Hill; 2009.

24. d

The MRA shown in Figure 2.7 demonstrates absence of the ICA on the left side. The left MCA is still partially seen and is being supplied via the anterior communicating artery.

Both vertebral arteries are seen, and the basilar artery is also present, branching at its top into both PCAs. Fetal PCAs originate from the anterior circulation (distal internal carotid arteries) and not from the basilar artery, and this can be seen in the normal population. This is not the case in this MRA.

Ropper AH, Samuels MA. Adams and Victor's Principles of Neurology, 9th ed. New York, NY: McGraw-Hill; 2009.

25. c

The anterior choroidal artery does not supply the anterior limb of the internal capsule, which is supplied by the recurrent artery of Heubner and deep penetrating branches of the ACA.

The anterior choroidal artery arises from the ICA just above the origin of the posterior communicating artery, and supplies the internal segment of the globus pallidus, part of the posterior limb of the internal capsule, and part of the geniculocalcarine tract. As it penetrates the temporal horn of the lateral ventricle, it supplies the choroid plexus and then joins the posterior choroidal artery from the posterior circulation.

Ropper AH, Samuels MA. Adams and Victor's Principles of Neurology, 9th ed. New York, NY: McGraw-Hill; 2009.

26. a

Figure 2.8 shows a conventional angiogram demonstrating occlusion of the main trunk of the left MCA, which is not filling with contrast. The ICA is visualized up to its terminus, and the ACA is also well visualized. In this case, the injection of contrast was performed on the left ICA, and therefore the vertebral artery cannot be assessed.

Ropper AH, Samuels MA. Adams and Victor's Principles of Neurology, 9th ed. New York, NY: McGraw-Hill; 2009.

27. d

Figure 2.9 demonstrates restricted diffusion almost linearly between vascular boundaries, consistent with a watershed infarction, in this case between the superficial and deep territories of the MCA. Watershed infarcts occur when there is reduction of blood supply to two vascular territories; these regions are most susceptible to ischemia. This reduction of blood flow can occur in the setting of systemic hypotension, especially with an underlying stenosis proximal to both territories, in this case, hypotension and a left carotid stenosis.

The distribution of the stroke in the MRI is consistent with a watershed infarct, and not likely an embolic stroke, lacunar strokes, or venous infarct.

Blumenfeld H. Neuroanatomy Through Clinical Cases, 1st ed. Sunderland, MA: Sinauer Associates; 2002.

28. c

This patient has left-sided Horner's syndrome as well as findings suggesting a left fifth cranial nerve lesion, left cerebellar, and vestibular nuclei involvement. This can occur at the level of the brainstem, more specifically in the lateral medulla. Therefore, the most likely cause is a left vertebral artery dissection.

A left carotid artery dissection may cause left-sided Horner's syndrome by affecting the fibers running along the carotid artery walls but will not explain brainstem findings depicted in this case. A right MCA stroke will not produce these clinical manifestations.

Goetz CG. Textbook of Clinical Neurology, 3rd ed. Philadelphia, PA: Saunders Elsevier; 2007.

Ropper AH, Samuels MA. Adams and Victor's Principles of Neurology, 9th ed. New York, NY: McGraw-Hill; 2009.

29. e

Figure 2.10 shows a hyperdense left MCA sign. In a patient with a presumed stroke, the hyperdense MCA sign has good specificity and positive predictive value for atheroembolic occlusions of the affected vessel, and it is associated with poor prognosis. This sign lacks sensitivity but is helpful when a strong clinical suspicion exists. Mimics of hyperdense MCA sign, also known as pseudohyperdense sign, include vascular calcification, increased hematocrit, and intravenous contrast.

Other early signs (within 6 hours) of ischemic stroke on CT scan include the loss of the insular ribbon, the attenuation of the lentiform nucleus, and the hemispherical sulcal effacement.

This patient does not have a hypertensive hemorrhage. There is no evidence on CT scan of SAH to suspect the development of vasospasm. An MCA occlusion is a large vessel occlusion and does not represent a lacunar stroke. Large MCA occlusions with large strokes may require hemicraniectomy, but not suboccipital craniectomy, which is used in cerebellar strokes.

Jha B, Kothari M. Pearls & Oysters: Hyperdense or pseudohyperdense MCA sign. A Damocles sword? Neurology. 2009; 72:e116–e117.

Koga M, Saku Y, Toyoda K, et al. Reappraisal of early CT signs to predict the arterial occlusion site in acute embolic stroke. J Neurol Neurosurg & Psychiatry. 2003; 74:649–653.

30. d

This patient suffered a watershed infarct affecting the right hemisphere, likely secondary to reduction of blood supply from hypotension in the setting of a right internal carotid stenosis.

Watershed infarcts manifest clinically with proximal weakness, affecting the proximal upper and proximal lower extremities, with weakness at the shoulder and at the hip. This occurs because the watershed regions correlate with the homuncular representation of the proximal limbs and trunk. In severe cases of bilateral watershed infarcts, a "person-in-a-barrel" syndrome occurs, in which the patient can only move the distal extremities.

The clinical history of hypotension and subsequent neurologic findings correlates with watershed ischemic events.

Given the unilateral involvement and the clinical history, this is not a myopathy. An infarct in the internal capsule will not produce the clinical picture that this patient has. A cardioembolic event is also less likely given the clinical presentation. Given the left side weakness, it is likely that there is a stenosis in the right and not the left carotid.

Blumenfeld H. Neuroanatomy Through Clinical Cases, 1st ed. Sunderland, MA: Sinauer Associates; 2002.

31. b

This patient has a medial medullary syndrome with a lesion on the left side. This syndrome is caused by occlusion of the vertebral artery or one of its medial branches, producing an infarct affecting the pyramid, medial lemniscus, and emerging hypoglossal fibers. The patient will have contralateral arm and leg weakness sparing the face (from corticospinal tract involvement prior to its decussation), contralateral loss of sensation to position and vibration, and ipsilateral tongue weakness.

Neither a lateral medullary syndrome, nor a pontine infarct will produce these clinical manifestations.

Goetz CG. Textbook of Clinical Neurology, 3rd ed. Philadelphia, PA: Saunders Elsevier; 2007.

Ropper AH, Samuels MA. Adams and Victor's Principles of Neurology, 9th ed. New York, NY: McGraw-Hill; 2009.

32. e

This patient may have temporal arteritis or giant cell arteritis, and given the visual manifestations, she should be treated with steroids as soon as possible.

Giant cell arteritis is a disease seen in older adults, typically older than 50 years of age. It is characterized by inflammation of the temporal artery predominantly but may also affect other branches of the ECA. These patients complain of headaches, associated with generalized constitutional symptoms, jaw claudication, and tenderness of the scalp around the temporal artery. This condition may overlap with polymyalgia rheumatica, and patients will also present with proximal muscle pain and achiness. Laboratory studies demonstrate leukocytosis and very elevated sedimentation rates and C-reactive protein levels. The diagnosis is based on a biopsy of the temporal artery demonstrating granulomatous inflammation.

Blindness may occur from ocular ischemia, and these patients should be treated as soon as possible with steroids while arranging for a temporal artery biopsy.

Cerebral angiogram and CT angiogram are not helpful in the diagnosis of this condition. Anticoagulation is not indicated.

Ropper AH, Samuels MA. Adams and Victor's Principles of Neurology, 9th ed. New York, NY: McGraw-Hill; 2009.

33. a

This patient has a Millard-Gubler syndrome, which is manifested by contralateral hemiplegia with ipsilateral facial palsy. The lesion is localized in the pons, and affects the corticospinal tract before its decussation at the level of the pyramids, as well as the VII cranial nerve nuclei. When there is also conjugate gaze paralysis toward the side of the brainstem lesion it is called Foville syndrome.

Infarcts in the other locations do not cause this constellation of findings.

Ropper AH, Samuels MA. Adams and Victor's Principles of Neurology, 9th ed. New York, NY: McGraw-Hill; 2009.

Silverman IE, Liu GT, Volpe NJ, et al. The crossed paralyses. Arch Neurol. 1995; 52:635–638.

34. c

Anterior circulation aneurysms have a lower risk of rupture when compared with posterior circulation aneurysms.

Intracranial aneurysms are most often acquired and sporadic; however, there are associations with various conditions, including AVMs, polycystic kidney disease, aortic coarctation, fibromuscular dysplasia, Marfan's syndrome, and Ehlers-Danlos syndrome. Aneurysms can also be familial.

Cerebral aneurysmal rupture leads to SAH, which is a serious, often fatal event. In a patient with an unruptured cerebral aneurysm, the presence of certain factors promotes a higher risk of rupture and influences treatment decisions. Risk of rupture and SAH depends on various factors. Size is important, and larger aneurysms have a higher risk of rupture, especially those larger than 10 mm. Some studies have suggested that the risk of rupture is significantly higher with diameters of 7 mm or higher; however, this topic is still controversial. Aneurysm location is also important, and posterior circulation aneurysms are at higher risk for rupture than anterior circulation aneurysms. Smoking and uncontrolled hypertension are also risk factors for aneurysmal rupture, and these conditions should be treated. Patients with previous aneurysmal rupture are at higher risk for SAH.

Unruptured aneurysms could be treated conservatively (observation in those patients with low risk of aneurysmal rupture), by endovascular management (coiling), or by surgical management (clipping). Selection of endovascular management or surgical treatment depends on the age of the patient and other comorbidities, size of the aneurysm, location and morphology, as well as the experience of the center where the patient is being treated.

Brisman JL, Song JK, Newell DW. Cerebral aneurysms. N Engl J Med. 2006; 355:928–939.

Wiebers DO, Piepgras DG, Meyer FB, et al. Pathogenesis, natural history and treatment of unruptured intracranial aneurysms. Mayo Clin Proc. 2004; 79:1572–1583.

35. e

Expressive aphasia will not be expected with this infarct. Figure 2.11 shows a left occipital infarct, in the distribution of the left PCA, which will likely cause a homonymous hemianopia in the contralateral side, in this case in the right visual hemifield. Typically, PCA strokes spare central vision because of collateral blood supply to macular cortical representation.

Occipital strokes in the dominant hemisphere may manifest with alexia (inability to read), anomia, achromatopsia (color anomia), and other visual agnosias. Patients with left occipital infarcts involving the splenium of the corpus callosum may present with the classical alexia without agraphia. This syndrome occurs because the patient cannot see what is placed in the right visual hemifield, and whatever can be seen in the left visual hemifield will be represented in the right occipital cortex, but due to corpus callosum involvement, this information will not be transmitted to language centers in the left hemisphere.

Expressive aphasia is caused by lesions in Broca's area in dominant frontal lobe and is not seen with occipital infarcts.

Ropper AH, Samuels MA. Adams and Victor's Principles of Neurology, 9th ed. New York, NY: McGraw-Hill; 2009.

36. a

This patient has an infarction in the right mesencephalic tegmentum in its ventral portion, involving the ventral part of the red nucleus, the brachium conjunctivum, and the fascicle of the third cranial nerve. This lesion produces a constellation of findings including an ipsilateral third nerve palsy with contralateral involuntary movements such as tremor and choreoathetosis. The combination of this manifestations have been called Benedikt's syndrome.

The lesions in the other locations do not cause these clinical manifestations.

Bradley WG, Daroff RB, Fenichel GM, Jankovic J. Neurology in Clinical Practice, 5th ed. Philadelphia, PA: Elsevier; 2008.

37. c

This patient has a left MCA distribution infarct, which in this case is a dominant hemispheric infarct. Dominant hemispheric strokes will manifest with aphasias, depending on the region affected. Superior division MCA strokes predominantly involve the frontal lobe and will manifest with Broca's aphasia. Inferior division MCA strokes predominantly involve the temporal lobe and will manifest with Wernicke's aphasia. In this case, given the extent of the lesion, the patient will most likely have a global aphasia.

With MCA strokes, the frontal eye fields may be involved, and patients will have gaze deviation toward the hemisphere involved. This occurs because the contralateral frontal eye fields will be unopposed, "pushing" the eyes to the side of the infarct. Given that optic radiations are also involved during their course within the territory of the MCA, a contralateral homonymous hemianopia is expected. In this case a right homonymous hemianopia.

Patients with MCA strokes present with contralateral hemiparesis. If the stroke predominantly involves the cortex, the weakness will be more prominent in the face and arm than in the leg, as the cortical leg area is supplied by the ACA. If the infarct extends to the subcortical region affecting the corona radiata or internal capsule, the patient could have a dense hemiplegia involving face, arm, and leg equally. Weakness that involves the leg more than the face and arm is characteristic of anterior cerebral infarctions, and not typically seen with MCA infarctions.

Neglect, anosognosia, and other visual-spatial disturbances are seen more frequently with nondominant hemispheric lesions.

Ropper AH, Samuels MA. Adams and Victor's Principles of Neurology, 9th ed. New York, NY: McGraw-Hill; 2009.

38. c

A 52-year-old patient with hyperthyroidism and intracranial atherosclerotic stenosis should be managed with antiplatelet agents. The other cases should be managed with oral anticoagulation.

Results of the Warfarin-Aspirin Symptomatic Intracranial Disease (WASID) trial suggested that oral anticoagulation with warfarin was associated with more adverse events and provided no benefit over aspirin in the prevention of cerebrovascular events in the setting of intracranial atherosclerotic disease. Use of oral anticoagulation is indicated in the prevention of strokes from a cardioembolic source, and this therapy is not indicated or is controversial in the setting of atherothrombotic etiologies. A patient with intracardiac thrombus should also be treated with anticoagulation. In the setting of anterior wall myocardial infarction with anterior wall akinesis and depressed ejection fraction, the use of anticoagulation should be contemplated, since the risk of formation of intramural thrombus is high in these patients. In general, oral anticoagulation should target an INR between 2.0 and 3.0, except in the setting of mechanical valves, in which the target INR is 2.5 to 3.5.

Treatment with oral anticoagulation should also be considered in patients with atrial fibrillation, and in these cases, the CHADS2 score (discussed in question 58) should be calculated to evaluate if treatment with warfarin is indicated, or if antiplatelet agents would suffice depending on the stroke risk. Other considerations such as risk of hemorrhage (as in patients with high fall risk) should be assessed. Certainly in patients with atrial fibrillation, heart rate control is required, and as suggested by the AFFIRM (Atrial Fibrillation Follow-up Investigation of Rhythm Management) trial, rhythm control does not confer benefit when compared with rate control.

Chimowitz MI, Lynn MJ, Howlett-Smith H, et al. Comparison of Warfarin and Aspirin for symptomatic intracranial arterial stenosis. N Engl J Med. 2005; 352:1305–1316.

Ropper AH, Samuels MA. Adams and Victor's Principles of Neurology, 9th ed. New York, NY: McGraw-Hill; 2009.

Wyse DG, Waldo AL, DiMArco JP, et al. A comparison of rate control and rhythm control in patients with atrial fibrillation. N Engl J Med. 2002; 347:1825–1833.

39. a

This patient has a stroke from an occlusion of the trunk of the left MCA before the bifurcation, affecting not only the cortex but also the deep subcortical structures provided by lenticulostriate branches.

The hemiparesis affecting face, arm, and leg is explained by involvement of the internal capsule, which is supplied by the lenticulostriate arteries that originate from the stem of the MCA prior to the bifurcation.

An occlusion at this site also explains the cortical findings such as the aphasia. In superior division left MCA strokes, a Broca's aphasia is more common, whereas Wernicke's aphasia is seen more often with inferior division left MCA strokes. In this case, the global aphasia is better explained by an MCA trunk occlusion affecting both divisions.

Gaze deviation to the left is caused by unopposed action of the right frontal eye fields. The right homonymous hemianopsia is caused by interruption of the geniculocalcarine radiations running in the left hemisphere.

A stroke localized to the left lenticulostriate branches will not explain the aphasia and the other neurologic findings except the hemiparesis.

An infarct isolated to the individual MCA segments after the first bifurcation will not explain the hemiparesis affecting also the lower extremity, nor the global aphasia.

A pontine stroke will not present with aphasia, and furthermore the eyes will deviate toward the hemiparetic side and not toward the side of the lesion.

Blumenfeld H. Neuroanatomy Through Clinical Cases, 1st ed. Sunderland, MA: Sinauer Associates; 2002.

Goetz CG. Textbook of Clinical Neurology, 3rd ed. Philadelphia, PA: Saunders Elsevier; 2007.

Ropper AH, Samuels MA. Adams and Victor's Principles of Neurology, 9th ed. New York, NY: McGraw-Hill; 2009.

40. d

The lenticulostriate arteries arise from the trunk of the MCA before its bifurcation.

The circle of Willis is an arterial ring that interconnects the anterior and posterior circulation as well as the right and left arterial systems (Figure 2.21).

The anterior circulation is provided by the ACA and the MCA, which are the terminal branches of the ICA. In the anterior circulation, the right and left sides connect via the anterior

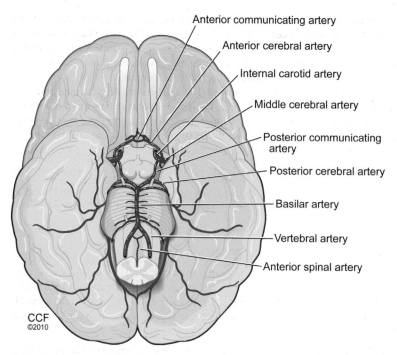

Anterior communicating artery

Anterior cerebral artery

Internal carotid artery

Middle cerebral artery

Posterior communicating
artery

Posterior cerebral artery

Basilar artery

Vertebral artery

Anterior spinal artery

CCF
©2010

FIGURE 2.21   Circle of Willis (Illustration by David R. Schumick, BS, CMI. Reprinted with permission of the Cleveland Clinic Center for Medical Art and Photography. © 2010. All rights reserved.)

communicating arteries. The posterior circulation is constituted by the vertebrobasilar system, with the PCAs being the terminal branches originating from the top of the basilar. The anterior and posterior circulations connect via the posterior communicating arteries.

The ACAs connect through the anterior communicating artery. Beyond this point, the ACA will continue around the genu of the corpus callosum, and it will give rise to various small branches, including the recurrent artery of Heubner, and the pericallosal artery, which runs along the corpus callosum.

The MCA originates from the ICA. The MCA main trunk before the bifurcation gives off many small vessels called the lenticulostriate arteries, which supply large regions of the basal ganglia and the internal capsule. The MCA will bifurcate into superior and inferior divisions that will supply the lateral convexity.

The PCA comes off the top of the basilar, and will run toward the back of the midbrain, along the lateral aspect of the quadrigeminal cistern and around the pulvinar, dividing into smaller branches at the calcarine fissure.

Blumenfeld H. Neuroanatomy Through Clinical Cases, 1st ed. Sunderland, MA: Sinauer Associates; 2002.

Morris P. Practical Neuroangiography, 1st ed. Baltimore, MD: Williams & Wilkins; 1997.

41. a

Statins reduce the risk of cerebrovascular events.

This patient had a TIA with negative cardioembolic work up. The Stroke Prevention by Aggressive Reduction in Cholesterol Levels (SPARCL) trial studied the effect of atorvastatin at a dose of 80 mg daily in patients with a recent (within 6 months) TIA or stroke, with low density lipoprotein (LDL) between 100 and 190 mg/dL. The conclusion was that 80 mg of atorvastatin daily reduces the overall incidence of strokes and cardiovascular events.

Warfarin and heparin are not indicated in this case and are used for the prevention of cardioembolic events. Thrombolysis with tissue plasminogen activator (tPA) is used for the treatment of acute ischemic stroke, but not for prevention of cerebrovascular events. The use of hormone replacement therapy is not indicated, and may be associated with an increased risk of stroke. The severity of stroke may also be increased in patients on hormone replacement therapy.

Amarenco P, Bogousslavsky J, Callahan A III, et al. High-dose atorvastatin after stroke or transient ischemic stroke. N Engl J Med. 2006; 355:549–559.

Bath PM, Gray LJ. Association between hormone replacement therapy and subsequent stroke: a meta-analysis. BMJ. 2005; 330:342.

42. e

This patient has Parinaud's syndrome, in which there is supranuclear paralysis of eye elevation, defect in convergence, convergence-retraction nystagmus, light-near dissociation, lid retraction, and skew deviation of the eyes. The lesion is localized in the dorsal midbrain, and is classically seen with pineal tumors compressing the quadrigeminal plate; however, it can occur from midbrain infarcts.

Goetz CG. Textbook of Clinical Neurology, 3rd ed. Philadelphia, PA: Saunders Elsevier; 2007.

Ropper AH, Samuels MA. Adams and Victor's Principles of Neurology, 9th ed. New York, NY: McGraw-Hill; 2009.

43. e

CT scan of the brain showing no evidence of acute infarct is not a contraindication for intravenous tissue plasminogen activator (tPA).

Patients presenting with an acute ischemic stroke within the time window for intravenous tPA should have a brain CT scan to rule out hemorrhage. The CT scan also helps to determine if there are already established signs of ischemia. Evidence of infarcted tissue on CT scan may suggest a longer time from the onset of symptoms than initially thought.

Exclusion criteria for treatment with intravenous tPA in the original trial by the National Institute of Neurological Disorders and Stroke (NINDS) include the following:

– Another stroke or serious head trauma within the prior 3 months
– Major surgery within the prior 14 days
– History of intracranial hemorrhage (ICH)
– Blood pressure above 185/110 mm Hg
– Rapidly improving or minor symptoms
– Symptoms suggestive of SAH
– Gastrointestinal or urinary tract hemorrhage within 21 days
– Arterial puncture at a noncompressible site within 7 days
– Seizure at the onset of the stroke
– Use of anticoagulants
– Patients who received heparin within 48 hours of the onset of stroke and have an elevated activated partial thromboplastin time

– Prothrombin time greater than 15 seconds
– Platelet count below 100,000/mm^3
– Glucose less than 50 mg/dL or more than 400 mg/dL

The ECASS3 (discussed in question 3) showed that intravenous tPA, when given between 3 and 4.5 hours after the onset of symptoms, can improve clinical outcomes in patients with acute ischemic stroke. Additional exclusion criteria for this group of patients include National Institutes of Health Stroke Scale (NIHSS) score of 25 or higher, age > 80, any anticoagulant use regardless of INR or prothrombin time, and history of prior stroke and/or diabetes.

Hacke W, Kaste M, Bluhmki E, et al. Thrombolysis with alteplase 3 to 4.5 hours after acute ischemic stroke. N Engl J Med. 2008; 359:1317–1329.

The National Institute of Neurological Disorders and Stroke rt-PA Stroke Study Group. Tissue plasminogen activator for acute ischemic stroke. N Engl J Med. 1995; 335:1581–1587.

44. e

At the time this book is published, aspirin is the only option with evidence to support its use in intracranial stenosis.

The Warfarin-Aspirin Symptomatic Intracranial Disease (WASID) trial randomized patients with a recent TIA or stroke with a 50% to 99% stenosis of a major intracranial artery to warfarin or aspirin, and concluded that warfarin was associated with higher rates of adverse events and provided no benefit over aspirin.

Endovascular procedures have evolved, and angioplasty and intracranial stenting have been used for the treatment of intracranial atherosclerotic stenosis; however, as of 2011, there is no clear evidence to support their use. At the time this book was published, there was an ongoing trial comparing the use of intracranial stent placement versus medical therapy.

Surgical bypass has fallen out of favor since it does not improve clinical outcomes, and patients who undergo such procedures may actually do worse. Surgical bypass may be considered in selected cases.

Chimowitz MI, Lynn MJ, Howlett-Smith H, et al. Comparison of warfarin and aspirin for symptomatic intracranial arterial stenosis. N Engl J Med. 2005; 352:1305–1316.

The EC/IC Bypass Study group. Failure of extracranial-intracranial arterial bypass to reduce the risk of ischemic stroke. Results of an international randomized trial. N Engl J Med. 1985; 313:1191–1200.

45. d

The Alberta Stroke Program Early CT Score (ASPECTS) is calculated based on findings on standard CT scan of the brain and provides a reproducible grading system to assess early ischemic changes in patients with acute ischemic strokes of the anterior circulation. This can be used to guide treatment with intravenous tPA by helping identify patients who will unlikely make an independent recovery.

To obtain the ASPECT score, two axial cuts are obtained on the CT, one at the level of the basal ganglia and thalamus, and another superior cut where these structures are not appreciated. On these sections, there are 10 regions of interest, of which 4 are deep and defined as the caudate, the internal capsule, the lentiform nucleus, and the insular region, and 6 regions are cortical. These regions are assigned a point, which is subtracted if there is early ischemic change in that specific region. A normal looking CT scan will obtain a maximum of 10 points, and a score of 0 is consistent with diffuse ischemic injury of the entire MCA territory.

The ASPECTS correlates inversely with the severity of the stroke, and patients with low scores should not be treated with thrombolytic agents. An ASPECTS score of 7 or less correlates with increased dependence and death.

Warwick Pexman JH, Barber PA, Hill MD, et al. Use of the Alberta Stroke Program Early CT Score (ASPECTS) for assessing CT scans in patients with acute stroke. Am J Neuroradiol. 2001; 22:1534–1542.

46. e

The anterior choroidal artery is a branch of the ICA and arises from the communicating segment.

Various classifications have been proposed for the segments of the ICA, with that by Bouthillier et al., being one of the most widely used and the basis for the following discussion.

The cervical (C1) segment of the ICA, beginning at the level of the common carotid artery and ending where the ICA enters the carotid canal in the petrous bone. It has no branches.

The petrous (C2) segment of the ICA runs within the carotid canal in the petrous bone. Vidian and caroticotympanic branches arise from this segment.

The lacerum (C3) segment of the ICA runs between where the carotid canal ends and the superior margin of the petrolingual ligament. This ligament runs between the lingula of the sphenoid bone and the petrous apex and is a continuation of the periosteum of the carotid canal.

The cavernous (C4) segment begins at the superior margin of the petrolingual ligament, runs within the cavernous sinus, and ends at the proximal dural ring formed by the junction of the medial and inferior periosteum of the anterior clinoid process. Meningohypophyseal trunk, inferolateral trunk, and capsular arteries arise from this segment.

The clinoid (C5) segment runs between the proximal dural ring and the distal dural ring where the ICA becomes intradural. This small segment has no branches.

The ophthalmic (C6) segment begins at the distal dural ring ending proximal to the origin of the posterior communicating artery. Two major branches originate at this level, the ophthalmic artery and the superior hypophyseal artery.

The communicating (C7) segment begins proximal to the origin of the posterior communicating artery extending to the ICA bifurcation. This segment gives off the posterior communicating artery and the anterior choroidal artery.

Blumenfeld H. Neuroanatomy Through Clinical Cases, 1st ed. Sunderland, MA: Sinauer Associates; 2002.

Bouthillier A, van Loveren HR, Keller J. Segments of the internal carotid artery: a new classification. Neurosurgery. 1996; 38:425–433.

47. e

A patient with left carotid stenosis of more than 70% may benefit from carotid endarterectomy (CEA) in this case.

In this case, the right carotid is the one that is producing symptoms, and therefore if a right carotid stenosis is detected, it is symptomatic carotid disease. On the other hand, a left carotid stenosis in this case will be asymptomatic.

Patients with extracranial ICA atherosclerotic disease can be treated medically or surgically to prevent cerebrovascular events. One of the most important factors in deciding if CEA will be beneficial is determination whether a lesion is symptomatic or asymptomatic, along with other patient characteristics.

According to the North American Symptomatic Carotid Endarterectomy Trial (NASCET), in patients with 70% to 99% symptomatic carotid stenosis, the 2-year ipsilateral stroke rate was 26% with medical treatment versus 9% with CEA. Therefore, a symptomatic carotid stenosis of

70% to 99% should be treated surgically. Patients with symptomatic stenosis of 50% to 69% will also benefit from CEA, with greater impact in men versus women, in those with previous strokes versus TIAs, and with hemispheric versus retinal symptoms. In patients with stenosis of less than 50%, there is no evidence that surgical treatment is better than aspirin. The same applies for carotid occlusions, in which the treatment should be medical management.

Regarding asymptomatic carotid disease, CEA has proven benefit over medical treatment in patients with more than 60% stenosis as demonstrated in the Asymptomatic Carotid Atherosclerosis Study (ACAS), and in the Asymptomatic Carotid Surgery Trial (ACST), however, the numbers needed to treat are high, and the benefit may not be significant in the real world, depending also on the experience of the surgeon. In ACAS, the absolute risk reduction was 1.2% per year with a number needed to treat of 85 favoring the surgical group. In the ACST, the absolute risk reduction was 1.1% with a number needed to treat of 93 favoring surgery over medical therapy.

Brott TG, Brown RD, Meyer FB. Carotid revascularization for prevention of stroke: carotid endarterectomy and carotid artery stenting. Mayo Clin Proc. 2004; 79:1197–1208.

48. e

This patient had a TIA, which is a brief episode of focal neurologic dysfunction caused by ischemia without cerebral infarction. It is important to recognize TIAs and evaluate them, since patients who have TIAs are at higher risk of stroke. Around 10% to 15% of patients who suffer a TIA will have a stroke within 3 months, and the risk is higher sooner after the TIA, with 50% of the strokes occurring within 48 hours. Therefore, patients presenting with TIAs should be urgently assessed, with a detailed analysis of their risk factors for stroke. Work up should be obtained to evaluate the vascular origin of the symptoms, to exclude alternative nonischemic causes, and to assess prognostic factors.

The current proposed definition of TIA is based on tissue damage and the presence of infarcted tissue. Brain imaging with MRI and diffusion-weighted imaging (DWI) is helpful in detecting the presence of infracted tissue.

Guidelines recommend the following:

- Neuroimaging within 24 hours, preferably an MRI with DWI
- Noninvasive vascular imaging of the extracranial arteries
- Noninvasive imaging of the intracranial vasculature if it is considered that this will alter management
- Patients should be evaluated as soon as possible.

Given that in the acute presentation a TIA is undistinguishable from an acute stroke, all patients presenting with acute neurologic symptoms should be assessed similarly, and considered candidates for intravenous tPA until proven contraindication is determined. No period of observation should be allowed in this setting, since on acute presentation these two spectrums of the disease cannot be differentiated.

Easton JD, Saver JL, Albers GW, et al. Definition and evaluation of transient ischemic attack. Stroke. 2009; 40:2276–2293.

49. d

Figure 2.13 shows a deep intracerebral hemorrhage, most likely caused by hypertension. Intracranial hemorrhage (ICH) can be primary or secondary (in which it complicates a preexisting lesion). Primary ICH accounts for approximately 10% of all strokes, and is a significant cause of morbidity and mortality. The most common cause of ICH is hypertension which is responsible for 75% of cases, followed by cerebral amyloid angiopathy.

Hypertensive ICH commonly originates in deep subcortical structures such as the putamen, caudate, and thalamus, as well as in the pons, cerebellum, and periventricular deep white matter. This occurs from rupture of deep perforating arteries, which suffer changes caused by chronic hypertension, leading to lipohyalinosis, making these vessels susceptible to sudden closure (causing lacunar infarctions) or rupture (causing hemorrhage).

Amyloid angiopathy is the deposition of congophilic material in the media and adventitia of cerebral vessels, especially cortical and leptomeningeal vessels. This process is associated with cortical and lobar hemorrhages. This condition is seen more commonly in the elderly, and MRI with gradient echo sequences can detect multiple small areas of hemorrhages in the brain, helping to make the diagnosis.

Anticoagulation can be associated with any type of hemorrhage; however, hypertension is a more common cause, and the most likely etiology in this case given the location. Patients on anticoagulation may have hemorrhages showing a fluid-fluid level.

Intracranial aneurysmal rupture presents with SAH rather than intraparenchymal hemorrhage.

Sinus venous thrombosis is associated with hemorrhagic infarcts, usually in the distribution of the thrombosed sinus.

Badjatia N, Rosand J. Intracerebral hemorrhage. Neurologist. 2005; 11:311–324.

Manno EM, Atkinson JL, Fulgham JR, Widjdicks EFM. Emerging medical and surgical management strategies in the evaluation and treatment of intracerebral hemorrhage. Mayo Clin Proc. 2005; 80:420–433.

50. e

Treatments of Moyamoya disease have not been satisfactory, and anticoagulation has not proven to be of benefit, being usually avoided given the hemorrhagic risk in these patients.

Moyamoya is a noninflammatory, nonatherosclerotic vasculopathy that affects the intracranial circulation, leading to arterial occlusions and prominent arterial collateral circulation. It presents most commonly in children and adolescents, with a second peak in the fourth decade of life, but in a much lower frequency. Clinical manifestations include TIAs and strokes, as well as intracranial hemorrhages (ICHs). In childhood the presentation is predominantly ischemic, with strokes and TIAs, which may be precipitated by hyperventilation. In adults, the presentation is most frequently ICH. Other manifestations seen in Moyamoya disease include headaches, seizures, movement disorders, and mental deterioration.

The diagnosis is based on the neuroangiographic findings, characterized by progressive bilateral stenosis of the distal internal carotid arteries, extending to proximal ACAs and MCAs, and the development of extensive collateral circulation at the base of the brain, with the "puff of smoke" appearance. Histopathologically, there is intimal thickening by fibrous tissue of the affected arteries, with no inflammatory cells or atheromas.

There is no curative treatment for this condition. Revascularization procedures may improve perfusion, angiographic appearance, and ischemic manifestations; however, they may not impact the frequency of hemorrhagic events.

Medications such as antiplatelets, vasodilators, calcium channel blockers, and steroids have been used with equivocal results. Anticoagulation is not helpful and usually avoided given the hemorrhagic complications.

Bradley WG, Daroff RB, Fenichel GM, Jankovic J. Neurology in Clinical Practice, 5th ed. Philadelphia, PA: Elsevier; 2008.

Ropper AH, Samuels MA. Adams and Victor's Principles of Neurology, 9th ed. New York, NY: McGraw-Hill; 2009.

51. a

This patient has a lobar hemorrhage likely associated with amyloid angiopathy. MRI of the brain shown in Figure 2.14 demonstrates multiple small rounded areas of gradient echo susceptibility throughout the brain, representing microhemorrhages with hemosiderin deposition.

Amyloid angiopathy is a condition that causes deposition of amyloid material in the cerebral vessels, especially in the cortex and leptomeninges, and is associated with lobar hemorrhages in the elderly. Since the angiopathy is diffuse, there are recurrent and multiple hemorrhages, and commonly MRI with gradient echo sequences will show multiple small areas of hypointensity suggesting prior hemosiderin deposition from prior hemorrhages, such as in this case.

Histologically, there is deposition of Congo-red positive amyloid material in the media and adventitia of small- and medium-sized vessels. This causes weakening of the vessel walls. There are associations of amyloid angiopathy with apolipoprotein $\epsilon 4$ and $\epsilon 2$, as well as with Alzheimer's disease.

Hypertension does not produce this pattern of microhemorrhages seen on gradient echo sequences.

Intracranial aneurysmal rupture presents with SAH rather than intraparenchymal hemorrhage.

Anticoagulation can be associated with any type of hemorrhage; however, the hemorrhage locations and clinical characteristics of this patient are more consistent with amyloid angiopathy. Patients with amyloid angiopathy are more susceptible to have intracranial hemorrhage (ICH) in the setting of anticoagulation.

Sinus venous thrombosis is associated with hemorrhagic infarcts, usually in the distribution of the thrombosed sinus.

Bradley WG, Daroff RB, Fenichel GM, Jankovic J. Neurology in Clinical Practice, 5th ed. Philadelphia, PA: Elsevier; 2008.

Ropper AH, Samuels MA. Adams and Victor's Principles of Neurology, 9th ed. New York, NY: McGraw-Hill; 2009.

52. e

This patient has Dejerine-Roussy syndrome, caused by a thalamic infarct, in which the lesion affects the sensory relay nuclei. These patients present with severe deep and cutaneous sensory loss of the contralateral hemibody, usually the entire hemibody and up to the midline. In some cases, there may be dissociation of sensory loss, affecting more pain and temperature sensation than touch, vibration, or proprioception. With time, some sensation returns, but the patient may develop severe pain, allodynia, and paresthesias of the affected body part.

Infarcts in the other structures will not produce the clinical manifestations depicted in this case.

Goetz CG. Textbook of Clinical Neurology, 3rd ed. Philadelphia, PA: Saunders Elsevier; 2007.

Ropper AH, Samuels MA. Adams and Victor's Principles of Neurology, 9th ed. New York, NY: McGraw-Hill; 2009.

53. b

The anterior choroidal arteries arise from the anterior circulation, more specifically from the ICA. The posterior choroidal arteries arise from the posterior circulation, more specifically from the posterior cerebral arteries.

The vertebral arteries originate from the subclavian arteries on their respective sides. The V1 segment extends from the subclavian artery to the transverse foramen of C5-C6. The V2 segment runs within the transverse foramina of the cervical vertebra from C5-C6 to C2. The V3 segment extends from the transverse foramen of C2 and turns posterolaterally around the arch of C1, between the atlas and the occiput. This segment is extracranial. The V4 segment begins where the vertebral artery enters the dura at the foramen magnum and joins the contralateral vertebral artery to form the basilar artery. The vertebral artery, at the V4 segment gives off the posterior inferior cerebellar artery (PICA) and the anterior spinal artery. Both vertebral arteries will join to form the basilar artery. The posterior circulation provides the vascular supply to the brainstem, cerebellum, the thalamus, and the occipital lobes.

Blumenfeld H. Neuroanatomy Through Clinical Cases, 1st ed. Sunderland, MA: Sinauer Associates; 2002.

Shin JH, Suh DC, Choi CG, et al. Vertebral artery dissection: spectrum of imaging findings with emphasis on angiography and correlation with clinical presentation. RadioGraphics. 2000; 20:1687–1696.

54. d

Based on the history and MRI findings in Figure 2.15, this patient most likely has a hemorrhagic infarct from sinus venous thrombosis, in this case, a left transverse sinus thrombosis. Occlusion of the venous sinuses will lead to venous infarction and localized edema. The affected tissue becomes engorged, swollen, and the parenchyma will suffer ischemia, leading to infarct and hemorrhage. Given the occlusion of venous drainage and in the setting of parenchymal edema, the content of the intracranial volume will rise, leading to intracranial hypertension.

Clinical presentation is characterized by the presence of headache, and depending on the extent of the disease, focal neurologic deficits, altered mental status, seizures, and coma will be present, sometimes progressing to herniation and death.

Risk factors are often encountered including prothrombotic states, either genetic or acquired, such as antiphospholipid antibody syndrome, pregnancy, and the use of oral contraceptives. Other causes include infections (otitis, mastoiditis, sinusitis, meningitis), inflammatory conditions, trauma, dehydration, and neoplastic processes.

The diagnosis should be considered in young patients with prothrombotic risk factors presenting with clinical manifestations suggestive of this condition. CT scan and MRI of the brain will show hemorrhagic infarcts that are not in a strictly arterial distribution (as in Figure 2.15, in which the infarct seems to involve both the left MCA and PCA territories). MRV will demonstrate the absence of signal in the thrombosed venous sinus.

Treatment involves stabilization of the patient and anticoagulation to stop the thrombotic process. Treatment of intracranial hypertension may be needed, sometimes requiring surgical decompression and removal of the hemorrhagic infarct. In some cases, endovascular intervention for thrombolysis and clot removal is required.

This is not an arterial infarct since it does not follow the distribution of an arterial vascular territory. This patient does not have a history of hypertension, and the characteristics of the MRI are not typical of hypertensive hemorrhage. This patient is not in the age group for amyloid angiopathy-related intracranial hemorrhage, and the history suggests an alternative diagnosis such as venous sinus thrombosis. The hemorrhage in this patient is not in the subarachnoid space.

Ropper AH, Samuels MA. Adams and Victor's Principles of Neurology, 9th ed. New York, NY: McGraw-Hill; 2009.

Stam J. Thrombosis of the cerebral veins and sinuses. N Engl J Med. 2005; 352:1791–1798.

55. a

The use of warfarin is less warranted based on the available evidence. The Warfarin-Aspirin Symptomatic Intracranial Disease (WASID) trial randomized patients with a recent TIA or stroke with a 50% to 99% stenosis of a major intracranial artery to warfarin or aspirin. The primary end point was ischemic stroke, intracranial hemorrhage (ICH), or death from vascular causes other than stroke. At the end of the study, it was concluded that warfarin was associated with higher rates of adverse events and provided no benefit over aspirin in these patients.

Antiplatelet agents have been the mainstay of therapy for this patient population, and aspirin was the one assessed in the WASID trial. The American Heart Association/American Stroke Association (AHA/ASA) recommends aspirin monotherapy, aspirin/dipyridamole, or clopidogrel monotherapy as acceptable options for the prevention of noncardioembolic strokes.

On the basis of the Stroke Prevention by Aggressive Reduction in Cholesterol Levels (SPARCL) trial, the AHA/ASA recommends statin therapy for patients with atherosclerotic ischemic stroke and TIA, to reduce the risk of subsequent cerebrovascular events.

Amarenco P, Bogousslavsky J, Callahan A III, et al. High-dose atorvastatin after stroke or transient ischemic stroke. N Engl J Med. 2006; 355:549–559.

Chimowitz MI, Lynn MJ, Howlett-Smith H, et al. Comparison of warfarin and aspirin for symptomatic intracranial arterial stenosis. N Engl J Med. 2005; 352:1305–1316.

Qureshi AI, Feldmann E, Gomez CR, et al. Intracranial atherosclerotic disease: an update. Ann Neurol. 2009; 66:730–738.

Sacco RL, Adams R, Albers G, et al. Guidelines for prevention of stroke in patients with ischemic stroke or transient ischemic attack. Stroke. 2006; 37:577–617.

56. c

This patient has Claude's syndrome, manifested by ipsilateral third nerve palsy, and contralateral ataxia and tremor. The lesion affects the dorsal red nucleus and the third nerve fascicle and is in the midbrain tegmentum more dorsally located than the lesion seen in Benedikt's syndrome, which is caused by a ventral mesencephalic tegmental lesion. Patients with Claude's syndrome, as compared to Benedikt's syndrome, have more ataxia but no involuntary choreoathetotic movements.

Lesions in the other locations will not present with the clinical features depicted in this case.

Bradley WG, Daroff RB, Fenichel GM, Jankovic J. Neurology in Clinical Practice, 5th ed. Philadelphia, PA: Elsevier; 2008.

Goetz CG. Textbook of Clinical Neurology, 3rd ed. Philadelphia, PA: Saunders Elsevier; 2007.

57. c

This patient has a left transverse sinus thrombosis, as seen in the MRV in Figure 2.16, in which the signal is lost in the left transverse sinus.

In patients with venous sinus thrombosis, an etiologic factor should be investigated, since it may be a treatable condition. Possible causes include oral contraceptives, pregnancy and puerperium, cancer, nephrotic syndrome, antiphospholipid syndrome, connective tissue disorders, hematologic conditions, trauma, and genetic prothrombotic conditions such as protein C and S deficiency, antithrombin deficiency, factor V Leiden mutation, prothrombin mutation, and homocysteinemia. Infectious causes may also lead to thrombosis in nearby venous structures, and middle ear infections as well as mastoiditis have been associated with transverse sinus thrombosis.

Diabetes and hypertension are typical risk factors for arterial strokes, but further search for prothrombotic risk factors should be done in cases of venous thrombosis. Since this is a venous thrombosis and not an arterial stroke, an embolic source does not need to be investigated, and therefore, an echocardiogram with bubble study and Holter monitor are not required.

In sinus venous thrombosis, anticoagulation is important to stop the thrombotic process. In cerebral venous thrombosis, studies comparing anticoagulation with placebo have shown no increased or new cerebral hemorrhages with anticoagulation, even in patients with the presence of hemorrhagic infarcts before the treatment.

Endovascular thrombolysis with pharmacological agents or mechanical clot removal can be performed but should be restricted to patients with severe neurologic impairment. However, there is no clear evidence comparing the results of this therapy with anticoagulation.

Ropper AH, Samuels MA. Adams and Victor's Principles of Neurology, 9th ed. New York, NY: McGraw-Hill; 2009.

Stam J. Thrombosis of the cerebral veins and sinuses. N Engl J Med. 2005; 352:1791–1798.

58. e

Renal disease is not a risk factor routinely taken into account for the assessment of stroke risk in patients with TIA.

Patients with atrial fibrillation are at risk for ischemic stroke; however, this population is heterogenous and the risk may vary depending on other risk factors. It is known that warfarin is beneficial to prevent strokes in patients with atrial fibrillation, especially when the stroke risk is high. However, the use of aspirin may be favored for low-risk patients. This is one of the reasons why the estimation of stroke risk in atrial fibrillation is important. The CHADS2 score has been validated for this purpose, in which 1 point is assigned for the presence of each of the following: congestive heart failure, history of hypertension, age of 75 years or older, diabetes mellitus, prior stroke, or TIA. Two points will be given for a history of stroke or TIA. The total score will range from 0 to 6 and will correlate with an expected stroke rate per 100 patient-years, with higher CHADS2 scores correlating with higher stroke rates.

This patient is aged 67 years, with history of diabetes and hypertension, and a recent TIA. All these factors will give him a CHADS2 score of 4, and therefore the stroke rate per 100 patient-years for this patient is approximately 8.5.

Gage BF, Waterman AD, Shannon W, et al. Validation of clinical classification schemes for predicting stroke. Results from the National Registry of Atrial Fibrillation. JAMA. 2001; 285:2864–2870.

59. d

In the brain, drainage of venous blood occurs through veins into dural venous sinuses, which eventually drain into the internal jugular veins. The dural venous sinuses are venous channels enclosed between dural layers, and they have no valves. The major venous sinuses are the superior sagittal sinus, the inferior sagittal sinus, the straight sinus, the transverse sinus, sigmoid sinus, and the cavernous sinus (Figure 2.22).

The superior sagittal sinus runs along the superior margin of the falx cerebri in the inter-hemispheric fissure, toward the confluence of the sinuses where it encounters the straight sinus and the transverse sinuses, which will continue as the sigmoid sinuses, draining into the internal jugular veins. The inferior sagittal sinus runs above the corpus callosum in the interhemispheric fissure.

The deep venous system is composed of the internal cerebral veins, which will empty into the great cerebral vein of Galen. The basal vein of Rosenthal is a deep vein that drains the base

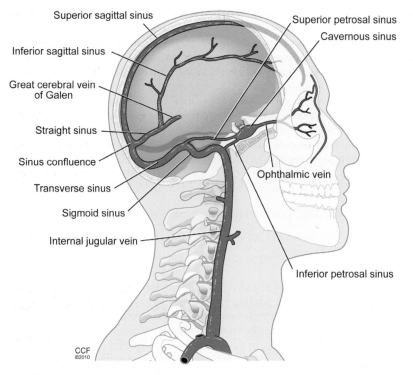

Superior sagittal sinus

Inferior sagittal sinus

Great cerebral vein of Galen

Straight sinus

Sinus confluence

Transverse sinus

Sigmoid sinus

Internal jugular vein

Superior petrosal sinus

Cavernous sinus

Ophthalmic vein

Inferior petrosal sinus

CCF
©2010

FIGURE 2.22   Venous sinuses (Illustration by David R. Schumick, BS, CMI. Reprinted with permission of the Cleveland Clinic Center for Medical Art and Photography. © 2010. All rights reserved)

of the forebrain, and also empties into the great cerebral vein of Galen, located beneath the splenium of the corpus callosum. The great cerebral vein of Galen joins the inferior sagittal sinus at the straight sinus, which will then run toward the confluence of the sinuses.

The cavernous sinuses are on both sides of the sella turcica and receive blood from facial and orbital structures, including the ophthalmic veins. The cavernous sinuses drain into the superior and inferior petrosal sinuses, which then drain into the sigmoid sinus.

The convexity of the brain has multiple superficial veins that drain into the superior sagittal sinus, the transverse sinus, or the middle cerebral vein, which runs along the Sylvian fissure. Between these structures there are anastomotic veins: the superior anastomotic vein of Trolard and the inferior anastomotic vein of Labbe.

Emissary veins connect scalp veins with the dural venous sinuses.

Blumenfeld, H. Neuroanatomy Through Clinical Cases, 1st ed. Sunderland, MA: Sinauer; 2002.

Morris P. Practical Neuroangiography, 1st ed. Baltimore, MD: Williams & Wilkins; 1997.

60.   C

This patient has cerebral autosomal dominant arteriopathy with subcortical infarcts and leukoencephalopathy (CADASIL), which can be suspected based on the history of multiple strokes without traditional vascular risk factors, a history of migraines, subsequent development of dementia, and a family history of strokes and dementia suggesting a hereditary condition. The diagnosis is confirmed with the histopathologic specimen shown in Figure 2.17, demonstrating a blood vessel with a thick wall, which contains a basophilic granular material. This pathologic finding is characteristic of CADASIL.

This condition is associated with a mutation in the gene *NOTCH3* on chromosome 19. The gene product is a transmembrane receptor expressed mainly in vascular smooth muscle, and the mutation leads to accumulation of this protein in the vascular walls, especially in small arteries and capillaries.

CADASIL is inherited in an autosomal dominant fashion, and patients present with migraines with aura, stroke episodes, seizures, pseudobulbar palsy, and progressive cognitive decline leading to the development of dementia. The strokes are recurrent and predominantly lacunes, caused by small vessel disease. Some patients present with psychiatric manifestations, especially depression and emotional lability. Parkinsonism is not a typical feature of CADASIL.

The MRI typically shows T2 hyperintensities in the subcortical white matter and basal ganglia. The diagnosis could be made based on detection of the *NOTCH3* mutation, or with skin biopsy demonstrating pathologic changes.

Currently, there is no treatment for this condition.

Bradley WG, Daroff RB, Fenichel GM, Jankovic J. Neurology in Clinical Practice, 5th ed. Philadelphia, PA: Elsevier; 2008.

61. b

This patient has a Weber's syndrome, which is a combination of an ipsilateral third nerve palsy with contralateral hemiplegia. This is caused by a midbrain lesion, in this case a left midbrain infarct.

Brainstem infarcts manifest with crossed syndromes, in which there are ipsilateral cranial nerve abnormalities and contralateral long tract signs.

This patient has a left third nerve palsy, manifested by limited adduction and upward movements of the left eye, therefore presenting with diplopia on upward gaze and when looking to the right side. The contralateral hemiplegia is caused by the lesion affecting the corticospinal tract before its decussation at the level of the pyramids, in this case at the cerebral peduncle. An ipsilateral third nerve palsy with contralateral hemiplegia localizes the lesion to the midbrain.

Bradley WG, Daroff RB, Fenichel GM, Jankovic J. Neurology in Clinical Practice, 5th ed. Philadelphia, PA: Elsevier; 2008.

Goetz CG. Textbook of Clinical Neurology, 3rd ed. Philadelphia, PA: Saunders Elsevier; 2007.

62. b

Intracranial vascular malformations include arteriovenous malformations (AVMs), cavernous malformations, venous angiomas, capillary telangiectasias, and dural arteriovenous fistulas (DAVF).

Cavernous malformations are clusters of vascular channels, composed of dilated thin-walled vessels, with no smooth muscle or elastic fibers, and with no intervening brain parenchyma separating the vascular structures. On MRI, they have the typical "popcorn-like" appearance, with a dark rim on T2 consistent with hemosiderin; gradient echo images (see Figure 2.18) may show evidence of cavernous malformations when not evident on T2-weighted images.

AVMs are congenital vascular lesions in which arteries and veins communicate without an intervening normal capillary bed in between. This lesion can be seen on CT, and CT angiogram (CTA) provides better vascular visualization. MRI demonstrates the vascular lesion with flow voids and regions of previous hemorrhage, as well as its relationship with the parenchyma. Conventional angiography is the standard to evaluate the vascular structure, pattern of vascular feeders, and drainage.

Venous angiomas are thin-walled venous structures with normal intervening brain tissue. These are asymptomatic with a very low risk of hemorrhage. MRI demonstrates a conglomerate of vessels in a "caput medusae pattern."

Capillary telangiectasias are abnormally dilated capillaries that are separated by normal brain tissue. They are typically found incidentally and rarely become symptomatic.

This is not a DAVF (discussed in question 64).

Bradley WG, Daroff RB, Fenichel GM, Jankovic J. Neurology in Clinical Practice, 5th ed. Philadelphia, PA: Elsevier; 2008.

Brown RD, Flemming KD, Meyer FB, et al. Natural history, evaluation and management of intracranial vascular malformations. Mayo Clin Proc. 2005; 80:269–281.

Prayson RA, Goldblum Jr. Neuropathology, 1st ed. Philadelphia, PA: Elsevier; 2005.

63. e

The common carotid artery ascends in the neck and divides into external and internal carotid arteries at the level of C4, below the angle of the jaw.

The arterial supply to the brain is divided into two main territories, the anterior and posterior circulation. The two internal carotid arteries provide perfusion to the anterior circulation, and the two vertebral arteries provide perfusion to the posterior circulation.

The aortic arch has three main branches, the innominate (brachiocephalic) artery, the left common carotid artery, and the left subclavian artery. Several normal variants exist in both the extracranial and intracranial circulation; the most common anatomy is described below.

The right ICA originates from the right common carotid artery, which is a branch of the innominate artery that comes off the aortic arch. The right vertebral artery comes off the right subclavian artery, which also branches off the innominate artery, and eventually joins the left vertebral artery to form the basilar artery.

The left common carotid artery originates directly from the aortic arch, and divides into left internal and left external carotid arteries. A small percentage of the population have what is called a "bovine aortic arch," in which the left common carotid has the same origin as the innominate artery, and in some cases the left common carotid will branch off the innominate artery.

The left subclavian artery originates from the aortic arch and gives off the left vertebral artery, which then ascends in the neck to join the right vertebral artery to form the basilar artery.

Blumenfeld H. Neuroanatomy Through Clinical Cases, 1st ed. Sunderland, MA: Sinauer Associates; 2002.

Ropper AH, Samuels MA. Adams and Victor's Principles of Neurology, 9th ed. New York, NY: McGraw-Hill; 2009.

64. c

This patient has a spinal dural arteriovenous fistula (DAVF), which is the most common type of spinal vascular malformation. This lesion can be fed by one or multiple arteries and is a low pressure and low flow vascular lesion. DAVF is more frequent in men and above 50 years of age. The typical location is in the lower thoracic and lumbar regions, and this type of lesion rarely produces hemorrhage. Patients present with pain, weakness, and sensory symptoms below the level of the lesion. The myelopathic syndrome is usually gradually progressive and caused by venous hypertension and congestion. MRI of the spine shows enlargement of the cord with hyperintensity on T2 seen over several levels, with intradural flow voids suggesting this pathology (Figure 2.19). Spinal angiogram is the gold standard diagnostic test to detect this abnormality.

Treatment involves angiographic embolization and/or surgical removal of the lesion. The radiographic findings in this case are consistent with an expanding lesion with T2 hyperintensity in the cord. The presentation is gradually progressive and consistent with DAVF.

Epidural hematoma and spinal cord infarct have a more acute presentation and do not show the MRI findings seen in this case. This is not a cavernous malformation or a venous angioma, which are not common in this location.

Bradley WG, Daroff RB, Fenichel GM, Jankovic J. Neurology in Clinical Practice, 5th ed. Philadelphia, PA: Elsevier; 2008.

65. d

This patient has intracranial hemorrhage (ICH) in the right anterior temporal lobe as seen in the brain CT as a hyperdense area (Figure 2.20). The MRI can be helpful to estimate the timing of the hemorrhage on the basis of the characteristics of the blood and the composition. Initially hemorrhage is composed of plasma and red blood cells, with the presence of intracellular oxyhemoglobin, which is then converted to deoxyhemoglobin, subsequently oxidized to methemoglobin. Later, cell lysis occurs with the presence of extracellular hemoglobin, which is then converted to hemosiderin.

Estimation of the timing of the hemorrhage is based on the presence of these different types of blood products, and is as follows:

– Between 0 and 24 hours: The predominant blood product is oxyhemoglobin and is seen on MRI as isointense on T1 sequences, and hyperintense on T2 sequences.
– Between 1 and 3 days: Deoxyhemoglobin is the predominant blood product, seen as isointense on T1 and hypointense on T2.
– Between 3 and 7 days: Intracellular methemoglobin, seen as hyperintense on T1 and hypointense on T2.
– One week up to probably a month: There is extracellular methemoglobin, seen as hyperintense on T1 and T2 sequences.
– After 1 or 2 weeks, and probably for years: There is hemosiderin, seen as isointense or hypointense on T1, and hypointense on T2 sequences.

Based on these estimates, this patient's hemorrhage is approximately 1 week old.

Bradley WG, Daroff RB, Fenichel GM, Jankovic J. Neurology in Clinical Practice, 5th ed. Philadelphia, PA: Elsevier; 2008.

Buzz Phrases	Key Points
Ipsilateral third nerve palsy and contralateral hemiplegia	Weber's syndrome (midbrain lesion)
Ipsilateral third nerve palsy and contralateral involuntary movements	Benedikt's syndrome (lesion in the ventral portion of the mesencephalic tegmentum)
Ipsilateral third nerve palsy and contralateral ataxia and tremor	Claude's syndrome (lesion in the dorsal portion of the mesencephalic tegmentum)
Ipsilateral sixth and seventh nerve palsies with contralateral hemiplegia	Millard-Gubler syndrome (lesion in the pons)

(*continued*)

Buzz Phrases	Key Points
Limited upward gaze, convergence retraction nystagmus, light-near dissociation, lid retraction, and skew deviation of the eyes	Parinaud's syndrome (lesion affecting the quadrigeminal plate)
Quadriplegia, inability to speak, limited horizontal gaze, with preserved consciousness, vertical gaze, and blinking	Locked-in syndrome
Vertigo, nystagmus, nausea, hiccups, hoarseness, dysphagia, ipsilateral paralysis of the palate and vocal cord, decreased gag reflex, impaired sensation on the ipsilateral hemiface, loss of sensation to pain and temperature in the contralateral hemibody, ipsilateral ataxia and lateropulsion, and ipsilateral Horner's syndrome	Wallenberg's syndrome Caused by a lateral medullary infarction (associated with posterior inferior cerebellar artery or vertebral artery occlusion)
Ipsilateral hearing loss, vertigo, ipsilateral ataxia, ipsilateral Horner's syndrome, sensory deficit in the ipsilateral hemiface, and contralateral hemibody	Anterior inferior cerebellar artery infarct
Contralateral hemibody sensory loss with subsequent development of pain, allodynia, and paresthesias. Results from a thalamic lesion.	Dejerine-Roussy syndrome
Finger agnosia, right-left disorientation, agraphia, and acalculia	Gerstmann's syndrome
Normal variant with vascular supply to both medial thalami	Artery of Percheron
Deep branch from ACA that supplies anterior limb of the internal capsule, inferior part of head of caudate nucleus, and anterior part of globus pallidus	Recurrent artery of Heubner
Caused by chronic hypertension, and associated with the pathogenesis of lacunar strokes	Lipohyalinosis
Infarct between two vascular territories. Produces the "person-in-a-barrel" syndrome, characterized by proximal weakness	Watershed infarcts
Infarct in the posterior circulation from thrombus lodging in the distal basilar. Symptoms: behavioral abnormalities, altered level of consciousness, and abnormalities of ocular motion	Top of the basilar syndrome
Right hemiparesis, right homonymous hemianopsia, and aphasia	Left MCA syndrome
Left hemiparesis, left homonymous hemianopsia, and left hemineglect	Right MCA syndrome
Thalamus, contralateral hemisensory loss	Pure sensory lacunar syndrome
Posterior limb of internal capsule, contralateral motor deficits. Also described with ventral pons lacunes	Pure motor lacunar syndrome
Paramedian pons, "clumsy hand," and dysarthria	Clumsy-hand dysarthria lacunar syndrome
Pons, midbrain, or internal capsule, weakness with ataxia out of proportion to weakness	Ataxic hemiparesis lacunar syndrome
NOTCH3	CADASIL: Cerebral autosomal dominant arteriopathy with subcortical infarcts and leukoencephalopathy

(*continued*)

Buzz Phrases	Key Points
Dilated thin-walled vessels, with no smooth muscle or elastic fibers, and no intervening brain parenchyma Popcorn appearance on MRI	Cavernous malformation
Thin-walled venous structure with normal intervening brain tissue	Venous angioma
Abnormally dilated capillaries, normal intervening brain tissue	Capillary telangiectasia
Arteries and veins communicate without an intervening normal capillary bed in between	Arteriovenous malformation
Hemorrhage in the putamen, caudate, thalamus, pons, cerebellum, and deep white matter Associated with lipohyalinosis	Hypertensive intracranial hemorrhage
Lobar hemorrhages Multiple microhemorrhages on MRI gradient echo Congo-red positive amyloid material, seen as apple-green birefringence with polarized light	Cerebral amyloid angiopathy
"Puff of smoke"	Extensive collateral circulation seen in Moyamoya disease, in which there is bilateral stenosis of the distal internal carotid arteries and intracranial arteries of the circle of Willis

Chapter 3

Neurocritical Care

Questions

Questions 1–2

1. A 57-year-old man presents with sudden onset of headache, nausea, vomiting, and change in mental status. A scan is obtained and is shown in Figure 3.1. The patient had a normal CT scan obtained 3 months earlier as part of a workup for headaches. Brain edema occurring in the setting of the condition shown in the scan has which of the following characteristics?

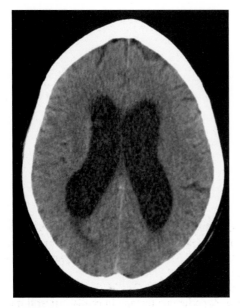

FIGURE 3.1 Axial CT

a. It is interstitial edema
b. It occurs from N-K ATPase pump failure
c. It is cytotoxic edema
d. It is vasogenic edema
e. The pathogenesis is associated with blood-brain barrier disruption

2. A 62-year-old patient is found to have a brain mass. An image of his MRI is shown in Figure 3.2. What are the characteristics of the surrounding cerebral edema?

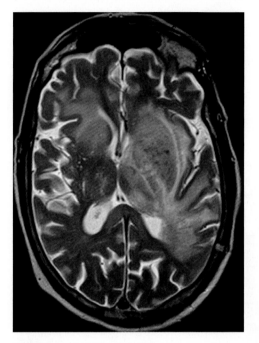

FIGURE 3.2   Axial T2-weighted MRI

a. It is caused by disruption of the CSF flow
b. It occurs from N-K ATPase pump failure
c. It is cytotoxic edema
d. It is vasogenic edema
e. It is caused by obstructive hydrocephalus

3. A 52-year-old man suffered a cardiac arrest associated with ventricular fibrillation and required cardiopulmonary resuscitation (CPR) for 10 minutes. On arrival to the hospital, the patient is unconscious. He gets intubated and is admitted to the ICU. Which of the following is incorrect?
a. The patient should be treated with hypothermia for 12 to 24 hours
b. The target temperature with hypothermic therapy should be 32°C to 34°C
c. There is strong evidence to support the use of hypothermic therapy in cardiac arrest from ventricular fibrillation, pulseless electrical activity, and asystole

d. Temperatures lower than 28°C can be harmful without significant benefit
e. In a patient such as the one depicted in this case, neurologic outcome improves with hypothermic therapy

4. A patient suffers a large intracranial hemorrhage. On examination, he has a right fixed dilated pupil and seems to be hemiparetic on the left side. Which type of herniation does this patient have?
   a. Uncal herniation
   b. Subfalcine herniation
   c. Tonsillar herniation
   d. Central transtentorial herniation
   e. Transcalvarial herniation

5. Which of the following is not a cause of cerebral edema?
   a. Prolonged cardiac arrest
   b. Hypernatremia
   c. Liver failure
   d. Lead intoxication
   e. Rapid ascent into high altitude

6. A patient is admitted to the neurocritical care unit with an acute neurological condition and a Glasgow Coma Scale score of 7. His brain CT scan is shown in Figure 3.3. A decision is made to place an ICP monitor. Which device is the best option in this case?

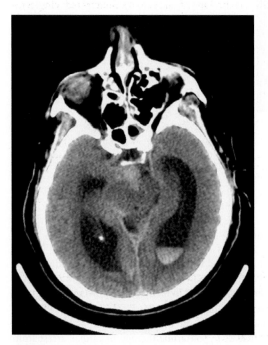

FIGURE 3.3 Axial CT.

a. A parenchymal catheter
b. An epidural device
c. A subarachnoid bolt
d. An intraventricular catheter
e. Based on the images, an ICP monitor should not be placed

Questions 7–8

7. A 20-year-old man was involved in a motor vehicle accident and suffered traumatic brain injury. He is intubated and admitted to the neurocritical care unit. An ICP monitor is placed measuring an ICP of 35 mm Hg. Hyperventilation is started, and 60 g of mannitol are given intravenously. Which of the following is correct regarding therapies for increased ICP?
   a. Hyperventilation will produce a change in the CSF osmolarity, favoring the shift of fluid from neurons into the CSF
   b. Hyperventilation is a short-lived therapy, and a rebound increase in the ICP may occur
   c. Hyperventilation should target a partial pressure of CO_2 of 15 to 20 mm Hg
   d. Mannitol increases CSF osmolarity, creating an osmotic gradient that will drive fluid from the intravascular compartment into the CSF
   e. Mannitol can be given in a continuous infusion and should be used to target a serum osmolarity of more than 330 mOsm/L

8. The patient described in question 7 deteriorates, and his ICP remains persistently elevated. He is currently sedated on propofol and receiving hypertonic saline. Barbiturate coma is induced. Regarding these therapies, which of the following is correct?
   a. Barbiturates decrease the ICP by reducing cerebral metabolic activity, thereby reducing cerebral blood flow and blood volume
   b. Barbiturates should be titrated to an EEG pattern of continuous β activity
   c. Hypertonic saline reduces the ICP by producing vasoconstriction and a reduction in cerebral blood flow
   d. Complications of propofol use include hypertension and metabolic alkalosis
   e. Propofol has a long half-life and has no effects on the ICP

9. A patient is found in a "sleep-like" state, not responsive to verbal stimuli, and poorly responsive to tactile stimuli, but he can be aroused by constant and continuous stimulation. When aroused, his cognitive function is significantly impaired. Which of the following states of consciousness correlates with the findings on this patient?
   a. Coma
   b. Stupor
   c. Locked-in state
   d. Persistent vegetative state
   e. Delirium

10. A 48-year-old man is found comatose after not being seen for at least 2 days. He requires endotracheal intubation on the way to the hospital and is admitted to the neurocritical care unit. His CT scan is shown in Figure 3.4 Which of the following is correct regarding the treatment of this patient?
    a. Endovascular reperfusion therapy is the next step in treatment
    b. Anticoagulation with intravenous heparin is indicated to prevent expansion of the stroke

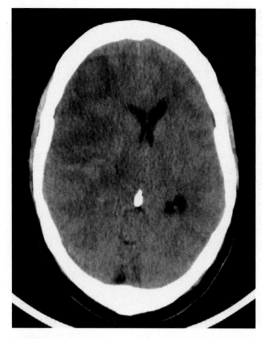

FIGURE 3.4   Axial CT.

   c. Early hemicraniectomy improves survival
   d. An intraventricular catheter should be placed
   e. Dexamethasone should be started at a dose of 4 mg intravenously every 6 hours

Questions 11–12

11. A 45-year-old patient with history of hypertension and end stage renal disease on hemodialysis presents with altered mental status and a blood pressure of 210/118 mm Hg. While in the emergency room he has a generalized tonic clonic seizure and requires endotracheal intubation. He is then admitted to the neurocritical care unit. His brain MRI is shown in Figure 3.5. Which of the following is the most likely diagnosis?
   a. Embolic strokes
   b. Acute disseminated encephalomyelitis
   c. Intracerebral hemorrhage
   d. Viral encephalitis
   e. Posterior reversible encephalopathy syndrome

12. Which of the following is incorrect regarding the condition of the patient depicted in question 11?
   a. Specific immunosuppressive therapies have been implicated in the etiology of this condition
   b. There has been an association with cancer chemotherapy and this condition
   c. Hyperlipidemia is intimately linked with this condition
   d. This condition is seen in association with eclampsia
   e. Hypertensive encephalopathy is intimately linked with this condition

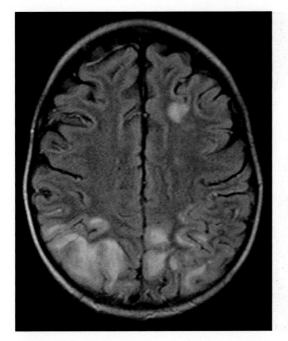

FIGURE 3.5   Axial FLAIR MRI.

13. A patient with severe hypertension is treated with an intravenous infusion of sodium nitroprusside. Which of the following is correct regarding this medication?
    a. It lowers the ICP and improves cerebral perfusion pressure
    b. It improves renal perfusion, and therefore is useful in patients with renal disease
    c. Sodium thiosulfate is used to treat the toxicity from one of its metabolites
    d. It is a calcium channel blocker resulting in direct vasodilation and negative cardiac chronotropism and inotropism
    e. Cyanide and thiocyanate are depleted with the use of sodium nitroprusside

14. Corticosteroids are used for the treatment of intracranial hypertension associated with which of the following etiologies?
    a. Traumatic brain injury
    b. Intracerebral hemorrhage
    c. Ischemic stroke
    d. Acute obstructive hydrocephalus
    e. Brain tumors

15. A patient is admitted after suffering head trauma. His head CT is shown in Figure 3.6. Regarding this condition, which of the following is correct?
    a. The hemorrhage originates from tearing of cerebral surface bridging veins
    b. The hemorrhage originates from rupture of the middle meningeal artery
    c. It is associated with Charcot Bouchard aneurysms
    d. Lipohyalinosis is present in cerebral vessels in this condition
    e. Coiling or clipping of the culprit aneurysm will prevent rebleeding

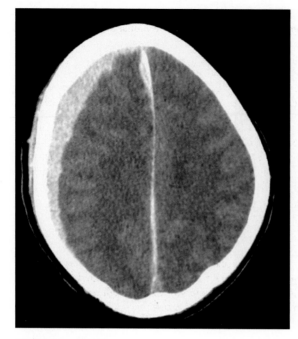

FIGURE 3.6 Axial CT.

16. A patient presents with nontraumatic SAH. On admission, he is drowsy and confused but moving all four extremities, with slight weakness on the right side. He is found to have a left MCA aneurysm and undergoes endovascular coiling on day 2. About 6 days later, his mental status declines and his right arm and leg become weaker. Which of the following is the most likely cause of his new symptoms?
    a. Acute hydrocephalus
    b. Rebleeding
    c. Mass effect from the hematoma
    ' d. Vasospasm
    e. Uncal herniation

17. A 32-year-old man went whitewater rafting with his friends. They did not hire a tour guide, and there were not enough helmets. On the last rapid he fell out of the boat and hit his head on a rock. His friends brought him back on the boat and noticed that he was slightly confused, but minutes later he came back to normal and finished the ride. Six hours later he became lethargic and his left side was not moving properly. He was taken to the emergency room of a local hospital. The CT scan showed an epidural hematoma. What is the vessel ruptured and through which foramen does it enter the skull?
    a. Jugular vein, through the jugular foramen
    b. Middle meningeal artery, through the foramen lacerum
    c. Jugular vein, through the foramen spinosum
    d. Carotid artery, through the carotid canal
    ` e. Middle meningeal artery, through the foramen spinosum

18. An 18-year-old man is involved in a motor vehicle accident. By the time emergency medical services arrive, he is dead. His autopsy shows evidence of diffuse axonal injury. Regarding this pathology, which of the following is correct?

    a. Contusion is the main cause of diffuse axonal injury

    b. It is more often seen in the site of contrecoup

    c. Evidence of intracranial hemorrhage is required to make the diagnosis

    d. Histopathologically, there is evidence of destroyed axonal cytoskeleton and retraction bulbs

    e. The outcome is invariably fatal

19. Which of the following is incorrect regarding ICP monitor waveforms?

    a. Lundberg A waves are associated with intracranial hypertension

    b. B waves have amplitudes of 20 to 50 mm Hg

    c. C waves last for 4 to 5 minutes and have amplitudes of less than 20 mm Hg

    d. A waves last 1 to 2 minutes and are less sustained than B and C waves

    e. B and C waves are seen in normal individuals

Questions 20–21

20. A 16-year-old girl is involved in a motorcycle accident while riding with her boyfriend. She was not wearing a helmet. On examination, she is comatose, has bruising around her eyes and behind her right ear, and drainage of clear fluid from the nose and the right ear. Based on the findings, which of the following is most likely present in this case?

    a. Epidural hematoma

    b. Skull base fracture

    c. Intraparenchymal hemorrhage

    d. SAH

    e. Subdural hematoma

21. The boyfriend of the patient in question 20 was wearing a helmet. However, he suffered lung contusions, left sided pneumothorax, multiple fractures, and splenic laceration. He remained comatose, and his examination a few days after admission demonstrated multiple petechial hemorrhages throughout the skin, particularly in the axillary region. The patient died a few days later. On autopsy, the brain showed multiple diffuse petechial hemorrhages. Which of the following causes explain the neuropathologic findings?

    a. Fat embolization

    b. Diffuse axonal injury

    c. Meningococcal meningitis

    d. Coup and contrecoup injury

    e. SAH

22. A 34-year-old man presents with ascending paralysis occurring 2 weeks after a diarrheal illness. On examination he has weakness of all four limbs, more distally than proximally, and deep tendon reflexes are absent. Analysis of CSF shows 1 μL WBCs (normal up to 5 lymphocytes/μL) and a protein level of 114 mg/dL (normal up to 45 mg/dL). Regarding this condition, which of the following is incorrect?

    a. Corticosteroids are not indicated

    b. Vital capacity should be measured frequently

    c. Hypercapnia on arterial blood gas is the most sensitive indicator of the need for intubation

    d. Blood pressure and heart rate monitoring is necessary in these patients

    e. Intravenous immunoglobulin therapy or plasmapheresis can be used in this case

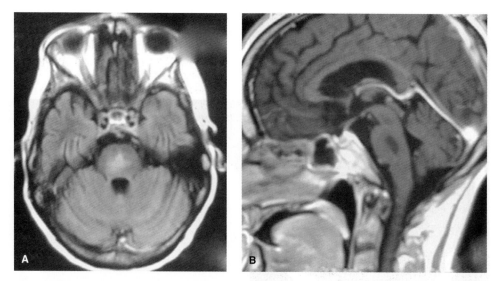

FIGURE 3.9   A. Axial FLAIR MRI; **B.** Sagittal T1-weighted MRI.

    a. Myasthenic crisis
    b. Botulism
    c. Cholinergic crisis
    d. Adrenergic crisis
    e. Thyrotoxicosis

28. Which of the following is correct regarding the treatment of patients with SAH?
    a. Hypertensive therapy should be avoided until the aneurysm is secure
    b. Prophylaxis with antiepileptic agents is not indicated
    c. Hypotonic fluids should be used for hemodilution
    d. Nifedipine is the calcium channel blocker of choice to prevent vasospasm
    e. Intraventricular catheter is standard of care for SAH Fisher grade 2

Questions 29–30

29. Which of the following findings will be seen in a comatose patient with a brainstem lesion and pinpoint pupils?
    a. No response to pain on motor examination and ataxic breathing
    b. Apneustic breathing pattern
    c. Hyperventilation pattern with decorticate posture
    d. Cheyne Stokes breathing(*cerebral hemisplan*)
    e. Hyperventilation

30. Which of the following conditions is associated with ataxic breathing (irregular gasping respiration)?
    a. Hepatic coma
    b. Pontine lesions
    c. Medullary lesions
    d. Forebrain impairment
    e. Uremia

31. Which of the following is correct regarding diagnostic tests used for SAH?

    a. The sensitivity of CT scan increases with time, being higher at 7 days than at 3 days from onset of hemorrhage

    b. A four-vessel angiogram should be performed in all cases of nontraumatic SAH

    c. The brain MRI is more sensitive than the CT scan in detecting the hemorrhage

    d. The presence of xanthochromia in the CSF decreases with time, and this study is more sensitive in the first 6 hours from onset of hemorrhage

    e. A lumbar puncture should be performed in all cases

Questions 32–33

32. A 60-year-old man with history of hypertension and atrial fibrillation on warfarin, suffers a sudden onset of headache and left hemiparesis. On arrival to the emergency room his initial blood pressure is 230/136 mm Hg and his Glasgow Coma Scale score is 6. His CT scan is shown in Figure 3.10. There is no living will and the family wants "everything done." Which is the next step in the treatment of this patient?

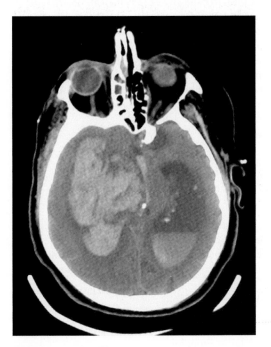

FIGURE 3.10 Axial CT

    a. Decompressive hemicraniectomy

    b. External ventricular drain

    c. Blood pressure control

    d. Endotracheal intubation

    e. Vitamin K and fresh frozen plasma

33. The patient depicted in question 32 has an INR of 6. Regarding the treatment of warfarin-related intracranial hemorrhage, which of the following is incorrect?

a. Vitamin K should be given intravenously
b. Fresh frozen plasma should be given
c. The use of recombinant Factor VIIa is associated with thromboembolic events
d. Recombinant Factor VIIa reduces hematoma expansion and accelerates correction of the INR
e. Protamine sulfate should be given

34. Which of the following is the best means of monitoring respiratory function in a patient with Guillain-Barré syndrome?
a. Arterial partial pressure of oxygen (pO_2)
b. Negative inspiratory force and vital capacity
c. Asking the patient if he is dyspneic
d. Pulse oximetry
e. Arterial partial pressure of carbon dioxide (pCO_2)

35. A 63-year-old woman who is admitted to the medical ICU with asthma exacerbation and pneumonia, develops septic shock. She is intubated and sedated, and given her bronchial constriction and difficulty ventilating she is administered paralytics. Broad-spectrum antibiotics are started, and bronchodilators are used along with steroids. She develops acute respiratory distress syndrome and her hospital course is complicated and prolonged. Over the next 3 weeks she improves; however, neurologic consultation is requested because the patient has severe weakness and areflexia in all four limbs, as well as difficulty weaning from the ventilator. A nerve conduction study is performed, showing normal latencies and conduction velocities and reduced compound motor and SNAP. Needle EMG shows numerous trains of fibrillation potentials and positive sharp waves in proximal muscles. What is the most likely diagnosis?
a. Acute inflammatory demyelinating polyneuropathy
b. Amyotrophic lateral sclerosis
c. Chronic inflammatory demyelinating polyneuropathy
d. Critical illness polyneuropathy and myopathy
e. Polymyositis

36. A 20-year-old man is noted to be febrile and have a depressed level of consciousness. His roommate brings him to the emergency room in his car, and while en route, he has a generalized tonic clonic seizure. By the time he reaches the emergency room, he has been seizing for 35 minutes. Besides ventilatory and hemodynamic support, the treatment of this patient should have the following sequence:
a. Lorazepam → Levetiracetam → Pentobarbital → Phenytoin
b. Fosphenytoin → Lorazepam → Phenobarbital → Repeat Fosphenytoin
c. Lorazepam → Midazolam → Pentobarbital → Fosphenytoin
d. Lorazepam → Fosphenytoin → Pentobarbital → Propofol
e. Lorazepam → Fosphenytoin → Propofol → Pentobarbital

37. Which of the following is the best predictor of outcome after cardiac arrest?
a. Bilateral absence of the N20 response on somatosensory-evoked potentials with median nerve stimulation
b. Creatine kinase BB isoenzyme
c. Duration of cardio-pulmonary resuscitation
d. Absent ocular movements within the first 24 hours
e. Absence of brain edema on CT scan

38. A 71-year-old man suffers a massive intracranial hemorrhage, and no brainstem reflexes are present on examination. The following is not consistent with a diagnosis of brain death:
   a. Apnea test with no respiratory movements observed at a partial pressure of carbon dioxide (pCO_2) level of 45 mm Hg with a core body temperature of 31°C
   b. Absent brainstem reflexes
   c. Cerebral angiography showing absent filling of contrast in the Circle of Willis
   d. No cerebral electrical activity on an EEG recorded for 30 minutes
   e. Absent signals on transcranial doppler

39. Which of the following correlates with decorticate rigidity?
   a. Associated with pinpoint pupils
   b. Lesion below the vestibular nucleus with facilitation of the rubrospinal tract
   c. Lesion below the level of the red nucleus with facilitation of the vestibulospinal tract
   d. Disinhibition of the red nucleus with facilitation of the rubrospinal tracts and lateral vestibulospinal tracts
   e. Decreased activity of the rubrospinal tracts

40. Based on the CT scan shown in Figure 3.11, what type of herniation does this patient have?

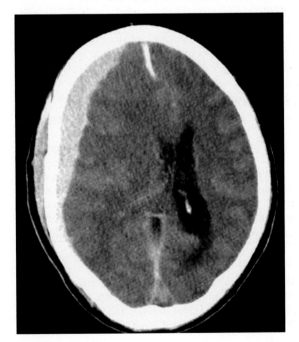

FIGURE 3.11 Axial CT

   a. Uncal herniation
   b. Subfalcine herniation
   c. Tonsillar herniation
   d. Central transtentorial herniation
   e. Transcalvarial herniation

41. Which of the following is incorrect regarding ICP volume and flow dynamics?
   a. Hypercapnia produces an increase in ICP
   b. Mean arterial pressure and ICP determine the cerebral perfusion pressure
   c. The relation between intracranial volume and ICP is linear
   d. Cerebral blood flow autoregulation is effective between mean arterial pressures of 60 and 150 mm Hg
   e. A decrease in the hematocrit favors cerebral blood flow

42. Which of the following is incorrect regarding decompressive hemicraniectomy for ischemic stroke?
   a. Outcomes are worse in patients older than 60 years of age
   b. Hemispheric language dominance should be taken into account when discussing outcome with the family
   c. Patients operated on earlier have better outcomes than those operated on later
   d. Smaller and narrower bone flaps have better clinical results than larger bone flaps
   e. This surgical procedure improves survival in patients with large hemispheric strokes

43. Which of the following is the most common cause of status epilepticus in adults?
   a. Noncompliance with antiepileptic drugs
   b. Central nervous system infection
   c. Febrile seizures
   d. Stroke
   e. Tumors

44. Which of the following statements regarding principles of medical ethics is incorrect?
   a. Beneficence is the principle of offering to patients diagnostic testing or interventions that would be of benefit to them
   b. Nonmaleficence, or "do no harm," is the principle of refraining from providing patients with treatments that will be harmful
   c. In medicine, practicing beneficence and nonmaleficence often entails weighing risks against benefits, since some medical interventions, while perceived as being beneficial, carry potential risks
   d. Justice is the principle of fair and equitable distribution of benefits to individuals
   e. Autonomy is the principle of providing patients with limited options so that they are not confused by all the possibilities

45. A 40-year-old woman on no medications at home undergoes open cholecystectomy. About 45 minutes into the surgery, the end tidal partial pressure of carbon dioxide (PCO_2) is increased in spite of increasing the respiratory rate. Her heart rate is also elevated, and her blood pressure becomes labile. Her temperature increases, reaching 104°F and generalized muscle rigidity is noticed. Which of the following is correct?
   a. Inhaled anesthetic should be increased
   b. Bromocriptine is the treatment of choice
   c. This patient most likely has neuroleptic malignant syndrome
   d. This patient most likely has serotonin syndrome
   e. Dantrolene is the treatment of choice

Answer key

1. a	**9.** b	**17.** e	**25.** c	**33.** e	**41.** c
2. d	**10.** c	**18.** d	**26.** d	**34.** b	**42.** d
3. c	**11.** e	**19.** d	**27.** c	**35.** d	**43.** a
4. a	**12.** c	**20.** b	**28.** a	**36.** e	**44.** e
5. b	**13.** c	**21.** a	**29.** b	**37.** a	**45.** e
6. d	**14.** e	**22.** c	**30.** c	**38.** a	
7. b	**15.** a	**23.** d	**31.** b	**39.** d	
8. a	**16.** d	**24.** b	**32.** d	**40.** b	

Answers

1. a, 2. d

The patient depicted in question 1 has hydrocephalus, a condition associated with interstitial edema.

The patient depicted in question 2 has a brain tumor, a condition associated with vasogenic edema.

There are three types of cerebral edema: vasogenic, cytotoxic, and interstitial.

The patient depicted in question 1 has an acute onset of symptoms suggestive of increased ICP, and a CT scan of the brain showing hydrocephalus. Given the rapid progression of the symptoms, the patient most likely has an acute obstructive hydrocephalus, in which there is disturbance in the normal flow of CSF within the ventricular system and/or from the ventricles to the subarachnoid space. The type of edema seen in acute obstructive hydrocephalus is interstitial edema, as the CSF is forced by hydrostatic pressure to move from the ventricular spaces to the interstitium of the parenchyma. Transependymal edema is another term used for this type of edema.

The patient depicted in question 2 has a brain tumor with surrounding vasogenic edema. Vasogenic edema is an extracellular accumulation of fluid that is usually associated with a disruption in the blood-brain barrier, leading to the extravasation of fluid out of the intravascular space. Multiple factors play a role in extravasation of fluid, including hydrostatic forces, inflammatory mediators, and endothelial permeability, leading to the opening of the endothelial tight junctions and subsequent formation of the edema. Vasogenic edema is usually seen surrounding neoplastic lesions.

In cytotoxic edema there is intracellular accumulation of fluid. This type of edema is most commonly seen in hypoxic-ischemic insult, in which there is a lack of energy to the cells, leading to depletion of adenosine triphosphate (ATP) and subsequent failure of the Na-K ATPase, causing an alteration in the selective permeability of cellular membranes. Cytotoxic edema may also be seen with alterations in the systemic osmolality, leading to intracellular edema.

Suarez JI. Critical Care Neurology and Neurosurgery, 1st ed. Totowa, NJ: Humana Press; 2004.

3. c

There is evidence to support the use of hypothermic therapy in cardiac arrest from ventricular fibrillation, but not in pulseless electrical activity or in asystole.

Patients with out-of-hospital cardiac arrest have a very high mortality rate, and those who survive have a significant risk of cerebral and cognitive dysfunction caused by damage from the absence of blood flow.

106   Chapter 3

Based on recent studies, management recommendations for unconscious adult patients with spontaneous circulation after out-of-hospital cardiac arrest when the initial rhythm is ventricular fibrillation have been proposed. These patients should be treated with hypothermia targeting a temperature of 32°C to 34°C for 12 to 24 hours. This therapy may also be beneficial for patients with other types of cardiac arrest, such as pulseless electrical activity or asystole; however, as of 2011 there is not strong evidence to support its use in these latter cases.

Mild hypothermia with temperatures between 32°C and 34°C has been used safely. However, lower temperatures may not provide extra benefit and may be harmful.

Sanders A. Therapeutic hypothermia after cardiac arrest. Curr Opin Crit Care. 2006; 12:213–217.

4. a

Uncal herniation produces mass effect and pressure over the ipsilateral midbrain, affecting the ipsilateral cranial nerve III nucleus, and the corticospinal fibers. The mass effect compresses parasympathetic fibers that mediate miosis, resulting in mydriasis. Since the corticospinal tract has not decussated at the level of the midbrain, patients have a contralateral hemiparesis. Occasionally, the uncal herniation will lead to displacement of the midbrain against the contralateral Kernohan's notch, resulting in a contralateral compression of the corticospinal tract, and therefore an ipsilateral hemiparesis.

The other types of herniation syndromes do not include an ipsilateral dilated pupil with contralateral hemiparesis.

Posner JB, Saper CB, Schiff ND, Plum F. Plum and Postern's Diagnosis of Stupor and Coma, 4th ed. New York, NY: Oxford University Press; 2007.

5. b

Hypernatremia is not a cause of cerebral edema.

There are different types of cerebral edema—Vasogenic edema, in which there is accumulation of fluid in the extracellular space, and cytotoxic edema, in which the fluid accumulates in the intracellular space.

In hyponatremia, there is a decrease in the osmolarity of the extracellular fluid, leading to the entry of water into the cells, especially when hyponatremia develops rapidly. On the other hand, in hypernatremia water moves from the intracellular space to the extracellular space; therefore, there is no cerebral edema. To that end, hypertonic saline and other hyperosmolar agents are used for the treatment of cerebral edema.

Prolonged cardiac arrest leading to hypoxic-ischemic encephalopathy is associated with diffuse cytotoxic edema, likely caused by the lack of energy supply and failure of the Na-K ATPase pumps in cellular membranes.

Rapid ascent into high altitude, lead intoxication, and liver failure are other conditions associated with cytotoxic cerebral edema.

Suarez JI. Critical Care Neurology and Neurosurgery, 1st ed. Totowa, NJ: Humana Press; 2004.

6. d

An intraventricular catheter should be placed. The CT scan depicts hydrocephalus with intraventricular blood. To measure the ICP, a surgically placed device is required. In general, an ICP-measuring device may be used in patients with a Glasgow Coma Scale score of 7 or less, and should be placed if the following conditions are met:

– The patient has a condition leading to ICP elevation amenable to treatment.
– The ICP measurement will have an impact on the decisions made for the treatment of the patient.
– The benefits of the device outweigh the risks.

If there is a need for ventricular CSF drainage, an intraventricular device is preferred. This patient has hydrocephalus with intraventricular blood and needs an intraventricular catheter. This device is inserted through a burr hole into the ventricular system, providing the capability to transduce the ICP and allowing the possibility of CSF drainage, which can help decrease ICP. Intraventricular catheters have a 1% to 6% risk of hemorrhage and a 2% to 22% risk of infection.

Parenchymal devices are inserted into the brain parenchyma and provide pressure measurements. However, these do not allow CSF drainage and may be susceptible to pressure gradients across the parenchyma.

Epidural devices are placed between the dura and the calvarium and have lower rates of hemorrhage and infection, but their accuracy is low. Subarachnoid bolts are placed in continuity with subarachnoid space. The accuracy is not optimal, but their placement is relatively technically simple and the risks of infection and hemorrhage are not as high as with intraventricular devices.

Suarez JI. Critical Care Neurology and Neurosurgery, 1st ed. Totowa, NJ: Humana Press; 2004.

7. b

Hyperventilation is a short-lived therapy, and a rebound increase in the ICP may occur.

This patient has increased ICP, which normally ranges between 5 and 15 mm Hg. Intracranial hypertension is deleterious since it produces a decrease in the cerebral perfusion pressure and therefore cerebral blood flow, resulting in cerebral ischemia. The care of the patient with increased ICP includes general measures and more specific therapy. The general measures are used in every patient and include head position (the head should be elevated above 30 degrees), maintenance of normothermia, glucose control, blood pressure control, adequate nutrition, and prevention of complications.

Specific interventions to reduce ICP include hyperventilation, use of osmotic agents, use of hypertonic solutions, use of corticosteroids in select cases, CSF drainage, surgical decompression in select cases, and barbiturate coma, pharmacologic paralysis, and hypothermia in refractory cases. Some of these therapies are controversial.

Hyperventilation has a rapid effect; however, it lasts for 10 to 20 hours and subsequently a rebound phase with increased ICP may be seen. Hyperventilation produces a reduction in partial pressure of CO_2 (pCO_2), and this hypocapnia leads to cerebral vasoconstriction, reducing cerebral blood volume and therefore reducing ICP. This therapy should be used to target a reduction of 10 mm Hg of the pCO2, and/or to a target of approximately 30 mm Hg of pCO2, and should be reversed slowly. Hyperventilation does not act by changing the CSF osmolarity.

Mannitol is an osmotic agent and acts by raising the serum osmolarity and producing an osmotic gradient driving the flow of water from the interstitium to the intravascular compartment. It is usually given in boluses of 0.5 to 1 g/kg and not as a continuous infusion. While on this medication, serum osmolarity should be checked at regular intervals targeting a level closer to 320 mOsm/L. Mannitol as an osmotic agent will also produce diuresis and may produce hypotension and hypovolemia. It is associated with depletion of potassium, magnesium, and phosphorus. If there is damage to the blood-brain barrier, mannitol can leak into the interstitium, worsening vasogenic edema.

Suarez JI. Critical Care Neurology and Neurosurgery, 1st ed. Totowa, NJ: Humana Press; 2004.

8. a

Barbiturates decrease the ICP by reducing cerebral metabolic activity and thereby reducing cerebral blood flow and blood volume.

Propofol is a commonly used sedative agent in the neurocritical care unit since it has a short half-life permitting prompt neurologic examinations soon after it is discontinued. It produces sedation within a few minutes, it has a drug effect that lasts between 5 and 10 minutes, and awakening may occur 10 to 15 minutes after discontinuation (depending on the baseline neurologic function). Propofol also has been shown to reduce the ICP in patients with normal intracranial dynamics and preserved cerebral perfusion pressure, which makes this attractive in the care of patients with increased ICP. Unfortunately, Propofol is not free of side effects, and a prominent hypotensive effect is frequently encountered. Other complications include hypertriglyceridemia and infections. Propofol infusion syndrome is a lethal complication seen rarely, mainly in patients on high doses for long periods of time, and manifests with hypotension, bradycardia, lactic acidosis, hyperlipidemia, and rhabdomyolysis.

Hypertonic saline reduces the ICP by drawing water out from brain cells via an osmotic gradient. It can be used as a continuous infusion targeting a serum sodium concentration of 150 mmol/L. Serum sodium concentration should be monitored closely during administration of hypertonic saline, and changes should occur very gradually.

Barbiturates may be used when the ICP is elevated and refractory to other measures. These agents reduce the ICP by lowering cerebral metabolic activity, leading to a decrease in cerebral blood flow and blood volume. Patients on barbiturate coma should have continuous EEG monitoring to titrate to burst-suppression. Continuous β activity is seen with benzodiazepines and is not a treatment goal. Pentobarbital is the barbiturate of choice and is usually started with a bolus followed by a continuous infusion. Its discontinuation should be gradual. Unfortunately, barbiturate coma has multiple complications, including hypotension, myocardial depression, predisposition to infections, and hypothermia.

Marino PL. The ICU Book, 3rd ed. Philadelphia, PA: Lippincott Williams & Wilkins; 2007.

Suarez JI. Critical Care Neurology and Neurosurgery, 1st ed. Totowa, NJ: Humana Press; 2004.

9. b

This patient is stuporous. The following are the definitions for these terms:

Stupor: state of pathologically reduced consciousness from which the patient can be aroused to purposeful response only with external stimulation.
Coma: state of unresponsiveness, in which the patient cannot be aroused even with vigorous stimulation. There may be a grimace response or stereotyped withdrawal movement of the limbs to noxious stimulation, but the patient does not localize to the stimulus.
Locked-in state: occurs in brainstem lesions, in which the patient is awake and conscious, but quadriplegic, with paralysis of the lower cranial nerves, and with horizontal gaze palsy. The patient can typically blink and move his eyes vertically (because of sparing of the vertical gaze centers) and may be able to communicate with vertical eye movements and blinking.
Persistent vegetative state (PVS): a vegetative state that last for more than 30 days. Vegetative state is characterized by return of sleep-wake cycles in an unresponsive patient (usually previously comatose), with apparent lack of cognitive function.
Delirium: a disturbance of consciousness, with poor attention and reduced ability to focus. This state develops over a short period of time and tends to fluctuate.
Obtundation: this term is not defined in neurology and should not be used.

Bradley WG, Daroff RB, Fenichel GM, Jankovic J. Neurology in Clinical Practice, 5th ed. Philadelphia, PA: Elsevier; 2008.

Posner JB, Saper CB, Schiff ND, Plum F. Plum and Postern's Diagnosis of Stupor and Coma, 4th ed. New York, NY: Oxford University Press; 2007.

10. C

This patient has a large right MCA infarct that affects almost the entire MCA vascular territory, with evidence of cerebral edema and midline shift. Reperfusion therapy in acute ischemic stroke either with intravenous tissue plasminogen activator (tPA) or intraarterial therapies is used within the first few hours since the onset of symptoms, and when there is brain tissue at risk for ischemia. In this patient, a large portion of the brain tissue in the affected vascular territory has already infarcted, since the CT scan shows hypodensity, and there is very little, if any, salvageable tissue in this vascular distribution. Therefore, reperfusion therapy should not be contemplated.

Cerebral edema in ischemic stroke develops within hours of stroke onset, with a peak of maximal swelling at days 2 to 5 poststroke. Malignant cerebral edema, which occurs in complete MCA infarctions, is associated with up to 80% mortality with conservative therapy. It is most commonly seen in strokes with occlusions at the ICA terminus and most proximal (M1) segment of the MCA. Other predictors of malignant cerebral edema include high National Institute of Health Stroke Scale (NIHSS) score (greater than 15), hypertension, early hypodensity of more than 50% of the MCA territory on CT, and younger age. The initial management of these patients is based on supportive care, along with tight control of blood glucose, blood pressure, and temperature. General measures for the treatment of increased ICP, such as hyperventilation, hypertonic saline, and mannitol, are also used. In the appropriate patient (see discussion in question 42), the plan for early hemicraniectomy (<48 h from symptom onset) should be discussed soon with the family, since this intervention improves survival.

Anticoagulation should not be used and may increase the risk of hemorrhage.

An intraventricular catheter is not indicated, since there is no hydrocephalus or intraventricular blood on CT, and there are no clear indications for ICP measurement in this case (see question 6). Steroids play no role in the treatment of cerebral edema in the setting of ischemic stroke.

Bershad EM, Humphreis WE, Suarez JI. Intracranial hypertension. Semin Neurol. 2008; 28:690–702.

Suarez JI. Critical Care Neurology and Neurosurgery, 1st ed. Totowa, NJ: Humana Press; 2004.

Subramaniam S, Hill MD. Decompressive hemicraniectomy for malignant middle cerebral artery infarction: An update. Neurologist. 2009; 15:178–184.

11. e, 12. C

This patient has posterior reversible encephalopathy syndrome (PRES), also known as reversible posterior leukoencephalopathy syndrome (RPLS), and this condition is not associated with hyperlipidemia.

The diagnosis of PRES is usually based on neuroimaging demonstrating a characteristic pattern of vasogenic edema predominantly in the posterior cerebral region, especially in the occipital and parietal lobes (though more anterior areas can also be involved in PRES). Risk factors and causative factors associated with PRES include hypertension, renal failure, organ transplantation, autoimmune diseases, immunosuppressive drugs (particularly cyclosporine), cancer chemotherapy, preeclampsia, and eclampsia. Hyperlipidemia is not associated with PRES.

Clinical manifestations include headache, nausea, visual changes, focal neurologic symptoms, altered mental status, coma, and seizures. Most patients present with severe hypertension, and some theories suggest that PRES is a manifestation in the spectrum of hypertensive encephalopathy. The pathophysiology is not well understood, but it is thought to be related to a disruption in autoregulation of the posterior circulation, which associated with hypertension and hyperperfusion results in alteration of the blood-brain barrier and vasogenic edema. Endothelial injury and dysfunction also play a role.

The treatment of this condition consists of aggressive blood pressure control. Supportive care is part of the treatment, and many times these patients need intensive care observation. Treating the underlying condition and/or withdrawing the offending etiologic factor is a central part of the treatment.

Bartynski WS. Posterior reversible encephalopathy syndrome, part 1: Fundamental imaging and clinical features. Am J Neuroradiol. 2008; 28:1036–1042.

13. c

Sodium nitroprusside is a vasodilator that produces arterial and venous dilation and reduces blood pressure rapidly. It is used in a continuous infusion; while it is not the first line of treatment for hypertension, it may be indicated in severe hypertension. When sodium nitroprusside enters the circulation, nitric oxide and cyanide are produced. Nitrous oxide then acts through the guanylate cyclase pathway, increasing cyclic guanosine monophosphate (GMP) and producing vasodilation. The vasodilation occurs in both cerebral and systemic vessels, causing an increase in cerebral blood flow and volume, and increasing the ICP, which along with a decrease in the mean arterial pressures can compromise cerebral perfusion pressure. Therefore, sodium nitroprusside should be used cautiously in patients with increased ICP. With continuous and prolonged infusion of sodium nitroprusside, cyanide and thiocyanate toxicity can occur. Cyanide originates from the nitroprusside molecule and can be cleared by binding to methemoglobin, or when thiosulfate donates a sulfur group, transforming the cyanide into thiocyanate. Cyanide intoxication manifests by behavioral changes, obtundation, coma, seizures, and lactic acidosis. The accumulation of cyanide can be treated with sodium thiosulfate, which provides sulfur groups favoring the conversion to thiocyanate, which can be cleared by the kidneys. However, thiocyanate can also produce toxicity, and the risk of this intoxication is increased in patients with renal disease; therefore, sodium nitroprusside should not be used in this patient population. Manifestations of thiocyanate toxicity include anxiety, confusion, pupillary constriction, tinnitus, hallucinations, and seizures. This intoxication can be treated with dialysis.

Marino PL. The ICU Book, 3rd ed. Philadelphia, PA: Lippincott Williams & Wilkins; 2007.

Suarez JI. Critical Care Neurology and Neurosurgery, 1st ed. Totowa, NJ: Humana Press; 2004.

14. e

Corticosteroids are used for the treatment of intracranial hypertension associated with primary brain tumors and metastasis to the brain. Corticosteroids are beneficial in vasogenic cerebral edema as is seen with intracranial tumors, either primary or metastatic. However, the exact mechanism of action of steroids in vasogenic edema is not well understood. Available evidence suggests that corticosteroids are not useful in the management of other conditions commonly associated with cerebral edema such as traumatic brain injury, intracerebral hemorrhage, or ischemic stroke. This is explained in part by the difference in the type of edema seen in the latter conditions (see questions 1 and 2). Acute obstructive hydrocephalus requires a neurosurgical intervention.

Suarez JI. Critical Care Neurology and Neurosurgery, 1st ed. Totowa, NJ: Humana Press; 2004.

15. a

The CT scan in Figure 3.6 shows a subdural hematoma, in which blood accumulates in the subdural space adopting a crescentic or concave shape over the cerebral convexity. The most common cause is trauma, by producing an acceleration force, thereby tearing and causing rupture of the cerebral surface bridging veins that drain into the dural venous sinuses. Patients usually present with headache, change in mental status, and focal neurologic deficits. Surgical evacuation is indicated if the subdural hematoma is more than 1 cm or if there is midline shift. If the subdural hematoma is small it may be observed without the need for surgical evacuation.

Rupture of the middle meningeal artery (usually associated with skull fracture) causes an epidural hematoma, in which the CT scan shows a lenticular-shaped biconvex hyperdensity. Lipohyalinosis and Charcot-Bouchard aneurysms are seen in chronic hypertension and may be associated with intraparenchymal hemorrhage. Subdural hematomas are not caused by aneurysmal rupture; therefore, coiling or clipping of an aneurysm is not indicated in this case.

Suarez JI. Critical Care Neurology and Neurosurgery, 1st ed. Totowa, NJ: Humana Press; 2004.

16. d

The cause of the new symptoms in the patient depicted in question 16 is likely vasospasm. Vasospasm causing ischemia and delayed infarcts is the leading case of morbidity and mortality in patients who survive initial SAH. Vasospasm can occur between 3 and 15 days from the onset of the bleeding, with a peak between days 6 and 8. The pathophysiology is not understood, but there is evidence of an inflammatory basis. Symptoms of vasospasm include headache, nausea, vomiting, altered mental status, and focal neurologic deficits. Transcranial doppler ultrasonography provides information by detecting the velocity of the flow in the intracranial vessels and should be performed daily to follow up the trends of these velocities. CT angiograms and conventional angiograms are helpful in the diagnosis of vasospasm.

Acute hydrocephalus, rebleeding, and vasospasm are complications of SAH. If a hematoma forms, it can produce mass effect and lead to uncal herniation. Acute hydrocephalus occurs from obstruction of the cerebral aqueduct associated with intraventricular extension of blood. Clinical manifestations include worsening headache, change in mental status, and coma. Treatment is placement of an intraventricular catheter. Rebleeding usually occurs early on, when the aneurysm has not been secured.

Suarez JI. Critical Care Neurology and Neurosurgery, 1st ed. Totowa, NJ: Humana Press; 2004.

17. e

Epidural hematoma is most commonly caused by head trauma, leading to rupture of the middle meningeal artery, which passes through the foramen spinosum. Rupture of this artery results in accumulation of blood in the epidural space. The appearance on CT is lenticular shaped or biconvex. Clinically, patients may present with a brief loss of consciousness followed by a lucid interval and subsequent deterioration over hours.

The jugular vein passes through the jugular foramen; however, injury to it is not the cause of epidural hematomas. The carotid artery passes through the carotid canal and runs in the foramen lacerum; however, injury to this structure is not the cause of epidural hematomas.

Blumenfeld H. Neuroanatomy Through Clinical Cases, 1st ed. Sunderland, MA: Sinauer; 2002.

Suarez JI. Critical Care Neurology and Neurosurgery, 1st ed. Totowa, NJ: Humana Press; 2004.

18. d

Diffuse axonal injury occurs from disruption of intracerebral axons and is caused by the effect of angular accelerations and shear injury, and not from direct contusion. Patients with diffuse axonal injury typically have loss of consciousness and amnesia that lasts for longer than 6 hours. Coma with long-term disability may occur, but in general, patients with isolated diffuse axonal injury have good outcomes at 3 months in 15% to 65% of cases. Neuropathologically, there is evidence of destruction of axonal cytoskeletons, with the presence of retraction bulbs, typically at the gray-white junction or along white matter fiber tracts.

Along the same spectrum of diffuse axonal injury is brain concussion, in which there is alteration of consciousness with confusion and amnesia in the setting of brain trauma, but with no evidence of contusion, and the prognosis is good.

Suarez JI. Critical Care Neurology and Neurosurgery, 1st ed. Totowa, NJ: Humana Press; 2004.

19. d

A waves last between 5 to 20 minutes and are more sustained than B and C waves.

ICP can be reliably assessed using invasive ICP monitors that will display several waveforms. Lundberg A waves or "plateau waves" are pathologic and associated with decreased intracranial compliance and intracranial hypertension, with the risk of cerebral ischemia. These waves are sustained with duration between 5 and 20 minutes. Their amplitude is high, in the range of 50 100 mm Hg. B waves are normal, with duration of 1 to 2 minutes and amplitudes in the range of 20 to 50 mm Hg. C waves are also normal and last for 4 to 5 minutes with less than 20 mm Hg of amplitude.

Along with the above-mentioned waves, the cardiac cycle and respirations also influence ICP monitor tracings.

Suarez JI. Critical Care Neurology and Neurosurgery, 1st ed. Totowa, NJ: Humana Press; 2004.

20. b

Signs of skull fracture include periorbital ecchymoses or hematoma (raccoon eyes), postauricular ecchymosis (Battle's sign), CSF rhinorrhea, and otorrhea.

Patients with head trauma may have a broad variety of injuries, including scalp injury, cervical injury, linear or depressed skull fractures, basal skull fractures, epidural hemorrhage, subdural hemorrhage, intraparenchymal hemorrhages, cerebral contusions, and SAH. All these can be potentially present in the patient depicted in this case; however, given the clinical findings, skull fracture is most likely to be present.

Patients with head trauma should be initially stabilized at the scene, with subsequent ICU care to prevent secondary injuries from hypoxia, increased ICP, and brain edema. ICU care includes not only management of increased ICP but also blood glucose control, blood pressure control, temperature control, prevention of deep venous thrombosis and infections, nutrition, and ventilatory and hemodynamic support. Surgery may be needed in some cases. In the case of basal skull fracture, nasogastric tubes should be avoided, and antibiotics should be used prophylactically since there may be an external access to the CSF.

Suarez JI. Critical Care Neurology and Neurosurgery, 1st ed. Totowa, NJ: Humana Press; 2004.

21. a

This patient has had fat embolism, which results from fat droplets entering the circulation usually in the setting of surgery or trauma, and most frequently after fractures of long bones such as the femur. Fat microparticles from the bone marrow travel in the venous system to the lungs and spread systemically. Patients will present with agitation, delirium, coma, respiratory distress, anemia, thrombocytopenia, and generalized petechial rash, often concentrated in the axilla, subconjunctival area, and palate. Multiple petechial hemorrhages can be seen in the gray and white matter of the brain on autopsy.

The clinical presentation and finding of petechial hemorrhages after multiple fractures is not consistent with the other options.

Posner JB, Saper CB, Schiff ND, Plum F. Plum and Postern's Diagnosis of Stupor and Coma, 4th ed. New York, NY: Oxford University Press; 2007.

22. c

Hypercapnia on arterial blood gas is not a sensitive indicator of the need for intubation in this setting.

This patient has a progressive ascending paralysis after a diarrheal illness and albumino-cytologic dissociation evidence from CSF analysis, which is consistent with Guillain Barré syndrome (GBS), an acute inflammatory demyelinating polyneuropathy. Patients with this disorder should be hospitalized and may need intensive unit care, since they may develop respiratory failure, inability to protect the airway, and autonomic dysfunction, with labile blood pressure and cardiac arrhythmias. Therefore, these patients should have close cardiac and ventilatory monitoring with frequent evaluations of negative inspiratory force and vital capacity. Arterial blood gases are not accurate predictors of the need for intubation and mechanical ventilation, since hypoxia and hypercapnia occur late in the course of respiratory failure, once the patient is decompensating.

The care of these patients include general supportive care, prevention of complications, rehabilitation, and specific therapies for the inflammatory process, which include plasmapheresis and intravenous immunoglobulin. Steroids play no role in the treatment of GBS.

Hughes RA, Wijdicks EF, Barohn R, et al. Practice parameter: Immunotherapy for Guillain-Barre syndrome: Report of the Quality Standards Subcommittee of the American Academy of Neurology. Neurology. 2003; 61:736–740.

Suarez JI. Critical Care Neurology and Neurosurgery, 1st ed. Totowa, NJ: Humana Press; 2004.

23. d

This patient suffered head trauma with coup and contrecoup injury. Figure 3.7 shows a left frontal lobe hematoma from direct contusion (coup) as well as a right occipito-temporal hematoma (contrecoup injury). The scalp laceration in this patient indicates that the initial impact was in the left frontal region. As deceleration occurs, the frontal lobe strikes the frontal bone and the falx, leading to formation of a hematoma. The countrecoup also seen in this patient is the result of injury that occurs distant from the site of initial impact and is usually seen in the frontal or temporal lobes, as these are in close relationship with the frontal bone and the sphenoid ridge, respectively.

With cerebral contusions there may be loss of consciousness and focal deficits, and subsequent rapid deterioration from mass effect. Multiple contusions can predispose to the rapid development of cerebral edema and elevated ICP.

The CT scan findings do not correlate with SAH from aneurysmal rupture, subdural hematoma, fat embolization, or diffuse axonal injury.

Suarez JI. Critical Care Neurology and Neurosurgery, 1st ed. Totowa, NJ: Humana Press; 2004.

24. b, 25. c

This patient has SAH, most likely caused by aneurysmal rupture. This patient's SAH is graded as Hunt Hess of 3. This patient has a clinical presentation and CT scan findings of a SAH,

TABLE 3.1	SAH grading scales
Hunt and Hess Grading Scale	1. Asymptomatic or minimal headache and slight nuchal rigidity 2. Moderate-severe headache, nuchal rigidity, no neurologic deficit other than cranial nerve palsy 3. Drowsiness, confusion, or mild focal neurologic deficit 4. Stupor, moderate-severe hemiparesis, possible early decerebrate rigidity and vegetative disturbances 5. Deep coma, decerebrate rigidity, moribund appearance
World Federation of Neurological Surgeons Grading Scale	1. Glasgow coma scale (GCS) score of 15, no motor deficit 2. GCS score of 13 to 14, no motor deficit 3. GCS score of 13 to 14, with motor deficit 4. GCS score of 7 to 12, with or without motor deficit 5. GCS score of 3 to 6, with or without motor deficit
Fisher Grading Scale	1. No SAH on CT 2. Diffuse or vertical layers <1 mm thick 3. Localized clot and/or vertical layer ≥1 mm 4. Intracerebral or intraventricular clot with diffuse or no SAH

which seems to be denser in the left Sylvian fissure, likely associated with rupture of a left MCA aneurysm, as seen in Figure 3.8.

Overall, the most common cause of SAH is trauma, and aneurysmal rupture is the most common nontraumatic cause. Hypertension and smoking are the most important risk factors for aneurysmal SAH. Family history, heavy alcohol use, atherosclerosis, and oral contraceptives are other risk factors for this condition.

The diagnosis of SAH can be suspected based on a clinical presentation of sudden onset severe headache (thunderclap headache, the "worst headache of my life"), sometimes accompanied by nausea, vomiting, photophobia, and neck stiffness. Altered mental status, coma, and focal neurologic findings are also common.

Whenever a SAH is suspected, a brain CT should be performed, demonstrating the hemorrhage in more than 95% of the cases when the scan is performed within 48 hours. If the CT scan is negative, a lumbar puncture should be performed in order to detect blood in the subarachnoid space, evidenced by elevated RBC count and xanthochromia. A negative CT scan does not rule out SAH.

Clinical and radiologic grading systems have been developed for SAH and include the Hunt and Hess Grading Scale, World Federation of Neurological Surgeons Grading Scale, and the Fisher Scale (Table 3.1).

Drake CG, Hun WE, Sano K, et al. Report of World Federation of Neurological Surgeons Committee on a universal subarachnoid hemorrhage grading scale. J Neurosurg. 1988; 68:985–986.

Fisher CM, Kistler JP, Davis JM. Relation of cerebral vasospasm to subarachnoid hemorrhage visualized by computerized tomographic scanning. Neurosurgery. 1980; 6:1–9.

Hunt WE, Hess RM. Surgical risk as related to time of intervention in the repair of intracranial aneurysms. J Neurosurg. 1968; 28:14–20.

Rosen DS, Macdonald RL. Subarachnoid hemorrhage grading scales. Neurocrit Care. 2005; 2:110–118.

Suarez JI. Critical Care Neurology and Neurosurgery, 1st ed. Totowa, NJ: Humana Press; 2004.

26. d

The history and images are consistent with central pontine myelinolysis (CPM), which is a disorder seen after rapid and aggressive correction of hyponatremia. This condition is not limited to the pons and could affect other areas of the central nervous system.

Because of the risk of CPM, the rate of correction of hyponatremia should be no more than 12 mEq/L per day, or 0.5 mEq/L per hour. Patients may develop CPM after rapid correction of hyponatremia, and the manifestations are evident within 3 to 10 days, with progressive paraparesis or quadriparesis, pseudobulbar palsy, dysphagia, dysarthria, and altered mental status. Progressive extension of the demyelination may lead to locked-in syndrome. Most patients who survive will have clinical disabilities.

Pathologically, there is bilateral symmetric focal destruction of myelin in the ventral pons, sparing axons and neuronal cell bodies. The myelin disruption is not limited to the pons, and extrapontine myelinolysis has been observed in the cerebellum, thalamus, external and extreme capsules, basal ganglia, deep layers of the cerebral cortex and adjacent white matter, and sometimes even in the fornix, subthalamic nucleus, amygdala, optic tract, and spinal cord.

Other conditions associated with CPM are severe alcoholism, chronic liver disease and liver transplantation, and extensive burns.

Aminoff MJ. Neurology and General Medicine, 4th ed. Philadelphia, PA: Elsevier; 2008.

27. c

This patient is in cholinergic crisis. Patients with myasthenia gravis taking excessive amounts of acetylcholinesterase inhibitors such as pyridostigmine may be at risk for a cholinergic crisis (also discussed in Chapter 10). It is sometimes difficult to differentiate this from a true myasthenic crisis; when patients start experiencing symptoms of worsening myasthenia, they may increase the frequency and dose of their pyridostigmine, putting themselves at risk for a cholinergic crisis.

The following include manifestations of a cholinergic crisis: small and even pinpoint pupils, excessive secretions, diarrhea, sweating, bradycardia, muscle weakness, and fasciculations. The symptoms will subside with cessation of the acetylcholinesterase inhibitor. The presence of pinpoint pupils and increased cholinergic activity suggest a cholinergic crisis and not a myasthenic crisis. A patient with adrenergic crisis or thyrotoxicosis may have similar manifestations but will have mydriasis and tachycardia. The clinical picture does not correlate with botulism (discussed in Chapter 17).

Suarez JI. Critical Care Neurology and Neurosurgery, 1st ed. Totowa, NJ: Humana Press; 2004.

28. a

In SAH, hypertensive therapy should be avoided until the aneurysm is secure. The goals of therapy in SAH are initial stabilization, prevention of complications such as rebleeding and vasospasm, and specific aneurysmal treatment.

Patients who are comatose or cannot protect the airway should be intubated. Blood pressure should be controlled, and hypertension should be avoided in the first few hours, and until the aneurysm has been secured (either by clipping or coiling). Intravenous isotonic fluids are aggressively administered, and hypotonic fluids should be avoided. Until the aneurysm is secured, prophylactic antiepileptic agents are given, since a generalized seizure may be catastrophic in a patient with an unsecured aneurysm. Mild sedation should be generally provided, and pain control should be optimal.

Nimodipine (not Nifedipine) is a calcium channel blocker that is utilized in a dose of 60 mg every 4 hours for 21 days following aneurysmal SAH and has been shown to improve outcomes from vasospasm. Pravastatin therapy has also been shown to improve outcomes and reduce delayed ischemic deficits from vasospasm.

Specific aneurysmal treatment includes isolation of the aneurysm from the circulation, either by surgical clips or endovascular coils. Once the aneurysm is secure, blood pressure can be liberalized, and hypertensive therapy can be used in case of vasospasm. "Triple H therapy" is used for the treatment of vasospasm, and it consists of hypervolemia, hypertension, and hemodilution. This is achieved by expanding the intravascular volume using isotonic fluids, and sometimes colloids such as albumin. Vasopressors can also be utilized. The risk of triple H therapy includes rebleeding from an unsecured aneurysm, pulmonary edema, congestive heart failure, and cerebral edema. If vasospasm is refractory, endovascular therapies may play a role, including intraarterial papaverine or nicardipine, or direct angioplasty. The use of intraventricular catheters is reserved for acute hydrocephalus, or intraventricular extension of blood (Fisher grade 4).

Suarez JI. Critical Care Neurology and Neurosurgery, 1st ed. Totowa, NJ: Humana Press; 2004.

29. b, 30. c

Apneustic breathing pattern is seen in patients with pontine lesions (patients with pontine lesions have pinpoint pupils). Medullary lesions are associated with ataxic breathing.

Breathing is a complex action that is integrated by circuits in the brainstem, with connections at different neural levels in the brain and upper cervical cord, and under the influence of chemical and mechanical input that enter via the vagus and the glossopharyngeal nerves. Respiratory rhythm is an intrinsic function of a group of neurons in the ventrolateral medulla, but under the control of a pontine cell group that integrates breathing with other functions, reflexes, and metabolic input.

Apneusis is a respiratory pause at full inspiration and occurs from bilateral pontine lesions. Since pinpoint pupils are seen in pontine lesions, it is most likely that this patient will have an apneustic breathing pattern, and likely decerebrate posture.

Cheyne Stokes respiration is a pattern of periodic breathing in which hyperpnea alternates with apnea and the depth of breathing increases and decreases gradually. It is seen in patients with forebrain impairment in the setting of intact brainstem respiratory reflexes, but it is also present in patients with cardiopulmonary disease.

Hyperventilation may be seen in metabolic encephalopathies such as in uremia and hepatic encephalopathy, but has also been reported in patients with midbrain lesions.

Ataxic breathing is an irregular and gasping respiration seen with lesions damaging the respiratory rhythm generator in the upper medulla.

Posner JB, Saper CB, Schiff ND, Plum F. Plum and Posner's Diagnosis of Stupor and Coma, 4th ed. New York, NY: Oxford University Press; 2007.

31. b

A four-vessel angiogram should be performed in all cases of SAH.

All patients with suspected SAH should have a brain CT scan, which will detect hemorrhage in 95% of the cases within 48 hours of the bleed. As days pass, the sensitivity of the CT will drop, being approximately 50% by day 7 posthemorrhage. If the CT does not show the hemorrhage, but there is high clinical suspicion, a lumbar puncture should be performed. CSF RBC count that does not decrease in subsequent tubes and xanthochromia are findings consistent with SAH. The appearance of xanthochromia requires the presence of RBCs in the CSF for some time; therefore, it may not be present in the first few hours following the hemorrhage.

A lumbar puncture is not required in all cases, and actually is rarely performed if the CT scan shows the hemorrhage. Brain MRI is less sensitive for SAH, and therefore is less helpful in the acute setting.

To determine the presence of aneurysm, a CT angiogram or MR angiogram can be performed; however, conventional cerebral angiography is the gold standard, and a four-vessel angiogram should be performed in all cases of SAH, since about 15% of the patients will have multiple aneurysms in different territories.

Suarez JI. Critical Care Neurology and Neurosurgery, 1st ed. Totowa, NJ: Humana Press; 2004.

32. d

The first step in the treatment of this patient is endotracheal intubation.

This patient has a massive intracranial hemorrhage, likely originating from the basal ganglia and extending to the ventricles. As in every patient who is in a critical condition, an initial survey should be performed, addressing the "ABC" (airway, breathing, circulation). Therefore, this patient should be intubated first in order to receive ventilatory support and maintain oxygenation. Second, hemodynamic support should be addressed, and in this case, blood pressure control is paramount. Once the patient is stable from the ventilatory and hemodynamic standpoint, specific therapies to address his neurologic condition should be started, such as correction of coagulopathy if this is present, an external ventricular drain, and surgical decompression, if needed.

It is important to always address the goals of therapy, code status, and end-of-life care with the family. This should be done early to avoid nondesired treatment against the patient's wishes and his family.

Suarez JI. Critical Care Neurology and Neurosurgery, 1st ed. Totowa, NJ: Humana Press; 2004.

33. e

Protamine sulfate does not correct warfarin-related coagulopathy. Protamine sulfate is utilized to reverse anticoagulation due to heparin, and it plays no role in the treatment of warfarin-related intracranial hemorrhage.

Coagulation factors II, VII, IX, and X and the anticoagulant proteins C and S require γ-carboxylation in the liver for their activation, and this process requires the reduced form of vitamin K. Warfarin is a vitamin K antagonist. Warfarin is rapidly absorbed in the gastrointestinal tract, highly bound to proteins, and metabolized in the liver. The use of this medication causes a prolongation in the prothrombin time (PT). However, to standardize the measure, the INR is used for this purpose.

Patients presenting with warfarin-related intracranial hemorrhage and a high INR need various therapies to reverse the anticoagulation and arrest the bleeding process. Administration of vitamin K is effective in reversing the effects of warfarin, and it can be used by oral, subcutaneous, or intravenous route. The intravenous route is preferred for urgent reversal of anticoagulation, with the rare risk of anaphylaxis. However, even with intravenous vitamin K, it may take between 6 hours and sometimes more than 24 hours to reverse the coagulopathy.

Fresh frozen plasma (FFP) provides the factors depleted by warfarin and is a fast way to reverse coagulopathy from warfarin. However, the use of FFP may result in delays in the process of compatibility testing and administration, and it may lead to fluid overload, allergic reactions, and transfusion-related complications. Furthermore, the reversal of anticoagulation from warfarin with FFP may be only transient. Recombinant factor VIIa (rFVIIa) is a procoagulant agent approved for bleeding complications in patients with hemophilia. It has been used in warfarin-related intracranial hemorrhage, and a study demonstrated reduction in hematoma expansion and rapid correction of the INR. A subsequent study showed no improvement in mortality or functional outcome. Recombinant FVIIa has been associated with increased incidence of thromboembolic events.

Ansell J, Hirsh J, Hylek E, et al. Pharmacology and management of the vitamin K antagonists. Chest. 2008; 133(6 Suppl):160S–198S.

Elijovich L, Patel PV, Hemphill JC. Intracerebral hemorrhage. Semin Neurol. 2008; 28:657–667.

Mayer SA, Brun NC, Broderick J, et al. Safety and feasibility of recombinant factor VIIa for acute intracerebral hemorrhage. Stroke. 2005; 36:74–79.

Mayer SA, Brun NC, Begtrup K, et al. Efficacy and safety of recombinant activated factor VII for acute intracerebral hemorrhage. N Engl J Med. 2008; 358:2127–2137.

34. b

Negative inspiratory force and vital capacity are the best methods of assessing the ventilation of patients with Guillain Barré syndrome (GBS) (discussed in Chapter 9).

Indications for intubation in GBS include the following:

– Clinical evidence of fatigue
– Severe oropharyngeal weakness
– Respiratory function: vital capacity less than 15 to 20 mL/kg, or less than 1 L, or a reduction of more than 30% of the baseline and/or negative inspiratory force less than 30 cm H_2O

Other parameters associated with the possible need for intubation include bulbar weakness or the presence of cranial nerve palsies, autonomic dysfunction, short period from onset to peak of symptoms, and the presence of abnormalities on chest x-ray, such as infiltrates or atelectasis.

Arterial partial pressure of oxygen (pO_2) and partial pressure of carbon dioxide (pCO_2) are not good predictors of need for early intubation, since abnormalities in these parameters occur when the patient is already decompensating. A subjective sensation of dyspnea and pulse oximetry are not adequate means of assessing ventilation.

Suarez JI. Critical Care Neurology and Neurosurgery, 1st ed. Totowa, NJ: Humana Press; 2004.

35. d

Critical illness polyneuropathy and myopathy is a neuromuscular disorder seen in patients admitted to the ICU. It is a cause of failure to wean patients from ventilatory support. There are multiple risk factors for this condition, such as sepsis, systemic inflammatory response syndrome, use of neuromuscular blocking agents, use of steroids, poor nutrition, abnormal glucose levels, and low albumin levels. The patient depicted in this question was critically ill, septic, and received sedatives, paralytics, and steroids, all of which are risk factors for critical illness polyneuropathy and myopathy.

The pathophysiology of the neuropathy is related to an inflammatory response and nerve microcirculatory dysfunction and hypoxia, leading to primary axonal degeneration and muscle tissue damage. NCS demonstrate normal latencies and conduction velocities, with reduced compound motor and SNAP. In the presence of critical illness myopathy, needle EMG will demonstrate myopathic motor unit potentials, creatine kinase levels may be elevated, and muscle biopsy demonstrates a myosin loss myopathy.

There is no evidence to support the other diagnoses provided in the options.

Suarez JI. Critical Care Neurology and Neurosurgery, 1st ed. Totowa, NJ: Humana Press; 2004.

36. e

Status epilepticus is a neurologic emergency. Classically, it has been defined as seizures lasting more than 30 minutes, or recurrent seizures without recovery in between. This definition is outdated and may not be useful in clinical practice, since patients presenting with ongoing seizures should be treated rapidly without waiting for a 30-minute time limit.

The goal of treatment is to stabilize the patient, abolish the seizures, and treat the underlying cause. Initial therapy should always begin with "ABC" (airway, breathing, circulation). Benzodiazepines are the first line of therapy to stop ongoing seizures, and lorazepam is the most commonly used, based on its rapid onset of action, and preferred to diazepam based on its relative longer half-life. It is usually given intravenously at a dose of 0.1 mg/kg. Following benzodiazepines, the second line of treatment is phenytoin and/or fosphenytoin, for which maximal effects peak at around 15 to 20 minutes. Fosphenytoin is preferred since it can be infused faster, with fewer infusion-related side effects and cardiovascular reactions. The usual loading dose is 20 mg/kg intravenously.

If the patient continues seizing, a second dose of phenytoin or fosphenytoin can be attempted, or a second antiepileptic agent can be administered, such as phenobarbital or valproic acid. At the time of this publication, levetiracetam had not been assessed in clinical trials yet for the treatment of status epilepticus; however, given its availability as an intravenous agent, it has become widely used.

Data from clinical trials suggest that if one drug fails, successful termination of status epilepticus becomes subsequently difficult. Therefore, many advocate endotracheal intubation (if it has not already been done) and the use of propofol or midazolam drips if a loading dose of phenytoin/fosphenytoin fails to abort the seizure. If after continuous infusion of propofol or midazolam the patient continues to seize, barbiturate coma is the next step, usually with pentobarbital, with titration of the dose to burst-suppression on the EEG.

Manno EM. New management strategies in the treatment of status epilepticus. Mayo Clin Proc. 2003; 78:508–518.

Suarez JI. Critical Care Neurology and Neurosurgery, 1st ed. Totowa, NJ: Humana Press; 2004.

37. a

From the options listed, bilateral absence of the N20 response on somatosensory-evoked potentials with median nerve stimulation is the best predictor of outcome after cardiac arrest.

A low percentage of patients survive after cardiac arrest, and of those who survive, a large number will have long-term cognitive and neurologic deficits. Prediction of outcome after cardiac arrest is important to guide treatment for these patients, as well as to provide useful information to the family.

In general, the circumstances surrounding the cardiac arrest and CPR do not have good predictive value and should not be used alone for this purpose. Physical examination findings are helpful, and there is good predictive value for poor outcome if there is no pupillary response at 24 to 72 hours from the cardiac arrest, or no corneal reflexes and eye movements at 72 hours after the cardiac arrest. Before these time frames, the predictive values of physical examination findings are not accurate.

Ancillary tests are useful in the prediction of outcome of patients after cardiac arrest. Brain edema on CT scan may occur, but its predictive value is poor for prognostication. EEG showing

responses and metabolic factors govern autoregulation by producing cerebral vasodilatation or vasoconstriction. The major metabolic factor is CO_2, and increases in pCO_2 cause vasodilatation resulting in increased ICP. Blood rheologic factors are also important for cerebral blood flow. Lower hematocrit and lower blood viscosity are associated with increased cerebral blood flow.

Suarez JI. Critical Care Neurology and Neurosurgery, 1st ed. Totowa, NJ: Humana Press; 2004.

42. d

Larger and wider bone flaps and duraplasty may be required for better clinical results as compared with smaller bone flaps.

In malignant cerebral edema, intracranial volume increases in the compartment of the infarcted tissue, and the ICP rises. Usual measures to reduce the ICP are usually not enough, and herniation syndromes may occur. Decompressive hemicraniectomy involves removal of a large bone flap and opening of the dura, permitting the swollen tissue to herniate outward, thereby decreasing the ICP. A successful intervention requires a large and wide bone flap and duraplasty; otherwise compression of the swollen brain will occur at the borders of cranial vault.

Several studies have shown the benefit of this intervention in terms of survival, with some controversy in terms of the functional outcome; however, better neurologic outcomes were seen in patients treated surgically.

The age of the patient, timing of the surgery, and the hemispheric dominance are factors to take into account when making the decision to intervene. Patients older than 60 years of age have lower survival rates and poorer functional outcomes than those younger than 60 after this procedure. The optimal timing of surgery is unknown, but earlier hemicraniectomy is associated with better outcomes. Most compressive hemicraniectomies are performed for nondominant hemispheric infarctions, and it is thought that functional outcome will be worse if performed for dominant hemispheres, since language will be disrupted. However, there is still some controversy regarding this issue. All these aspects should be discussed clearly with the family, making sure that they understand that this surgery is a life-saving measure, with the potential of survival with significant disability.

Bershad EM, Humphreis WE, Suarez JI. Intracranial hypertension. Semin Neurol. 2008; 28:690–702.

Subramaniam S, Hill MD. Decompressive hemicraniectomy for malignant middle cerebral artery infarction: An update. Neurologist. 2009; 15:178–184.

43. a

Status epilepticus is a neurological emergency and should be treated as such. The most frequent cause of status epilepticus is antiepileptic medication noncompliance in patients with known epilepsy. Central nervous system infections, strokes, and tumors can also cause seizures and status epilepticus. Febrile seizures are not seen in adults, though fever can lower the threshold in patients with epilepsy.

Manno EM. New management strategies in the treatment of status epilepticus. Mayo Clin Proc. 2003; 78:508–518.

Suarez JI. Critical Care Neurology and Neurosurgery, 1st ed. Totowa, NJ: Humana Press; 2004.

44. e

Four principles of medical ethics include beneficence (providing patients with care that will be of benefit to them), nonmaleficence (doing no harm or malice to the patient), justice (ensuring equitable and fair distribution of resources), and autonomy, or self-determination, with patients as the ultimate decision maker. In order for a patient to practice autonomy, all available feasible options should be provided to the patient. Because any intervention could have potential harms, practicing nonmaleficence in practicality often means weighing the potential harms against the risks.

ABIM Foundation, American Board of Internal Medicine, ACP-ASIM Foundation. American College of Physicians-American Society of Internal Medicine, European Federation of Internal Medicine. Medical professionalism in the new millennium: A physician charter. Ann Intern Med. 2002; 136(3):243–246.

Jonsen A, Siegler M, Winslade W. Clinical Ethics: A Practical Approach to Ethical Decisions in Clinical Medicine, 6th ed. New York, NY: McGraw-Hill; 2006.

45. e

This patient has malignant hyperthermia, which is an uncommon syndrome seen during general anesthesia. It is an autosomal dominant disorder, in which there is an excessive release of calcium from the sarcoplasmic reticulum in the skeletal muscle in response to halogenated inhaled anesthetics and depolarizing muscle relaxants (more commonly succinylcholine). A mutation in the ryanodine receptor gene has been found, and patients with central core disease (a myopathy resulting from a mutation in the ryanodine receptor gene) are at increased risk of malignant hyperthermia.

Malignant hyperthermia presents with an initial rise in the end-tidal partial pressure of carbon dioxide (PCO_2) during anesthesia, muscle rigidity, increased body temperature, altered consciousness, and autonomic instability. Rhabdomyolysis occurs, leading to myoglobinuric renal failure.

In patients developing malignant hyperthermia, the culprit anesthetics should be stopped and alternative anesthetics not associated with malignant hyperthermia should be used instead, ventilatory support and oxygenation should be optimized, intravenous fluids should be increased, and physical measures to reduce the temperature should be attempted. Dantrolene is a specific treatment that blocks release of calcium from the sarcoplasmic reticulum and should be administered early on.

This patient does not have a history of being on antipsychotics or serotonin reuptake inhibitors. These are related to neuroleptic malignant syndrome (NMS) and serotonin syndrome, respectively. NMS is similar to malignant hyperthermia and is characterized by increased body temperature, muscle rigidity, altered mental status, and autonomic instability. It is induced by antipsychotics, but other drugs that inhibit dopaminergic transmission may also be implicated. Management includes discontinuation of the antipsychotic and use of Dantrolene and bromocriptine. The latter plays no role in the management of malignant hyperthermia.

Serotonin syndrome starts abruptly and is characterized by mental status changes, hyperthermia, autonomic hyperactivity, hyperkinesis, hyperactive deep tendon reflexes, clonus, and muscle rigidity. The treatment is supportive, along with benzodiazepines and discontinuation of the causative drug.

Ropper AH, Samuels MA. Adams and Victor's Principles of Neurology. 9th ed. New York, NY: McGraw-Hill; 2009.

Suarez JI. Critical Care Neurology and Neurosurgery, 1st ed. Totowa, NJ: Humana Press; 2004.

Buzz Phrases	Key Points
Vasogenic edema	Extracellular edema. Blood-brain barrier damage (brain tumor)
Cytotoxic edema	Intracellular edema. Associated with cellular membrane damage (ischemia)
Plateau waves or Lundberg A waves	Increased intracranial pressure
Crescentic hematoma	Subdural hematoma. Rupture of the bridging veins
Biconvex hematoma	Epidural hematoma. Rupture of the middle meningeal artery
Angular acceleration and shear injury	Diffuse axonal injury
CSF with xanthochromia	SAH
Pinpoint pupils, apneustic breathing pattern	Pontine lesion
Ataxic breathing pattern	Medullary lesion
Decorticate posture	Lesion above the red nucleus
Decerebrate posture	Lesion between the red nucleus and the vestibular nucleus
Petechial hemorrhages in the brain	Fat embolism
State of pathologically reduced consciousness from which the patient can be aroused to purposeful response only with external stimulation	Stupor
"Deep sleep," cannot be aroused, may grimace or have stereotyped movements but does not localize to the stimulus	Coma
Awake and conscious, but quadriplegic, paralysis of lower cranial nerves and horizontal gaze. Preserved vertical gaze and blinking	Locked-in state
Previously comatose, but with return of the sleep-wake cycles. Lack cognitive function	Vegetative state
Alteration of consciousness with poor attention, and fluctuation	Delirium

Chapter 4

Headache

Questions

Questions 1–2

1. An overweight 36-year-old woman presents with three to four severe, debilitating headaches per month for the last 2 years. The headaches last 1 to 2 days. They are sometimes localized bifrontally, but more often localized to the right temple, right frontal region, and behind the right eye. There is often rhinorrhea and congestion associated with her headaches. She denies any prodrome or auras. The pain is usually a deep ache, but throbbing when severe. She sometimes gets some nausea, but no vomiting. She has to wear sunglasses and go to a quiet room because she "can't function." What is the most likely diagnosis?
   a. Cluster headache
   b. Intermittent sinus headache
   c. Episodic tension headache
   d. Idiopathic intracranial hypertension (IIH; pseudotumor cerebri)
   e. Episodic migraine

2. Which of the following is not included in the International Classification of Headache Disorders—II (ICHD-II) criteria for episodic migraine?
   a. Nausea/vomiting
   b. Photophobia/phonophobia
   c. Osmophobia
   d. Worsening with activity
   e. Pain severity/characterization

3. A 41-year-old man presents with what you suspect to be tension-type headache. Which one of the following symptoms is included in the International Classification of Headache Disorders—II (ICHD-II) criteria for this disorder?
   a. Photophobia
   b. Throbbing/pulsating pain
   c. Aggravation by routine physical activity

  d. Nausea

  e. Vomiting

4. Which of the following would be the earliest step in the proposed pathophysiology of migraine?

  a. Release of vasoactive neuropeptides from trigeminal sensory nerves

  b. Meningeal blood vessel dilation

  c. Activation of trigeminal sensory afferents in the meningeal vessels

  ✓ d. Cortical spreading depression

  e. Meningeal blood vessel constriction

Questions 5–6

5. A 34-year-old overweight woman presents with a severe migraine that began 2 days ago, but is now nearly gone. She has not identified any triggers since these headaches began 2 years ago, has tried to avoid stress, and has kept a headache diary prior to her visit with you today. She averages about five migraines per month, each lasting 1 to 2 days. What is the best choice of treatment at this time, assuming there are no contraindications?

  a. Prescribe sumatriptan and a NSAID to take immediately today to stop her resolving headache

  b. Prescribe a preventative agent

  c. Give her a dihydroergotamine (DHE) infusion today in the office

  d. Follow her over the next couple of months before prescribing anything

  ι e. Prescribe sumatriptan to use as needed, as well as a preventative agent

6. The patient depicted in question 5 returns 1 week later. She is currently in a prolonged, severe headache phase that began 4 days ago and has missed 2 days of work. She recently got a new job at a law firm, and these headaches are beginning to interfere with her job. Her last triptan dose was 1 day ago. As you examine her head, you find that her right temporal and right frontal regions are exquisitely sensitive to touch. What is the best choice of treatment at this time, assuming there are no contraindications?

  a. Increase her preventative medication dose and have her take another triptan

  b. Change her preventative agent because it does not appear to be working

  ι c. Give an IV dihydroergotamine (DHE) infusion

  d. Change her triptan therapy and have her to take one now

  e. Noncontrast brain CT to investigate the dysesthesia found on examination

7. A 22-year-old mildly overweight woman presents to the emergency department with increasing frequency of previously diagnosed migraines. Other medical history is unremarkable with exception of mild asthma and recurrent constipation. The attacks are occurring 4 days per week and are lasting the entire day. What would be the best preventive medication to start in this patient?

  a. Amitriptyline

  b. Propranolol

  c. Sumatriptan

  ι d. Topiramate (MA Ø↓ weight.

  e. Verapamil

8. During an office visit, a 46-year-old man with a long-standing history of recurrent headaches is diagnosed for the first time with migraine. He has a history of anxiety, hypertension, hyperlipidemia, tobacco abuse, and is noncompliant with medications. Family history is significant for his mother having migraine and his father dying from a "heart attack" in his mid-fifties. If this

patient presented to the emergency department at the very onset of a migraine, what would be the least optimal choice of treatment?

a. Sumatriptan — *Contraindicated in pt w/ known coronary artery dx*
b. Ketorolac
c. Valproic acid
d. Prochlorperazine
e. IV magnesium

9. A 39-year-old man presents to your office with the abrupt onset of severe holocephalic headache, nausea, and blurred vision about 4 hours ago. When asked, he admits that this is the worst headache he has ever had. He also reports some neck pain and says it feels stiff. He has a history of migraine, but says this headache is not like his normal migraine. What would be the next best course of action?
   a. Dihydroergotamine (DHE) infusion to try to break this headache early
   b. Intramuscular injection of ketorolac and consider prochlorperazine for nausea
   c. Arrange for an urgent lumbar puncture (LP)
   d. Obtain an urgent noncontrast brain CT
   e. Subcutaneous injection of sumatriptan

10. The triptan medications are effective in treatment of migraine because they work at which of the following subreceptors?
    a. Agonism at $5HT\text{-}2_B$, $5HT\text{-}2_D$
    b. Antagonism at $5HT\text{-}1_B$, $5HT\text{-}1_D$
    c. Agonism at $5HT\text{-}1_B$, $5HT\text{-}2_D$
    d. Antagonism at $5HT\text{-}2_B$, $5HT\text{-}2_D$
    e. Agonism at $5HT\text{-}1_B$, $5HT\text{-}1_D$

11. A 24-year-old woman with depression presents with a daily headache for the past 2 years. The headache began suddenly on November 14, 2008. She recalls it was on her birthday, but otherwise nothing out of the ordinary had happened. She reports being healthy, other than a mild sore throat the day before the onset of the headache, which is described as a daily, pressing, moderate, holocephalic pain. There is photophobia when the headache is exacerbated, but no visual or other neurologic symptoms. There is no postural component to the headache. She has had an MRI without and with contrast and an MRV, both normal. On the basis of the history, how would you classify this headache?
    a. Tension-type headache
    b. New daily persistent headache
    c. Migraine without aura
    d. Psychogenic headache disorder
    e. Aseptic meningitis

12. The autonomic features of lacrimation, rhinorrhea, and nasal congestion seen in the trigeminal autonomic cephalalgias are due to the activation of which nucleus?
    a. Parasympathetic outflow from the superior salivatory nucleus
    b. Sympathetic outflow from the superior salivatory nucleus
    c. Parasympathetic outflow from the nucleus solitarius
    d. Parasympathetic outflow from the trigeminal nucleus caudalis (TNC)
    e. Sympathetic outflow from the TNC

Questions 13–14

13. A 39-year-old woman presents with a 4-month history of headache. She reports it is only right sided, daily, and continuous since onset, with occasional lacrimation of the right eye. The pain is described as moderate, although exacerbations of severe pain occur. She also notes a sensation of grit in her right eye, and occasional paroxysmal and brief jabs and jolts on the right side of her head. She denies photophobia, phonophobia, nausea, vomiting, visual changes, or other neurologic features. How would you classify this headache?

  a. Cluster headache
  b. Paroxysmal hemicrania
  c. Hemicrania continua
  d. New daily persistent headache
  e. Migraine without aura

14. What would be your first treatment of choice in this patient, assuming there are no contraindications?

  a. Sumatriptan
  b. Amitriptyline
  c. Propranolol
  d. Indomethacin
  e. Topiramate

Questions 15–17

15. A 58-year-old man who does not typically get headaches presents to your office. He has a history of melanoma, which had been successfully treated. His headache has been worsening over the last month and has been constant. The pain is a deep ache around the left temporal and left frontal regions. He admits to mild intermittent low-grade fever and slight weight loss. He describes one episode in which he had some trouble seeing out of the left eye. He is worried because his mother had "some type of brain tumor." Which of the following is not considered a "red flag" in evaluation of this headache?

  a. Age
  b. Family history of brain tumor
  c. Fever
  d. Weight loss
  e. History of malignancy

16. On further questioning, he mentions that over the last 3 weeks he has been experiencing a cramp in his jaw while chewing and talking. On examination, you note that he is very sensitive to touch in the left temporal and scalp regions. What is the most likely diagnosis that should be first considered?

  a. Tension-type headache
  b. Brain tumor
  c. Episodic migraine
  d. Cluster headache
  e. Temporal arteritis

17. What would be the next step in step in management?

  a. β-blocker
  b. Prednisone
  c. Triptan

d. Temporal artery biopsy

e. Tricyclic antidepressant

18. A patient with a history of paroxysmal hemicrania (PH) has been reading about cluster headache on the internet and asks if that is what he has. You begin educating him on cluster headache. According to the International Classification of Headache Disorders—II (ICHD-II) criteria, the duration of a cluster headache is:

    a. 4 to 72 hours

    b. 1 to 60 minutes

    c. 1 to 60 seconds

    d. 15 to 180 minutes

    e. 1 to 12 hours

Questions 19–20

19. A 42-year-old woman presents with episodic headaches. Her headaches are described as severe attacks of unilateral periorbital pain lasting 10 minutes and associated with ipsilateral ptosis, lacrimation, conjunctival injection, and nasal congestion. She has more than five attacks daily for the majority of the time, and they usually occur during waking hours. There are no symptoms suggestive of an aura. What would be the best medication to try first?

    a. High-flow oxygen during an attack

    b. Sumatriptan

    c. Verapamil

    d. Indomethacin

    e. Lithium

20. On the basis of the above history, how would you classify this headache?

    a. Short-lasting unilateral neuralgiform headache with conjunctival injection and tearing (SUNCT)

    b. Migraine without aura

    c. Paroxysmal hemicrania (PH)

    d. Cluster headache

    e. Hemicrania continua

21. Which of the following headache types is not currently considered a trigeminal autonomic cephalalgia by the International Classification of Headache Disorders—II (ICHD-II) criteria?

    a. Paroxysmal hemicrania (PH)

    b. Trigeminal neuralgia

    c. Cluster headache

    d. Short-lasting unilateral neuralgiform headache with conjunctival injection and tearing (SUNCT)

    e. Probable trigeminal autonomic cephalalgia

Questions 22–26

22. A 62-year-old man presents with episodes of left-sided facial pain. The episodes are brief and shock-like, lasting anywhere from several seconds up to a minute. They are located in the left cheek and are triggered by brushing his teeth and touching the area. What do you suspect on the basis of this history?

    a. Short-lasting unilateral neuralgiform headache with conjunctival injection and tearing (SUNCT)

    b. Paroxysmal hemicrania (PH)
    c. Cluster headache
    d. Trigeminal neuralgia
    e. Hemicrania continua

23. What would be the first-line treatment for this patient?
    a. Lamotrigine
    b. Carbamazepine
    c. Lithium
    d. Topiramate
    e. Gabapentin

24. On the basis of your choice of treatment, which of the following adverse effects should be monitored for closely, especially when starting the medication?
    a. Diabetes insipidus
    b. Hypernatremia
    c. Hyperkalemia
    d. Hyponatremia
    e. Metabolic acidosis

25. Which of the following medications could lead to an increased possibility of the adverse effect you are concerned about with your choice of treatment selected above?
    a. Furosemide
    b. Propranolol
    c. Levetiracetam
    d. Warfarin
    e. Potassium supplementation

26. If this same presentation occurred in a 22-year-old woman with type I diabetes mellitus, what would be the most likely etiology that should be evaluated for?
    a. Aneurysm
    b. Arterial compression
    c. Multiple sclerosis
    d. Sarcoidosis
    e. Neoplasm

27. A 42-year-old man complains of facial pain. He estimates about 100 attacks daily of severe, stabbing, periorbital pain, lasting about 20 seconds per attack. There is also prominent conjunctival injection and lacrimation associated with these attacks. What do you tell him you suspect as his diagnosis?
    a. Cluster headache
    b. Short-lasting unilateral neuralgiform headache with conjunctival injection and tearing (SUNCT)
    c. Trigeminal neuralgia
    d. Paroxysmal hemicrania (PH)
    e. Hemicrania continua

28. A 29-year-old woman with a history of depression presents with frequent headaches fitting the description of chronic tension-type. The location of her pain is occipital, slightly greater than frontal, and she has tenderness throughout the neck and shoulder musculature. There are no visual or neurologic symptoms or findings on examination. There are no exacerbating factors, such as postural changes or cough. She had an MRI of the brain 6 months ago, which reported a 4 mm Chiari I malformation. She is asking you if her symptoms are all from her Chiari I malformation and what should be done for it. What is the most appropriate next step in your evaluation and treatment plan?

a. Lumbar spine MRI to evaluate for spina bifida or other spinal malformations

b. Referral to neurosurgery to evaluate the possible role of suboccipital craniectomy and decompression

c. Repeat brain MRI to see if there has been progression of the Chiari malformation

, d. Send her for physical therapy for the neck and shoulders and begin a preventative agent

e. Lumbar puncture (LP) for opening pressure and routine analysis

Questions 29–32

29. A 52-year-old man fell 5 ft from a ladder and landed on his back. His history is significant for recurrent pneumonia, and atrial fibrillation for which he takes warfarin. Later in the day, he began experiencing a bothersome headache located bifrontally. Other symptoms included stiff neck, nausea, photophobia, tinnitus, worsening on standing, and improvement on lying down. He has recently been healthy other than a worsening upper respiratory infection. Which of the following would be the most common diagnostic finding of your suspected diagnosis?

a. Lumbar puncture (LP) revealing significant leukocytosis

b. Brain CT showing cisternal blood

, c. Brain MRI with gadolinium showing pachymeningeal enhancement

d. Neck CT angiogram showing an intramural hematoma in a carotid artery

e. Brain CT showing bifrontal crescentic hematomas

30. He is evaluated further with MRI of the brain. Using the MRI shown in Figures 4.1 and 4.2, what is the most likely diagnosis?

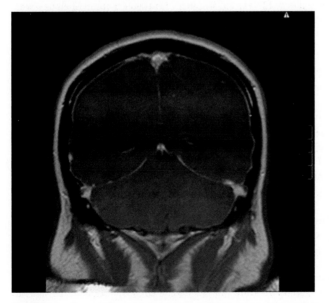

FIGURE 4.1 Coronal T1-weighted postcontrast MRI (Courtesy of Dr. Krishe Menezes)

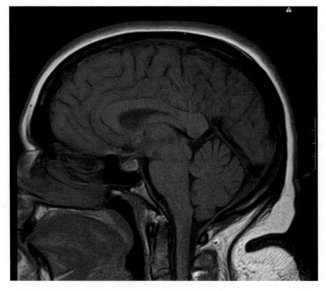

FIGURE 4.2 Sagittal T1-weighted precontrast MRI (Courtesy of Dr. Krishe Menezes)

    a. Early meningitis
    b. SAH
    c. Subdural hematoma
    d. Carotid dissection
    e. Low CSF pressure headache

31. Where is the most common location for the pathology leading to this type of headache?
    a. Subdural space
    b. Cervical spine
    c. Thoracic spine
    d. Distal ICA
    e. Intracranial circulation, especially at an aneurysmal location

32. What is the most appropriate treatment of this patient?
    a. Aneurysmal coiling if an endovascular approach is possible
    b. Bed rest, hydration, caffeine, and epidural blood patch if conservative measures fail
    c. Antibiotics and sending CSF for infectious etiologies
    d. Neurosurgical evaluation and close monitoring for possible hematoma decompression
    e. Anticoagulation

33. Which of the following treatments would be the least useful to use as an abortive agent in cluster headache?
    a. Sumatriptan subcutaneous injection
    b. Dihydroergotamine (DHE) subcutaneous injection
    c. Zolmitriptan nasal spray
    d. Frovatriptan tablets
    e. Intranasal lidocaine

34. Which of the following treatments would be the least useful for cluster headache prevention during a cluster period?
    a. Verapamil
    b. Propranolol
    c. Valproic acid
    d. Lithium
    e. Melatonin

Questions 35–40

35. A 26-year-old obese woman with borderline hypertension presents with worsening headache, which she describes as a bifrontal and bioccipital band-like pressure and pain. Occasionally, she experiences brief visual loss or graying, especially with straining, which lasts only seconds, but no photophobia or phonophobia. She sometimes gets nauseated and vomits when the pain is severe and she feels her vision is becoming increasingly blurred. What do you suspect may be the diagnosis?
    a. Migraine
    b. Tension-type headache
    c. New daily persistent headache
    d. Idiopathic intracranial hypertension (IIH)
    e. Posterior fossa mass

36. Her fundoscopic examination of the left eye is shown in Figure 4.3. These findings are most consistent with which of the following?

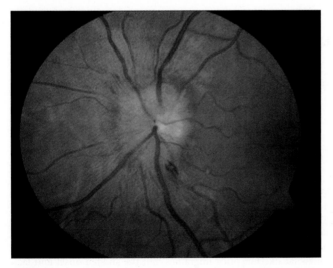

FIGURE 4.3 Fundoscopy of left eye (Courtesy of Anne Pinter). Shown also in color plates

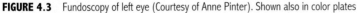

    a. Acute optic neuritis
    b. Normal examination
    c. Posterior ischemic optic neuropathy
    d. Papilledema
    e. Anterior ischemic optic neuropathy

37. Topiramate is one treatment frequently used for this condition. What is the specific mechanism of action that makes <u>topiramate</u> useful as a treatment in this condition?
    a. Sodium channel inhibition
    b. NMDA antagonist
    c. GABA_A agonist
    d. Kainate/AMPA antagonist
    e. Carbonic anhydrase inhibitor

 # the other is acetazolamide

38. Which of the following is not a proposed mechanism in the pathogenesis of this condition?
    a. Aqueduct stenosis
    b. Decreased CSF absorption
    c. Increased venous pressure
    d. Increased CSF formation
    e. Congenital stenosis of venous sinuses

39. Which of the following is not a treatment option for this condition?
    a. Weight loss
    b. Lumboperitoneal shunt
    c. Ventriculoperitoneal shunt
    d. Optic nerve fenestration
    e. Hydrochlorothiazide

40. Which of the following would you not expect to find on physical examination in this condition?
    a. Papilledema
    b. Facial nerve palsy
    c. Abducens nerve palsy
    d. Visual loss (enlarging blind spot)
    e. Elevated opening pressure

41. An overweight 41-year-old woman with hypertension, recurrent kidney stones, and increasing migraine frequency wishes to begin a preventive medication. Which of the following would be a poor choice to use?
    a. Propranolol
    b. Topiramate
    c. Verapamil
    d. Neurontin
    e. Magnesium

Questions 42–45

42. A 47-year-old perimenopausal woman with a history of episodic migraine and prior idiopathic deep venous thrombosis in the right leg presents with a sudden-onset predominantly left-sided headache. She says it feels somewhat like her prior migraines, but the sudden onset and lack of photophobia and phonophobia are atypical for her. You notice on examination that venous pulsations are absent. What is this finding concerning for?
    a. Diminished flow to the anterior circulation
    b. Increased intracranial pressure
    c. Diminished flow to the posterior circulation
    d. Carotid cavernous fistula
    e. Vasospasm

43. What is your suspected diagnosis on the basis of this information?
 a. Episodic migraine with atypical features related to hormonal changes
 b. SAH
 c. Cerebral sinus venous thrombosis
 d. Carotid dissection
 e. Vertebral dissection

44. What test do you order next on the basis of your clinical suspicion?
 a. Four-vessel angiogram
 b. Brain and neck CT angiogram
 c. Hypercoagulable profile
 d. Brain MRV and MRI
 e. Noncontrast brain CT

45. After your evaluation confirms the diagnosis, what is the standard therapy that should be started?
 a. Aneurysmal coiling if endovascular approach is possible
 b. Sumatriptan injection
 c. Heparin
 d. Decrease blood pressure with close monitoring of mean arterial pressure
 e. Stenting the vessel

Questions 46–50

46. A 30-year-old man with a history of frequent migraine with aura has had several unclear TIAs. Family history reveals that his father also had migraine with aura and later developed an unknown neurologic disease. When questioned further, the patient says his father developed dementia in his fifties, had multiple strokes and TIAs, and lost the ability to walk, requiring a wheelchair shortly before his death at age 61. What diagnosis do you suspect?
 a. Mitochondrial encephalopathy with lactic acidosis and stroke-like episodes (MELAS)
 b. Recurrent migrainous cerebral infarction
 c. Cerebral autosomal dominant arteriopathy with subcortical infarcts and leukoencephalopathy (CADASIL)
 d. Primary CNS angiitis
 e. Moyamoya disease

47. What chromosome is affected in this disorder?
 a. 21
 b. 3
 c. 17
 d. 19
 e. 11

48. What is the mode of genetic transmission for this disorder?
 a. Autosomal recessive
 b. X-linked dominant
 c. Sporadic
 d. Autosomal dominant
 e. X-linked recessive

49. What would you expect to see on an MRI of the brain of a patient affected with this disorder?
  a. Benign nonspecific white matter changes
  b. Extensive intracranial stenosis with "puff of smoke" appearance
  c. Extensive confluent deep white matter changes extending to the anterior temporal lobes
  d. Alternating beading of intracranial vessels due to "skip" areas of stenosis
  e. Ischemic areas throughout the basal ganglia

50. What gene is affected in this disorder?
  a. *NOTCH1* gene
  b. Transfer RNA gene at mt3243
  c. P/Q-type calcium channel receptor gene
  d. *NOTCH3* gene
  e. *CACNA1A* gene

51. A 26-year-old woman has a history of migraine with aura that is often associated with hemiplegia lasting up to a day. Her mother has similar episodes with her migraine. Abnormalities in which of the following channels or channel subunits have not been associated with this disorder?
  a. P/Q calcium channel subunit
  b. Chloride channel subunit
  c. A1A2 sodium–potassium ATPase channel
  d. Presynaptic voltage-gated sodium channel
  e. Postsynaptic voltage-gated sodium channel

52. A 43-year-old man comes to your clinic. He has had a 6-month persistent headache that is pounding and worse with bending down. He has had occasional episodes of confusion, but otherwise, is neurologically intact. An MRI of the brain shows diffuse leptomeningeal enhancement. CSF and blood testing have been negative for fungi, tuberculosis (TB), HIV, lupus, Lyme disease, and tumor cells. C- and P-ANCA (anti-neutrophil cytoplasmic antibodies) tests are negative. His CSF shows a mild lymphocytic pleocytosis. A leptomeningeal biopsy shows some perivascular inflammation, but no granulomas. You suspect that he has:
  a. Wegener's granulomatosis
  b. Malignant angioendotheliomatosis
  c. A remote effect of cancer
  d. Idiopathic cranial pachymeningitis
  e. Chemical meningitis

Answer key

1. e	10. e	19. d	28. d	37. e	46. c
2. c	11. b	20. c	29. c	38. a	47. d
3. a	12. a	21. b	30. e	39. e	48. d
4. d	13. c	22. d	31. c	40. b	49. c
5. e	14. d	23. b	32. b	41. b	50. d
6. c	15. b	24. d	33. d	42. b	51. b
7. d	16. e	25. a	34. b	43. c	52. d
8. a	17. b	26. c	35. d	44. d	
9. d	18. d	27. b	36. d	45. c	

Answers

1. e, 2. c

This patient fits the International Classification of Headache Disorders—II (ICHD-II) criteria for episodic migraine. She does not have aura, so this is episodic migraine without aura. Only 15% to 20% of patients with migraine have aura (classic migraine) as opposed to 80% to 85% who have migraine without aura (common migraine). Rhinorrhea and nasal congestion frequently coexist with migraine due to trigeminal cross-activation of the parasympathetics via stimulation of the superior salivatory nucleus of the facial nerve. Migraine is frequently misdiagnosed as sinus headache because of these "sinus-like" signs and symptoms. Primary headache disorders are not associated with an underlying pathologic process and include migraine, tension, cluster, and other trigeminal autonomic cephalalgias. Baseline neurologic examination is normal, and diagnostic workup is negative with primary headaches. Osmophobia is not included in the ICHD-II criteria for episodic migraine. The ICHD-II criteria for episodic migraine without aura include at least five headaches, each lasting 4 to 72 hours. The headache must have two of the four following criteria: unilateral location, pulsating quality, moderate-to-severe pain intensity, and worsening with physical activity. The headache must also be associated with one of the two following features: nausea and/or vomiting, *or* photophobia and phonophobia. Lastly, the symptoms cannot be attributable to another disorder.

Headache Classification Subcommittee of the International Headache Society. The international classification of headache disorders: 2nd edition. Cephalalgia. 2004; 24(Suppl. 1):9–160.

3. a

The International Classification of Headache Disorders—II (ICHD-II) criteria for episodic tension-type headache include at least 10 attacks of headache lasting 30 minutes to 7 days. The headache must have two of the four following features: bilateral location, pressing/tightening (nonpulsating), mild-to-moderate pain intensity, and not worsened by routine physical activity. It must also have both of the following: no nausea/vomiting (anorexia may occur); no more than one of photophobia or phonophobia (either or neither, not both). Symptoms are not attributable to another disorder. Photophobia is the only option that is included in the criteria for tension-type headache in this patient. All others listed are criteria for migraine.

Headache Classification Subcommittee of the International Headache Society. The international classification of headache disorders: 2nd edition. Cephalalgia. 2004; 24(Suppl. 1):9–160.

4. d

Of the choices listed, cortical spreading depression is felt to occur first. However, it is uncertain whether the trigger for cortical spreading depression occurs in the brain stem or within the cortex.

The pathophysiology of migraine is as follows:

1. Activation of hypersensitive "central generator" (it is debated whether the initiating trigger for migraine occurs in the cortex or in the brain stem) →
2. Disrupted ion homeostasis, release of neurochemicals, and transient dysfunction of neuronal function →
3. Meningeal blood vessel dilation and activation of trigeminovascular system →
4. Release of vasoactive neuropeptides (calcitonin gene-related peptide (CGRP), neurokinins, prostaglandins, substance P, etc.) from activated trigeminal sensory nerves leads to sterile neurogenic inflammation →
5. Worsening vasodilation, increasing firing of trigeminal afferents causing pain intensification →

6. Trigeminal nociceptive afferents carry pain signals to trigeminal nucleus caudalis (TNC) for processing and ascent through thalamus to cortex →

7. Continuous ascending pain signals activate more neurons leading to associated symptoms such as photo/phonophobia, nausea, and vomiting →

8. Continuous TNC firing, leads to central sensitization if activated pathways are not stopped

Silberstein SD, Lipton RB, Dodick D, et al. Wolff's Headache and Other Head Pain, 8th ed. New York: Oxford University Press; 2008.

5. e, 6. c

In the scenario depicted in question 5, this patient should have a triptan prescribed for abortive treatment at the earliest symptom identified for best effect. The abortive treatment should be combined with an NSAID for early treatment aimed at decreasing neurogenic sterile inflammation. If she still had a severe headache, dihydroergotamine (DHE) infusion would be an option, but unnecessary at this time because her headache is nearly resolved. It is crucial to treat migraine at the earliest symptoms identified. Optimal abortive treatment in the absence of vascular contraindications begins with a triptan. Concurrent administration of NSAIDs with the triptan decreases the neurogenic inflammation, the cause of worsening migraine symptoms. The purpose of the triptan is to reverse meningeal vasodilation, prevent release of vasogenic neuropeptides from the trigeminovascular system, and interfere with return of pain signals to the brain stem. The longer a patient waits to treat migraine, the less effective the acute treatments in reversing the entire complex of symptoms.

In addition, her headaches are severe, debilitating, occurring up to 10 days per month, and interfering with her job, so she should also be prescribed a preventative agent. Preventive therapy, if not previously started, should be initiated in migraine if the attacks are debilitating, severe (including presence of uncommon migraine findings, such as hemiplegic migraine, basilar migraine, and migrainous infarction), interfering with daily activities/jobs, and if there are greater than four migraines or ten headache-days per month. Preventive medication should be picked on the basis of comorbidities. In her case, she is overweight, so topiramate would be a reasonable choice because weight loss can be a side effect. Other examples would be a tricyclic antidepressant in depressed patients, β-blockers, or calcium-channel blockers in hypertensive patients.

In question 6, the patient now has had a migraine for more than 72 hours, so she is considered to be in status migrainosus and needs more aggressive therapy. The paresthesias represent cutaneous allodynia as a result of central sensitization related to the prolonged headache phase. IV DHE infusion would be reasonable and safe at this point because she has not had a triptan within the last 24 hours. Other IV medications commonly infused with DHE for additional benefit include antiemetics, magnesium, ketorolac, valproate sodium, and steroids. DHE, steroids, promethazine, and ketorolac can all be administered intramuscularly in the absence of infusion capability. Inhaled DHE is also available.

Raskin NH. Modern pharmacotherapy of migraine. Neurol Clin. 1990; 8:857–865.

Saper JR, Silberstein S. Pharmacology of dihydroergotamine and evidence for efficacy and safety in migraine. Headache. 2006; 46(Suppl. 4):S171–181.

Silberstein SD, Lipton RB, Dodick D, et al. Wolff's Headache and Other Head Pain, 8th ed. New York: Oxford University Press; 2008.

7. d

Topiramate would be the best option and is the least contraindicated in this patient. The possible weight loss and appetite suppression side effect of topiramate would be beneficial for her. Other side effects to instruct the patient to be aware of when using topiramate include paresthesias in the digits, cognitive slowing, word-finding difficulty, kidney stone formation, and rarely, acute angle-closure glaucoma. The side effects of the remaining medications make them less desirable. Amitriptyline could cause weight gain in an already overweight patient. Propranolol and other β-blockers are contraindicated in patients with asthma, and can also cause weight gain and reduced exercise tolerance. Verapamil could worsen her constipation. Sumatriptan is used as an acute treatment of migraine, not as a preventive therapy.

Silberstein SD, Lipton RB, Dodick D, et al. Wolff's Headache and Other Head Pain, 8th ed. New York: Oxford University Press; 2008.

8. a

Sumatriptan is contraindicated in patients with known coronary heart disease and should only be used after a cardiac workup if a patient has multiple cardiac risk factors. This patient has several cardiovascular risk factors, such as uncontrolled hypertension, hyperlipidemia, tobacco abuse, gender, age, and a family history of early heart disease. This patient would require a full cardiac evaluation (including a stress test), prior to any use of triptans, and they would still be used only cautiously with the first dose administered in the office if his risk factors were controlled and cardiac evaluation showed no evidence of cardiac ischemia. Combinations of various antiemetics, anti-inflammatories, anticonvulsants, and magnesium are all commonly used as acute treatments of migraine, especially when the preferred treatment with triptans is not an option. A new class of migraine medication called calcitonin gene-related peptide (CGRP) inhibitors is proposed to be safe for the acute treatment of migraine in those with cardiac risk factors, in which triptans would otherwise be contraindicated.

Silberstein SD, Lipton RB, Dodick D, et al. Wolff's Headache and Other Head Pain, 8th ed. New York: Oxford University Press; 2008.

Tepper SJ. Safety and rational use of the triptans. Med Clin North Am. 2001; 85:959–970.

9. d

This man gives the history of an abrupt-onset thunderclap headache. Patients usually admit that it is the "worst headache of their life." The current headache does not reflect his normal migraine pattern or quality and warrants further investigation. A noncontrast brain CT scan is necessary to evaluate for SAH. If brain CT scan is negative but suspicion remains high, a lumbar puncture (LP) should be performed. CT sensitivity for detecting SAH is highest in the first 12 hours after SAH (nearly 100%), is about 92% sensitive for SAH within 24 hours, and it falls to around 58% by the end of day 5 postbleed. LP is best performed at least 6 hours after symptom onset and becomes very low yield at 3 weeks. If LP is obtained, an opening pressure should be measured, and the CSF should be sent for cell counts in tubes 1 and 4, protein, glucose, xanthochromia, and gram stain.

Latchaw RE, Silva P, Falcone SF. The role of CT following aneurysmal rupture. Neuroimaging Clin N Am. 1997; 7:693–708.

Sames TA, Storrow AB, Finkelstein JA, et al. Sensitivity of new-generation computed tomography in subarachnoid hemorrhage. Acad Emerg Med. 1996; 3:16–20.

Sidman R, Connolly E, Lemke T. Subarachnoid hemorrhage diagnosis: lumbar puncture is still needed when the computed tomography scan is normal. Acad Emerg Med. 1996; 3:827–831.

Silberstein SD, Lipton RB, Dodick D, et al. Wolff's Headache and Other Head Pain, 8th ed. New York: Oxford University Press; 2008.

10. e

The triptans work as agonists at the serotonin receptor subtypes 5HT-1_B and 5HT-1_D. Agonism at 5-HT$_{1B}$ receptors constricts the pain-producing intracranial, extracerebral blood vessels in the meninges. Agonism at 5-HT_{1D} receptors presynaptically inhibits trigeminal peptide release and interferes with central trigeminal nucleus caudalis (TNC) nociceptive transduction and processing, whereas those of the nucleus tractus solitarius in the brain stem are thought to inhibit nausea/vomiting. Ultimately, these effects result in reversal of vasodilation, decrease in neurogenic inflammation, reduction of central nociceptive signal transmission to the thalamus and cortex, and cessation of other ascending pathways to the cortex, which result in associated migrainous symptoms, such as photophobia and phonophobia.

Tepper SJ. Safety and rational use of the triptans. Med Clin North Am. 2001; 85:959–970.

Tepper SJ, Millson D. Safety profile of the triptans. Expert Opin Drug Saf. 2003; 2:123–132.

11. b

This headache fits the criteria for new daily persistent headache (NDPH). This primary headache typically begins abruptly, and patients often recall the exact date it started. Examination and evaluations are normal. It does not fit criteria for the other headache types listed. A psychogenic etiology is a diagnosis of exclusion, and aseptic meningitis would not be this prolonged. Other considerations for abrupt onset of daily headache include a CSF leak, excluded by a lack of pain with postural changes and absence of pachymeningeal enhancement on MRI; and venous sinus thrombosis, excluded by the normal MRV.

The International Classification of Headache Disorders—II (ICHD-II) criteria for NDPH include a headache that, within 3 days of onset, is present daily, and is unremitting, for more than 3 months. It must have at least two of the four following criteria: bilateral location, pressing/tightening (nonpulsating) quality, mild-to-moderate pain intensity, and not worsened by routine physical activity, such as walking or climbing. In addition, it must also have both of the following: no more than one of photophobia, phonophobia, or mild nausea; neither moderate or severe nausea nor vomiting. Lastly, symptoms are not attributable to another disorder.

Headache Classification Subcommittee of the International Headache Society. The international classification of headache disorders: 2nd edition. Cephalalgia. 2004; 24(Suppl. 1):9–160.

12. a

Parasympathetic outflow from the superior salivatory nucleus of cranial nerve VII leads to activation of lacrimal and nasal mucosal glands. Parasympathetic fibers travel with the greater superficial petrosal nerve of cranial nerve VII to the sphenopalatine ganglion, synapse, and then travel with the maxillary division of cranial nerve V to the lacrimal glands. Parasympathetic fibers also travel in the lesser superficial petrosal nerve of cranial nerve VII to the otic ganglia. There is a brainstem connection between the trigeminal nucleus caudalis and the superior salivatory nucleus causing the trigeminal-autonomic reflex. This reflex is activated by a noxious stimulus applied to the trigeminal distribution. For example, getting hit in the face with a ball will cause lacrimation and rhinorrhea.

Silberstein SD, Lipton RB, Dodick D, et al. Wolff's Headache and Other Head Pain, 8th ed. New York: Oxford University Press; 2008.

Tubbs RS, Menendez J, Loukas M, et al. The petrosal nerves: anatomy, pathology, and surgical considerations. Clin Anat. 2009; 22:537–544.

13. c, 14. d

This patient's history is consistent with hemicrania continua. This primary headache is more common in women and is one of several "indomethacin-responsive" headaches, with others being paroxysmal hemicrania (PH), primary cough headaches, primary stabbing headaches, and for some patients, primary headaches associated with sexual activity. Therefore, indomethacin should be the first medication tried. In order to rule out incomplete response, indomethacin should be used in a dose of ≥150 mg daily orally for at least a week, but for maintenance, smaller doses are often sufficient. It is reasonable to obtain an MRI and MRA of the brain with and without gadolinium with thin cuts through the cerebellopontine angle and Meckel's cave in patients presenting with suspected involvement of the trigeminal nerve, as in hemicrania continua, trigeminal neuralgia, or any of the trigeminal autonomic cephalalgias.

The International Classification of Headache Disorders—II (ICHD-II) criteria for hemicrania continua consist of a headache for more than 3 months. It must have all of the following criteria: unilateral pain without side shift, daily and continuous without pain-free periods, and moderate intensity, but with exacerbations of severe pain. It must have at least one of the following autonomic features during exacerbations and ipsilateral to the side of pain: conjunctival injection and/or lacrimation, nasal congestion and/or rhinorrhea, and ptosis and/or miosis. A complete response to therapeutic doses of indomethacin should be seen, and the headache is not attributable to another disorder.

Cluster headache and paroxysmal hemicrania (PH) are discussed in further questions. Migraine was discussed in questions 1 and 2, and new daily persistent headache (NDPH) in question 11.

Headache Classification Subcommittee of the International Headache Society. The international classification of headache disorders: 2nd edition. Cephalalgia. 2004; 24(Suppl. 1):9–160.

Silberstein SD, Lipton RB, Dodick D, et al. Wolff's Headache and Other Head Pain, 8th ed. New York: Oxford University Press; 2008.

15. b, 16. e, 17. b

Headache red flags include systemic symptoms (fever, chills, and weight loss), history of prior cancer or immunodeficiency, focal neurologic signs or symptoms, new headache with onset to peak of seconds to minutes (thunderclap), "first or worst headache," new-onset headache after age 50, precipitation by exertion, strain, or positional changes, increasing headache frequency and severity, and new-onset seizures. Secondary headache disorders have many possible etiologies and are related to an underlying pathologic process. They are associated with an abnormal neurologic examination and/or abnormal diagnostic workup. A family history of brain tumor is not considered a typical "red flag." A common mnemonic used for headache red flags is SNOOP:

Systemic symptoms (fever, chills, and weight loss) or secondary headache risk factors (HIV and cancer)
Neurologic symptoms or signs (confusion, impaired consciousness, and focal findings)
Older: new-onset or progressive headache, especially >50 years old (temporal arteritis)
Onset: sudden, abrupt (thunderclap)
Progression of headache (change in frequency, severity, or clinical features)

Temporal arteritis (giant-cell arteritis) often presents in persons older than 50 years of age. It is associated with jaw claudication and headache usually localized to the temple region, although it may be nonlocalized. Constitutional symptoms are often present, such as fever and weight loss. The patient may also complain of visual disturbances, including visual loss. Patients with suspected temporal arteritis should have an ESR checked. ESR is usually greater than 50 to 60 mm/h in temporal arteritis. Diagnosis is confirmed by temporal artery biopsy. On suspicion of this diagnosis, prednisone 60 to 80 mg daily should be started to prevent permanent visual loss, even before biopsy confirmation. It is also worth noting that this patient has a previous history of melanoma, which can recur and commonly metastasize to the brain. For that reason, MRI with and without contrast should be obtained (melanoma metastases are notoriously vascular). See discussion to question 18 for cluster headache, question 3 for tension-type headache, and questions 1 and 2 for migraine.

Dodick DW. Clinical clues and clinical rules: primary vs secondary headache. Adv Stud Med. 2003; 3(6 C):S550–S555.

Silberstein SD, Lipton RB, Dodick D, et al. Wolff's Headache and Other Head Pain, 8th ed. New York: Oxford University Press; 2008.

Silberstein SD, Stiles MA, Young WB. Atlas of Migraine and Other Headaches, 2nd ed. London and New York: Taylor and Francis Group; 2005.

18. d

The duration of a cluster headache is 15 to 180 minutes. The International Classification of Headache Disorders—II (ICHD-II) criteria for cluster headache require at least five attacks fulfilling the following: severe or very severe unilateral orbital, supraorbital, and/or temporal pain lasting 15 to 180 minutes if untreated. The headache must be associated with at least one of the following: ipsilateral conjunctival injection and/or lacrimation, ipsilateral nasal congestion and/or rhinorrhea, ipsilateral eyelid edema, ipsilateral forehead and facial sweating, ipsilateral miosis and/or ptosis, a sense of restlessness, or agitation. Attacks occur at a frequency of 1 every other day to 8 per day, and symptoms are not attributable to another disorder.

Headache Classification Subcommittee of the International Headache Society. The international classification of headache disorders: 2nd edition. Cephalalgia. 2004; 24(Suppl. 1):9–160.

19. d, 20. c

This is paroxysmal hemicrania (PH), one of the "indomethacin-responsive" headaches (see question 13). Therefore, indomethacin should be the first medication tried. In order to rule out incomplete response, indomethacin should be used in a dose of ≥150 mg daily orally for at least a week, but for maintenance, smaller doses are often sufficient. As with hemicrania continua, PH is more common in women. Of note, PH often gets confused with cluster headache. Differentiating features of PH include shorter-lasting and more frequent attacks, as well as a complete response to indomethacin.

The International Classification of Headache Disorders—II (ICHD-II) criteria for PH require at least 20 attacks of severe unilateral orbital, supraorbital, or temporal pain lasting 2 to 30 minutes. The headache is accompanied by at least one of the following: ipsilateral conjunctival injection and/or lacrimation, ipsilateral nasal congestion and/or rhinorrhea, ipsilateral eyelid edema, ipsilateral forehead and facial sweating, ipsilateral miosis and/or ptosis. The attacks have a frequency of more than 5 per day for more than half of the time, although periods with lower frequency may occur. The attacks are prevented completely by therapeutic doses of indomethacin, and the headache is not attributable to another disorder. See discussion to question 27 for short-lasting unilateral neuralgiform headache with conjunctival injection and tearing (SUNCT), question 1 for migraine, question 18 for cluster headache, and question 13 for hemicrania continua.

Headache Classification Subcommittee of the International Headache Society. The international classification of headache disorders: 2nd edition. Cephalalgia. 2004; 24(Suppl. 1):9–160.

Silberstein SD, Lipton RB, Dodick D, et al. Wolff's Headache and Other Head Pain, 8th ed. New York: Oxford University Press; 2008.

21. b

Trigeminal neuralgia is not associated with autonomic features and is therefore not classified as a trigeminal autonomic cephalalgia. It is currently classified in the International Classification of Headache Disorders—II (ICHD-II) criteria as one of the "cranial neuralgias, facial pain and other headaches." The headaches that are classified as one of the "cluster headache and other trigeminal autonomic cephalalgias" include cluster headache, paroxysmal hemicrania (PH), short-lasting unilateral neuralgiform headache with conjunctival injection and tearing (SUNCT), and probable trigeminal autonomic cephalalgia.

Headache Classification Subcommittee of the International Headache Society. The international classification of headache disorders: 2nd edition. Cephalalgia. 2004; 24(Suppl. 1):9–160.

Silberstein SD, Lipton RB, Dodick D, et al. Wolff's Headache and Other Head Pain, 8th ed. New York: Oxford University Press; 2008.

22. d, 23. b, 24. d, 25. a, 26. c

This is a classic presentation of trigeminal neuralgia. The first-line treatment is carbamazepine, although the other choices have been reported as beneficial (except for lithium) if carbamazepine is contraindicated or ineffective. Hyponatremia is the most common side effect seen with carbamazepine. If the patient is taking diuretics such as furosemide, the risk of hyponatremia will increase. Serum sodium levels should be monitored for the first few months of treatment. If a young woman presented with the same symptoms, multiple sclerosis should be evaluated for, especially with bilateral trigeminal neuralgia.

The International Classification of Headache Disorders—II (ICHD-II) criteria for trigeminal neuralgia include paroxysmal attacks of pain lasting from a fraction of a second to 2 minutes, affecting one or more divisions of the trigeminal nerve. The pain has at least one of the following characteristics: intense, sharp, superficial, or stabbing, and precipitated from trigger areas or by trigger factors. Attacks are stereotyped, there is no clinically evident neurologic deficit, and symptoms are not attributable to another disorder. See discussion to question 27 for short-lasting unilateral neuralgiform headache with conjunctival injection and tearing (SUNCT), question 18 for cluster headache, question 13 for hemicrania continua, and question 19 for paroxysmal hemicrania (PH).

Headache Classification Subcommittee of the International Headache Society. The international classification of headache disorders: 2nd edition. Cephalalgia. 2004; 24(Suppl. 1):9–160.

Silberstein SD, Lipton RB, Dodick D, et al. Wolff's Headache and Other Head Pain, 8th ed. New York: Oxford University Press; 2008.

27. b

This patient is describing episodes of short-lasting unilateral neuralgiform headache with conjunctival injection and tearing (SUNCT). This is a very rare primary headache disorder, more common in males, and can easily be confused with trigeminal neuralgia and other trigeminal autonomic cephalalgias. Trigeminal neuralgia does not have associated autonomic features and is discussed in question 22. Following a painful paroxysm in trigeminal neuralgia, there is usually a refractory period during which pain cannot be triggered, whereas this refractory period is not seen in SUNCT. SUNCT is rare enough that an MRI without and with contrast to rule out secondary causes, especially pituitary tumors, is mandatory.

The International Classification of Headache Disorders—II (ICHD-II) criteria for SUNCT must include at least 20 attacks characterized by the following: attacks of unilateral orbital, supraorbital, or temporal stabbing or pulsating pain lasting 5 to 240 seconds, the pain is accompanied by ipsilateral conjunctival injection and lacrimation, attacks occur with a frequency from 3 to 200 per day, and symptoms are not attributable to another disorder.

Headache Classification Subcommittee of the International Headache Society. The international classification of headache disorders: 2nd edition. Cephalalgia. 2004; 24(Suppl. 1):9–160.

Silberstein SD, Lipton RB, Dodick D, et al. Wolff's Headache and Other Head Pain, 8th ed. New York: Oxford University Press; 2008.

28. d

It is very unlikely that this patient's headaches are related to her Chiari I malformation. Chiari I is defined as tonsillar herniation below the level of foramen magnum, and it may be associated with syringomyelia (50%-70%) and hydrocephalus. When headaches are related to Chiari malformation, it is due to compression of neural tissues and alteration of CSF dynamics. The headaches are usually in the occipital region and precipitated paroxysmally by cough, bending forward, and valsalva maneuvers. When symptomatic, there are other symptoms of brainstem compression or cervical cord compression, such as ataxia, visual disturbances, hoarseness, dysphagia, vertigo, nystagmus, hearing loss, and cervical myelopathy. The upper limits of normal for tonsillar descent by age are as follows: 6 mm for ages 0 to 10 years, 5 mm for ages 10 to 30 years, 4 mm for ages 30 to 80 years, and 3 mm for ages older than 80 years. This patient has no neurologic features or symptoms consistent with a symptomatic Chiari, and her imaging is within the acceptable range. Her neck and shoulder musculature tenderness may be contributing to her tension-type headache, and physical therapy should be arranged. In addition, contributors such as stress, depression, and caffeine overuse should be assessed and addressed. She might benefit from preventive therapy at this time, and an antidepressant, such as amitriptyline, would be a good consideration.

Mikulis DJ, Diaz O, Egglin TK, et al. Variance of the position of the cerebellar tonsils with age: preliminary report. Radiology. 1992; 183:725–728.

Silberstein SD, Lipton RB, Dodick D, et al. Wolff's Headache and Other Head Pain, 8th ed. New York: Oxford University Press; 2008.

29. c, 30. e, 31. c, 32. b

Although all of the mentioned options are included in the differential diagnosis, the history of trauma and positional quality to the headache suggest traumatic CSF leak and subsequent low-CSF-pressure headache, which is what this patient has. Some causes of low-CSF-pressure headache include lumbar puncture (LP), neurosurgical procedures, dural tear from spondylosis, and meningeal diverticuli. The most common location of spontaneous CSF leaks is at the level of the thoracic spine. An MRI of the brain with gadolinium will often show pachymeningeal enhancement (as seen in Figure 4.1) and downward displacement of the brain and crowding of the posterior fossa due to the sagging and traction of intracranial structures and dura, which may mimic Chiari I malformation (as seen in Figure 4.2). Neuroimaging may also reveal subdural hematomas or hygromas, engorgement of cerebral venous sinuses, pituitary enlargement, flattening of the optic chiasm, increased anteroposterior diameter of the brainstem, and decrease in the size of cisterns and ventricles. Other evaluations helpful in the diagnosis include low opening pressure on spinal tap, radioisotope cisternography, and CT myelography. Conservative measures include bed rest, hydration, and caffeine. If these measures fail, an epidural blood patch should be performed. Surgical repair of the dural defect is done as a last resort.

The International Classification of Headache Disorders—II (ICHD-II) criteria for headache attributed to spontaneous low CSF pressure consist of a diffuse and/or dull headache that worsens within 15 minutes after sitting or standing. The headache must also have at least one of the following criteria: neck stiffness, tinnitus, hypacusia, photophobia, or nausea. It must also have at least one of the following: evidence of low CSF pressure on MRI (e.g., pachymeningeal enhancement), evidence of CSF leakage on conventional myelography, CT myelography or cisternography, or CSF opening pressure <60 mm H_2O in sitting position. There should be no history of dural puncture or other cause of CSF fistula, and the headache resolves within 72 hours after epidural blood patching.

Chung SJ, Lee JH, Kim SJ, et al. Subdural hematoma in spontaneous CSF hypovolemia. Neurology. 2006; 67:1088–1089.

Headache Classification Subcommittee of the International Headache Society. The international classification of headache disorders: 2nd edition. Cephalalgia. 2004; 24(Suppl. 1):9–160.

Marcelis J, Silberstein SD. Spontaneous low cerebrospinal fluid pressure headache. Headache. 1990; 30:192–196.

Schievink WI. Spontaneous spinal cerebrospinal fluid leaks and intracranial hypotension. JAMA. 2006; 295:2286–2296.

Spelle L, Boulin A, Tainturier C, et al. Neuroimaging features of spontaneous intracranial hypotension. Neuroradiology. 2001; 43:622–627.

33. d

Frovatriptan would be a poor choice for acute treatment of cluster headache, although it has been used for preventive purposes during cluster periods. Frovatriptan has a half-life of around 26 hours and a slower onset of action than sumatriptan, zolmitriptan, rizatriptan, almotriptan, and eletriptan. Any medication taken by mouth is a poor choice for acute treatment of cluster headache because cluster attacks peak very rapidly, so a fast onset of action is needed to abort the headache quickly. Triptans can be used, but the choice would need to be a formulation with a rapid onset of action, such as sumatriptan subcutaneous injections, sumatriptan nasal spray, or zolmitriptan nasal spray. Sumatriptan subcutaneous needle-free drug delivery system may also be used. Oxygen is very effective as an abortive for cluster and is often used as a first-line treatment. All of the other choices listed above, except for frovatriptan, are used for acute treatment of cluster.

Silberstein SD, Lipton RB, Dodick D, et al. Wolff's Headache and Other Head Pain, 8th ed. New York: Oxford University Press; 2008.

Silberstein SD, Stiles MA, Young WB. Atlas of Migraine and Other Headaches, 2nd ed. London and New York: Taylor and Francis Group; 2005.

34. b

Cluster headache preventive therapy should be started immediately at the beginning of a cluster period in episodic cluster. If the cluster periods become chronic (<1 month headache-free period per year) or are significantly increasing in duration, preventive therapy should be continued indefinitely. Preventive therapy should be thought of as "verapamil plus." In other words, verapamil should be first line and other agents added to it. All of the choices except for propranolol are used as cluster preventives. Melatonin levels have been shown to be decreased during cluster periods, so melatonin can also be used in high doses (up to 15 mg) during cluster periods, although positive randomized-controlled studies are lacking.

Silberstein SD, Lipton RB, Dodick D, et al. Wolff's Headache and Other Head Pain, 8th ed. New York: Oxford University Press; 2008.

Silberstein SD, Stiles MA, Young WB. Atlas of Migraine and Other Headaches, 2nd ed. London and New York: Taylor and Francis Group; 2005.

35. d, 36. d, 37. e, 38. a, 39. e, 40. b

This patient's history suggests idiopathic intracranial hypertension (IIH) or pseudotumor cerebri. It occurs most commonly in young, overweight women. Topiramate is used because of its carbonic anhydrase inhibitor effect; it decreases CSF production. Acetazolamide is the classic carbonic anhydrase inhibitor used, unless the patient has a sulfa allergy, which would make topiramate a better choice. Of the possible etiologies listed, aqueductal stenosis is not a cause of idiopathic intracranial hypertension (IIH), although it would be a secondary cause of hydrocephalus. Treatment typically begins conservatively with measures such as weight loss, cessation of vitamin A (if toxicity is suspected), weaning steroids, and minimizing other potential risks. If there is no evidence of visual loss, some feel that treatment of the headache alone is sufficient. If there is evidence of visual loss, a carbonic anhydrase inhibitor such as acetazolamide or topiramate should be started. Hydrochlorothiazide is not a typical treatment for IIH.

The fundoscopic examination is consistent with papilledema. An early finding of increased intracranial pressure preceding papilledema is loss of spontaneous venous pulsations, although this can also be a normal variant. Disc margin splinter hemorrhages may be seen early also. Eventually, the disc becomes elevated, the cup is lost, and the disc margins become indistinct. Blood vessels appear blurred as they course the disc. Engorgement of retinal veins lead to a hyperemic disc. As the edema progresses, the optic nerve head appears enlarged and may be associated with flame hemorrhages and cotton wool spots, as a result of nerve fiber infarction. The photograph does not show optic neuritis (see Chapter 1), anterior ischemic optic neuropathy (AION) (see Chapter 1), or posterior ischemic optic neuropathy (see Chapter 1).

Procedures should generally be performed when there is progressive visual field defect, visual acuity loss from papilledema, and intractable headache while on maximal pharmacotherapy. Optic nerve fenestration can be done if visual loss is progressive on pharmacotherapy. Serial high-volume lumbar puncture (LP) has fallen out of favor because of the short-lasting effect and unnecessary patient discomfort and inconvenience. There are no studies suggesting clinical benefit from weight loss, although this is commonly recommended. Procedures performed as a last resort include lumboperitoneal or ventriculoperitoneal shunt. Most patients with idiopathic intracranial hypertension (IIH) have a headache, but not all. They may complain of transient visual obscurations (seconds), graying of vision (especially with straining), diplopia (cranial nerve VI palsy), bilateral pulsatile tinnitus, nausea, and vomiting. Examination findings may include those listed in question 40, especially papilledema, visual field loss, or decreased venous pulsations. Facial nerve palsy would not be an associated finding.

The International Classification of Headache Disorders—II (ICHD-II) criteria for IIH include a progressive headache with at least one of the following characteristics: daily occurrence, diffuse and/or constant (nonpulsating) pain, aggravated by coughing or straining. Intracranial hypertension in an alert patient should demonstrate a neurologic examination that either is normal or shows any of the following abnormalities: papilledema, enlarged blind spot, visual field defect (progressive if untreated), or abducens nerve palsy. There should be increased CSF pressure (>200 mm H_2O in the nonobese, >250 mm H_2O in the obese) measured by LP in the recumbent position or by epidural or intraventricular pressure monitoring. There should be normal CSF chemistry (low CSF protein is acceptable) and cellularity. Intracranial diseases (including venous sinus thrombosis) are ruled out by appropriate investigations, and no metabolic, toxic, or hormonal cause of intracranial hypertension should be present. The headache develops in close temporal relation to increased intracranial pressure, and the headache improves after withdrawal of CSF to reduce pressure to 120 to 170 mm H_2O and resolves within 72 hours of persistent normalization of intracranial pressure.

Acheson JF, Green WT, Sanders MD. Optic nerve sheath decompression for the treatment of visual failure in chronic raised intracranial pressure. J Neurol Neurosurg Psychiatry. 1994; 57:1426–1429.

Burgett RA, Purvin VA, Kawasaki A. Lumboperitoneal shunting for pseudotumor cerebri. Neurology. 1997; 49:734–739.

Headache Classification Subcommittee of the International Headache Society. The international classification of headache disorders: 2nd edition. Cephalalgia. 2004; 24(Suppl. 1): 9–160.

Silberstein SD, Lipton RB, Dodick D, et al. Wolff's Headache and Other Head Pain, 8th ed. New York: Oxford University Press; 2008.

41. b

Topiramate is often used in overweight patients because it can be associated with weight loss, but given that this patient has a history of recurrent kidney stones, topiramate becomes a poor choice. All of the other choices have been shown to be beneficial for preventive purposes and are commonly used. Because she is hypertensive, a β-blocker or calcium-channel blocker would be a good treatment option. Preventive therapy should always be targeted not only for headache prevention, but also for any comorbidities that are present.

Peikert A, Wilimzig C, Kohne-Volland R. Prophylaxis of migraine with oral magnesium: results from a prospective, multi-center, placebo-controlled and double-blind randomized study. Cephalalgia. 1996; 16:257–263.

Silberstein SD, Lipton RB, Dodick D, et al. Wolff's Headache and Other Head Pain, 8th ed. New York: Oxford University Press; 2008.

42. b, 43. c, 44. d, 45. c

This patient's history is concerning for a cerebral venous sinus thrombosis, especially in the setting of prior idiopathic deep venous thrombosis (DVT), which may suggest an underlying hypercoagulable state. Absent venous pulsations suggests elevated intracranial pressure, which can be the result of cerebral venous sinus thrombosis. Besides headache, other symptoms may include seizures, encephalopathy, focal neurologic findings, papilledema, and vomiting. Although a hypercoagulable panel should be checked, the more immediate testing should be a brain MRV and MRI to look for venous sinus filling defects. If imaging confirms the diagnosis, heparin should be started with transition to warfarin. It is important to obtain the hypercoagulable workup prior to starting warfarin, because this medication may alter the results of these blood tests. Other risk factors include oral contraceptive use (especially in conjunction with smoking), pregnancy, infection, head trauma, and malignancy. Treatment duration varies between 3 and 6 months, but if the hypercoagulable workup is positive, lifelong anticoagulation may be needed.

Bousser MG, Russell RR. Cerebral venous thrombosis. In: Major Problems in Neurology, Warlow CP, Van Gijn, J (Eds), London, UK: WB Saunders; 1997.

Ferro JM, Canhão P, Stam J, et al; ISCVT Investigators. Prognosis of cerebral vein and dural sinus thrombosis: results of the International Study on Cerebral Vein and Dural Sinus Thrombosis (ISCVT). Stroke. 2004; 35:664–670.

Silberstein SD, Lipton RB, Dodick D, et al. Wolff's Headache and Other Head Pain, 8th ed. New York: Oxford University Press; 2008.

46. c, 47. d, 48. d, 49. c, 50. d

This patient's history and family history are suggestive of cerebral autosomal dominant arteriopathy with subcortical infarcts and leukoencephalopathy (CADASIL). This disorder presents with migraine with aura, stroke or stroke-like episodes, progressive dementia, and other neurodegenerative findings. This is an autosomal dominant disorder most often due to a missense mutation in the *NOTCH3* gene, on chromosome 19q13.1, although splice site mutations and small in-frame deletions have also been reported. The *NOTCH3* gene encodes a transmembrane protein thought to be involved in cell signaling during embryonic development. It can be diagnosed by genetic testing or skin biopsy. MRI of the brain will show confluent deep white matter changes. These deep white matter changes may characteristically affect the anterior temporal lobes.

Dichgans M, Mayer M, Uttner I, et al. The phenotypic spectrum of CADASIL: clinical findings in 102 cases. Ann Neurol. 1998; 44:731–739.

Joutel A, Vahedi K, Corpechot C, et al. Strong clustering and stereotyped nature of Notch3 mutations in CADASIL patients. Lancet. 1997; 350:1511–1515.

Peters N, Opherk C, Bergmann T, et al. Spectrum of mutations in biopsy-proven CADASIL: implications for diagnostic strategies. Arch Neurol. 2005; 62:1091–1094.

Silberstein SD, Lipton RB, Dodick D, et al. Wolff's Headache and Other Head Pain, 8th ed. New York: Oxford University Press; 2008.

51. b

This patient's presentation and history suggest hemiplegic migraine. Although there are sporadic forms, she likely falls into the category of familial hemiplegic migraine (FHM) given her mother's history. There are three types of FHM that are all autosomal dominant with variable penetrance. FHM1 is linked to chromosome 19p13 (*CACNA1A* gene), resulting in a defect in P/Q calcium-channel subunit. Additional FHM1 symptoms may include cerebellar involvement, such as gaze-evoked nystagmus or ataxia, also attacks of coma, prolonged hemiplegia, or both, but full recovery is the rule. Transient cerebral edema and cerebral atrophy are less commonly seen. FHM2 is linked to 1q23 (*ATP1A2* gene), resulting in a defect in the A1A2 sodium–potassium ATPase channel. Additional FHM2 symptoms may include recurrent coma, frequent and long-lasting hemiplegia, or seizures with mental retardation. Cerebellar ataxia is not associated with FHM2. FHM3 is linked to chromosome 2q24 (*SCN1A* gene), resulting in defects of presynaptic and postsynaptic voltage-gated sodium channels.

Dichgans M, Freilinger T, Eckstein G, et al. Mutation in the neuronal voltage-gated sodium channel SCN1 A in familial hemiplegic migraine. Lancet. 2005; 366:371–377.

Jen JC, Kim GW, Dudding KA, et al. No mutations in CACNA1 A and ATP1A2 in probands with common types of migraine. Arch Neurol. 2004; 61:926–928.

Silberstein SD, Lipton RB, Dodick D, et al. Wolff's Headache and Other Head Pain, 8th ed. New York: Oxford University Press; 2008.

52. d

This patient has an idiopathic cranial pachymeningitis. In this syndrome, patients experience headache as well as other neurologic symptoms such as hemiparesis, ataxia, aphasia, and confusion. Patients have prominent leptomeningeal enhancement. CSF findings are variable but may show a lymphocytic pleocytosis. Leptomeningeal biopsy may show perivascular inflammation. This may be associated with rheumatoid arthritis or idiopathic CNS vasculitis. It is essentially a diagnosis of exclusion when other infectious or inflammatory conditions are ruled out.

Bruggemann N, Gottschalk S, Holl-Ulrich K, et al. Cranial pachymeningitis. Clin Exp Rheum. 2009; 27:S10–S13.

Buzz Phrases	Key Points
Thunderclap headache, "worst headache of my life"	SAH
Indomethacin-responsive headache	Hemicrania continua, paroxysmal hemicrania (PH)
Headache red flags	Systemic symptoms (fever, chills, weight loss), history of prior cancer, immunodeficiency, focal neurologic signs or symptoms, thunderclap headache, new-onset headache after age 50, precipitation by exertion, strain, or positional changes, increasing headache frequency and severity, and new-onset seizures
Headache with jaw claudication, scalp sensitivity, visual complaints in age >50, with ESR >50	Temporal (giant-cell) arteritis
Bilateral trigeminal neuralgia or trigeminal neuralgia in a young patient	Multiple sclerosis, sarcoidosis, Lyme disease
Cerebral autosomal dominant arteriopathy with subcortical infarcts and leukoencephalopathy (CADASIL)	Autosomal dominant, chromosome 19, *NOTCH3* mutation
FHM1	Autosomal dominant, chromosome 19p13, *CACNA1A* gene, defective P/Q calcium channel
FHM2	Autosomal dominant, chromosome 1q23, *ATP1A2* gene, defective A1A2 sodium–potassium ATPase channel
FHM3	Autosomal dominant, chromosome 2q24, *SCN1A* gene, defective pre- and postsynaptic voltage-gated sodium channels

Chapter 5

Adult and Pediatric Epilepsy and Sleep

Questions

1. If an AED is required in pregnancy, the safest choice of the following would be:
   a. Phenytoin
   b. Primidone
   c. Lamotrigine
   d. Valproic acid (worst).
   e. Phenobarbital

2. Which of the following AEDs is associated with weight loss?
   a. Pregabalin
   b. Gabapentin
   c. Topiramate
   d. Carbamazepine
   e. Valproic acid

3. A 36-year-old male with a prior history of HSV infection presents with new-onset epilepsy that you suspect is due to his prior encephalitis affecting the temporal lobes. The clinical features of seizures in mesial temporal lobe epilepsy may have all of the following characteristic symptoms, except:
   a. Olfactory hallucinations
   b. Altered consciousness
   c. Complex partial seizures
   d. Automatisms
   e. Tonic posturing of one limb (fencer's posture)

4. Which of the following AEDs would have the least drug–drug interactions?
   a. Gabapentin
   b. Carbamazepine
   c. Valproic acid

  d. Lamotrigine
  e. Phenytoin

5. In a young child with generalized epilepsy refractory to multiple antiepileptic medications, what would be the next best choice of treatment, if tolerated?
  a. Corpus callosotomy
  b. Ketogenic diet
  c. Vagus nerve stimulation
  d. Phenytoin
  e. Carbamazepine

6. Which of the following is the best treatment option for simple febrile seizures?
  a. IV lorazepam
  b. Rectal diazepam
  c. Supportive management
  d. Phenobarbital
  e. Intranasal midazolam

7. Which of the following mutations has not been associated with generalized epilepsy with febrile seizures plus (GEFS+)?
  a. *SCN1D*
  b. *SCN1A*
  c. *SCN1B*
  d. *SCN2A*
  e. *GABRD*

8. A 13-year-old girl is being evaluated for epilepsia partialis continua. Rasmussen's syndrome is suspected. What would be the most common finding on brain MRI in Rasmussen's syndrome?
  a. Lissencephaly
  b. Schizencephaly
  c. Cortical atrophy
  d. Pachygyria
  e. Porencephaly

9. A 12-year-old boy presents to your office with a history of progressively worsening frequency and severity of daily myoclonic seizures. His mitochondrial testing has so far been negative, although you suspect a progressive myoclonic epilepsy (PME) of some type. What would be the best antiepileptic medication to try first, given there are no contraindications?
  a. Carbamazepine
  b. Phenytoin
  c. Oxcarbazepine
  d. Valproic acid
  e. Gabapentin

10. The benefits of fosphenytoin over phenytoin include all of the following, except:
  a. Can be given intramuscularly
  b. Less cardiovascular side effects
  c. Achieves therapeutic plasma concentrations faster

    d. Faster rate of IV administration possible

    e. Less infiltration reactions (purple glove syndrome)

11. Which of carbamazepine the following has not been associated with worsening of myoclonic seizures?

    a. Topiramate

    b. Carbamazepine

    c. Lamotrigine

    d. Pregabalin

    e. Vigabatrin

12. Which of the following antiepileptic medications is a hepatic enzyme inhibitor?

    a. Phenytoin   +All other – inducer.

    b. Carbamazepine

    c. Valproic acid

    d. Phenobarbital

    e. Primidone

13. Which of the following EEG findings would be associated with the highest incidence of seizures?

    a. Small sharp spikes

    b. 6-Hz spike and wave

    c. Wicket spikes

    d. 3-Hz spike and wave

    e. 14 and 6 positive spikes

14. At what age do human beings attain the predominant α-frequency (posterior background) that is seen in adults?

    a. 6 to 8 years

    b. 8 to 10 years

    c. 10 to 12 years

    d. 12 to 14 years

    e. 14 to 16 years

15. A 47-year-old woman presents with confusion, fever, and seizures. CSF studies are positive for HSV infection. What would be the most likely finding on an EEG in this patient?

    a. Triphasic waves

    b. Wicket spikes

    c. Periodic lateralized epileptiform discharges (PLEDs) (ö-ʒ M7)

    d. Polyspikes

    e. Fast spike–wave complexes

16. In a patient with absence epilepsy, absence status epilepticus can be precipitated by all of the following antiepileptic medications, except:

    a. Phenytoin

    b. Topiramate

    c. Carbamazepine

    d. Lamotrigine

    e. Gabapentin

17. Which of the following antiepileptic medications is the most likely to have an effect on steroid hormone concentration in the blood in patients taking oral contraceptive pills and, therefore, lead to contraceptive failure?
    a. Levetiracetam
    b. Gabapentin
    c. Topiramate (dose <200 mg/day)
    ʾ d. Oxcarbazepine
    e. Zonisamide

18. An 8-year-old boy is brought to your office by his parents. They tell you that his teacher suggested the boy should see a neurologist for inattention. His EEG is shown in Figure 5.1 and is characteristic of what type of epilepsy?

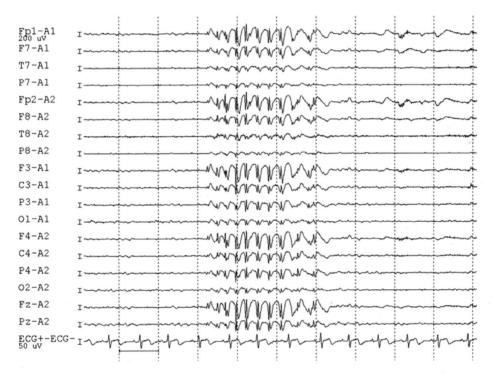

FIGURE 5.1   EEG (Courtesy of Dr. Andreas Alexopoulos)

    a. Juvenile myoclonic epilepsy (JME)
    b. Absence epilepsy
    c. Myoclonic epilepsy
    d. Benign childhood epilepsy with centrotemporal spikes (benign rolandic epilepsy of childhood)
    e. Lennox–Gastaut epilepsy

Questions 19–20

19. A 12-year-old boy with complaints of early morning falls, clumsiness, and dropping objects presents with a generalized tonic–clonic (GTC) seizure. His EEG shown in Figure 5.2 suggests which of the following?

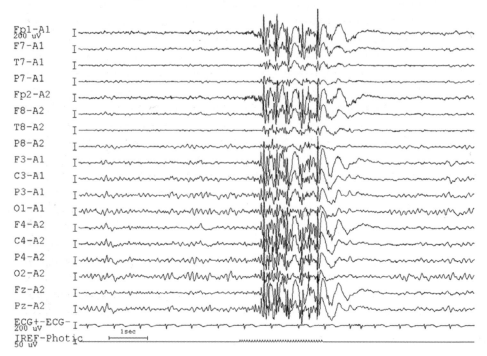

FIGURE 5.2   EEG (Courtesy of Dr. Andreas Alexopoulos)

    a. Juvenile myoclonic epilepsy (JME)
    b. Absence epilepsy
    c. Myoclonic epilepsy
    d. Benign childhood epilepsy with centrotemporal spikes (benign rolandic epilepsy of childhood)
    e. Lennox–Gastaut epilepsy

20. Which of the following antiepileptic drugs would typically be the first-line treatment for this patient?
    a. Carbamazepine
    b. Phenytoin
    c. Phenobarbital
    d. Valproic acid
    e. Topamax

Questions 21–22

21. A 7-year-old boy has recurrent nocturnal events, which awaken his parents, because they hear "his bed shaking." They have witnessed him "shaking uncontrollably" on entering his bedroom on occasion. They have also seen only his face and arm twitching before or after the convulsions. His EEG is shown in Figure 5.3 and suggests which of the following?

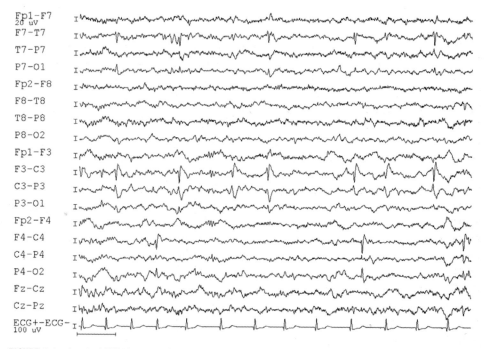

FIGURE 5.3   Interictal EEG (Courtesy of Dr. Andreas Alexopoulos)

    a. Juvenile myoclonic epilepsy (JME)
    b. Metabolic encephalopathy
    c. Myoclonic epilepsy
    d. Benign childhood epilepsy with centrotemporal spikes (benign rolandic epilepsy of childhood)
    e. Periodic lateralized epileptiform discharges (PLEDs)

22. When necessary, what is the antiepileptic of choice in this condition, given no contraindications?
    a. Phenytoin
    b. Valproic acid
    c. Topiramate
    d. Carbamazepine
    e. Ethosuximide

23. A 56-year-old man presents with confusion and seizures. His EEG is shown in Figure 5.4 and is characteristic of which of the following?
    a. Juvenile myoclonic epilepsy (JME)
    b. Metabolic encephalopathy
    c. Myoclonic epilepsy

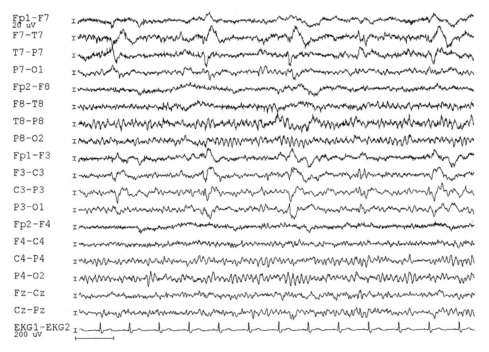

FIGURE 5.4 EEG (Courtesy of Dr. Andreas Alexopoulos)

   d. Benign childhood epilepsy with centrotemporal spikes (benign rolandic epilepsy of child-
      hood)
   e. Periodic lateralized epileptiform discharges (PLEDs)

Questions 24–25

24. A 6-month-old baby boy is brought to your office by his parents. They describe sudden tonic
   flexion of limbs and body occurring in clusters after waking. His EEG is shown in Figure 5.5.
   What is your diagnosis?
   a. Juvenile myoclonic epilepsy (JME)
   b. Hypsarrhythmia of infantile spasms
   c. Myoclonic epilepsy
   d. Benign childhood epilepsy with centrotemporal spikes (benign rolandic epilepsy of child-
      hood)
   e. Absence epilepsy

25. Which of the following is the most accepted treatment for this disorder?
   a. Lamotrigine
   b. Phenytoin
   c. Phenobarbital
   d. ACTH
   e. Carbamazepine

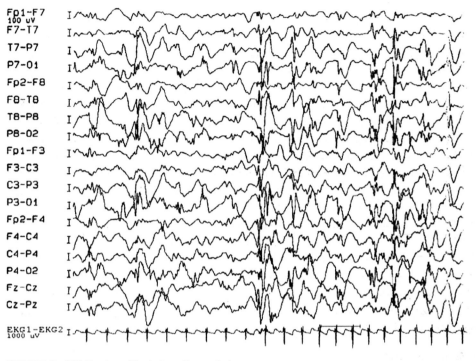

FIGURE 5.5   EEG (Courtesy of Dr. Andreas Alexopoulos)

Questions 26–28

Inhibits Nat Channels, Hepatic metabolism — inducer
— non-linear zero order kinetics.

26. Regarding the pharmacokinetics of phenytoin, which of the following is correct?
    a. It is predominantly renally metabolized
    b. It is exclusively metabolized by the liver
    c. It has zero-order (nonlinear) kinetics
    d. It is a hepatic enzyme inhibitor
    e. It has first-order (linear) kinetics

27. Which of the following is not a common long-term side effect of chronic phenytoin use?
    a. Hirsutism
    b. Osteoporosis
    c. Gingival hyperplasia
    d. Cortical atrophy
    e. Coarse facial features

28. A patient with known epilepsy on phenytoin presented to the emergency department with a breakthrough seizure. His total phenytoin level is 10 μg/mL, but when you look back at his prior levels, it is usually around 15 μg/mL. Assuming a volume of distribution of 0.8 L/kg, which of the following would be the best IV dose to boost him to his baseline level if he weighs 75 kg (assuming that the patient does not have any comorbidities that are known to modify phenytoin kinetics, such as uremia or hypoalbuminemia)?

= (Target level - Actual level) × (BW (kg)) × volume of distribution kinetics

a. 1000 mg
b. 600 mg
c. 300 mg
d. 150 mg
e. 50 mg

Questions 29–31

29. A 43-year-old male on valproic acid for long-standing epilepsy presents to the emergency department with a breakthrough seizure. He is 70 kg and his total valproic acid level is 70 μg/mL, although he normally has levels around 100 μg/mL. Assuming a volume of distribution of 0.2 L/kg, what will be your correcting IV bolus?
   a. 120 mg   *— some formula or above*
   b. 220 mg
   c. 320 mg
   d. 420 mg
   e. 520 mg

30. Which of the following is not a possible long-term side effect of valproic acid ?
   a. Hair loss
   b. Cerebellar atrophy
   c. Polycystic ovarian syndrome
   d. Tremor
   e. Weight gain

31. The neurologist is called to see this patient as a consult in the emergency department. The emergency department physician asks if lamotrigine could be added as an additional antiepileptic agent to his valproic acid. Which of the following best describes the interaction between these two medications?
   a. Lamotrigine significantly increases the half-life of valproic acid
   b. Valproic acid significantly decreases the half-life of lamotrigine
   c. Valproic acid significantly increases the half-life of lamotrigine
   d. Lamotrigine significantly decreases the half-life of valproic acid
   e. Lamotrigine and valproic acid do not have any significant interaction

Questions 32–35

32. Which of the following is not a known side effect of carbamazepine?
   a. Dizziness
   b. Nystagmus
   c. Drowsiness
   d. Hypernatremia *(Hypo)*
   e. Nausea

33. Which of the following is true regarding carbamazepine?
   a. It inhibits its own metabolism
   b. For new-onset, frequent seizures, carbamazepine is a good option as initial antiepileptic therapy
   c. It has no effect on its own metabolism
   d. It induces its own metabolism
   e. It has no hepatic metabolism

34. A 34-year-old man being treated with carbamazepine presents with dizziness and nystagmus after valproic acid was recently added for his epilepsy. These symptoms are likely related to:
   a. Elevated levels of carbamazepine
   b. Elevated levels of valproic acid
   c. Elevated levels of 10,11-carbamazepine epoxide
   d. Withdrawal symptoms from increased carbamazepine metabolism
   e. Valproic acid itself, as his body adjusts to a second antiepileptic

35. Oxcarbazepine is a structural derivative of carbamazepine. Which of the following is true about oxcarbazepine in comparison to carbamazepine?
   a. Is not a hepatic enzyme inducer
   b. No risk of hyponatremia
   c. Is not metabolized to an epoxide
   d. Indicated in both partial and generalized epilepsy
   e. No risk of rash as seen with carbamazepine

36. Which of the following is a mechanism of action of benzodiazepines?
   a. Chloride channel antagonism
   b. Chloride channel agonism
   c. $GABA_A$ antagonism
   d. $GABA_A$ agonism
   e. $GABA_B$ agonism

Questions 37–38

37. Which of the following is the least likely side effect of lamotrigine?
   a. Stevens–Johnson syndrome
   b. Blurred vision
   c. Ataxia
   d. Dizziness
   e. Cognitive complaints

38. Which of the following is incorrect regarding lamotrigine and hormonal interactions?
   a. Oral contraceptives containing only ethinylestradiol increase lamotrigine clearance
   b. Oral contraceptives containing both ethinylestradiol and progesterone increase lamotrigine clearance
   c. Oral contraceptives containing only progesterone increase lamotrigine clearance
   d. Lamotrigine clearance is increased significantly during pregnancy
   e. Hormone replacement therapy increases lamotrigine clearance

Questions 39–40

39. Which of the following is false regarding topiramate?
   a. It is metabolized predominantly by the liver
   b. It is a sodium channel antagonist
   c. It is an NMDA-glutamate antagonist
   d. It is a $GABA_A$ agonist
   e. It is a carbonic anhydrase inhibitor

40. Which of the following is not a side effect of topiramate?
   a. Word-finding difficulty
   b. Increased appetite

    c. Paresthesias

    d. Kidney stones

    e. Acute angle-closure glaucoma

41. Which of the following is incorrect regarding the mechanism of action of lacosamide?

    a. Selectively enhances fast inactivation of voltage-dependent sodium channels

    b. Stabilizes hyperexcitable neuronal membranes

    c. Inhibits repetitive neuronal firing

    d. Enhances slow inactivation of voltage-dependent sodium channels

    e. Binds to the collapsin response mediator protein 2 (CRMP2)

42. Which of the following is incorrect regarding rufinamide?

    a. It modulates activity at neuronal sodium channels

    b. It is FDA-approved as an adjunct for Lennox–Gastaut syndrome

    c. It prolongs the inactive state of neuronal sodium channels

    d. Elimination of rufinamide occurs primarily through renal excretion

    e. It is metabolized by the cytochrome P450 system

43. A 21-year-old man comes to the clinic because he has been having spells in which he suddenly stops what he was previously doing and stares for about a minute, sometimes picking at his nose and his shirt. He cannot recall what happens during the spell itself. He says, however, that he knows when a spell is going to happen because he experiences a warm sensation in his epigastric region, followed by a sensation of fear and a rapid recollection of episodes of past life experiences along with palpitations. He may have postictal confusion. His EEG shows focal spikes. Which of the following best describes the type of seizure this patient has?

    a. Temporal lobe seizures

    b. Frontal lobe seizures

    c. Absence seizures

    d. Occipital lobe seizures

    e. Parietal lobe seizures

44. An 18-year-old man presents for a second opinion regarding seizures, which occur multiple times per day, starting with eye deviation to the left. He then emits a loud "cry-like" sound, his head turns left, and his left arm adopts a tonic posture with shoulder external rotation and abduction with arm extension, while his right arm is flexed. These seizures last for about 30 seconds, and sometimes generalize. Which of the following is the most likely origin of his seizures?

    a. Right temporal lobe

    b. Right supplementary motor area

    c. Left temporal lobe

    d. Left supplementary motor area

    e. Right parietal lobe

45. A 5-month-old boy with developmental delay is brought for evaluation of repeated clusters of spasms characterized by bilateral arm flexion along with neck, trunk, and leg flexion. His EEG is shown in Figure 5.5. Which of the following is incorrect regarding this condition?

    a. MRI should be done in every patient with this condition

    b. Diagnosis of tuberous sclerosis should be considered and ruled out

    c. ACTH is used for treatment

    d. These types of seizures do not need treatment and the prognosis is good

    e. Vigabatrin may be effective to treat this condition

46. A 2-month-old girl has blindness, infantile spasms, and an abnormal retinal examination. Her *chorioretinal lacunae.* brain MRI shows agenesis of the corpus callosum. Which of the following is the most likely cause?

    a. West syndrome

    b. Ohtahara syndrome

    c. Severe myoclonic epilepsy of infancy (Dravet syndrome)

    d. Aicardi syndrome

    e. Myoclonic–astatic epilepsy (Doose syndrome)

47. A 4-year-old boy with normal cognitive development is brought in after a generalized tonic-clonic (GTC) seizure. Over the past couple of months he has been having episodes of falls, suffering multiple injuries. His mother describes episodes in which he loses tone, causing him to fall, and episodes of rapid "jerk-like" symmetric movements of the upper extremities that may also lead to falls. There is no clear loss of consciousness with these brief events. His interictal EEG shows parietal rhythmic θ and bilateral synchronous irregular 2- to 3-Hz spike and wave complexes. Which of the following is the most likely diagnosis?

    a. Severe myoclonic epilepsy of infancy (Dravet syndrome)

    b. Ohtahara syndrome

    c. Benign myoclonic epilepsy of infancy

    d. Generalized epilepsy with febrile seizures plus (GEFS+)

    e. Myoclonic–astatic epilepsy (Doose syndrome)

48. A 2-year-old boy with a history of developmental delay and a prolonged febrile seizure at age 1 is admitted with frequent seizures of multiple types. He initially began having myoclonic seizures; however, he has now also developed absence seizures, as well as unilateral and generalized tonic-clonic (GTC) seizures. Which of the following is the most likely diagnosis?

    a. Severe myoclonic epilepsy of infancy (Dravet syndrome)

    b. Ohtahara syndrome

    c. Benign myoclonic epilepsy of infancy

    d. Generalized epilepsy with febrile seizures plus (GEFS+)

    e. Myoclonic–astatic epilepsy (Doose syndrome)

49. You see a 15-day-old baby with severe hypotonia and frequent tonic spasms occurring in clusters of more than 100 times/day. The EEG shows burst suppression, present when the patient is either awake or asleep. Which is the most likely diagnosis?

    a. Severe myoclonic epilepsy of infancy (Dravet syndrome)

    b. Ohtahara syndrome

    c. Benign myoclonic epilepsy of infancy

    d. Generalized epilepsy with febrile seizures plus (GEFS+)

    e. Myoclonic–astatic epilepsy (Doose syndrome)

50. A 2.5-year-old child comes for a follow-up appointment. At the age of 8 months he began having brief generalized myoclonic seizures, associated with fast (>3-Hz) spike–wave and polyspike and wave discharges on the EEG. Interictal EEG is normal. His seizures are well controlled on valproic acid and his development has been normal. Which of the following is the most likely diagnosis?

a. Severe myoclonic epilepsy of infancy (Dravet syndrome)
b. Ohtahara syndrome
c. Benign myoclonic epilepsy of infancy
d. Generalized epilepsy with febrile seizures plus (GEFS+)
e. Myoclonic–astatic epilepsy (Doose syndrome)

51. A newborn is being evaluated for seizures, which are characterized by apneic spells associated with unilateral or bilateral clonic movements. Starting on day 5 of life he has been having multiple spells per day. His neurologic examination is otherwise normal in between seizures. His interictal EEG is normal. Which of the following is the most likely diagnosis?
    a. West syndrome
    b. Benign neonatal seizures
    c. Aicardi syndrome
    d. Ohtahara syndrome
    e. Benign myoclonic epilepsy of infancy

52. A 4-year-old boy presents for evaluation of spells. Apparently, the episodes begin with some visual phenomena, which he cannot describe, followed by eye deviation and vomiting. He has had a total of three of these spells. His EEG shows a normal background with high-voltage occipital spikes, which disappear with eye opening. Which of the following is the most likely diagnosis?
    a. Ohtahara syndrome
    b. Late-onset or Gastaut-type childhood occipital epilepsy
    c. Early-onset or Panayiotopoulos-type childhood occipital epilepsy
    d. Dravet syndrome
    e. Doose syndrome

53. A 3-year-old boy with mental retardation is brought for evaluation of his seizures. He began having drop attacks about a year ago, but progressively has developed multiple seizure types, including absences, tonic seizures, and clonic seizures. Multiple antiepileptic agents have been tried with mild improvement, but he still has multiple seizures per day. His EEG shows 2-Hz spike–wave discharges. Which of the following is the most likely diagnosis?
    a. Panayiotopoulos syndrome
    b. West syndrome
    c. Landau–Kleffner syndrome
    d. Lennox–Gastaut syndrome
    e. Seizures associated with mesial temporal lobe sclerosis

54. The parents of a 5-year-old boy report that he seems to be more withdrawn over the past several months. One year ago he began having seizures, initially myoclonic seizures and later generalized tonic-clonic (GTC) seizures. About 9 months ago he was noticed to have some problems understanding verbal communication, and he now appears to be aphasic. His EEG shows multifocal spikes. Which of the following is the most likely diagnosis?
    a. Panayiotopoulos syndrome
    b. West syndrome
    c. Landau–Kleffner syndrome
    d. Lennox–Gastaut syndrome
    e. Seizures associated with mesial temporal lobe sclerosis

55. An 11-year-old girl is brought to the epilepsy monitoring unit for evaluation of possible "pseu-doseizures." Her spells occur only at night, and are described as large-amplitude and violent movements of all four limbs and her trunk. Given the hyperkinetic bizarre movements and a normal awake EEG, her seizures were thought to be nonepileptic by a local neurologist. In the epilepsy monitoring unit a seizure is captured during non-REM sleep. Which of the following is the most likely diagnosis?
   a. Electrical status epilepticus during sleep (ESES)
   b. Lennox–Gastaut syndrome
   c. Landau–Kleffner syndrome
   d. Autosomal dominant nocturnal frontal lobe epilepsy (ADNFLE)
   e. Panayiotopoulos syndrome

Questions 56–59

56. A 15-year-old girl has seizures that begin with eye and head deviation toward the left, with subsequent generalization. Where is the most likely location of the seizure focus?
   a. Hypothalamus
   b. Right frontal lobe
   c. Left frontal lobe
   d. Right temporal lobe
   e. Left temporal lobe

57. An 18-year-old man has seizures that begin with asymmetric tonic posturing in which his right arm is extended at the elbow with the fist clenched, while the left arm is flexed at the elbow. He subsequently has generalized tonic-clonic (GTC) seizures. Where is the most likely location of the seizure focus?
   a. Right temporal lobe
   b. Left temporal lobe
   c. Right supplementary motor area
   d. Left supplementary motor area
   e. Right occipital lobe

58. A 32-year-old woman has seizures in which her left arm becomes dystonic, while she exhibits automatisms with the right arm. Where is the most likely location of the seizure focus?
   a. Right temporal lobe
   b. Left temporal lobe
   c. Left frontal lobe
   d. Hypothalamus
   e. Left supplementary motor area

59. A 7-year-old boy has seizures that are characterized by uncontrollable episodes of laughter. Where is the most likely origin of his seizures?
   a. Hypothalamus
   b. Right frontal lobe
   c. Left frontal lobe
   d. Right temporal lobe
   e. Left temporal lobe

60. A 56-year-old woman has a history of coronary disease, atrial fibrillation, and seizures secondary to a stroke she suffered last year, which are well controlled on phenytoin. Two weeks ago she was diagnosed with a urinary tract infection and was placed on trimethoprim–sulfamethoxazole and fluconazole. She is now admitted with unsteady gait and frequent falls. On examination she is lethargic and dysarthric, with nystagmus and ataxia. Which of the following tests you should order first?

a. MRI of the brain
b. EEG
c. Free and total phenytoin level
d. Urine culture
e. CT of the brain

Question 61–62

61. A 2-year-old girl without a significant past medical or family history has a generalized seizure lasting 5 minutes in the setting of a fever of 39°C. The patient recovered without any residual neurologic deficit. The mother would like to know the risk of recurrence. Which of the following is not a predictor of recurrence of febrile seizures (FS)?

a. Family history of FS
b. Age younger than 18 months at the time of FS
c. Shorter duration of fever prior to FS
d. Lower peak temperature at the time of FS
e. Complex FS

62. In a patient who suffered a febrile seizure (FS), which of the following is not a risk to develop subsequent epilepsy?

a. Family history of FS
b. Complex FS
c. Developmental delay
d. Family history of epilepsy
e. Neurologic abnormality

63. A 14-year-old boy is brought to the clinic for evaluation. He has had stimulus-sensitive myoclonus noticed about 4 years ago, which has become more frequent lately. Over the past 3 months he has been having generalized tonic-clonic (GTC) seizures, and he is clumsier and having frequent falls and problems with hand coordination. The neurologic examination demonstrates ataxia. His MRI is unremarkable and the EEG shows generalized spikes and waves. Genetic testing demonstrated an *EPM1* gene mutation. Which of the following is the most likely diagnosis?

a. Lafora body disease
b. Unverricht Lundborg syndrome
c. Sialidosis
d. Juvenile myoclonic epilepsy
e. Neuronal ceroid lipofuscinosis

64. A 12-year-old boy with a history of migraines has short stature, ataxia, proximal weakness, mild cognitive impairment, deafness, and various types of seizures. He is admitted after a viral illness, becomes dehydrated, and is found to have lactic acidosis. He has been diagnosed with a progressive myoclonic epilepsy (PME); a muscle biopsy has been obtained and shown in Figure 5.6. Which of the following is a feature of this patient's condition?

a. Mutation affecting cystatin B
b. Cherry red spot on the fundoscopic examination

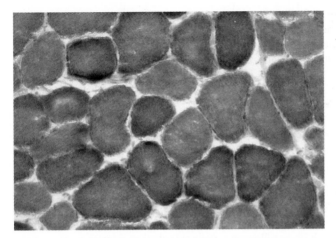

FIGURE 5.6 Muscle specimen (Courtesy of Dr. Richard A. Prayson). Shown also in color plates

c. This is a mitochondrial disorder
d. *EPM2 A* mutation
e. Lafora bodies on skin biopsy

65. A 21-year-old man presents with progressive myoclonic jerks and generalized tonic-clonic (GTC) seizures. He has also had a mild and gradual onset of gait instability, ataxia, hyperreflexia, and decreased visual acuity, which is worse at night. His fundoscopic examination shows a cherry red spot. Which of the following is the most likely diagnosis?
    a. Unverricht Lundborg syndrome
    b. Lafora body disease
    c. Sialidosis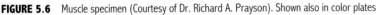
    d. Juvenile myoclonic epilepsy
    e. Neuronal ceroid lipofuscinosis

66. A 14-year-old boy with progressive cognitive decline and ataxia has a history of myoclonic epilepsy and multiple seizure types. His EEG shows spikes and waves with predominance in the occipital region. A diagnosis was made on the basis of skin biopsy, which showed periodic-acid-Schiff (PAS)-positive intracellular inclusions. Which of the following is the most likely finding in this patient?
    a. Mutation affecting cystatin B
    b. Cherry red spot on fundoscopic examination
    c. Ragged red fibers on muscle biopsy
    d. *EPM1* mutation
    e. *EPM2 A* mutation

67. A 12-year-old boy with intractable epilepsy is being evaluated for surgical treatment of Rasmussen's encephalitis. He has progressive cognitive decline, left hemiparesis, left visual field defect, and the EEG shows status epilepticus arising from the right hemisphere. Which of the following is incorrect regarding this condition?
    a. There are autoantibodies against the glutamate receptor subunit GluR3
    b. The seizures are typically well controlled with AED monotherapy

c. Histopathology shows perivascular cuffs of lymphocytes and monocytes, as well as glial nodules in the gray and white matter
d. There is spongy tissue degeneration in the long term
e. Hemispherectomy is a treatment option

68. Regarding the use of AEDs in the elderly, all the following statements are correct, except:
a. The distribution of hydrophilic drugs decreases
b. The distribution of lipophilic drugs decreases
c. Hepatic blood flow, bile flow, and protein synthesis decrease along with hepatic metabolism
d. Renal blood flow and glomerular filtration rate decrease
e. Gastric acidity may increase, making weakly basic drugs easily absorbed, and weakly acidic drugs less easily absorbed

69. An 18-year-old woman is diagnosed with juvenile myoclonic epilepsy, and her neurologist plans to start valproic acid for this type of epilepsy. She would like to know about the potential side effects of this medication. Which of the following is not a side effect of valproic acid?
a. Tremor
b. Hepatotoxicity
c. Hyperammonemia
d. Hyponatremia
e. Neural tube defects in children of mothers who take this medication

70. A 67-year-old man with a history of bipolar disorder and epilepsy is brought to the clinic by his wife. Over the past 6 months, since he was started on a new medication, he has become "meaner" and his wife states that she cannot stand him anymore, he yells all the time, and has become abusive and very aggressive. Which of the following medications is the patient most likely taking that would explain his behavior?
a. Lamotrigine
b. Valproic acid
c. Carbamazepine
d. Levetiracetam
e. Phenytoin

71. A 59-year-old man presents for evaluation of partial seizures and is prescribed an antiepileptic agent. About 2 weeks later he wakes up with a painful red eye and decreased visual acuity. He is diagnosed with acute closed-angle glaucoma. Which of the following is the most likely antiepileptic agent that he was prescribed recently?
a. Valproic acid
b. Levetiracetam
c. Phenytoin
d. Lamotrigine
e. Topiramate

72. A 42-year-old man with a history of hyperlipidemia and no prior history of epilepsy is brought to the emergency department after a seizure that witnesses described as generalized tonic–clonic, associated with tongue biting and urinary incontinence. The seizure lasted for less than a minute, and the patient was confused for about 20 minutes after the event. His neurologic examination is unremarkable. Which of the following statements is incorrect?

a. There is evidence in the literature to support the need for an EEG
b. Brain imaging is recommended
c. There are strong data to support the need to order routine blood count, glucose, and electrolytes
d. There is not enough evidence to support or refute the need for toxicology screen
e. An abnormal EEG may predict the risk of recurrence

73. Which of the following is correct regarding the EEG in Figure 5.7?

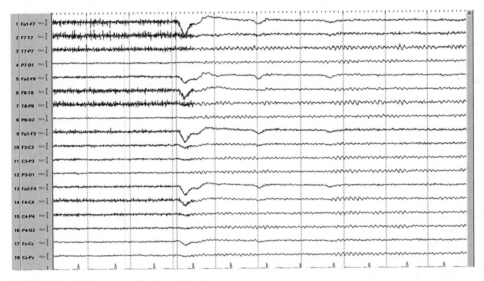

FIGURE 5.7   EEG (Courtesy of Dr. Joanna Fong)

a. There is poor reactivity of the posterior background
b. The patient has an occipital seizure
c. The posterior background shows δ-frequencies
d. An eye closure is recorded during this EEG page
e. The patient is sleeping

74. Which of the following is correct regarding EEG frequencies?
a. α-frequency is >13 Hz
b. β-frequency is 8 to 13 Hz
c. δ-frequency is <4 Hz
d. θ-frequency is 2 to 3 Hz
e. All of the above

75. Which of the following is not an activation procedure that is used during EEG recording to increase the diagnostic yield?
a. Hyperventilation
b. Sleep deprivation prior to the EEG
c. Noxious stimulation
d. Photic stimulation
e. Recording during sleep

76. Which of the following is the most likely diagnosis on the basis of the EEG shown in Figure 5.8?

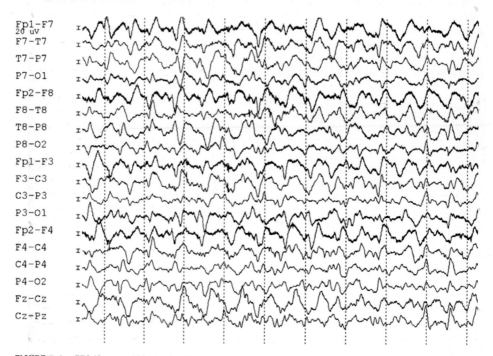

FIGURE 5.8   EEG (Courtesy of Dr. Joanna Fong)

   a. Hepatic encephalopathy
   b. Generalized periodic pattern
   c. A generalized seizure
   d. Postcardiac arrest anoxia
   e. Infantile spasms

77. Which of the following is consistent with the EEG shown in Figure 5.9?
   a. Burst suppression
   b. Triphasic waves
   c. Hypsarrhythmia
   d. Periodic lateralized epileptiform discharges (PLEDs)
   e. A generalized seizure

78. Which of the following is consistent with the EEG shown in Figure 5.10?
   a. Burst suppression
   b. Triphasic waves
   c. Generalized periodic pattern
   d. Periodic lateralized epileptiform discharges (PLEDs)
   e. Sharp waves

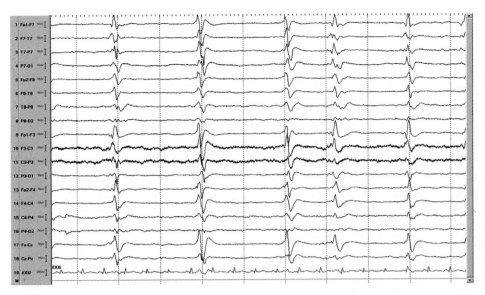

FIGURE 5.9   EEG (Courtesy of Dr. Joanna Fong)

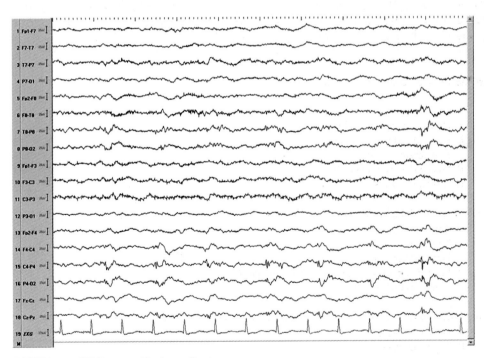

FIGURE 5.10   EEG (Courtesy of Dr. Joanna Fong)

Questions 79–81

79. K complexes are seen predominantly in which stage of sleep?
   a. Stage 1 sleep
   b. Stage 2 sleep
   c. Stage 3 sleep
   d. Stage 4 sleep
   e. REM sleep

80. How long after sleep onset does the first REM period normally occur?
   a. 15 minutes
   b. 30 minutes
   c. 45 minutes
   d. 60 minutes
   e. 90 minutes

81. Which of the following is considered to be the circadian pacemaker?
   a. Pineal gland
   b. Suprachiasmatic nucleus in the anterior hypothalamus
   c. Intralaminar thalamic nucleus
   d. Suprachiasmatic nucleus in the posterior hypothalamus
   e. Dorsolateral hypothalamus

82. Which of the following apnea–hypopnea indices (AHI) are diagnostic of moderate obstructive sleep apnea (OSA)?
   a. 0 to 5/hour
   b. 5 to 15/hour
   c. 15 to 30/hour
   d. 30 to 45/hour
   e. 45 to 60/hour

83. A 43-year-old man presents with excessive daytime sleepiness. During a polysomnogram he has at least 9 episodes/hour, in which he stops breathing for approximately 10 seconds. Sometimes these are associated with arousals. Despite absent airflow he has respiratory effort during these episodes. Which of the following is correct?
   a. This patient has central sleep apnea syndrome
   b. Polysomnogram is not helpful for the diagnosis
   c. This condition is associated with an increased risk of cardiovascular events
   d. Alcohol and sedatives do not worsen this condition
   e. Oxygen desaturation is rarely associated with these events

84. A 42-year-old obese woman presents with excessive daytime sleepiness. She has frequent arousals during the night and her husband reports that sometimes she stops breathing. A polysomnogram is performed and shows about 8 apneas/hour associated with desaturations. During these apneas in addition to no airflow there is no respiratory effort. Which of the following is correct regarding this condition?
   a. This patient has partial or complete airway obstruction that results in hypopneas and apneas
   b. There is a transient central cessation of respiratory drive
   c. Some cases need surgical interventions to reduce the airway obstruction

d. This is the most common form of sleep disorder of breathing

e. All of the above

85. A 10-year-old boy has been reported to have episodes during which he wakes up screaming, hyperventilating, and is tachycardic and diaphoretic. He appears to be asleep during the episode, and when he awakens he is confused and does not recall the event. Which of the following is correct regarding his sleep disorder? *✓ sleep terror.*

    a. This is a REM parasomnia

    b. This occurs out of sleep stage II

    c. This is a nightmare

    • d. This occurs out of slow-wave sleep

    e. This occurs more often during the last third of the night

86. A 16-year-old boy is reported to have episodes in which he walks around his house in the middle of the night. Once, during such an episode, he took the garbage out of his house and placed it in front of his neighbor's door. His neighbor tried to talk to him, but he did not respond. When the neighbor shook him, the patient suddenly changed his behavior, started to scream, and became violent and confused. A sleep disorder was later diagnosed. Which of the following is correct?

    a. This patient has a REM parasomnia

    b. This patient has confusional arousals

    c. This patient has narcolepsy

    • d. During these episodes, the EEG shows slow-wave sleep

    e. This patient has sleep terrors

87. A 12-year-old boy wakes up in the middle of the night with frightening dreams of a big clown eating his parents. On awaking, he recalls the dream well and does not look confused. Which of the following is the most likely diagnosis?

    ı a. Nightmares

    b. Confusional arousals

    c. Sleep terrors

    d. REM sleep behavior disorder

    e. Non-REM parasomnia

88. A 75-year-old man with a history of Parkinson's disease is brought for evaluation by his wife who reports that he frequently has very vivid dreams, in which he screams, kicks, and punches. She is concerned because she has been punched at least twice. Which of the following is not correct? *(Pts try to act out their dream or fight back).*

    a. This patient has a REM parasomnia

    b. This condition can be seen in patients with multisystem atrophy

    • c. Polysomnogram demonstrates the absence of muscle tone during REM sleep

    d. This patient has REM sleep behavior disorder (RBD)

    e. This condition can be seen in patients with dementia with Lewy bodies

89. Which of the following statements regarding sleep phenomena is not correct?

    a. Sleep paralysis is a feature of narcolepsy

    b. Hypnagogic hallucinations occur on falling asleep

    c. Hypnopompic hallucinations occur on waking up from sleep

    d. Patients have recollection of nightmares

    ɪ e. REM sleep behavior disorder (RBD) is associated with excessive atonia during REM sleep

90. A 14-year-old obese boy has recurrent episodes lasting up to 10 days, in which he sleeps almost continuously throughout the day and night, waking up only to eat and go to the bathroom. His mother reports that during these episodes he is in a bad mood. In between episodes he is a normal child. Which of the following is the most likely diagnosis?
   a. Idiopathic hypersomnia
   b. Narcolepsy
   c. Kleine–Levine syndrome
   d. Untreated obstructive sleep apnea syndrome
   e. Delayed sleep phase syndrome

91. An 18-year-old woman is referred for evaluation of possible pseudoseizures. During the episodes she loses muscle tone and falls to the floor suddenly, being unable to move for about 40 to 50 seconds. These episodes are often preceded by emotional triggers, frequently laughter. On further questioning, she reports being conscious during these events. She also reports being very sleepy during daytime, having multiple episodes of falling asleep during the day, after which she feels refreshed. Which of the following is the most likely diagnosis?
   a. Pseudoseizures
   b. Gelastic seizures
   c. Kleine–Levin syndrome
   d. Narcolepsy with cataplexy
   e. Idiopathic hypersomnia

92. Regarding narcolepsy with cataplexy, which of the following is incorrect?
   a. CSF hypocretin levels are increased
   b. During cataplexy, muscle tone is lost and patients are hyporeflexic or areflexic
   c. Sleep paralysis is frequent
   d. Mean sleep latency test (MSLT) needs to be performed to help make the diagnosis
   e. γ-hydroxybutyrate is approved for the treatment of narcolepsy with cataplexy

93. A 16-year-old girl complains of excessive sleepiness during the day, with difficulty waking up to go to school in the morning. At night, she has difficulty falling asleep and tosses and turns for a long time. On the weekends, even though she usually goes out with her friends and sleeps late at night, she wakes up without problems late in the day and feels refreshed. Which of the following is the most likely diagnosis?
   a. Psychophysiologic insomnia
   b. Delayed sleep phase syndrome
   c. Advanced sleep phase syndrome
   d. Jet lag syndrome
   e. Shift work sleep disorder

94. A 62-year-old man comes for evaluation of difficulty sleeping. He reports that he wakes up on his own every day at 4 AM, and cannot fall asleep again. He usually eats dinner at 5 PM and is very sleepy by 7 PM. Which of the following is the most likely diagnosis?
   a. Psychophysiologic insomnia
   b. Delayed sleep phase syndrome
   c. Advanced sleep phase syndrome
   d. Jet lag syndrome
   e. Shift work sleep disorder

95. A 45-year-old female who works at the nursing unit desk comes for evaluation of sleepiness during the daytime and episodes of insomnia. She usually works between 11 PM and 7 AM 3 days/week, and between 7 AM and 3 PM 2 days/week. During vacations, she tends to sleep well. Which of the following is the most likely diagnosis?
   a. Psychophysiologic insomnia
   b. Delayed sleep phase syndrome
   c. Advanced sleep phase syndrome
   d. Jet lag syndrome
   e. Shift work sleep disorder

96. A 32-year-old woman comes for evaluation of excessive daytime sleepiness and insomnia. She reports that she cannot fall asleep well despite going to bed early every day and attempts to fall asleep by reading or watching television while in her bed. She says that as the night advances she gets more anxious and continuously thinks about falling asleep. Which of the following is the most likely diagnosis?
   a. Psychophysiologic insomnia
   b. Delayed sleep phase syndrome
   c. Advanced sleep phase syndrome
   d. Jet lag syndrome
   e. Shift work sleep disorder

97. A 32-year-old woman complains of insomnia and excessive daytime sleepiness. She reports that when she goes to bed at night, she experiences an abnormal leg sensation that is hard to describe and is associated with an irresistible urge to move her legs. The urge to move her legs is temporarily relieved by moving them. Which of the following is the most likely diagnosis?
   a. Restless legs syndrome (RLS)
   b. Periodic limb movements of sleep (PLMS)
   c. Psychophysiologic insomnia
   d. Delayed sleep phase syndrome
   e. Advanced sleep phase syndrome

98. Which of the following is incorrect regarding restless legs syndrome (RLS)?
   a. Can be seen in patients with chronic renal failure
   b. Can be associated with folate deficiency
   c. Low ferritin levels are implicated in the pathophysiology of this condition
   d. Low hypocretin levels are implicated in the pathophysiology of this condition
   e. Dopamine agonists are used for the treatment of this condition

Answer Key

1. c	10. c	19. a	28. c	37. e	46. d
2. c	11. a	20. d	29. d	38. c	47. e
3. e	12. c	21. d	30. b	39. a	48. a
4. a	13. d	22. d	31. c	40. b	49. b
5. b	14. b	23. e	32. d	41. a	50. c
6. c	15. c	24. b	33. d	42. e	51. b
7. a	16. b	25. d	34. c	43. a	52. c
8. c	17. d	26. c	35. c	44. b	53. d
9. d	18. b	27. d	36. d	45. d	54. c

5. b

The ketogenic diet has been reported to be effective in refractory cases of epilepsy in childhood, even when multiple antiepileptic trials have failed. It is typically initiated in the hospital by starvation for 1–2 days in order to induce ketosis. This is followed by a strict diet in which 80% to 90% of calories are derived from fat. Surgical procedures such as vagus nerve stimulation and even more invasive procedures such as corpus callosotomy should be used as the last resort in select cases. Resective surgical therapies do not play a significant role in the treatment of generalized epilepsies. Carbamazepine and phenytoin can frequently worsen generalized epilepsy and are unlikely to be useful.

Bough KJ, Rho JM. Anticonvulsant mechanisms of the ketogenic diet. Epilepsia. 2007; 48:43–58.

Hartman AL, Vining EP. Clinical aspects of the ketogenic diet. Epilepsia. 2007; 48:31–42.

6. c

Supportive care is the general recommendation for the management of a simple febrile seizure (FS). It is estimated that about 3% to 5% of children aged 5 months to 5 years have simple FS. Ninety percent of these events occur in the first 3 years of life. One-third of patients have at least one additional seizure. Risk factors for having a simple FS include family history of FS, prolonged neonatal ICU stay, developmental delay, and day care. Incidence does not increase in proportion to increase in temperature. No risk factors are found in 50% of children with an FS. The risk of afebrile epilepsy after FS is increased in children with developmental delay, abnormal neurologic examination, complex FS (defined below), and a family history of afebrile seizures. There is a <5% risk that patients with a simple FS will develop epilepsy. It is estimated that approximately 15% of patients with epilepsy have a history of FS.

Simple FS are characterized by the following: <15 minutes in duration, generalized seizure, lack of focality, neurologically normal examination, no persistent deficits, and negative family history for seizures. Complex FS occur in approximately 20% of FS and are characterized by the following: >15 minutes in duration, focal features, abnormal neurologic examination, seizure recurrence in <24 hours, postictal signs (Todd's paralysis), and are more likely to be due to meningitis, encephalitis, or an underlying seizure disorder.

Prophylaxis is generally not needed, but can be considered for recurrent or prolonged seizures, afebrile seizures, after complex FS, and with an abnormal neurologic examination and developmental delay. Chronic prophylaxis commonly includes phenobarbital and valproic acid, whereas short-term prophylaxis could include diazepam and antipyretics, though definitive data on the use of antipyretics for the prevention of FS are lacking. Furthermore, the potential toxicities associated with available antiepileptic agents outweigh the relatively minor risks associated with simple FS. After reviewing the potential risks and benefits of available effective therapies for short- and long-term prophylaxis, the American Academy of Pediatrics concluded (in its clinical practice guideline on long-term management of children with FS) that neither continuous nor intermittent anticonvulsant therapy is recommended for children with one or more simple FS.

Berg AT, Shinnar S. Complex febrile seizures. Epilepsia. 1996; 37:126–133.

Knudsen FU. Febrile seizures: treatment and prognosis. Epilepsia. 2000; 41(1):2–9.

Steering Committee on Quality Improvement and Management, Subcommittee on Febrile Seizures American Academy of Pediatrics. Febrile seizures: clinical practice guideline for the long-term management of the child with simple febrile seizures. Pediatrics. 2008; 121:1281–1286.

7. a

Generalized epilepsy with febrile seizures plus (GEFS+) is considered to be a familial syndrome and *SCN1D* mutations are not a recognized cause. In contrast to febrile seizures (FS), which occur most commonly between 6 months and 5 years of age, the phenotype of "febrile seizures plus" includes patients in whom FS continue past the defined upper limit of age. GEFS+ may also be associated with afebrile generalized tonic-clonic (GTC) seizures. One-third of patients have other seizure types as well. The pattern of inheritance is usually complex, although initial genetic discoveries first identified an autosomal dominant familial pattern. Mutations of a number of ion channel genes have been identified in GEFS+ kindreds. These include sodium channel (SCN) subunits (*SCN1A*, *SCN1B*, and *SCN2A*) and GABA$_A$ receptor subunit genes (GABRD and GABRG2). The result is increased sodium channel activity or impaired GABA activity, ultimately leading to increased cortical hyperexcitability. The most frequently reported mutation is *SCN1A*, which encodes the pore-forming α-subunit of the sodium channel and comprises four transmembrane domains. The EEG usually shows generalized spike–wave or polyspikes.

Scheffer IE, Zhang YH, Jansen FE, et al. Dravet syndrome or genetic (generalized) epilepsy with febrile seizures plus? Brain Dev. 2009; 31(5):394–400.

Zucca C, Redaelli F, Epifanio R, et al. Cryptogenic epileptic syndromes related to SCN1A: twelve novel mutations identified. Arch Neurol. 2008; 65(4):489–494.

8. c

Rasmussen's syndrome is a rare, but severe, inflammatory brain disorder characterized by progressive unilateral hemispheric atrophy, associated progressive neurologic dysfunction (hemiparesis and cognitive deterioration), and intractable focal seizures (epilepsia partialis continua). Imaging reveals slowly progressive development of focal cortical atrophy, which correlates to the clinical findings. It has been postulated that antibodies to glutamate receptor-3 (GLUR3) may play a pathogenic role, although the available data are conflicting and the specificity of GLUR3 antibodies in the pathogenesis of Rasmussen's encephalitis has been challenged in recent years. The focal cortical atrophy is progressive and eventually spreads to the surrounding cortical areas in the same hemisphere, and thus, the best treatment option for the patient's intractable seizures is the surgical approach with hemispherectomy. The other listed options are all developmental cortical malformations, with porencephaly often resulting from an ischemic insult in utero.

Bien CG, Granata T, Antozzi C, et al. Pathogenesis, diagnosis and treatment of Rasmussen encephalitis: a European consensus statement. Brain. 2005; 128:454–471.

Bien CG, Urbach H, Deckert M, et al. Diagnosis and staging of Rasmussen's encephalitis by serial MRI and histopathology. Neurology. 2003; 58:250–257.

9. d

Most progressive myoclonic epilepsies are due to either lysosomal storage disorders and/or mitochondrial disorders. They are characterized by progressive cognitive decline, myoclonus (epileptic and nonepileptic), seizures (tonic–clonic, tonic, and myoclonic), and may be associated with ataxia or movement disorders. Examples include Lafora body disease, Unverricht Lundborg syndrome, neuronal ceroid lipofuscinosis, myoclonic epilepsy with ragged red fibers (MERRF), and sialidosis. Valproic acid is often the first-line treatment for myoclonic epilepsy. Caution is advised with use of valproic acid in patients with mitochondrial mutations, such as *POLG* gene mutations, because fulminant hepatic failure may result. Other treatments include clonazepam, levetiracetam, topiramate, and zonisamide. Lamotrigine is sometimes used, but caution is advised because it rarely may worsen myoclonic seizures. Gabapentin, carbamazepine, pregabalin, and vigabatrin are also known to exacerbate some myoclonic epilepsies.

Genton P, Gelisse P. Antimyoclonic effect of levetiracetam. Epileptic Disord. 2000; 2:209–212.

Malphrus AD, Wilfong AA. Use of the newer antiepileptic drugs in pediatric epilepsies. Curr Treat Option Neurol. 2007; 9(4):256–267.

10. c

Fosphenytoin is an IV prodrug of phenytoin. It is composed of a disodium phosphate ester that is water soluble and less alkaline than phenytoin. It does not include propylene glycol and ethyl alcohol as a solvent vehicle as is the case with IV phenytoin. Fosphenytoin can be loaded at a faster rate, but because the fosphenytoin needs to be converted into phenytoin in plasma, the rate of rise of serum levels is approximately equal to that of phenytoin. Compared to phenytoin, fosphenytoin is not associated with purple glove syndrome, it can be given more rapidly intravenously, its administration is associated with a lower occurrence of cardiovascular side effects, such as hypotension, and it can be given intramuscularly. Purple glove syndrome may ensue when phenytoin infiltrates into the subcutaneous tissue, resulting in swelling, pain, and discoloration of the extremity because of blood vessel leakage. The most common side effects of IV fosphenytoin include pruritus, as well as the other less problematic and typical phenytoin side effects, such as dizziness, nystagmus, and drowsiness.

Bradley WG, Daroff RB, Fenichel GM, et al. Neurology in Clinical Practice, 5th ed. Philadelphia, PA: Elsevier; 2008.

Fischer JH, Patel TV, Fischer PA. Fosphenytoin: clinical pharmacokinetics and comparative advantages in the acute treatment of seizures. Clin Pharmacokinet. 2003; 42(1):33–58.

11. a

Topiramate is typically not associated with myoclonic seizure exacerbation. Lamotrigine, gabapentin, carbamazepine, pregabalin, and vigabatrin are known to exacerbate some myoclonic epilepsies.

Guerrini R, Belmonte A, Parmeggiani L, et al. Myoclonic status epilepticus following high-dosage lamotrigine therapy. Brain Dev. 1999; 21:420–424.

Welty TE. Juvenile myoclonic epilepsy: epidemiology, pathophysiology, and management. Paediatr Drugs. 2006; 8(5):303–310.

12. c

Valproic acid is the only antiepileptic medication listed that is a hepatic enzyme inhibitor. All others listed are hepatic enzyme inducers. This information is important to know in order to safely prescribe a concurrent antiepileptic or other medications. Concurrent use of valproic acid with medications that undergo the same hepatic enzyme metabolism, may result in dangerously elevated serum levels of these medications because their metabolism is inhibited. An example would be concurrent valproic acid and warfarin, which could result in elevated INR levels and, thus, increased bleeding risk.

Wyllie E, Gupta A, Lachhwani DK (Eds). The Treatment of Epilepsy: Principles and Practice, 4th ed. Philadelphia, PA: Lippincott Williams & Wilkins; 2005.

13. d

-Hz spike and wave is characteristic for absence epilepsy. The other options are benign EEG patterns unassociated with seizures (also known as normal variants). Absence epilepsy has a peak age around 6 years and more often affects girls (70%). These patients are generally normal neurologically. Absence epilepsy is characterized by multiple daily spells lasting a few seconds. They begin and end abruptly and interrupt whatever activity is being carried out. During a seizure, there will often be a blank stare; automatisms such as lip smacking, nose rubbing, and picking at clothes may also be present, especially with longer episodes. These seizures are classically provoked by hypoglycemia and hyperventilation. Mild ictal jerks of eyelids, eyes, and eyebrows may occur at the onset of the seizure. The thalamus is implicated in the generation and sustainment of absence epilepsy with the low-threshold (T-type) calcium channels of thalamic neurons playing a central role in thalamocortical interactions. First-line treatment includes ethosuximide (which acts via T-type calcium channel inhibition). Valproic acid, lamotrigine, topiramate, and zonisamide are also used. Notably, the use of lamotrigine has been associated with aggravation of absence seizures on rare occasions. In a double-blind, randomized, controlled clinical trial, the efficacy, tolerability, and neuropsychologic effects of ethosuximide, valproic acid, and lamotrigine were compared in children with newly diagnosed childhood absence epilepsy. Ethosuximide and valproic acid were found to be more effective than lamotrigine. Notably, ethosuximide was also associated with fewer adverse attentional effects, and therefore, it is considered to be the best choice for initial empirical monotherapy in children with absence epilepsy.

Valproic acid or lamotrigine are often the drugs of choice when there are concurrent generalized tonic-clonic (GTC) and absence seizures. It is important to note that $GABA_B$ receptors promote activation of T-type calcium channels. Therefore, some GABAergic drugs can exacerbate absence seizures.

Antiepileptic medications can often be discontinued as the child grows older, if the EEG is normal, and there have been no seizures for 1 to 2 years. Absence epilepsy carries a good prognosis. Eighty percent of children have remission through adolescence and at least 90% eventually have remission overall.

Glauser TA, Cnaan A, Shinnar S, et al. Ethosuximide, valproic acid, and lamotrigine in childhood absence epilepsy. N Engl J Med. 2010; 362(9):790–799.

Wyllie E, Gupta A, Lachhwani DK (Eds). The Treatment of Epilepsy: Principles and Practice, 4th ed. Philadelphia, PA: Lippincott Williams & Wilkins; 2005.

14. b

The adult pattern of normal posterior dominant α-rhythm in older children and adults is usually seen by the age of 8 to 10 years. The following is a review of adult EEG frequencies:

$-\beta >13$ Hz
$-\alpha$ 8 to 13 Hz
$-\theta$ 4 to 7 Hz
$-\delta <4$ Hz

Bradley WG, Daroff RB, Fenichel GM, et al. Neurology in Clinical Practice, 5th ed. Philadelphia, PA: Elsevier; 2008.

Levin K, Luders H. Comprehensive Clinical Neurophysiology, Philadelphia, PA: WB Saunders Company; 2000.

15. c

Periodic lateralized epileptiform discharges (PLEDs) would be expected, and are also discussed in question 78. PLEDs consist of unilateral or bilateral, independent, high-amplitude, sharp, and slow-wave complexes at 0.5 to 3 Hz. Any destructive process such as anoxia, HSV encephalitis, stroke, and tumor can cause PLEDs. Triphasic waves are seen with hepatic coma, anoxia, drug toxicity, and other toxic and metabolic encephalopathies. Triphasic waves are generalized and maximal bifrontal, and consist of a prominent positive wave preceded and followed by minor negative waves at 0.5- to 2-Hz intervals. Wicket spikes belong to the benign normal variants. Polyspikes and fast spike–wave complexes are true epileptiform discharges.

Levin K, Luders H. Comprehensive Clinical Neurophysiology. Philadelphia, PA: WB Saunders Company; 2000.

16. b

Phenytoin, carbamazepine, gabapentin, and lamotrigine have all been associated with aggravation of absence seizures and even absence status epilepticus in children with absence epilepsy. Topiramate does not have this association.

Kaplan PW, Drislane FW (Eds). Nonconvulsive Status Epilepticus. New York: Demos Medical Publishing; 2009.

Manning JP, Richards DA, Bowery NG. Pharmacology of absence epilepsy. Trends Pharmacol Sci. 2003; 24(10):542–549.

Shorvon S, Walker M. Status epilepticus in idiopathic generalized epilepsy. Epilepsia. 2005; 46(Suppl 9):73–79.

17. d

Many enzyme-inducing antiepileptics (phenytoin, carbamazepine, phenobarbital, oxcarbazepine, and topiramate at doses >200 mg/day) increase metabolism of oral contraceptives. Antiepileptic medications with minimal oral contraceptive interaction include valproic acid, gabapentin, pregabalin, levetiracetam, zonisamide, tiagabine, and topiramate (at doses <200 mg/day).

Crawford P. Best practice guidelines for the management of women with epilepsy. Epilepsia 2005; 46(Suppl 9):117–124.

18. b

This EEG reveals a run of 3-Hz spike and wave discharges typically seen with absence seizures in childhood absence epilepsy. A paroxysmal 3-Hz spike and wave pattern emerges abruptly out of a normal background and suddenly ceases after a few seconds. Absence epilepsy is discussed further in question 13.

Levin K, Luders H. Comprehensive Clinical Neurophysiology, Philadelphia, PA: WB Saunders Company; 2000.

19. a, 20. d

The EEG in Figure 5.2 reveals polyspikes in a patient with juvenile myoclonic epilepsy (JME), and the history is also very suggestive of this disorder. Valproic acid is typically the first-line agent for JME. JME is one of the idiopathic generalized epilepsies. Onset is typically between 8 and 24 years (peaks in teens). Development is typically normal. Boys and girls seem to be equally affected. Myoclonic seizures constitute the most frequent seizure type. These are usually described as large-amplitude and bilateral simultaneous myoclonic jerks. Myoclonic seizures are predominantly seen on awakening, and the patient often complains about being "clumsy" in the morning and frequently dropping things. Falls are not infrequent. There is typically no loss of consciousness, although myoclonic seizures can occasionally be followed by a generalized tonic-clonic (GTC) seizure. Most patients have infrequent GTC seizures, which usually also occur on awakening. Some patients with JME also have typical absence seizures. The EEG reveals generalized 4- to 6-Hz polyspike and wave discharges interictally. Ictally, trains of spikes are seen, which are commonly triggered by photic stimulation (during EEG recordings). The first-line treatment is with valproic acid. Second-line treatments include lamotrigine, levetiracetam, topiramate, and zonisamide. Carbamazepine and phenytoin should be avoided because they may lead to worsening of myoclonic seizures, similar to the worsening of childhood absence epilepsy seen with these agents. Good control will generally require lifelong treatment and avoidance of triggers, such as alcohol intake and lack of sleep.

Auvin S. Treatment of juvenile myoclonic epilepsy. CNS Neurosci Ther. 2008; 14(3):227–233.

Levin K, Luders H. Comprehensive Clinical Neurophysiology, Philadelphia, PA: WB Saunders Company; 2000.

Ropper AH, Samuels MA. Adams and Victor's principles of Neurology, 9th ed. New York: McGraw-Hill; 2009.

21. d, 22. d

The history and EEG in Figure 5.3 suggest benign childhood epilepsy with centrotemporal spikes (benign rolandic epilepsy of childhood). The EEG classically reveals bilateral independent centrotemporal spikes on a normal background. The discharges on the two sides can be either independent or synchronized. They may extend beyond the centrotemporal regions. Although the spikes on the EEG appear in the centrotemporal area, the temporal lobe is not the generator of these spikes. Rather, they are felt to be generated in the base of the rolandic fissure.

Benign childhood epilepsy with centrotemporal spikes (benign rolandic epilepsy of childhood) is fairly common and accounts for about 25% of childhood seizures. Onset is usually between 2 and 13 years of age, and the condition typically resolves in the midteenage years. Seizures are characterized by focal motor, sensory, or autonomic manifestations involving predominantly the face, mouth, throat, or extremities, although secondary generalization can occur. These are seizures that classically occur nocturnally (70% only in sleep, 15% only awake, and 15% both). EEG is characterized by the presence of independent bilateral, repetitive, broad, centrotemporal interictal EEG spikes on a normal background. The discharges are thought to arise from the vicinity of the precentral and postcentral gyri in the lower suprasylvian region. The characteristic EEG spike pattern is inherited as an autosomal dominant trait with variable penetrance. Normal development, physical examination, and brain imaging is the rule, though there are exceptions. Seizures respond well to certain antiepileptic medication and carbamazepine is usually considered the first line of therapy in the United States. It is important to note that it is often not necessary to treat with AEDs unless seizures are prolonged or frequent; some advocate waiting for two or more seizures to occur before initiating treatment. If antiepileptic medications are started, they can generally be stopped after adolescence. (Only 10% continue to have seizures 5 years after onset.)

Bouma PA, Bovenkerk AC, Westendorp RG, et al. The course of benign partial epilepsy of childhood with centrotemporal spikes: a meta-analysis. Neurology. 1997; 48(2):430–437.

Heijbel J, Blom S, Rasmuson M. Benign epilepsy of childhood with centrotemporal EEG foci: a genetic study. Epilepsia. 1975; 16:285–293.

Levin K, Luders H. Comprehensive Clinical Neurophysiology, Philadelphia, PA: WB Saunders Company; 2000.

23. e

The EEG in Figure 5.4 reveals periodic lateralized epileptiform discharges (PLEDs). PLEDs occur in acute lateralized pathology, such as a stroke, HSV encephalitis, rapidly expanding tumor, or any other destructive process to the brain parenchyma. PLEDs are discussed further in question 15.

Levin K, Luders H. Comprehensive Clinical Neurophysiology, Philadelphia, PA: WB Saunders Company; 2000.

24. b, 25. d

The EEG in Figure 5.5 reveals hypsarrhythmia, which is the most common interictal EEG correlate of infantile spasms. Hypsarrhythmia is characterized by abnormal interictal high-amplitude slow waves on a background of irregular multifocal spikes. These waves and spikes have no consistent pattern or rhythm and vary in duration and size, resulting in a chaotic-appearing EEG record. Hypsarrhythmia disappears ictally during a cluster of spasms and/or REM sleep.

Infantile spasms occur during the first year of life (typically 3–8 months), and are discussed further in question 45. They are characterized by sudden tonic extension or flexion of limbs and axial body, often occurring in clusters, and especially shortly after awakening. West syndrome is a triad of infantile spasms, hypsarrhythmia, and mental retardation. This disorder often occurs due to pre/peri/postnatal insults, tuberous sclerosis, cerebral dysgenesis, and others. Treatment with ACTH is generally first line, but it is expensive, especially in the United States. Other treatments include corticosteroids, vigabatrin, clonazepam, levetiracetam, topiramate, pyridoxine, and valproic acid. Vigabatrin has been associated with retinal toxicity.

Levin K, Luders H. Comprehensive Clinical Neurophysiology. Philadelphia, PA: WB Saunders Company; 2000.

Mackay MT, Weiss SK, Adams-Webber T, et al. Practice parameter: medical treatment of infantile spasms: report of the American Academy of Neurology and the Child Neurology Society. Neurology. 2004; 62:1668–1681.

Ropper AH, Brown RH. Adams and Victor's Principles of Neurology, 8th ed. New York: McGraw-Hill; 2005.

Wong M, Trevathan E. Infantile Spasms. Pediatr Neurol. 2001; 24:89–98.

26. c, 27. d, 28. c

Phenytoin is used for the treatment of partial and/or generalized tonic-clonic (GTC) seizures (primary or secondary). Its primary mechanism of action is inhibition of voltage-dependent neuronal sodium channels. It undergoes predominantly liver metabolism, although there is also minimal renal metabolism. Patients who are in low-protein disease states (such as liver failure, etc.) need to be followed with free phenytoin levels because of less available protein for binding, making the total levels unreliable. It is important to understand that phenytoin exhibits nonlinear (zero-order) kinetics, as the metabolic pathways responsible for its metabolism become saturated. This means that when the dose of phenytoin is increased beyond a certain point, its plasma concentration at steady state will no longer increase in a proportionate manner, rather small dose changes may result in a large/toxic increment in plasma concentrations. In general, phenytoin approaches zero-order kinetics at total levels >10 to 15 μg/mL and small dose increments can potentially cause large increases in the serum level.

Idiosyncratic reactions caused by phenytoin include aplastic anemia, Stevens–Johnson syndrome, and hepatic failure. Other side effects include thrombocytopenia, lymphadenopathy, gingival hyperplasia, acne, coarse facial features (also called "phenytoin facies," from hypertrophy of subcutaneous facial tissue), hirsutism, purple glove syndrome (with intravenous administration), nystagmus, ataxia, dysarthria, diplopia, nausea, dizziness, and drowsiness. Phenytoin can also cause folate deficiency and increased vitamin D metabolism, resulting in premature osteoporosis. Chronically, its use has been associated with a usually mild peripheral neuropathy and with cerebellar, but not cortical atrophy. Acutely, the IV form can cause phlebitis, pain, burning, hypotension, and cardiac conduction abnormalities. Phenytoin is a liver enzyme inducer, so it can increase metabolism of many other drugs.

There are variations of calculating loading and correcting doses of phenytoin. A general simple formula for calculating a supplementing (or loading) IV bolus of phenytoin is as follows: (target total phenytoin level − current total phenytoin level) × (kilogram body weight × volume of distribution). The therapeutic range for phenytoin is 10 to 20 μg/mL. The range for volume of distribution for phenytoin is 0.5 to 1 L/kg, with an average of 0.8 L/kg often used. If we insert the numbers from the case into the formula, the calculation will be as follows: (15 − 10) × (75 × 0.8) = 300 mg. An accurate reassessment of new levels can be obtained by checking free and total levels approximately 2 hours after the IV load.

Ahn JE, Cloyd JC, Brundage RC, et al. Phenytoin half-life and clearance during maintenance therapy in adults and elderly patients with epilepsy. Neurology. 2008; 71(1):38–43.

Ropper AH, Samuels MA. Adams and Victor's Principles of Neurology, 9th ed. New York: McGraw-Hill; 2009.

Schachter SC. Review of the mechanisms of action of antiepileptic drugs. CNS Drugs. 1995; 4:469–477.

29. d, 30. b, 31. c

The correcting IV bolus for valproic acid is as follows: (target total valproic acid level − current total valproic acid level) × (kilogram body weight × volume of distribution). The therapeutic range for valproic acid is 50 to 100 μg/mL. The range for volume of distribution for valproic acid is 0.1 to 0.3 L/kg, with an average of 0.2 L/kg often used. If we apply this formula to the case, the result is as follows: (100 − 70) × (70 × 0.2) = 420 mg.

Valproic acid has broad-spectrum antiseizure activity and is commonly used in partial, generalized tonic-clonic (GTC), absence, myoclonic, and tonic seizures, as well as infantile spasms. Its mechanism of action is by sodium and T-type calcium channel antagonism, and it also works as an agonist at the GABA$_A$ receptor. It primarily undergoes liver metabolism and is a hepatic enzyme inhibitor. Side effects include cognitive and gastrointestinal complaints. Infrequently, it can cause increased liver enzymes and, rarely, idiosyncratic fatal hepatitis (most common in those <2 years of age). Chronically, it can cause weight gain, hair thinning, polycystic ovarian syndrome, acne, menstrual irregularities, tremor, pancreatitis, and thrombocytopenia. Cerebellar atrophy occurs with long-term phenytoin use, but not with valproic acid.

Valproic acid significantly increases the half-life of lamotrigine by 24 to 48 hours. Initiation of as little as 500 mg of valproic acid in chronic lamotrigine users may necessitate an immediate 50% reduction in the dose of lamotrigine.

Löscher W. Basic pharmacology of valproate: a review after 35 years of clinical use for the treatment of epilepsy. CNS Drugs. 2002; 16:669–694.

Ropper AH, Samuels MA. Adams and Victor's Principles of Neurology, 9th ed. New York: McGraw-Hill; 2009.

32. d, 33. d, 34. c, 35. c

Carbamazepine is used for partial or secondarily generalized tonic-clonic (GTC) seizures, although it is important to remember that it can rarely worsen some generalized epilepsies (including myoclonic and absence epilepsies), similar to phenytoin. Its primary mode of action is via blockade of sodium channels, which leads to a decrease/prevention of repetitive firing in depolarized neurons. Side effects include dizziness, vertigo, fatigue, drowsiness, diplopia, nystagmus, headache, nausea, vomiting, elevated liver function tests, hyponatremia, and ataxia. Serious idiosyncratic reactions include Stevens–Johnson syndrome, leukopenia, and aplastic anemia.

Carbamazepine undergoes liver metabolism with renal excretion of metabolites, so caution is advised with kidney or liver failure. Carbamazepine is also a hepatic enzyme inducer, and undergoes autoinduction. The dose must be titrated up gradually to allow tolerance to develop to its CNS side effects, but also to avoid early toxicity as carbamazepine "autoinduces" the hepatic enzymes responsible for its own metabolism. If carbamazepine is started at too high of a dose, or titrated too fast, the result would be elevated carbamazepine levels with accompanying toxicity early on, as the hepatic enzymes responsible for carbamazepine's metabolism have not been fully activated (autoinduced) yet. It is therefore important to remember that carbamazepine's half-life decreases from 30 hours to 10 to 20 hours after the first few days to weeks of use. Autoinduction is completed after 3 to 5 weeks of a fixed dosing regimen. Plasma concentrations decrease in the first 1 to 2 months, and during this time, the dose of carbamazepine should be gradually increased. Therefore, carbamazepine would not be a good option if quick control of new-onset, frequent seizures was desired. Of note, oxcarbazepine does not undergo autoinduction and can be titrated faster.

Oxcarbazepine is a structural derivative of carbamazepine, and is reduced to 10-monohydroxy-carbamazepine and unlike carbamazepine does not undergo oxidation to epoxide. Carbamazepine on the other hand is oxidized to 10,11-carbamazepine epoxide, which is the principal metabolite of carbamazepine. It is important to remember that the 10,11-carbamazepine epoxide is pharmacologically active and responsible for many of the side effects seen with carbamazepine use. Because of these differences, oxcarbazepine has less side effects, overall, as compared to carbamazepine. Oxcarbazepine has less liver enzyme induction, no autoinduction (and can thus be titrated more rapidly), and is used for the same seizure types as carbamazepine, having the same mechanism of action, metabolic pathways, and side-effect profile. Approximately 30% of patients who have a history of a rash with carbamazepine will also develop a rash when exposed to oxcarbazepine.

Valproic acid inhibits the metabolism of the pharmacologically active 10,11-carbamazepine epoxide (the principal metabolite of carbamazepine). Thus, although the carbamazepine level may be normal, the patient may experience toxicity because of elevated 10,11-carbamazepine epoxide levels. The 10,11-carbamazepine epoxide is not routinely measured, but can be ordered specifically if there are concerns about toxicity.

Koch MW, Polman SK. Oxcarbazepine versus carbamazepine monotherapy for partial onset seizures. Cochrane Database Syst Rev. 2009;CD006453.

Porter RJ. How to initiate and maintain carbamazepine therapy in children and adults. Epilepsia. 1987; 28(Suppl 3):S59–S63.

Purcell TB, McPheeters RA, Feil M, et al. Rapid oral loading of carbamazepine in the emergency department. Ann Emerg Med. 2007; 50(2):121–126.

Tudur SM, Marson AG, Clough HE, et al. Carbamazepine versus phenytoin monotherapy for epilepsy. Cochrane Database Syst Rev. 2002; (2):CD001911.

36. d

Benzodiazepines are broad-spectrum antiepileptic medications used most commonly for partial, generalized tonic-clonic (GTC), absence, and myoclonic seizures, as well as status epilepticus. They work as GABA$_A$ agonists. Binding to the GABA$_A$ receptor leads to subsequent activation of chloride channels and, as a result, hyperpolarization of the neuronal membrane and decreased neuronal excitability. Benzodiazepines, in general, undergo liver metabolism and renal excretion of their metabolites.

Brunton LL, Lazo JS, Parker KL, eds. Goodman and Gilmans' Pharmacological Basis of Therapeutics, 11th ed. New York: McGraw-Hill; 2005.

37. e, 38. c

Lamotrigine is typically well tolerated as long as it is introduced gradually with a slow titration, although dizziness, blurred vision, diplopia, and ataxia may be seen. Stevens–Johnson syndrome, or toxic epidermal necrolysis, is associated with concurrent use of valproic acid or rapid lamotrigine titration, and this risk appears to be increased in ages younger than 16 years. Cognitive disturbances are typically not seen with lamotrigine. Lamotrigine is a broad-spectrum antiepileptic medication and is used for partial and generalized tonic-clonic seizures (GTC), as well as generalized seizures of Lennox–Gastaut syndrome. It has also been used for absence and myoclonic seizures, although it is not the first line of therapy for these types of seizures. It works as a sodium channel antagonist and also inhibits glutamate release. It undergoes liver metabolism with renal excretion of metabolites.

Oral contraceptives and hormone replacement therapy increase lamotrigine clearance and, thus, decrease serum lamotrigine levels. This effect appears to be limited to contraceptives containing ethinylestradiol. Progesterone-only medications do not appear to have this effect. During pregnancy, lamotrigine clearance may increase up to 65%, which may result in breakthrough seizures. Therefore, monitoring of lamotrigine serum levels with dose adjustments is recommended during pregnancy and after delivery.

de Haan GJ, Edelbroek P, Segers J, et al. Gestation-induced changes in lamotrigine pharmacokinetics: a monotherapy study. Neurology. 2004; 63:571–573.

LaRoche SM, Helmers SL. The new antiepileptic drugs: scientific review. JAMA. 2004; 291:605–614.

Tran TA, Leppik IE, Blesi K, et al. Lamotrigine clearance during pregnancy. Neurology 2002; 59:251–255.

39. a, 40. b

Topiramate is a broad-spectrum antiepileptic used for partial, generalized tonic-clonic (GTC) and absence seizures, and for Lennox–Gastaut syndrome. It has multiple mechanisms of action, including voltage-dependent sodium channel antagonism, enhancement of GABA activity through a nonbenzodiazepine site on GABA$_A$ receptors, and antagonism of AMPA/kainate glutamate receptors. It is predominantly excreted unchanged in urine with minimal liver metabolism.

Similar to zonisamide, topiramate is also a weak carbonic anhydrase inhibitor, which explains the potential risk of renal stone formation in patients treated with these agents. Other side effects include paresthesias, decreased appetite, weight loss, dizziness, fatigue, and cognitive complaints, such as word-finding difficulty and slowed thinking. Acute angle-closure glaucoma has been reported, but is rare.

Glauser TA, Dlugos DJ, Dodson WE, et al. Topiramate monotherapy in newly diagnosed epilepsy in children and adolescents. J Child Neurol. 2007; 22:693–699.

Meldrum BS. Update on the mechanism of action of antiepileptic drugs. Epilepsia. 1996; 37(Suppl 6):S4–S11.

41. a

Lacosamide works by selective enhancement of slow inactivation of voltage-dependent sodium channels. The result is inhibition of repetitive neuronal firing and stabilization of hyperexcitable neuronal membranes. Lacosamide is also known to interfere with the activity of the collapsing response mediator protein-2 (CRMP-2), a cell protein involved in neuronal differentiation and axonal guidance. The nature of the interaction between lacosamide and CRMP-2 and its role in seizure control are unclear. Lacosamide is FDA approved as an adjunct for partial-onset seizures in patients aged 17 years and older. It is available in oral or IV formulation. It is eliminated primarily by renal excretion and has little drug–drug interaction with other antiepileptic medications. Dizziness and nausea are the most common side effects.

Beyreuther BK, Freitag J, Heers C, et al. Lacosamide: a review of preclinical properties. CNS Drug Rev. 2007; 13:21–42.

Perucca E, Yasothan U, Clincke G, et al. Lacosamide. Nat Rev Drug Discov. 2008; 7:973–974.

42. e

Rufinamide is not metabolized by the cytochrome P (CYP) 450 system. Rufinamide modulates the activity of neuronal sodium channels, resulting in prolongation of the inactive state of the channel. It is FDA approved as an adjunctive treatment of seizures associated with Lennox–Gastaut syndrome in children 4 years and older, and adults.

Rufinamide undergoes extensive metabolism, with only 4% excreted as parent drug. Rufinamide is primarily metabolized via enzymatic hydrolysis of the carboxylamide group to form carboxylic acid. This metabolic route is not CYP 450 dependent. There are no known active metabolites. Elimination of rufinamide is predominantly via urine. Plasma half-life of rufinamide is approximately 6 to 10 hours. Rufinamide shows little or no inhibition of most CYP 450 enzymes at clinically relevant concentrations, with weak inhibition of CYP 2E1. Rufinamide is a weak inducer of the CYP 3A4 enzyme.

Perucca E, Cloyd J, Critchley D, et al. Rufinamide: clinical pharmacokinetics and concentration-response relationships in patients with epilepsy. Epilepsia. 2008; 49:1123–1141.

43. a

This patient has complex partial seizures originating from the temporal lobe, most likely from the mesial temporal lobe region. These are often associated with mesial temporal lobe sclerosis. Complex partial seizures arise from a focal area of epileptogenicity, and unlike simple partial seizures, are associated with impairment of consciousness.

Mesial temporal lobe seizures are characterized by behavioral arrest, and may be preceded by an aura (a simple partial seizure), such as a rising epigastric sensation, nausea, olfactory and/or gustatory hallucinations, a sensation of fear and terror, or other emotional changes, as well as autonomic manifestations such as tachycardia, respiratory changes, face flushing, or pallor. Patients may also experience dysmnesic manifestations such as déjà vu (sensation of familiarity as if an experience has occurred before, although it has not), déjà entendu (if the experience is auditory), jamais vu (sensation that a familiar experience is new, although it is not), jamais entendu (if the latter experience is auditory), or panoramic vision (a rapid recollection of episodes from the past). During the seizure, the patient may also have automatisms, which are involuntary complex motor activities, such as nose picking, lip smacking, chewing, and picking with the hands. Typically patients have postictal confusion, which is not present in absence seizures.

Frontal lobe seizures are abrupt in onset, brief, and predominantly associated with elementary motor manifestations, but may include complex automatisms. They frequently occur in sleep, often in clusters. Parietal lobe seizures are predominantly associated with episodic sensory symptoms, although clinical localization may be difficult as parietal discharges propagate to other brain regions. Occipital lobe seizures usually present with visual phenomena. Given the focal discharges on the EEG and characteristic clinical features, this patient does not have absence seizures.

Bradley WG, Daroff RB, Fenichel GM, et al. Neurology in Clinical Practice, 5th ed. Philadelphia, PA: Elsevier; 2008.

Browne TR, Holmes GL. Handbook of Epilepsy. 4th ed. Philadelphia, PA: Lippincott Williams & Wilkins; 2008.

44. b

This patient has seizures coming from his frontal lobe, more specifically the right supplementary motor area (SMA). The typical semiology of these seizures has been referred to as "fencer's posture," a tonic posture in which the patient exhibits deviation of the eyes and head, as well as tonic arm extension to the side contralateral to the hemisphere where seizures are originating. These seizures are frequent, occurring in clusters or many times per day, and frequently arising during sleep. They are usually difficult to treat with medications.

Given the lateralization in this case, the left side is unlikely to be the origin of these seizures. Temporal lobe seizures are described in question 43. Parietal seizures are predominantly associated with episodic sensory symptoms, which include positive symptoms such as tingling or, less commonly, negative symptoms such as asomatognosia. In posterior parietal seizures, visual phenomena may occur.

Bradley WG, Daroff RB, Fenichel GM, et al. Neurology in Clinical Practice, 5th ed. Philadelphia, PA: Elsevier; 2008.

Browne TR, Holmes GL. Handbook of Epilepsy, 4th ed. Philadelphia, PA: Lippincott Williams & Wilkins; 2008.

45. d

This patient has infantile spasms with an EEG (Figure 5.5) that shows hypsarrhythmia. These patients usually have developmental arrest and a poor prognosis with respect to neurologic recovery, and this type of seizures should be treated.

Infantile spasms are better viewed as a type of seizure rather than an epilepsy syndrome, and are also discussed in questions 24 and 25. The triad of infantile spasms, hypsarrhythmia, and developmental arrest is known as West syndrome. This condition has been associated with multiple etiologies, such as hypoxic–ischemic injuries, brain malformations or structural abnormalities, congenital or acquired infections, chromosomal abnormalities, and inborn errors of metabolism. Infantile spasms are frequent in patients with tuberous sclerosis and this condition should be considered in this setting. Every patient presenting with infantile spasms should have an appropriate, thorough workup to look for the cause, including a brain MRI. In close to 30% of the cases, no specific etiology is found, and these cases are considered cryptogenic.

ACTH is commonly used for the treatment of infantile spasms. ACTH should be used carefully, given its potential side effects, which include hypertension, hyperglycemia, weight gain, electrolyte abnormalities, risk of infections, risk of avascular necrosis, and gastrointestinal bleeding. Vigabatrin may also be used for the treatment of infantile spasms, especially in patients with tuberous sclerosis. Vigabatrin should be used with caution as it carries the risk of retinal toxicity.

Bradley WG, Daroff RB, Fenichel GM, et al. Neurology in Clinical Practice, 5th ed. Philadelphia, PA: Elsevier; 2008.

Korff CM, Nordli DR. Epilepsy syndromes in infancy. Pediatr Neurol. 2006; 34:253–263.

46. d

This patient has Aicardi syndrome, which is a rare genetic disorder, usually associated with an X-linked dominant pattern of inheritance. Aicardi syndrome is characterized by the presence of infantile spasms, chorioretinal lacunae, and agenesis of the corpus callosum. Being an X-linked dominant disorder, it is encountered predominantly in girls, as the mutation is lethal in males. This syndrome is associated with various nonspecific ocular malformations, such as cataracts, microphthalmia, retinal detachment, and hypoplastic papilla. The presence of chorioretinal lacunae is pathognomonic for this syndrome. EEG shows multiple epileptiform abnormalities, such as burst suppression pattern with asynchrony between the two hemispheres and a disorganized background. West syndrome is described in question 45. Ohtahara syndrome is described in question 49. Dravet syndrome is described in question 48. Doose syndrome is described in question 47.

Rosser T. Aicardi Syndrome. Arch Neurol. 2003; 60:1471–1473.

47. e

This patient has Doose syndrome or myoclonic–astatic epilepsy. Typical onset is between 1 and 5 years of age. Children are normal prior to the onset of seizures, and many continue to have normal cognitive development. Seizures are predominantly generalized with myoclonic or astatic components, in which the patient loses postural tone and falls, sometimes resulting in injuries. There may be other seizure types, such as absence, generalized tonic-clonic (GTC), and tonic seizures, and/or nonconvulsive status epilepticus. The EEG demonstrates interictal bilateral synchronous irregular 2- to 3-Hz spike and wave complexes along with parietal rhythmic θ-activity. Myoclonic seizures are associated with irregular spikes and polyspikes. There may be a genetic predisposition, and a family history of epilepsy or abnormal EEGs is frequent.

Even though many patients remain normal, some have severe developmental delay and intractable seizures, and the prognosis may be variable. Valproic acid is commonly prescribed. Ethosuximide may help with absence seizures. Levetiracetam and ketogenic diet have also been reported to be beneficial in some cases.

Dravet syndrome is described in question 48. Ohtahara syndrome is described in question 49. Benign myoclonic epilepsy of infancy is described in question 50. Generalized epilepsy with febrile seizures plus (GEFS+) is described in question 7.

Bradley WG, Daroff RB, Fenichel GM, et al. Neurology in Clinical Practice, 5th ed. Philadelphia, PA: Elsevier, 2008.

Korff CM, Nordli DR. Epilepsy syndromes in infancy. Pediatr Neurol. 2006; 34:253–263.

48. a

This patient has Dravet syndrome or severe myoclonic epilepsy of infancy. This is a severe epilepsy syndrome, in which the patient has frequent seizures and various seizure types. The typical initial presentation is a febrile seizure (FS) in the first year of life; later, these patients develop other seizure types, including myoclonias, atypical absences, and tonic and tonic–clonic seizures, which could be generalized and/or unilateral. Given the initial presentation with an FS, the diagnosis may be delayed. Males are more affected than females, and there may be a family history of epilepsy or abnormal EEGs. In fact, Dravet syndrome may lie at the most severe end of the spectrum of generalized epilepsy with febrile seizures plus (GEFS+) and may commonly be associated with a mutation in the sodium channel *SCN1A*. The EEG may be normal initially in the interictal period, later showing generalized spike–wave complexes as well as focal and multifocal spikes. Developmental delay is the rule and neurologic abnormalities are common. The prognosis is poor, seizures are difficult to control, and there is sensitivity to hyperthermia.

Treatment options include valproic acid, topiramate, zonisamide, and ketogenic diet. Importantly, treatment with phenobarbital, phenytoin, carbamazepine, and lamotrigine may exacerbate the seizures.

Ohtahara syndrome is described in question 49. Benign myoclonic epilepsy of infancy is described in question 50. Generalized epilepsy with febrile seizures plus (GEFS+) is described in question 7. Doose syndrome is described in question 47.

Bradley WG, Daroff RB, Fenichel GM, et al. Neurology in Clinical Practice, 5th ed. Philadelphia, PA: Elsevier; 2008.

Korff CM, Nordli DR. Epilepsy syndromes in infancy. Pediatr Neurol. 2006; 34:253–263.

49. b

This patient has Ohtahara syndrome, also known as early infantile epileptic encephalopathy (EIEE). This is a rare severe neurologic condition in which seizures begin during early infancy (between 1 day and 3 months of age). Patients have epileptic tonic spasms occurring multiple times per day. The EEG typically shows a burst suppression pattern that is present during wakefulness or sleep. This is a catastrophic epileptic encephalopathy with intractable seizures and a very poor prognosis. In one series, 25% of patients died before 2 years of age. All survivors have severe disabilities and developmental impairment.

Dravet syndrome is described in question 48. Benign myoclonic epilepsy of infancy is described in question 50. Generalized epilepsy with febrile seizures plus (GEFS+) is described in question 7. Doose syndrome is described in question 47.

Bradley WG, Daroff RB, Fenichel GM, et al. Neurology in Clinical Practice, 5th ed. Philadelphia, PA: Elsevier; 2008.

Korff CM, Nordli DR. Epilepsy syndromes in infancy. Pediatr Neurol. 2006; 34:253–263.

50. c

This patient has benign myoclonic epilepsy of infancy (BMEI). This condition affects males more than females, between the ages of 4 months and 3 years. It is characterized by the presence of brief myoclonic seizures, which are easily treatable. These myoclonias are brief (1–3 seconds) and usually isolated, and are more prominent during drowsiness, photostimulation, and external stimulation. Unlike infantile spasms, the myoclonic seizures of BMEI do not occur in long series/clusters. During a myoclonic seizure, the EEG shows generalized spikes and waves or polyspikes and waves. The interictal EEG is normal. Neuroimaging is usually normal. Seizures respond well to valproic acid, and the prognosis is generally good with spontaneous resolution of seizures in less than a year. Neuropsychologic outcome is favorable, although a small minority of patients may have mild mental retardation.

Dravet syndrome is described in question 48. Ohtahara syndrome is described in question 49. Generalized epilepsy with febrile seizures plus (GEFS+) is described in question 7. Doose syndrome is described in question 47.

Bradley WG, Daroff RB, Fenichel GM, et al. Neurology in Clinical Practice, 5th ed. Philadelphia, PA: Elsevier; 2008.

Korff CM, Nordli DR. Epilepsy syndromes in infancy. Pediatr Neurol. 2006; 34:253–263.

51. b

This patient has benign neonatal seizures. In this syndrome, full-term, otherwise healthy, newborns develop seizures around day 5 of life (also referred to as "fifth day fits"), which are partial clonic seizures that may be unilateral and/or symmetric and may migrate to other regions of the body. These seizures are frequently associated with apneic spells. The EEG is normal, but may demonstrate the "θ pointu alternant" pattern, characterized by discontinuous, asynchronous, unreactive θ-activity with intermixed sharp waves. Patients are neurologically normal. In general, there is no need for treatment with antiepileptic agents, and seizures resolve spontaneously by 4 to 6 weeks of age.

Benign neonatal seizures and benign familial neonatal seizures should be diagnoses of exclusion, and workup to rule out symptomatic seizures is indicated. Benign familial neonatal seizures is an autosomal dominant disorder, characterized by seizures in the first few days of life, which resolve spontaneously within few weeks. Genetic linkage studies have mapped two disease loci, both associated with mutations in voltage-gated potassium channels, in the genes *KCNQ2* on chromosome 20 and *KCNQ3* on chromosome 8.

West syndrome is described in question 45. Aicardi syndrome is discussed in question 46. Ohtahara syndrome is described in question 49. Benign myoclonic epilepsy of infancy is described in question 50.

Bradley WG, Daroff RB, Fenichel GM, et al. Neurology in Clinical Practice, 5th ed. Philadelphia, PA: Elsevier; 2008.

Browne TR, Holmes GL. Handbook of Epilepsy, 4th ed. Philadelphia, PA: Lippincott Williams & Wilkins; 2008.

52. c

This child presents with an idiopathic occipital epilepsy, more specifically early-onset childhood occipital epilepsy or Panayiotopoulos syndrome. In this condition, the seizures begin between 4 and 8 years of age (with a peak incidence at 4–5 years), and are characterized by tonic eye deviation and vomiting. Visual auras are reported during wakefulness, characterized by elementary or complex visual hallucinations and illusions. Partial or generalized tonic-clonic (GTC) seizures may occur during sleep; in fact, in the majority of children, seizures occur predominantly or exclusively in sleep. The EEG shows high-voltage occipital spikes in 1- to 3-Hz bursts, which disappear with eye opening and reappear with eye closure or darkness. Treatment is generally not required. The prognosis is good, and this condition resolves within several years.

Late-onset childhood occipital epilepsy or Gastaut type occurs in older children at a mean age of 8 years (between the ages of 4 and 13 years) and consists of brief seizures with visual manifestations followed by hemiclonic convulsions and in some cases a postictal migraine. The EEG is similar to that seen in Panayiotopoulos syndrome. The prognosis is variable in the Gastaut type, but most patients have a benign course. However, pharmacologic therapy may be needed and seizures may be difficult to control in some cases.

Ohtahara syndrome is discussed in question 49. Dravet syndrome is discussed in question 48. Doose syndrome is discussed in question 47.

Bradley WG, Daroff RB, Fenichel GM, et al. Neurology in Clinical Practice, 5th ed. Philadelphia, PA: Elsevier; 2008.

Browne TR, Holmes GL. Handbook of Epilepsy, 4th ed. Philadelphia, PA: Lippincott Williams & Wilkins; 2008.

53. d

This patient has Lennox–Gastaut syndrome. This syndrome is characterized by the triad of seizures of multiple types, EEG with diffuse slow (1.5–2 Hz) spike–wave complexes, and mental retardation. The onset is between the ages of 1 to 8 years, with most children presenting at the age of 3 to 5 years. Less than half of these patients will have normal cognitive function before the onset of seizures, eventually deteriorating after the onset of seizures leading to severe psychomotor retardation. About 60% of the cases have an identified cause, but some are cryptogenic. Patients with Lennox–Gastaut syndrome will develop various seizure types, including atypical absence, tonic, atonic, myoclonic, and tonic–clonic seizures. Valproic acid and clonazepam are frequently used. Other medications that could be given include lamotrigine, felbamate, topiramate, and vigabatrin. Ketogenic diet may be considered. These seizures are often refractory to therapy.

Panayiotopoulos syndrome is described in question 52. West syndrome is described in question 45. Landau–Kleffner syndrome is described in question 54. Question 43 contains a description of seizures arising from the mesial temporal lobe.

Bradley WG, Daroff RB, Fenichel GM, et al. Neurology in Clinical Practice, 5th ed. Philadelphia, PA: Elsevier; 2008.

Fenichel GM. Clinical Pediatr Neurol: A Signs and Symptoms Approach, 6th ed. Philadelphia, PA: Saunders Elsevier; 2009.

54. c

This patient has Landau–Kleffner syndrome, also known as acquired epileptic aphasia. This syndrome is characterized by an acquired aphasia associated with epileptiform abnormalities on EEG and seizures of various types. The age of onset is between 2 and 11 years, with a peak onset between 5 and 7 years; these children may initially present with word deafness in the setting of normal hearing. The disorder of language progresses and both a receptive and expressive aphasia may eventually occur. The seizures are of various types, including atypical absence, myoclonic, tonic, and tonic–clonic. Furthermore, a small minority of patients do not have a history of clinical seizures. The EEG demonstrates multifocal cortical spikes, predominantly in the temporal and parietal lobes, most frequently bilaterally. Antiepileptic agents such as valproic acid and lamotrigine are usually effective in controlling the seizures. Recovery of speech on the other hand is variable, with some patients having significant improvement, but others not. Corticosteroids have been tried with variable success.

Panayiotopoulos syndrome is described in question 52. West syndrome is described in question 45. Lennox–Gastaut syndrome is described in question 53. Question 43 contains a description of seizures arising from the mesial temporal lobe.

Bradley WG, Daroff RB, Fenichel GM, et al. Neurology in Clinical Practice, 5th ed. Philadelphia, PA: Elsevier; 2008.

Fenichel GM. Clinical Pediatr Neurol: A Signs and Symptoms Approach, 6th ed. Philadelphia, PA: Saunders Elsevier; 2009.

55. d

This patient has autosomal dominant nocturnal frontal lobe epilepsy (ADNFLE). These seizures begin in childhood and frequently persist into adult life. Patients with ADNFLE present with bizarre episodic behaviors in the context of hypermotor seizures, that is, hyperkinetic seizures with prominent motor phenomena, such as thrashing and jerking. These seizures occur during non-REM sleep, and patients may experience sudden awakenings with motor manifestations. Some patients will be conscious and report auras with epigastric, sensory, or psychic components. Because of the unusual appearance of these seizures, they are often mistaken for psychogenic nonepileptic seizures ("pseudoseizures") or sleep-related disorders. The interictal EEG is usually normal, and the diagnosis is based on capturing the seizures on video EEG. These seizures usually respond well to carbamazepine or oxcarbazepine. Mutations in the genes that encode subunits of the nicotinic acetylcholine receptors, *CNRNA4* and *CHRNB2*, have been detected.

Electrical status epilepticus during slow-wave sleep (ESES) presents in children between ages 1 and 12 years (peak around 4–5 years) with psychomotor retardation and multiple seizure types that occur more often during sleep. The diagnosis is made with the EEG showing slow spike–wave complexes occurring during non-REM sleep occupying at least 85% of the slow-wave sleep time. This disorder has been linked to Landau–Kleffner syndrome (see question 54). Although there is an overlap between these two syndromes, children with ESES present with a more global regression and seizures that may be more difficult to treat.

Lennox–Gastaut syndrome is described in question 53. Landau–Kleffner syndrome is described in question 54. Panayiotopoulos syndrome is described in question 52.

Bradley WG, Daroff RB, Fenichel GM, et al. Neurology in Clinical Practice, 5th ed. Philadelphia, PA: Elsevier; 2008.

Browne TR, Holmes GL. Handbook of Epilepsy, 4th ed. Philadelphia, PA: Lippincott Williams & Wilkins; 2008.

56. b, **57.** d, **58.** a, **59.** a

Lateralizing semiological signs and symptoms during epileptic seizures are helpful to predict the side of the seizure focus, and this may have implications on the correct classification of the patient's epilepsy and for presurgical evaluation in patients whose seizures are difficult to control with AEDs. Auras preceding a seizure represent focal discharges, which activate the area responsible for generation of the patient's aura at the beginning of the clinical (but not necessarily the electrographic) seizure. Thus, auras may provide a clue with regard to the seizure origin. Some seizures do not start with an aura, but other semiological signs may point toward the origin of these seizures.

Eyes and head version, characterized strictly by a forced and involuntary movement leading to an unnatural position of the head toward one side, are associated with a seizure focus in the contralateral hemisphere, and more specifically in the frontal region in the frontal eye fields and motor areas anterior to the precentral gyrus. The association of version with the contralateral hemisphere is more robust if the version occurs immediately prior to the secondarily generalized tonic–clonic phase. Therefore the patient in question 56 has a seizure focus in the right frontal region.

Question 57 depicts a case of asymmetric tonic posturing during a seizure, which is characteristic of seizures arising from the supplementary motor area (SMA). This specific case describes the "figure of 4 sign," in which the extended arm is contralateral to the seizure focus. Therefore, this patient's seizures originate in the left SMA (see question 44).

Unilateral dystonic hand/arm posture during a seizure has important lateralizing value in temporal lobe epilepsies, suggesting that the seizure arises from the temporal lobe contralateral to the dystonic upper extremity. The suggested hypothesis is that the discharges originate in the hippocampus and amygdala, spreading via the fornix and through the basal ganglia, more specifically the ventral striatum, pallidum, and anterior cingulate gyrus. Patients with dystonic posture of one upper limb and automatisms in the opposite upper limb have seizures originating in the temporal lobe ipsilateral to the automatisms. In question 58, the seizure focus is in the right temporal lobe.

Gelastic seizures are characterized by uncontrollable episodes of laughter that occur in clusters, as depicted in question 59. These seizures are rare, and commonly originate in the hypothalamus, more specifically associated with hypothalamic hamartomas, although gelastic seizures arising from various cortical areas mainly in the frontal and temporal lobe have been well described in the literature. Hypothalamic hamartoma is a congenital malformation that may be asymptomatic in some cases, but commonly presents with precocious puberty and seizures. Seizures may progress and the patient may manifest other seizure types.

Harvey AS, Freeman JL. Epilepsy in hypothalamic hamartoma: clinical and EEG features. Semin Pediatr Neurol. 2007; 14(2):60–64.

Loddenkemper T, Kotagal P. Lateralizing signs during seizures in focal epilepsy. Epilepsy & Behavior. 2005; 7:1–17.

60. c

This patient has phenytoin toxicity, and free and total phenytoin levels should be checked. CT and MRI of the brain may need to be performed to rule out a new cerebrovascular event; however, the symptoms most likely correlate with the introduction of the two antimicrobial medications resulting in phenytoin toxicity. Given the patient's symptoms, the most likely cause can be determined by assessing the serum levels of phenytoin. There is no evidence to suggest a new seizure and therefore an EEG is not indicated. Urinalysis and urine culture may need to be obtained to rule out an infectious process; however, it is unlikely to be the cause of this patient's symptoms.

Phenytoin is a widely used medication for seizures. However, due to its narrow therapeutic index, nonlinear kinetics, and multiple interactions with other medications, toxicity can occur in patients treated with this medication. Phenytoin can be given orally or intravenously. It binds extensively to albumin (almost 90%); only unbound phenytoin is pharmacologically active. Medications (such as sulfamethoxazole) that displace phenytoin from albumin may increase free levels, producing manifestations of toxicity.

Phenytoin is metabolized by hepatic cytochrome (CYP) P450 enzymes to inactive metabolites, which are then excreted in the urine. Phenytoin follows zero-order kinetic metabolism (discussed in questions 26–28).

There is a long list of medications that could potentially interact with the metabolism of phenytoin, either increasing or decreasing its serum levels. Fluconazole and trimethoprim are substrates of the same CYP 450 pathway, and can therefore raise levels of this antiepileptic drug.

The clinical manifestations of phenytoin toxicity are usually neurologic in nature, and depending on the drug level, range from dizziness, nystagmus, ataxia, and other manifestations of cerebellar dysfunction to lethargy, confusion, and coma.

Bradley WG, Daroff RB, Fenichel GM, et al. Neurology in Clinical Practice, 5th ed. Philadelphia, PA: Elsevier; 2008.

Craig S. Phenytoin poisoning. Neurocrit Care. 2005; 3:161–170.

French JA, Pedley TA. Initial management of epilepsy. N Engl J Med. 2008; 359:166–176.

Toledano R, Gil-Nagel A. Adverse effects of antiepileptic drugs. Semin Neurol. 2008; 28:317–327.

61. e, 62. a

This patient had a simple febrile seizure (FS). FS is defined as a seizure that occurs in association with a febrile illness in the absence of CNS infection or acute electrolyte imbalance in children without prior afebrile seizures. These occur commonly between 6 months and 5 years of age, with a peak incidence at 18 months. FS can be simple or complex. Most FS represent simple FS, that is, generalized, usually isolated, seizures of relatively brief duration lasting less than 15 minutes. Complex FS on the other hand are prolonged, lasting more than 15 minutes, have focal features, and may occur multiple times in the course of the same febrile illness, or within the same 24-hour period.

A prior history of a complex FS is a known risk factor for subsequent development of epilepsy, whereas a family history of FS does not increase the risk of subsequent epilepsy. Interestingly, a prior history of a complex FS has not been found to be associated with a higher risk for recurrence of FS.

Risk factors to develop a first FS include a first- or second-degree relative with a history of FS, developmental delay, neonatal nursery stay for more than 30 days, and attendance of day care. Most patients will have only one FS without recurrence and without subsequent development of epilepsy. Recurrent FS may occur, especially in the presence of recognizable risk factors, which include a family history of FS, age younger than 18 months at the time of the first FS, lower peak temperature, and shorter duration of fever prior to the FS. Simple or complex FS carry similar risk of recurrence.

The risk of developing epilepsy following a single simple FS is not substantially different than the risk in the general population. On the other hand, patients with complex FS may be at risk of developing epilepsy in the future. The risk is even higher when the complex FS was very prolonged in duration (i.e., febrile status epilepticus). Other risk factors to develop epilepsy include the presence of a neurodevelopmental abnormality and/or family history of epilepsy. Importantly, a family history of FS does not predispose the patient to subsequent development of epilepsy.

The evaluation of patients with FS should be targeted at assessing the cause of the seizure and ruling out CNS infections or abnormalities. The exact pathophysiology of FS remains unclear. A relationship between prolonged FS and mesial temporal lobe sclerosis has been proposed; however, this association is controversial and has not conclusively been confirmed in prospective and population-based studies, which are ongoing.

Long-term prophylaxis and AEDs are not indicated for FS, but can be considered in some cases, especially if a high risk of recurrence exists. In these cases, phenobarbital or valproic acid can be considered on a case-by-case basis. Short-term prophylaxis may also be needed in some cases, and should be focused on temperature control during febrile illness and use of benzodiazepines, such as rectal diazepam gel.

Shinnar S, Glauser TA. Febrile Seizures. J Child Neurol. 2002; 17:S44–S52.

63. b

This patient has Unverricht Lundborg syndrome, one of the progressive myoclonic epilepsies. This group of disorders is characterized by myoclonic epilepsy and progressive neurologic deterioration, and includes Unverricht Lundborg syndrome, Lafora body disease, myoclonic epilepsy with ragged red fibers (MERFF), sialidosis, and neuronal ceroid lipofuscinosis. Unverricht Lundborg syndrome, also known as Baltic myoclonic epilepsy, is an autosomal recessive condition associated with mutations in the gene *EPM1* located on the chromosomal locus 21q22.3, which encodes for cystatin B, a cysteine protease inhibitor associated with the initiation of apoptosis. Patients with Unverricht Lundborg syndrome present between 6 and 15 years of age with stimulus-sensitive myoclonus, which is action related and worsens over time. Eventually, they develop various seizure types, including absences, focal motor, or generalized tonic–clonic seizures. These patients will deteriorate neurologically, presenting with ataxia, tremor, and intellectual decline. MRI is usually normal, and EEG shows generalized spike–waves and polyspikes. Treatment options include valproic acid, clonazepam, levetiracetam, and zonisamide. Certain AEDs may worsen the seizures, including phenytoin, carbamazepine, oxcarbazepine, vigabatrin, tiagabine, gabapentin, and pregabalin. These patients may worsen progressively, but in some cases, the disease stabilizes over the years.

Lafora body disease is discussed in question 66. Sialidosis is discussed in question 65. Juvenile myoclonic epilepsy is discussed in questions 19 and 20, and neuronal ceroid lipofuscinosis is discussed in Chapter 14.

Bradley WG, Daroff RB, Fenichel GM, et al. Neurology in Clinical Practice, 5th ed. Philadelphia, PA: Elsevier; 2008.

Delgado-Escueta AV, Ganesh S, Yamakawa K. Advances in the genetics of progressive myoclonus epilepsy. Am J Med Genet. 2001; 106:129–138.

64. c

This patient has myoclonic epilepsy with ragged red fibers (MERFF), which is a mitochondrial disorder.

The patient has various characteristics suggestive of a mitochondrial disorder, including migraines, short stature, ataxia, cognitive impairment, deafness, epilepsy, and elevated lactate. He has generalized proximal weakness suggesting a myopathy, and the muscle biopsy in Figure 5.6 demonstrates ragged red fibers, which supports the diagnosis.

Mitochondrial disorders are a heterogeneous group of disorders that can affect both the peripheral and central nervous system. MERRF is a mitochondrial disorder that usually starts in the second or third decade of life, and is maternally inherited (like other disorders of mitochondrial DNA). CSF studies will show elevation of pyruvate and lactate, and the serum creatine kinase may be elevated. MRI of the brain usually demonstrates cerebral atrophy. Point mutations in mitochondrial DNA have been detected in this disorder.

Mutation affecting cystatin B is seen with *EPM1* mutations in Unverricht Lundborg syndrome. Cherry red spot is seen in various conditions, including sialidosis, which is another progressive myoclonic epilepsy. *EPM2A* mutation is seen in Lafora body disease, in which Lafora bodies are also detected on skin biopsy.

Delgado-Escueta AV, Ganesh S, Yamakawa K. Advances in the genetics of progressive myoclonus epilepsy. Am J Med Genet. 2001; 106:129–138.

Schmiedel J, Jackson S, Schafer J, et al. Mitochondrial cytopathies. J Neurol. 2003; 250:267–277.

65. c

This patient has a progressive myoclonic epilepsy (PME), more specifically sialidosis. There are two types of sialidosis that can cause PME: Type I is caused by a deficiency of α-neuraminidase and presents in adolescents and adults with action myoclonus, and slowly progressive ataxia, tonic–clonic seizures, and vision loss. These patients do not have mental deterioration or dysmorphism, and characteristically, the fundoscopic examination demonstrates a cherry red spot. Type II is caused by deficiency of *N*-acetyl neuraminidase and β-galactosialidase, and begins between the neonatal period and the second decade of life. These patients have myoclonus, along with coarse facial features, corneal clouding, hepatomegaly, skeletal dysplasia, and learning disabilities. The sialidoses are autosomal recessive, and the gene implicated is *NEU1* in chromosome 6p21.3. The diagnosis is confirmed with the detection of high urinary sialyloligosaccharides and by confirmation of the lysosomal enzyme deficiency in leukocytes or cultured fibroblasts.

Unverricht Lundborg syndrome is discussed in question 63. Lafora body disease is discussed in question 66. Juvenile myoclonic epilepsy is discussed in questions 19–20, and neuronal ceroid lipofuscinosis is discussed in Chapter 14.

Delgado-Escueta AV, Ganesh S, Yamakawa K. Advances in the genetics of progressive myoclonus epilepsy. Am J Med Genet. 2001; 106:129–138.

Shahwan A, Farrel M, Delanty N. Progressive myoclonic epilepsies: a review of genetic and therapeutic aspects. Lancet Neurol. 2005; 4:239–248.

66. e

This patient has Lafora body disease, which is an autosomal recessive disorder associated with a mutation in the gene *EPM2A* on chromosome 6q, encoding laforin, a ribosomal protein with undetermined function. Patients with Lafora body disease present between 12 and 17 years of age. These patients have seizures of various types, including myoclonus, atypical absences, atonic, complex partial, and occipital seizures with transient blindness and visual hallucinations. These patients also have dysarthria, ataxia, as well as emotional disturbance, and cognitive decline leading to dementia. EEG shows an evolution, with multiple spike–wave discharges at the beginning, but progressively over months or years, the background deteriorates and multifocal epileptiform abnormalities appear, mainly in the occipital regions, in addition to generalized bursts. Lafora bodies are PAS-positive intracellular polyglucosan inclusion bodies found in neurons, cardiac muscle, skeletal muscle, hepatocytes, and sweat gland duct cells, making it possible to detect these bodies in skin biopsy specimens. Most patients die within 10 years of onset, and the treatment remains palliative.

Mutation in cystatin B and *EPM1* mutation are seen in Unverricht Lundborg syndrome. Cherry red spot in a patient with progressive myoclonic epilepsy (PME) suggests sialidosis. Ragged red fibers on muscle biopsy are seen in myoclonic epilepsy with ragged red fibers.

Delgado-Escueta AV, Ganesh S, Yamakawa K. Advances in the genetics of progressive myoclonus epilepsy. Am J Med Genet. 2001; 106:129–138.

Shahwan A, Farrel M, Delanty N. Progressive myoclonic epilepsies: a review of genetic and therapeutic aspects. Lancet Neurol. 2005; 4:239–248.

67. b

In Rasumussen's encephalitis, seizures are not typically well controlled with AED monotherapy.

Rasmussen's encephalitis is an inflammatory condition that affects one hemisphere, and is characterized by focal seizures, often epilepsia partialis continua, hemiparesis, and progressive neurologic deterioration. This condition most frequently affects children, though adolescents and adults may also be affected. The pathogenesis is not well understood; however, it is known that it is an inflammatory condition, and an antibody has been detected targeted against the GluR3 subunit of the AMPA receptor, which is a glutamate receptor. Histopathologic findings demonstrate perivascular cuffs of lymphocytes and monocytes, as well as glial nodules in the gray and white matter, and the continuous neuron loss leaves areas of spongy tissue degeneration. MRI demonstrates cortical atrophy that is progressive and focal areas of white matter hyperintensity. Seizures are usually intractable with AEDs. Anti-inflammatory agents such as corticosteroids and other immune modulating treatments including IV immune globulin and plasmapheresis have been tried with some promise, but variable success. Hemispherectomy is often needed, providing the possibility of cure of the seizures. Rasmussen's syndrome is also discussed in question 8.

Bradley WG, Daroff RB, Fenichel GM, et al. Neurology in Clinical Practice, 5th ed. Philadelphia, PA: Elsevier; 2008.

Granata T. Rasmussen's syndrome. Neurol Sci. 2003; 24:S239–243.

68. e

Absorption, distribution, metabolism, and excretion of AEDs are altered in the elderly. These patients tend to have lower gastric acidity, making the weakly basic drugs less easily absorbed and weakly acidic drugs more easily absorbed. Gastric emptying may be slowed and intestinal villi height may be reduced, making the absorption surface smaller. Given that lean body mass decreases with aging, total body water mass decreases, making the volume of distribution of hydrophilic drugs smaller. The proportion of fat also decreases with age, reducing lipophilic drug distribution volume. The metabolism of drugs is also affected, and hepatic metabolism decreases, given the reduction in liver volume, hepatic flow, and bile flow. Renal blood flow and glomerular filtration rate are lower in the elderly, and therefore, renal excretion is also decreased. Hepatic synthesis of protein is lower, and the free fraction of drug that binds to protein tends to increase. Therefore the measurement of free drug levels is recommended if available for that specific drug. The therapeutic window is also smaller in elderly patients. These patients tend to have multiple comorbidities and are usually on multiple medications that could potentially interact with AEDs. Therefore, careful selection of drugs and monitoring for side effects are strongly recommended in this group of patients.

Jetter GM, Cavazos JE. Epilepsy in the Elderly. Semin Neurol. 2008; 28(3):336–341.

69. d

Valproic acid is a broad-spectrum antiepileptic agent that can be used in various seizure types. Its acts by blocking sodium channels, but it may have other mechanisms of action, including effects on $GABA_A$ receptors and T-type calcium channels. This medication is widely used; however, it has various side effects. These include weight gain, alopecia, tremor, gastrointestinal symptoms, such as nausea and vomiting, and pancreatitis. It can be hepatotoxic and even produce fulminant hepatic failure and hyperammonemia, leading to encephalopathy. It can be undesirable in women, as it may produce a polycystic ovarian syndrome with menstrual irregularities, and it is teratogenic, specifically producing neural tube defects. Valproic acid is an enzyme inhibitor, and may lead to interactions with other medications, elevating the levels of many medications, including other AEDs. Osteoporosis from vitamin D deficiency is postulated to occur from enzyme-inducing antiepileptic agents; however, vitamin D deficiency is also seen in patients taking valproic acid monotherapy.

Hyponatremia is not a side effect of valproic acid and is more commonly seen with carbamazepine and oxcarbazepine.

Bradley WG, Daroff RB, Fenichel GM, et al. Neurology in Clinical Practice, 5th ed. Philadelphia, PA: Elsevier; 2008.

French JA, Pedley TA. Initial management of epilepsy. N Engl J Med. 2008; 359:166–176.

Toledano R, Gil-Nagel A. Adverse effects of antiepileptic drugs. Semin Neurol. 2008; 28:317–327.

70. d

Many antiepileptic agents produce cognitive and behavioral side effects, with levetiracetam being notorious for doing so. This medication in general has few side effects and does not interact with other medications; however, it can produce significant behavioral problems and emotional lability, sometimes agitation and even aggressiveness. Levetiracetam should be used carefully in the elderly and in patients with psychiatric disorders, with alternative medications used when possible.

Of the antiepileptic agents mentioned in the options, the one that presents most behavioral side effects is levetiracetam. Lamotrigine is a broad-spectrum AED that has no significant adverse impact on cognition and behavior and has few side effects if titrated slowly, with skin rash being the main side effect. Valproic acid, besides being used for epilepsy, is also used as a mood stabilizer. Carbamazepine and phenytoin can produce fatigue, dizziness, nystagmus, ataxia, and sedation, but usually not the behavioral problems seen with levetiracetam.

Bradley WG, Daroff RB, Fenichel GM, et al. Neurology in Clinical Practice, 5th ed. Philadelphia, PA: Elsevier; 2008.

French JA, Pedley TA. Initial management of epilepsy. N Engl J Med. 2008; 359:166–176.

Toledano R, Gil-Nagel A. Adverse effects of antiepileptic drugs. Semin Neurol. 2008; 28:317–327.

71. e

This patient has acute angle-closure glaucoma, which is a potential adverse effect of topiramate. This medication acts on voltage-dependent sodium channels, and also has an effect on GABA receptors as well as glutamate receptors. It is a carbonic anhydrase inhibitor. Topiramate has been used as an AED as well as for the treatment of migraines. Potential side effects from topiramate include drowsiness, fatigue, ataxia, word-finding difficulties, difficulty concentrating, paresthesias, weight loss, metabolic acidosis, nephrolithiasis, and acute angle-closure glaucoma.

Valproic acid, levetiracetam, phenytoin, and lamotrigine have not been associated with acute angle-closure glaucoma.

French JA, Pedley TA. Initial management of epilepsy. N Engl J Med. 2008; 359:166–176.

Toledano R, Gil-Nagel A. Adverse effects of antiepileptic drugs. Semin Neurol. 2008; 28:317–327.

72. c

This patient had a first, likely unprovoked, seizure. The International League Against Epilepsy defines this as a seizure occurring in a person older than 1 month of age with no prior history of unprovoked seizures. This definition excludes neonatal seizures, febrile seizures (FS), or seizures in the setting of an acute precipitating cause. The risk of recurrence of seizures is influenced by various parameters, including history suggesting an underlying abnormal brain, a focal neurologic examination, an abnormal EEG, or evidence of an underlying cause on brain imaging studies. A practice parameter guideline has been published by the American Academy of Neurology on the basis of available evidence. At the time of that publication, there was evidence to support the use of a routine EEG and brain imaging with CT or MRI in patients presenting with a first unprovoked seizure. Blood tests such as blood count, glucose, and electrolytes may be helpful in certain cases and are almost always performed; however, there was not enough evidence to support such testing in these patients. The same holds for CSF analysis and toxicology screens, which may be helpful in certain situations.

Not every patient with a first unprovoked seizure needs to be treated. The decision to treat is a complex one, and depends on the risk of recurrence on the basis of the factors mentioned, the risk–benefit ratio of treatment, and other patient-specific considerations.

Haut SR, Shinnar S. Considerations in the treatment of a first unprovoked seizure. Semin Neurol. 2008; 28(3):289–296.

Krumholz A, Wiebe S, Gronseth G, et al. Practice parameter: evaluating an apparent unprovoked first seizure in adults (an evidence-based review). Neurology. 2007; 69:1996–2007.

73. d

This is an EEG showing posterior background with reactivity demonstrated after an eye closure. Normal background rhythm is seen in the posterior head regions, with α-frequency (between 8 and 13 Hz), and is usually present in normal people when they are awake, more prominent with eye closure, and attenuating with eye opening. Failure of attenuation with eye opening and reactivity with eye closure may be a sign of abnormality. Usually an α-frequency of 8 Hz is seen by 3 years of age in normal children, and this frequency increases with age. A voltage asymmetry of >50% between sides is abnormal. The posterior background is the first feature usually analyzed when reading an EEG.

There are no spikes or other epileptiform discharges seen in Figure 5.7 and therefore no evidence of an occipital seizure. The posterior background has α-frequencies (in this case around 9 Hz) and not δ-frequencies. This patient has good reactivity of the background rhythm, suggesting an awake patient. There are no sleep structures visualized.

Tatum WO, Husain AM, Benbadis SR, et al. Handbook of EEG Interpretation. Demos Medical Publishing, LLC; 2008.

74. C

α-frequency is between 8 and 13 Hz, and is usually present in normal people when they are awake, more prominent with eye closure, and attenuating with eye opening. Failure of attenuation with eye opening and reactivity with eye closure may be a sign of abnormality. Usually an α-frequency of 8 Hz is seen by 3 years of age in normal children, and this frequency increases with age.

β-frequencies are those greater than 13 Hz, are normal, but may be enhanced by benzodiazepines or barbiturates, and may increase with drowsiness and light sleep.

θ-frequencies are those between 4 and 7 Hz, and are present in the frontal and frontocentral regions of one-third of young adults. These frequencies are enhanced with focused concentration, during mental tasks, by hyperventilation, drowsiness, and sleep.

δ-frequencies are those lesser than 4 Hz, and can be seen in normal infants, in sleep, and sometimes in the elderly. Generalized δ frequencies may indicate nonspecific encephalopathy, and if focal, may indicate a structural lesion.

Bradley WG, Daroff RB, Fenichel GM, et al. Neurology in Clinical Practice, 5th ed. Philadelphia, PA: Elsevier; 2008.

Tatum WO, Husain AM, Benbadis SR, et al. Handbook of EEG Interpretation. Demos Medical Publishing, LLC; 2008.

75. C

EEG represents the recording along the scalp of electrical activity that is produced by the firing of pyramidal neurons within the cerebral cortex. EEG recording is based on differential amplification, in which the difference in voltage between two sites is compared with each recording channel. This recording helps in the evaluation and diagnosis of abnormalities in brain electrical activity, but is also useful in the evaluation of other neurologic conditions. Patients undergoing an evaluation for "spells" will often have an EEG to determine the presence or absence of epileptogenic activity. During a routine recording, various procedures are utilized to enhance potentially abnormal electrical activity. These so-called activation procedures include hyperventilation, photic stimulation, sleep deprivation prior to the EEG, and recording during sleep. Noxious stimulation is not part of the EEG activation procedures.

Hyperventilation may produce generalized slowing or no effect in normal subjects; however, in certain epilepsies, such as absence epilepsy, hyperventilation may activate epileptiform discharges and even seizures. Photic stimulation is performed with various frequencies, and may be helpful to induce epileptiform activity and seizures, most commonly myoclonic seizures, in individuals with photosensitive epilepsies. Sleep deprivation may also enhance epileptogenic activity. Furthermore, seizures may occur predominantly (or exclusively) during sleep in certain epilepsy syndromes, and EEG abnormalities may not be seen in the awake patient. Therefore an EEG may be incomplete without a sleep recording.

Tatum WO, Husain AM, Benbadis SR, et al. Handbook of EEG Interpretation, Demos Medical Publishing, LLC; 2008.

76. a

The EEG in Figure 5.8 shows diffuse slowing and triphasic waves, suggesting a metabolic encephalopathy. Triphasic waves represent a special type of continuous generalized slow activity, with characteristic slow waves that consist of three phases, beginning with a small negative (upward) wave, followed by a prominent positive (downward) wave, and ending in a negative (upward) wave. These waveforms typically occur in a bilaterally symmetric, bisynchronous fashion with an anterior-to-posterior lag. They are seen in various types of toxic and/or metabolic encephalopathies that involve altered states of consciousness, most commonly in hepatic encephalopathy. Other common causes include uremia, hypoglycemia, and electrolyte disturbances, such as hyponatremia or hypercalcemia.

Generalized periodic patterns are characterized by the appearance of generalized sharp wave discharges occurring in a periodic fashion. A generalized periodic pattern with a 1 Hz frequency is a characteristic finding of CJD. Although triphasic waves may sometimes be difficult to distinguish from generalized epileptiform activity, especially when occurring in prolonged runs, the EEG pattern seen in this figure would not be typical of a generalized seizure. Postcardiac arrest anoxia can produce various EEG patterns, including α-coma, burst suppression, and electrocerebral silence in the case of brain death. It should be noted that triphasic-appearing waves are also seen in anoxic brain injury. Infantile spasms are associated with the EEG finding of hypsarrhythmia (see questions 24 and 25).

Tatum WO, Husain AM, Benbadis SR, et al. Handbook of EEG Interpretation. Demos Medical Publishing, LLC; 2008.

77. a

This EEG shows burst suppression, characterized by bursts of electrical activity at regular intervals separated by intervals of no electrical activity represented by the flat EEG line. Burst suppression signifies severe bilateral cerebral dysfunction. The etiology of burst suppression is nonspecific. This pattern may be iatrogenic, such as in general anesthesia or in barbiturate coma for status epilepticus, among others. It may have a good prognosis in intoxications, but typically signifies a poor prognosis when seen in patients with a hypoxic–ischemic insult. Patients with burst suppression are comatose, and usually show no reactivity to activation procedures. Patients in status epilepticus intractable to antiepileptic agents may need to be treated with pharmacologically induced coma, in which case the therapy is initially targeted to burst suppression.

There are no triphasic waves, hypsarrhythmia, periodic lateralized epileptiform discharges, or generalized seizures in this EEG.

Tatum WO, Husain AM, Benbadis SR, et al. Handbook of EEG Interpretation. Demos Medical Publishing, LLC; 2008.

78. d

This patient has periodic lateralized epileptiform discharges (PLEDs) in the right hemisphere. PLEDs are sharply contoured waveforms with various morphologies that appear at regular periodic intervals every 1 or 2 seconds and are lateralized to one hemisphere only or to a single region in one hemisphere. These are seen in structural brain lesions, usually in the acute or subacute setting, such as a stroke, hemorrhage, infection (importantly HSV encephalitis), brain abscess, or tumor, and are usually transient, disappearing with time as the patient recovers from the acute event. Typically patients with PLEDs are encephalopathic with a diffusely slow EEG background. Usually PLEDs are not thought to represent ongoing ictal activity and are considered among the interictal phenomena/patterns. It is important to remember, however, that seizures may be seen in a significant number of patients who are found to have PLEDs on EEG.

Burst suppression is described in question 77. Triphasic waves are described in question 76. The figure does not show a generalized periodic pattern or sharp waves.

Tatum WO, Husain AM, Benbadis SR, et al. Handbook of EEG Interpretation. Demos Medical Publishing, LLC; 2008.

79. b, **80.** e, **81.** b

Sleep stages are separated into four stages: stage 1 (N1), stage 2 (N2), stage 3 (N3), and REM sleep. Stages 3 and 4 sleep (previously separated) are now combined together and called slow-wave sleep. Normal sleep consists of 4 to 6 cycles/night of non-REM (NREM) sleep, with each cycle followed by REM sleep. The first REM period is normally around 90 minutes after sleep onset. The electrographic and other characteristics of the sleep stages per current grading criteria are as follows:

N1 (previously stage 1) (5% of sleep time):

- – Disappearance of occipital dominant α-rhythm
- – Increasing θ-frequency in all regions
- – Muscle artifact decreases
- – Diphasic sharp waves maximal at vertex may occur (vertex waves)
- – POSTS (positive occipital sharp transients of sleep) occur

N2 (previously stage 2) (45% of sleep time):

- – Sleep spindles—bursts of 12- to 14-Hz activity maximal over central regions lasting less than 2 seconds; first appear around 2 months, but do not reach adult appearance until 2 years
- – K complexes—high-voltage diphasic slow wave that may be preceded or followed by a sleep spindle, maximal over frontocentral regions
- – Lower voltage, mixed-frequency background activity
- – Vertex waves may still be seen
- – POSTS may still be seen
- – δ-activity less than 20% of sleep period

N3, or slow wave sleep (previously separated into stage 3 and stage 4) (20% to 25% of sleep time):

- – High-amplitude δ-activity 20% to 50% of sleep period and has increased voltage
- – Sleep spindles, K complexes, and POSTS rarely persist
- – Stage 4 is no longer scored as an independent sleep stage

REM (20% to 25% of sleep time):

- – Generally lower voltage, similar to stage 1
- – In some individuals runs of α-activity may appear in occipital leads identical to α-rhythm in awake tracing
- – Spontaneous REMs
- – Tonic motor activity suppression on EMG leads
- – Sawtooth waves in central regions
- – The percentage of sleep spent in REM decreases with increasing age
- – Selective serotonin reuptake inhibitors (SSRIs) reduce the length of time spent in REM

The suprachiasmatic nucleus in the anterior hypothalamus is known as the circadian pacemaker and regulates not only the sleep–wake cycle, but all biological circadian rhythms.

Iber C, Ancoli-Israel S, Chesson A, et al. The AASM Manual for the Scoring of Sleep and Associated Events: Rules, Terminology, and Technical Specification, 1st ed. Westchester, IL: American Academy of Sleep Medicine; 2007.

Levin K, Luders H. Comprehensive Clinical Neurophysiology. Philadelphia, PA: WB Saunders Company; 2000.

82. c

Obstructive sleep apnea (OSA) is diagnosed by the apnea-hypopnea index (AHI) observed during an overnight polysomnogram. The AHI counts how many apneas and hypopneas, on average, occur per hour. A similar although not exactly identical index of apneas and hypopneas is the so-called respiratory disturbance index (RDI), which in addition to apneas and hypopneas also accounts for respiratory-event-related arousals (RERAs). Apneas and hypopneas are characterized by complete cessation or reduction of airflow, respectively, for at least 10 seconds. Mild OSA is diagnosed by an AHI of 5 to 15/hour, moderate OSA by 15 to 30/hour, and severe OSA by more than 30/hour. In addition, apneas are associated with EEG arousal and oxygen desaturation of 2% to 4%.

Iber C, Ancoli-Israel S, Chesson A, et al. The AASM Manual for the Scoring of Sleep and Associated Events: Rules, Terminology, and Technical Specification, 1st ed. Westchester, IL: American Academy of Sleep Medicine; 2007.

83. c

This patient has obstructive sleep apnea (OSA). This syndrome is characterized by repetitive episodes of upper airway obstruction during sleep, associated with arousals or oxygen desaturations. Apneas should occur more than five times per hour and last at least 10 seconds, as detected by polysomnogram, which is a useful study for the diagnosis of this condition. During apneas, respiratory effort is present, differentiating this condition from central sleep apnea, in which there is no respiratory effort. OSAS is more frequently seen in obese patients and in those with small or crowded upper airways. The use of alcohol and sedatives may reduce airway tone, worsening OSAS.

Besides the clinical manifestations directly associated with OSAS, patients with this condition are at a higher risk of cardiovascular events. Patients with OSA are at higher risk to develop cardiac arrhythmias, hypertension, cor pulmonale, as well as myocardial infarctions and strokes. Management includes weight loss, avoidance of alcohol and sedatives, and use of positive airway pressure. Some patients may be candidates for upper airway surgery.

American Academy of Sleep Medicine. International Classification of Sleep Disorders, 2nd ed. Diagnostic and Coding Manual, Westchester, IL: American Academy of Sleep Medicine; 2005.

Bradley WG, Daroff RB, Fenichel GM, et al. Neurology in Clinical Practice, 5th ed. Philadelphia, PA: Elsevier; 2008.

Yaggi HK, Concato J, Kernan WN, et al. Obstructive sleep apnea as a risk factor for stroke and death. N Engl J Med. 2005; 353:2034–2041.

84. b

This patient has central sleep apnea syndrome (CSAS), characterized by recurrent episodes during which there is absent airflow along with a cessation of ventilatory effort during sleep. The clinical manifestations of CSAS are similar to those of obstructive sleep apnea (OSA), because patients will often experience insomnia, inability to maintain sleep, and excessive daytime sleepiness, as well as arousals, bradycardia or tachycardia, and desaturations during the apneas. The difference is that the main problem is a transient central cessation of respiratory drive, and airway obstruction does not occur. Polysomnogram is helpful in making the diagnosis, showing episodes of apnea, in which there is no respiratory effort. This type of sleep-disordered breathing is much less common than OSA. Given that there is no airway obstruction, surgical interventions are not indicated.

American Academy of Sleep Medicine. International Classification of Sleep Disorders, 2nd ed. Diagnostic and Coding Manual, Westchester, IL: American Academy of Sleep Medicine; 2005.

Bradley WG, Daroff RB, Fenichel GM, et al. Neurology in Clinical Practice, 5th ed. Philadelphia, PA: Elsevier; 2008.

85. d

This patient has a non-REM parasomnia, more specifically sleep terrors. Parasomnias have been classified into REM parasomnias, arousal disorders, sleep–wake transition disorders, and other parasomnias. Arousal disorders include confusional arousals, sleepwalking, and sleep terrors. The latter three are non-REM parasomnias arising from slow-wave sleep or stage III sleep (previously known as stage III and stage IV sleep; these two stages have more recently been combined into stage III sleep).

Sleep terrors are more common in children, usually between the ages of 5 and 7 years. These events are characterized by a sudden arousal with screaming or crying, associated with autonomic and behavioral manifestations of intense fear and some degree of confusion on awakening. Sleep terrors occur in the first third of the night. In nightmares, as opposed to sleep terrors, the patients usually remember the dream in detail, they occur in the last third of the night, and there is less autonomic activity. When awakened from nightmares, patients tend to have good intellectual function and are not confused.

American Academy of Sleep Medicine. International Classification of Sleep Disorders, 2nd ed. Diagnostic and Coding Manual, Westchester, IL: American Academy of Sleep Medicine; 2005.

Bradley WG, Daroff RB, Fenichel GM, et al. Neurology in Clinical Practice, 5th ed. Philadelphia, PA: Elsevier; 2008.

86. d

This patient has a non-REM parasomnia, specifically sleepwalking. Parasomnias have been classified into REM parasomnias, arousal disorders, sleep–wake transition disorders, and other parasomnias. Arousal disorders include confusional arousals, sleepwalking, and sleep terrors. The latter three are non-REM parasomnias arising from slow-wave sleep or stage III sleep (previously known as stage III and stage IV sleep; these two stages have more recently been combined into stage III sleep).

Sleepwalking consists of a series of complex behaviors resulting in walking during sleep. This condition occurs more commonly in children, but can present in adolescents and adults, and a positive family history has been reported in many cases. Sleepwalking occurs more commonly in the first third of the sleep, and patients have complex motor behaviors, with amnesia of the episode. These patients are difficult to arouse, and may become confused and exhibit violent behavior when this is attempted.

Confusional arousals are a non-REM parasomnia occurring in children, in which the patient is confused following an arousal from slow-wave sleep. The clinical presentation of this patient is not consistent with narcolepsy, nor with sleep terrors.

American Academy of Sleep Medicine. International Classification of Sleep Disorders, 2nd ed. Diagnostic and Coding Manual, Westchester, IL: American Academy of Sleep Medicine; 2005.

Bradley WG, Daroff RB, Fenichel GM, et al. Neurology in Clinical Practice, 5th ed. Philadelphia, PA: Elsevier; 2008.

87. a

This patient has had a nightmare, which is a complicated dream that becomes frightening toward the end. Nightmares should be differentiated from sleep terrors. Patients with nightmares usually recall the dream in detail, the event occurs in the last third of the night, and there is much less autonomic activity as compared to sleep terrors. When patients are awakened from nightmares, they tend to have good intellectual function and are not confused. Sleep terrors occur more commonly in children, and patients wake up screaming or crying, with prominent associated autonomic and behavioral manifestations of intense fear, as well as confusion on awakening. Sleep terrors occur in the first third of the night.

Confusional arousals are a non-REM parasomnia occurring in children, in which the patient is confused following an arousal from slow-wave sleep.

The clinical presentation of this patient is not consistent with REM sleep behavior disorder or a non-REM parasomnia.

American Academy of Sleep Medicine. International Classification of Sleep Disorders, 2nd ed. Diagnostic and Coding Manual, Westchester, IL: American Academy of Sleep Medicine; 2005.

Bradley WG, Daroff RB, Fenichel GM, et al. Neurology in Clinical Practice, 5th ed. Philadelphia, PA: Elsevier; 2008.

88. c

This patient has a REM parasomnia, specifically REM sleep behavior disorder (RBD).

Normally, there is atonia (loss of muscle tone) during REM sleep. RBD is characterized by intermittent loss of this normal REM atonia (REM without atonia) and by the appearance of complex motor activity during which the patient acts out dreams. Dream content is usually violent with associated movements (e.g., punching, kicking, and running). This can cause injuries to the patient or to the bed partner. RBD is seen in elderly patients, and may be associated with neurodegenerative conditions, more specifically α-synucleopathies such as Parkinson's disease, multisystem atrophy, and DLB. Polysomnography is helpful in making the diagnosis, demonstrating the presence of REM without atonia.

American Academy of Sleep Medicine. International Classification of Sleep Disorders, 2nd ed. Diagnostic and Coding Manual, Westchester, IL: American Academy of Sleep Medicine; 2005.

Bradley WG, Daroff RB, Fenichel GM, et al. Neurology in Clinical Practice, 5th ed. Philadelphia, PA: Elsevier; 2008.

89. e

REM sleep behavior disorder (RBD) is characterized by REM without atonia and by the appearance of complex motor activity during which the patient acts out dreams. Dream content is usually violent with associated movements (e.g., punching, kicking, and running).

Sleep paralysis is a feature of narcolepsy and is characterized by a transient paralysis during sleep onset or on awakening; the patient is fully conscious during these events.

Hypnagogic hallucinations occur at sleep onset and are seen in patients with narcolepsy, and hypnopompic hallucinations occur on awakening from sleep.

A nightmare is a complicated dream that becomes frightening toward the end. Patients with nightmares usually recall the dream in detail, the event occurs in the last third of the night, and there is much less autonomic activity as compared to sleep terrors. When patients are awakened from nightmares, they tend to have good intellectual function and are not confused.

American Academy of Sleep Medicine. International Classification of Sleep Disorders, 2nd ed. Diagnostic and Coding Manual, Westchester, IL: American Academy of Sleep Medicine; 2005.

Bradley WG, Daroff RB, Fenichel GM, et al. Neurology in Clinical Practice, 5th ed. Philadelphia, PA: Elsevier; 2008.

90. c

This patient has Kleine–Levin syndrome, which is a type of recurrent hypersomnia. This condition is characterized by recurrent episodes of hypersomnia that typically occur weeks or months apart. The onset is in early adolescence, typically in males, and the episodes can last for several days and sometimes weeks, appearing many times per year. Patients sleep for prolonged periods of time, 18 to 20 hours, waking only to eat and void. During these episodes, patients may have disrupted behaviors, such as irritability, aggressiveness, confusion, hypersexuality, and a voracious appetite. Disturbance of social life is significant during these episodes. In between episodes, patient sleep well and behave normally.

This patient does not have idiopathic hypersomnia, narcolepsy, obstructive sleep apnea (OSA), or delayed sleep phase syndrome.

Idiopathic hypersomnia is characterized by long-term inability to obtain adequate sleep, in which the patients have excessive sleepiness and the etiology is thought to be abnormal neurologic control of the sleep–wake system. Patients complain of insomnia, they sleep for long periods of time, but the sleep is not refreshing. The diagnosis is made only when no other medical or psychiatric condition can explain the hypersomnia.

Narcolepsy is a disorder that is characterized by excessive sleepiness, cataplexy, sleep paralysis, and hypnagogic and hypnopompic hallucinations. Patients with narcolepsy suffer sleep attacks, in which the patient has an irresistible desire to fall asleep during inappropriate circumstances. These sleep attacks are short, lasting 15 to 30 minutes, and the patient feels refreshed afterward.

OSA is characterized by repetitive episodes of upper airway obstruction during sleep, associated with arousals or oxygen desaturations.

In delayed sleep phase syndrome, the major sleep episode is delayed in relation to the desired clock time, resulting in symptoms of sleep-onset insomnia and difficulty awakening. When these patients are able to sleep when they would like, there is no problem with falling asleep or waking up.

American Academy of Sleep Medicine. International Classification of Sleep Disorders, 2nd ed. Diagnostic and Coding Manual, Westchester, IL: American Academy of Sleep Medicine; 2005.

Bradley WG, Daroff RB, Fenichel GM, et al. Neurology in Clinical Practice, 5th ed. Philadelphia, PA: Elsevier; 2008.

91. d

This patient has narcolepsy with cataplexy. Narcolepsy is a disorder that is characterized by excessive sleepiness, cataplexy, sleep paralysis, and hypnagogic and hypnopompic hallucinations. Patients with narcolepsy suffer sleep attacks, in which the patient has an irresistible desire to fall asleep during inappropriate circumstances. These sleep attacks are short, lasting 15 to 30 minutes, and the patient feels refreshed afterward. Even though cataplexy is associated with narcolepsy, not all patients with narcolepsy have cataplexy. Cataplexy is characterized by episodes of sudden loss of tone of voluntary muscles, except respiratory and ocular muscles. During these attacks, the patients may fall and be unable to move, and deep tendon reflexes are decreased or absent. Patients have preserved consciousness. Cataplectic attacks are triggered by emotional events, such as laughter or anger.

This patient does not have pseudoseizures, nor gelastic seizures.

This patient does not have Kleine–Levin syndrome, which is a type of recurrent hypersomnia, characterized by recurrent episodes of hypersomnia that typically occur weeks or months apart. The episodes can last several days and sometimes weeks, appearing many times per year, and these patients sleep for prolonged periods of time, 18 to 20 hours, waking only to eat and void. During these episodes, patients may have disrupted behaviors, such as irritability, aggressiveness, confusion, hypersexuality, and a voracious appetite. In between episodes, patients sleep well and behave normally.

This patient does not have idiopathic hypersomnia, which is characterized by long-term inability to obtain adequate sleep, in which the patients have excessive sleepiness and the etiology is thought to be abnormal neurologic control of the sleep–wake system. Patients complain of insomnia, they sleep for long periods of time, but the sleep is not refreshing. The diagnosis is made only when no other medical or psychiatric condition can explain the hypersomnia.

American Academy of Sleep Medicine. International Classification of Sleep Disorders, 2nd ed. Diagnostic and Coding Manual, Westchester, IL: American Academy of Sleep Medicine;, 2005.

Bradley WG, Daroff RB, Fenichel GM, et al. Neurology in Clinical Practice, 5th ed. Philadelphia, PA: Elsevier; 2008.

92. a

Narcolepsy with cataplexy is thought to be associated with a loss of hypocretin neurons in the lateral hypothalamus, and hypocretin CSF levels are low in these patients.

During cataplectic attacks, patients have loss of muscle tone and hypo- or areflexia. Sleep paralysis is a feature that commonly accompanies this condition. The diagnosis of narcolepsy with cataplexy can be suspected on clinical grounds; however, polysomnogram and mean sleep latency test (MSLT) can provide information to support the diagnosis by detecting a mean sleep latency of less than 8 minutes and two or more sleep-onset REM periods (SOREMPs). γ-hydroxybutyrate has been approved for the treatment of sleepiness and cataplexy that is associated with narcolepsy. Other treatment options for cataplexy include tricyclic antidepressants or serotonin reuptake inhibitors.

American Academy of Sleep Medicine. International Classification of Sleep Disorders, 2nd ed. Diagnostic and Coding Manual, Westchester, IL: American Academy of Sleep Medicine; 2005.

Bradley WG, Daroff RB, Fenichel GM, et al. Neurology in Clinical Practice, 5th ed. Philadelphia, PA: Elsevier; 2008.

93. b

This patient has a circadian rhythm sleep disorder, specifically delayed sleep phase syndrome. Circadian rhythm disorders are characterized by a misalignment between the patient's sleep pattern and the sleep pattern regarded as the societal norm. In delayed sleep phase syndrome, the major sleep episode is delayed in relation to the desired clock time, resulting in symptoms of sleep-onset insomnia and difficulty awakening. When these patients are able to sleep when they would like, there is no problem with falling asleep or waking up. This condition is more common in adolescents. Treatment may include chronotherapy or melatonin.

This patient does not have psychophysiologic insomnia, advanced sleep phase syndrome, jet lag syndrome, or shift work sleep disorder. In advanced sleep phase syndrome, the major sleep episode is advanced in relation to the desired clock time, resulting in excessive evening sleepiness and early sleep onset, as well as awakening earlier than desired. This condition is more common in the elderly. Jet lag syndrome is caused by the travel across multiple time zones. In shift work sleep disorder, patients experience symptoms of insomnia or excessive sleepiness that occur as transient phenomena in relation to work schedules. In psychophysiologic insomnia, patients worry about being unable to sleep and focus on their insomnia, which causes frustration and further inability to fall asleep.

American Academy of Sleep Medicine. International Classification of Sleep Disorders, 2nd ed. Diagnostic and Coding Manual, Westchester, IL: American Academy of Sleep Medicine; 2005.

Bradley WG, Daroff RB, Fenichel GM, et al. Neurology in Clinical Practice, 5th ed. Philadelphia, PA: Elsevier; 2008.

94. c

This patient has a circadian rhythm sleep disorder, specifically advanced sleep phase syndrome. Circadian rhythm sleep disorders are characterized by a misalignment between the patient's sleep pattern and the sleep pattern regarded as the societal norm. In advanced sleep phase syndrome, the major sleep episode is advanced in relation to the desired clock time, resulting in excessive evening sleepiness and early sleep onset, as well as awakening earlier than desired. This condition is more common in the elderly.

This patient does not have psychophysiologic insomnia, delayed sleep phase syndrome, jet lag syndrome, or shift work sleep disorder. In psychophysiologic insomnia, patients worry about being unable to sleep and focus on their insomnia, which causes frustration and further inability to fall asleep. In delayed sleep phase syndrome, the major sleep episode is delayed in relation to the desired clock time, resulting in symptoms of sleep-onset insomnia and difficulty awakening. Jet lag syndrome is caused by the travel across multiple time zones. In shift work sleep disorder, patients experience symptoms of insomnia or excessive sleepiness that occur as a transient phenomena in relation to work schedules.

American Academy of Sleep Medicine. International Classification of Sleep Disorders, 2nd ed. Diagnostic and Coding Manual, Westchester, IL: American Academy of Sleep Medicine; 2005.

Bradley WG, Daroff RB, Fenichel GM, et al. Neurology in Clinical Practice, 5th ed. Philadelphia, PA: Elsevier; 2008.

95. e

This patient has a circadian rhythm sleep disorder, specifically shift work sleep disorder. In shift work sleep disorder, patients experience symptoms of insomnia or excessive sleepiness that occur as transient phenomena in relation to work schedules. Also, given the need for social interaction with people maintaining regular working hours, individuals with shift work sleep disorder may restrict their sleeping hours, worsening the symptoms of insomnia and sleepiness.

This patient does not have psychophysiologic insomnia, delayed sleep phase syndrome, advanced sleep phase syndrome, or jet lag syndrome. In psychophysiologic insomnia, patients worry about being unable to sleep and focus on their insomnia, which causes frustration and further inability to fall asleep. In delayed sleep phase syndrome, the major sleep episode is delayed in relation to the desired clock time, resulting in symptoms of sleep-onset insomnia and difficulty awakening. In advanced sleep phase syndrome, the major sleep episode is advanced in relation to the desired clock time, resulting in excessive evening sleepiness and early sleep onset, as well as awakening earlier than desired. This condition is more common in the elderly. Jet lag syndrome is caused by the travel across multiple time zones.

American Academy of Sleep Medicine. International Classification of Sleep Disorders, 2nd ed. Diagnostic and Coding Manual, Westchester, IL: American Academy of Sleep Medicine; 2005.

Bradley WG, Daroff RB, Fenichel GM, et al. Neurology in Clinical Practice, 5th ed. Philadelphia, PA: Elsevier; 2008.

96. a

This patient has psychophysiologic insomnia. Patients with this condition have difficulty falling asleep at the desired bedtime, with frequent awakening. These patients "try to fall asleep," and are extremely concerned about and focus on their insomnia. There is frustration about being unable to initiate and maintain sleep. This worry about the need for sleep prevents these patients from falling asleep adequately, creating anxiety regarding sleepless. These patients do not meet criteria for a generalized anxiety disorder.

· This patient does not have delayed sleep phase syndrome, advanced sleep phase syndrome, jet lag syndrome, or shift work sleep disorder. In delayed sleep phase syndrome, the major sleep episode is delayed in relation to the desired clock time, resulting in symptoms of sleep-onset insomnia and difficulty awakening. In advanced sleep phase syndrome, the major sleep episode is advanced in relation to the desired clock time, resulting in excessive evening sleepiness and early sleep onset, as well as awakening earlier than desired. This condition is more common in the elderly. Jet lag syndrome is caused by the travel across multiple time zones. In shift work sleep disorder, patients experience symptoms of insomnia or excessive sleepiness that occur as a transient phenomena in relation to work schedules.

American Academy of Sleep Medicine. International Classification of Sleep Disorders, 2nd ed. Diagnostic and Coding Manual, Westchester, IL: American Academy of Sleep Medicine; 2005.

Bradley WG, Daroff RB, Fenichel GM, et al. Neurology in Clinical Practice, 5th ed. Philadelphia, PA: Elsevier; 2008.

97. a

This patient has restless legs syndrome (RLS), which is characterized by an urge to move the legs that may be associated with abnormal sensations that may be difficult to describe. The urge to move the legs is worse at rest and in the evening or nighttime. The urge to move the legs is partially or completely relieved by movement. This condition occurs more commonly in women, and although the pathophysiology is not well known, it has been associated with abnormalities in dopaminergic pathways, basal ganglia abnormalities, and decreased ferritin levels. Patients with RLS can have sleep disturbance and insomnia.

Periodic limb movements (PLMs) are a polysomnographic finding, in which there are recurrent limb movements during non-REM sleep, more commonly of the lower extremities. PLMs can produce arousals and sleep fragmentation, leading to insomnia and excessive daytime sleepiness. PLMs are often seen in patients with RLS, but in this case, the most likely diagnosis on the basis of the clinical information is RLS.

This patient does not have psychophysiologic insomnia, delayed sleep phase syndrome, or advanced sleep phase syndrome. In psychophysiologic insomnia, patients worry about being unable to sleep and focus on their insomnia, which causes frustration and further inability to fall asleep. In delayed sleep phase syndrome, the major sleep episode is delayed in relation to the desired clock time, resulting in symptoms of sleep-onset insomnia and difficulty awakening. In advanced sleep phase syndrome, the major sleep episode is advanced in relation to the desired clock time, resulting in excessive evening sleepiness and early sleep onset, as well as awakening earlier than desired. This condition is more common in the elderly.

American Academy of Sleep Medicine. International Classification of Sleep Disorders, 2nd ed. Diagnostic and Coding Manual, Westchester, IL: American Academy of Sleep Medicine; 2005.

Bradley WG, Daroff RB, Fenichel GM, et al. Neurology in Clinical Practice, 5th ed. Philadelphia, PA: Elsevier; 2008.

98. d

Low hypocretin levels have been associated with narcolepsy, but have not been implicated in the pathophysiology of restless legs syndrome (RLS).

RLS is associated with low ferritin levels and iron deficiency, and it is thought that these may be implicated in the pathophysiology of the disease, and therefore ferritin levels should be tested in patients with this disorder. In general, iron supplementation should be initiated for ferritin levels less than 50 ng/mL. Dopaminergic pathways have been also implicated in the pathophysiology, and dopamine agonists are part of the treatment options, including pramipexole and ropinirole.

Many other conditions can also be associated with RLS, including folate deficiency, chronic renal failure, neuropathies, myelopathies, multiple sclerosis, diabetes mellitus, amyloidosis, cancer, peripheral vascular disease, rheumatoid arthritis, hypothyroidism, and certain drugs.

American Academy of Sleep Medicine. International Classification of Sleep Disorders, 2nd ed. Diagnostic and Coding Manual, Westchester, IL: American Academy of Sleep Medicine; 2005.

Bradley WG, Daroff RB, Fenichel GM, et al. Neurology in Clinical Practice, 5th ed. Philadelphia, PA: Elsevier; 2008.

Buzz Phrases	Key Points
Periodic lateralized epileptiform discharges	HSV infection
Automatisms	Temporal lobe epilepsy
3-Hz spike and wave	Absence epilepsy
4- to 6-Hz polyspikes	Juvenile myoclonic epilepsy
Autoinduction	Carbamazepine
Nephrolithiasis	Topiramate and zonisamide
Stevens–Johnson syndrome	Lamotrigine
Hypsarrhythmia	Infantile spasms
Fencer's posture	Supplementary motor area
Figure of 4 sign	Supplementary motor area
Doose syndrome	Myoclonic–astatic epilepsy
Dravet syndrome	Severe myoclonic epilepsy of infancy
Ohtahara syndrome	Early infantile epileptic encephalopathy
West syndrome	Triad of infantile spasms, hypsarrhythmia, and mental retardation

(*continued*)

Buzz Phrases	Key Points
Panayiotopoulos syndrome	Occipital epilepsy with tonic eye deviation, ictal vomiting, and visual seizures
Lennox–Gastaut syndrome	Multiple seizure types, slow spike–wave complexes, and mental retardation
Landau–Kleffner syndrome	Epilepsy with multiple seizure types and acquired aphasia
Nocturnal hypermotor seizures (non-REM)	Autosomal dominant nocturnal frontal lobe epilepsy
Gelastic seizures	Hypothalamic hamartoma
Head version	Contralateral frontal lobe
Dystonic posture during seizure	Contralateral temporal lobe
EPM1	Unverricht Lundborg syndrome
Cystatin B	Unverricht Lundborg syndrome
EPM2A	Lafora body disease
PME and cherry red spot	Sialidosis
PME and mitochondrial disease	Myoclonic epilepsy with ragged red fibers
Antibodies to glutamate receptor-3	Rasmussen's encephalitis
α-rhythm frequency	8–13 Hz
β-rhythm frequency	>13 Hz
θ-rhythm frequency	4–7 Hz
δ-rhythm frequency	<4 Hz
Triphasic waves	Metabolic encephalopathy
Temporal periodic lateralized epileptiform discharges	HSV encephalitis
K complex and sleep spindles	Stage II sleep
REMs and atonia	REM sleep
Apnea with no respiratory effort	Central sleep apnea
Apnea with respiratory effort	Obstructive sleep apnea
Low hypocretin	Narcolepsy
Low ferritin	Restless legs syndrome
REM sleep behavioral disorders	α-synucleinopathies

Chapter 6

Movement Disorders

Questions

Questions 1–2

1. Regarding the anatomy of the basal ganglia, which of the following statements is incorrect?
   a. The striatum consists of the caudate and putamen
   b. The lenticular nucleus consists of the putamen and globus pallidus
   c. The majority of cortical projections to the basal ganglia are to the striatum and subthalamic nucleus
   d. The major outflow of the basal ganglia arises in the putamen
   e. The globus pallidus projects to the thalamus, which, in turn, projects to multiple cortical areas

2. Regarding basal ganglia circuits, which of the following statements is correct?
   a. The indirect pathway is excitatory: by increasing inhibition of the globus pallidus interna (GPi), it increases thalamic output
   b. The direct pathway is inhibitory: by increasing inhibition of the GPi, it decreases thalamic output
   c. Projections from the GPi to the thalamus are inhibitory
   d. Projections of the thalamus to the cortex are inhibitory
   e. Projections from the subthalamic nucleus to the GPi are inhibitory

Questions 3–4

3. Which of the following statements is correct regarding the direct and indirect circuits of the basal ganglia?
   a. Hyperkinetic movement disorders result from increased activity in the indirect pathway
   b. Hypokinetic movement disorders result from increased activity in the direct pathway
   c. The net effect of activity in the indirect pathway is to normally increase movement
   d. The net effect of activity in the direct pathway is to normally inhibit movement
   e. Hyperkinetic movement disorders result from reduced activity in the indirect pathway

211

4. Which of the following statements is incorrect?
   a. The substantia nigra pars compacta (SNc) normally inhibits the indirect pathway and excites the direct pathway
   b. Parkinson's disease (PD) results from degeneration of the SNc, which leads to reduced activity in the direct pathway and increased activity in the indirect pathway, leading to bradykinesia
   c. In Huntington's disease, a reduction of activity in the indirect pathway disinhibits the thalamus, leading to increased activity, in the form of chorea and other extraneous movements
   d. Abnormalities in the direct and indirect pathway do not account for all of the features of most movement disorders such as PD, in which both hyperkinetic and bradykinetic movements occur in combination
   e. Decreased thalamocortical activity results in hyperkinetic movement disorders and increased thalamocortical activity results in hypokinetic movement disorders

5. Regarding neurotransmission in the basal ganglia, which of the following statements is incorrect?
   a. Glutamate is the major excitatory neurotransmitter of the basal ganglia
   b. GABA is the major inhibitory neurotransmitter of the basal ganglia
   c. GABA is the major neurotransmitter released in striatal projections to the globus pallidus and in globus pallidus interna projections to the thalamus
   d. D_1 receptors are primarily found on neurons involved in the indirect pathway, and D_2 receptors on neurons involved in the direct pathway
   e. The substantia nigra pars compacta inhibits the indirect pathway via activity at D_2 receptors and excites the direct pathway via activity at D_1 receptors

Questions 6–7

6. A 52-year-old man presented to the clinic complaining of a tremor. His wife had noticed a tremor over the prior year, mainly while he was at rest, such as while watching television. He also complained of walking slower, and his wife reported that his voice was softer. On directed questioning, his handwriting had gotten smaller as well. He was otherwise healthy, and had no complaints of cognitive problems. On examination, he had a moderate frequency rest tremor in the right hand, with mild cogwheeling in the right arm. On gait examination, he had a slightly flexed posture and he swung his right arm less than the left. Finger tapping was slower on the right. Examination was otherwise unremarkable. What is the most likely diagnosis in this patient?
   a. Idiopathic Parkinson's disease
   b. DLB
   c. Vascular parkinsonism
   d. Drug-induced parkinsonism
   e. Corticobasal ganglionic degeneration

7. A 63-year-old woman presented to the clinic complaining of walking difficulties of 2 years' duration that had worsened over time. She had first noticed less agility of her right hand and felt her right foot was dragging slightly. She had always been a fast walker, but more recently, she had noticed that she had significantly slowed down. She also complained that she had a hard time projecting her voice, and her handwriting had gotten smaller. She denied having tremor. On examination, she had reduced facial expression, reduced blinking frequency, and moderate cogwheeling rigidity of the right upper extremities. There was mild cogwheeling in the left upper extremity with facilitation. On gait examination, she had a stooped posture, and reduced arm swing bilaterally, right more than left. She turned en bloc. On the pull test (pulled backward by examiner while stationary), she was able to take one step back and prevent herself from falling. No tremor was evident on examination. Finger tapping was slow bilaterally, right more than left. What is the most likely diagnosis in this patient?

   a. Idiopathic Parkinson's disease
   b. DLB
   c. Vascular parkinsonism
   d. Drug-induced parkinsonism
   e. Progressive supranuclear palsy

8. Regarding the clinical features of idiopathic Parkinson's disease (PD), which of the following statements is incorrect?

   a. The tremor is typically a resting tremor of moderate frequency, 4 to 6 Hz
   b. Postural tremor can occur; with assumption of a specific posture, there is usually a latency of a few seconds before the tremor reemerges
   c. Loss of postural reflexes does not occur in idiopathic PD; its presence suggests an alternative diagnosis
   d. Freezing is most often a feature of advanced disease
   e. The rigidity is often cogwheeling, and can be proximal or distal, involving both axial and limb muscles

9. Which of the following statements is correct regarding the nonmotor symptoms seen in patients with idiopathic Parkinson's disease (PD)?

   a. Shoulder pain in a patient with PD should prompt an extensive work-up for orthopedic problems, as the pain would not be attributable to the PD itself
   b. Urinary frequency, urgency, and nocturia occur only in male PD patients with prostatic hypertrophy
   c. In a patient with parkinsonism and orthostatic hypotension, the diagnosis cannot be idiopathic PD; it must be multiple-system atrophy
   d. Constipation is a prominent symptom in patients with PD, and may predate the motor symptoms for years
   e. REM sleep behavioral disorder in a patient with parkinsonism implies the diagnosis is DLB, not idiopathic PD

10. A 63-year-old woman with a 5-year history of idiopathic Parkinson's disease (PD) presents to her neurologist for routine follow-up. Her motor examination is stable, and she feels that her regimen of dopaminergic therapy is adequate. However, her affect is blunted and she describes multiple complaints, including loss of interest in social activities, reduced appetite, increased sleep, and a sense of hopelessness. Which of the following statements is correct in relation to this patient?

   a. She is suffering from depression, and should be treated with appropriate pharmacologic and nonpharmacologic measures targeted at the depression specifically
   b. These symptoms are part of her PD and are best treated by optimizing her dopaminergic regimen
   c. She is suffering from an adjustment disorder due to the diagnosis of PD, and just needs some encouragement
   d. Her affect is blunted only because of the hypomimia that occurs in PD
   e. Her symptoms are likely due to the sedating side effects of her dopaminergic therapy, and her dopaminergic therapy regimen should be reduced

11. A 72-year-old man diagnosed with idiopathic Parkinson's disease (PD) 15 years earlier presented for follow-up with his neurologist. He had bilateral asymmetric tremor, rigidity, and bradykinesia, all of which had worsened. He had been falling frequently recently, and had started using a walker. The patient's wife reported concerns about his memory; he was forgetting even basic things like his son's phone number, and he had forgotten his car engine turned on overnight in recent weeks. He was also somewhat more withdrawn and less sociable. The patient denied memory loss. He was referred for formal neuropsychologic evaluation, which showed markedly impaired memory and impaired visuospatial abilities. Word fluency was moderately impaired. There had been significant declines in performance as compared to neuropsychologic evaluation done 10 years prior; on that evaluation, the patient had normal or borderline impaired scores. What is the most likely diagnosis in this patient?
    a. FTD occurring concomitant with idiopathic PD
    b. He was misdiagnosed 15 years earlier; he has had DLB all along
    c. PD with dementia
    d. Normal-pressure hydrocephalus
    e. He was misdiagnosed 15 years earlier; he has corticobasal ganglionic degeneration

12. Which of the following statements is incorrect regarding the pathophysiology of idiopathic Parkinson's disease (PD)?
    a. Results from degeneration of dopaminergic neurons in the substantia nigra pars reticulata
    b. Pathologic changes occur in the olfactory regions, dorsal motor nucleus of the vagus, brain stem (locus coeruleus and raphe nuclei), and basal ganglia, as well as enteric nervous system
    c. A subset of patients have familial, monogenetic forms of PD
    d. The pathologic hallmark of idiopathic PD is deposition of Lewy bodies
    e. Idiopathic PD is a synucleinopathy

13. Which of the following Parkinson's disease medication-mechanism of action pairs is incorrect?
    a. Carbidopa–dopa-decarboxylase inhibitor
    b. Ropinirole–agonist at D_2 and D_3 receptors
    c. Rasagiline–monoamine oxidase type B inhibitor
    d. Entacapone–nonspecific monoamine oxidase inhibitor
    e. Trihexyphenidyl–anticholinergic

14. Which of the following statements regarding side effects of therapies for idiopathic Parkinson's disease is incorrect?
    a. Anticholinergic agents can cause significant cognitive dysfunction
    b. Dopamine agonists carry little risk of impulse control problems unless the patient has a prior history of impulse control problems
    c. Levodopa can cause extraneous movements, dyskinesias, and the risk increases with increasing dose and duration of therapy
    d. One of the metabolites of selegiline is methamphetamine, and side effects from it include insomnia
    e. Sedation is a prominent side effect of dopamine agonists

15. A 79-year-old male presents to the clinic complaining of tremor. On examination, he has moderate bradykinesia, and bilateral tremor and rigidity, both worse in the right arm. His wife reports

that he takes several naps during the day and that he is sometimes forgetful. The wife and the patient minimized his cognitive symptoms. What is the most appropriate treatment for this patient?

a. Ropinirole

b. Carbidopa-levodopa

c. Pramipexole

d. Trihexyphenidyl

e. Bromocriptine

16. Regarding the surgical treatment of idiopathic Parkinson's disease (PD), which of the following statements is incorrect?

a. If the motor symptoms are markedly asymmetric, with the less affected side being minimally involved, unilateral deep brain stimulation (DBS) can be done

b. DBS is effective in treating tremor and bradykinesia

c. DBS is effective in treating gait freezing and falls

d. Significant cognitive impairment is a contraindication to DBS

e. DBS targets for PD have included the subthalamic nucleus, globus pallidus interna, and the ventral intermediate nucleus of the thalamus

17. A 64-year-old woman presented to the clinic with a 2-year history of falling that had progressed over time. She reported she would just suddenly fall, without a trigger. She noticed difficulty going downstairs. On examination, in primary gaze, she had subtle jerk nystagmus. Her neck was hyperextended and she had difficulty flexing it. She had impaired vertical gaze, predominantly on downward gaze. However, on vertical oculocephalic maneuver, downward gaze was normal. There was mild bilateral rigidity in the upper extremities. On the pull test (examiner pulls the patient backward, instructing the patient to take a step back and prevent falling), she had significant retropulsion and would have fallen if not caught by the examiner. What is the most likely diagnosis in this patient?

a. Idiopathic Parkinson's disease with early falling

b. Multiple-system atrophy

c. Progressive supranuclear palsy

d. Normal-pressure hydrocephalus

e. Corticobasal ganglionic degeneration

Questions 18–19

18. A 54-year-old woman presents with a 1-year history of light-headedness when rising from a seated position. This had worsened over time, and she uses a wheelchair to get around for fear of having a syncopal episode. On directed questioning, she reports urinary urgency for several years, with urge incontinence for the past 6 months. On examination in the clinic, her sitting blood pressure is 120/80 mm Hg. Standing blood pressure is 80/60 mm Hg, associated with significant light-headedness. Examination also shows an involuntary flexed posture of her neck, bilateral rigidity in the upper and lower extremities, and a bilateral slight rest tremor of moderate frequency. What is the most likely diagnosis in this patient?

a. Idiopathic Parkinson's disease with associated dysautonomia

b. Multiple-system atrophy

c. Progressive supranuclear palsy

d. Primary autonomic failure

e. Corticobasal ganglionic degeneration

19. A 56-year-old man presented to the clinic with bilateral upper extremity rest tremor of 6 months' duration. On examination, he had bilateral moderate-frequency rest tremor, slightly worse in the right upper extremity compared to the left, and bilateral cogwheel rigidity that appeared to be equal in both extremities. He had significant bradykinesia affecting both sides of his body. He was prescribed levodopa, which had little effect on his symptoms. On follow-up 1 year later, he reported significant gait instability. Examination showed bilateral dysmetria and his gait was wide-based and slightly lurching. MRI is shown in Figure 6.1. What is the most likely diagnosis in this patient?

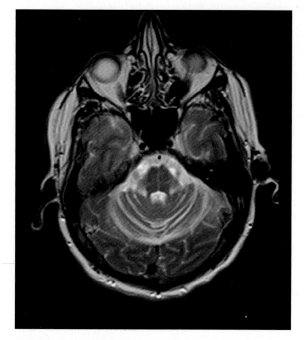

FIGURE 6.1 Axial T2-weighted MRI

    a. Idiopathic Parkinson's disease
    b. Multiple-system atrophy
    c. Progressive supranuclear palsy
    d. Primary autonomic failure
    e. Corticobasal ganglionic degeneration

20. A 62-year-old male presented to the clinic complaining of arm pain. He reported that his right arm felt stiff and painful, and it would tremor at rest. He also reported difficulty walking, but had not fallen. On examination, he had dystonia of the right arm with flexed posture at the elbow and wrist. He had occasional whole-body jerks. Sensation to light-touch, pinprick, and other primary sensory modalities was normal, but with his eyes closed, he could not identify objects placed in his right hand or numbers drawn on his palm. What is the most likely diagnosis in this patient?

    a. Idiopathic Parkinson's disease
    b. Multiple-system atrophy

c. Progressive supranuclear palsy
d. Normal-pressure hydrocephalus
e. Corticobasal ganglionic degeneration

21. Which of the following statements regarding secondary parkinsonism is incorrect?
    a. Postencephalitic parkinsonism has been seen following infection with influenza virus, West Nile virus, and Japanese encephalitis virus
    b. Vascular parkinsonism classically affects the lower extremities more than the upper extremities, and rigidity and bradykinesia predominate the picture, with little tremor
    c. Drug-induced parkinsonism is most commonly seen with antipsychotic agents
    d. Magnesium toxicity can lead to parkinsonism
    e. Parkinsonism can be a feature of normal-pressure hydrocephalus and other causes of chronic hydrocephalus

Questions 22–24

22. A 33-year-old overweight woman with asthma presents to the clinic complaining of tremor. She reports she had a tremor since her teenage years but it had not really bothered her until the prior year. Her handwriting was starting to be "shaky" and she was not able to eat soup without spilling. She worked in construction and often operated heavy machinery, and was concerned that her tremor was putting herself and others in danger. Her father and paternal grandfather had a similar tremor. On examination, there was no tremor at rest. With outstretched arms, or while pouring water from one cup to another, a prominent bilateral high-frequency tremor was observed. What is the most likely diagnosis in this patient?
    a. Enhanced physiologic tremor
    b. Essential tremor
    c. Dystonic tremor
    d. Task-specific tremor
    e. Rubral tremor

23. Regarding the disorder depicted in question 22, which of the following statements is incorrect?
    a. The tremor is typically high frequency, in the range of 4 to 8 Hz
    b. The tremor is typically most prominent with assumption of specific postures and with action
    c. Alcohol intake improves the tremor
    d. The tremor seen in this disorder persists during sleep
    e. There is typically a family history of tremor in patients with this disorder

24. What is the most appropriate long-term therapy for this patient given her medical history and occupation?
    a. Propranolol
    b. Clonazepam
    c. Ethanol
    d. Topiramate
    e. Levodopa

Questions 25–27

25. A 9-year-old boy is brought to the clinic by his parents. They reported that for the past 2 years, he had multiple gestures and behaviors. They were frustrated that he would not stop them.

His teachers at school complained that he was disruptive to his classmates, and many of his prior friends would no longer spend time with him. They reported frequent grunting, sniffing, and odd loud vocalizations that sounded like a chicken clucking. In addition, he had frequent eye blinking, arm flapping, and shoulder shrugging. The patient reported that he could suppress these sounds or movements, but only for a brief period, after which he would have to do them and would feel better after doing so. Besides the abnormal movements and vocalizations, his physical examination is otherwise normal. What is the most likely diagnosis in this patient?

  a. Tourette's syndrome
  b. Simple motor tic
  c. Simple vocal tic
  d. Complex motor tic
  e. Secondary tourettism

26. Which of the following statements regarding the disorder depicted in question 25 is incorrect?
  a. It is more common in males
  b. To make the diagnosis, symptoms have to start before the age of 18
  c. Common comorbidities include attention deficit/hyperactivity disorder and obsessive–compulsive disorder
  d. The symptoms commonly improve with age
  e. Its pathophysiology relates to dopamine deficiency

27. Which of the following management strategies is not typically used for treatment of patients with this disorder?
  a. Clonidine
  b. Risperidone or other atypical antipsychotics
  c. Haloperidol or other typical antipsychotics
  d. Levodopa
  e. Habit-reversal therapy

Questions 28–29

28. A 21-year-old woman presents with multiple abnormal movements, including a moderate-frequency rest and postural tremor and a twisting and in-turning of her right foot. Her history was also significant for depression with suicide attempt and significant anxiety. Her MRI is shown in Figure 6.2. Laboratory tests show elevated liver enzymes. What is the most likely diagnosis in this patient?
  a. Essential tremor
  b. Tardive dystonia and tremor
  c. Wilson's disease
  d. Early-onset Parkinson's disease
  e. A psychogenic disorder

29. Which of the following statements is correct regarding the disorder depicted in question 28?
  a. It is autosomal dominant in inheritance
  b. It results from a mutation in the gene encoding for the copper-binding protein ceruloplasmin
  c. Treatment includes copper supplementation
  d. Treatment includes low zinc diet
  e. Treatment includes low copper diet

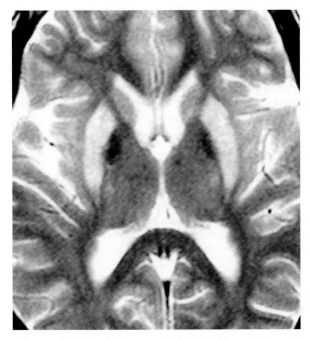

FIGURE 6.2   Axial T2-weighted MRI

Questions 30–31

30. A 32-year-old woman is brought to the clinic accompanied by her mother and brother. The patient had a 7-year history of depression with psychotic features and three suicide attempts. In recent months, she had started to have abnormal movements. The mother reported that the patient was "wiggly and jerky" all the time. On examination, she had rapid dance-like movements of all extremities. She could not protrude her tongue for a sustained period of time and move her eyes on a target while keeping her head still. The patient's psychiatrist had attributed these movements to antipsychotic therapy he had prescribed to her for psychotic depression, but the mother was concerned because the patient's father had similar symptoms before he died in a car accident a few years earlier. What is the most likely diagnosis in this patient?

   a. Tardive dyskinesia

   b. Wilson's disease

   c. Psychogenic disorder

   d. Huntington's disease

   e. Benign hereditary chorea

31. Which of the following statements is correct regarding the disorder depicted in question 30?

   a. It is autosomal recessive in inheritance

   b. It results from a mutation on chromosome 4

   c. Age of onset is stable over generations

   d. It results from a single-point mutation

   e. Atrophy of the brain stem is the most consistent imaging finding seen

32. Which of the following statements is incorrect regarding chorea?

    a. Chorea following streptococcal infection with rheumatic fever (Sydenham's disease) may occur months after the infection or may be the sole manifestation of rheumatic fever

    b. Occurrence of chorea during pregnancy (chorea gravidarum) may suggest prior history of rheumatic fever or presence of a connective tissue disorder, such as systemic lupus erythematosus

    c. Chorea may be the presenting feature of antiphospholipid antibody syndrome

    d. Sydenham's disease is best treated with dopaminergic therapies, such as levodopa

    e. Benign hereditary chorea results from a mutation in thyroid transcription factor

33. A 22-year-old man is brought to the clinic by his family for multiple symptoms. One year earlier, he had begun biting his lips to the point that they were macerated. He also was having forceful tongue protrusion, to the point where he could barely eat, and he had lost significant weight. He was having wavy, writhing movements as well as more rapid jerk-like movements of his extremities. His cognitive function had declined significantly, and his speech had become slow and slurred, barely intelligible. Serum cholesterol, vitamin E, and uric acid levels were normal. Retinal examination was also normal. What is the most likely diagnosis in this patient?

    a. Dentatorubral-pallidoluysian atrophy

    b. Neuroacanthocytosis

    c. Huntington's disease

    d. Abetalipoproteinemia

    e. Lesch-Nyhan syndrome

34. A 62-year-old man with diabetes, hypertension, and dyslipidemia presents to the emergency department with sudden onset of forceful, flinging movements of his right arm and involuntary jerking of his right leg. He reports that the day prior to the onset of these movements, he had transient weakness of the right arm and leg that had then resolved. A lesion in which of the following structures would explain this patient's symptoms?

    a. Ipsilateral subthalamic nucleus (STN)

    b. Ipsilateral medulla

    c. Contralateral STN

    d. Contralateral medulla

    e. Ipsilateral frontal lobe

35. A 52-year-old man with a 30-year history of schizophrenia that had been stable for 15 years since therapy with fluphenazine was initiated, presents to the clinic complaining of involuntary movements of his tongue, mouth, and jaw. On examination, he has almost constant jaw and lip movements and tongue protrusions. Which of the following statements is correct regarding this patient's disorder?

    a. He likely has an acute dystonic reaction to antipsychotics. His antipsychotic should be stopped immediately and he should be administered an anticholinergic agent

    b. He likely has tardive dyskinesia. His antipsychotic should be stopped immediately and he should be administered an anticholinergic agent

    c. He likely has a primary dystonia unrelated to his prior history of medication exposure

    d. He likely has tardive dyskinesia and he should be treated with higher doses of fluphenazine

    e. This disorder is more likely to occur with typical antipsychotics, but can occur with atypical antipsychotics as well

36. A 22-year-old man presents to the clinic on a wheelchair. At the age of 11 years, he had started having involuntary twisting posturing of his left foot that would occur while he was playing soccer. Over time, the twisting of his foot started to occur at rest and then his entire left leg became involved. Later, his trunk and other extremities became involved as well. By the age of 16, his limbs and trunk were so "contorted" that he could no longer walk without assistance, and in the prior year, had become wheelchair bound. He had two cousins affected with a similar disorder but of less severity; his sister, who was 33-years-old, had abnormal posturing of her left foot but was otherwise fine. The patient was given a trial of levodopa without benefit. What is the most likely diagnosis in this patient?

   a. Dopa-responsive dystonia (Segawa's syndrome)
   b. Primary generalized dystonia
   c. A segmental dystonia
   d. A psychogenic disorder, because he did not respond to levodopa
   e. Juvenile Parkinson's disease

37. A 52-year-old woman presents with head tremor and involuntary eyelid movements. She reports that for more than 10 years she had felt her head would pull to the right and slightly downward, causing pain. In recent years, she had begun to have a tremor in her head all the time, and the pain in her neck had worsened. Her head is now almost constantly pulled to the right and downward, and the only way she can relieve this is by resting her head on a pillow in a very specific position. More recently, she has begun to have involuntary eyelid closure that occurs most often when it is sunny and she is driving. She has no prior exposure to dopamine antagonists and is otherwise generally healthy. Which of the following statements is correct regarding this patient's condition?

   a. Botulinum toxin therapy is contraindicated in this disorder
   b. Botulinum toxin therapy is the mainstay of treatment for this disorder
   c. Her involuntary eyelid closure is likely a tic
   d. She has a rare form of focal dystonia
   e. The tremor in her head is likely from essential tremor

38. A 13-year-old girl is brought to the clinic by her parents, who complain that whenever it is time for the girl to participate in afterschool activities such as dance class, she starts to walk in a funny way and cannot participate in the activities. Some of the girl's teachers had suggested that she was "faking it" to get out of dance class. On examination, she has mild cogwheel rigidity of the upper extremities and slow finger tapping bilaterally, right more than left, and gait examination showed in-turning and dorsiflexion at the left ankle. Which of the following statements is incorrect?

   a. This patient likely has dopa-responsive dystonia
   b. This patient's disorder results from a mutation in the enzyme guanosine triphosphate cyclo-hydrolase I
   c. The occurrence of her symptoms in the afternoon suggests she is malingering to get out of dance class
   d. This disorder is more common in females
   e. This patient will likely improve with low doses of levodopa without significant risk of dyskinesias

39. A 52-year-old woman violinist presents to the clinic complaining of abnormal contractions of her fingers that occur while she is playing her violin. These began around 1 year earlier. These contractions have been interfering with her performance, and she is concerned about losing her position in the orchestra. These contractions occur only while she is playing the violin and never during other activities. On examination, no abnormalities are seen, but on a video she brings of herself playing the violin, her fourth and fifth digits are seen to contract briefly in initial extension and then flexion. Which of the following statements is incorrect regarding this patient's condition?

a. She has a task-specific dystonia
b. Focal botulinum toxin can be effective for this disorder
c. She is at high risk of developing generalized dystonia
d. She has a primary dystonia
e. The dystonia may overflow to more proximal areas over time

40. A 42-year-old man with congenital heart disease suffers a cardiac arrest. After 20 minutes of cardiopulmonary resuscitation, pulse is regained and blood pressure is stabilized. He remains in the ICU on mechanical ventilation for several days, but is finally extubated and discharged to a rehabilitation facility. Three months later, he presents with involuntary jerks of his arms and trunk and significant difficulty walking due to a sensation that his legs are suddenly giving out. Which of the following statements is incorrect regarding this patient's condition?

a. He has cortical myoclonus
b. He has a form of spinal segmental myoclonus
c. His gait disorder is likely resulting from involvement of his leg muscles with the myoclonus
d. An EEG employing specific electrophysiologic techniques would show a cortical discharge prior to the myoclonus
e. This is Lance-Adams syndrome that may be seen after hypoxic–ischemic brain injury

41. A 33-year-old woman presents to the clinic complaining of clicking in her ear. On examination, rhythmic contractions of her palate are seen. Which of the following statements is correct?

a. She likely has epileptic myoclonus
b. She has palatal myoclonus, and the contractions may persist during sleep in some cases
c. This disorder results from caudate atrophy
d. Inferior olive atrophy will be seen on an MRI of her brain
e. She is having auditory hallucinations and the rhythmic contractions are voluntary

42. A 62-year-old woman presents with involuntary facial contractions. When they had started 1 year earlier, there was just involuntary jerking of her eye, and people always thought she was winking at them. Later on, they began to involve her cheek and upper lip as well. There was no pain, but there was some discomfort, and the appearance bothered her. Which of the following statements regarding this patient's condition is incorrect?

a. A structural lesion is not identified on MRI of the brain in the majority of patients
b. This patient has hemifacial spasm
c. This patient has blepharospasm (only eyes).
d. Botulinum toxin injection is the mainstay of therapy for this disorder
e. Vascular compression of the facial nerve may be involved in some cases

43. A 7-year-old boy is brought to the clinic by his parents for concern of seizures. He has episodes during which he flaps his arms repeatedly against his sides and then against his head, sometimes for several minutes. During these episodes, he ignores everyone around him. These episodes most often occur when he is upset, but also in the evening around the time his father gets back

home from work, particularly when his father brings home ice cream or other treats. He has a history of delayed motor and language milestones, and has been recommended special classes at school. He does not have many friends and spends most of his free time playing with the same train set, assembling and disassembling it repeatedly. Which of the following statements is correct regarding the nature of this patient's episodes?

   a. He likely has seizures and he should undergo video-EEG monitoring

   b. He likely has a complex motor tic disorder

   c. This patient's history is consistent with Tourette's syndrome

   d. He has paroxysmal dyskinesias

   e. This patient likely has stereotypies

44. A 12-year-old boy has multiple attacks per day, characterized by dystonic posturing of his arm and leg. These episodes most often occur when he is playing with his friends, but can occur at anytime. He is an avid basketball player, but has not been participating as much in basketball lately because the attacks occur frequently during such activities, and he has fallen or dropped the ball several times during these attacks. They last about 15 to 30 seconds, and can occur multiple times a day, depending on his level of activity. They also occur if he is startled. In between episodes, he has an entirely normal examination. Which of the following statements is correct regarding this patient's condition?

   a. This disorder results from a mutation in the nicotinic acetylcholine receptor

   b. This patient has paroxysmal nonkinesigenic dyskinesia

   c. A good response to anticonvulsants is seen in this disorder

   d. A good response to acetazolamide is seen in this disorder

   e. This is an epileptic disorder

45. A 10-year-old boy is brought to the clinic by his mother for episodes of unsteadiness. The patient experiences episodes once every few days characterized by gait unsteadiness, "as if he was drunk," associated with "jiggling eyes," some double vision, mild slurring of speech, and a throbbing headache. These last around 4 hours on most days, but once lasted a whole day. In between episodes, he is normal. What is the most likely diagnosis in this patient?

   a. Episodic ataxia type I

   b. Episodic ataxia type II

   c. Episodic ataxia type III

   d. Episodic ataxia type IV

   e. Paroxysmal nonkinesigenic dyskinesias

46. A 45-year-old woman presents to the clinic complaining of difficulty walking. She had begun to have cramps in her arms and legs many years earlier and over the prior year, had noticed that her legs were very stiff and tight. She was having trouble walking and had fallen several times, and also reported difficulty leaning forward to pick things up off the floor. She felt "tight and stiff all over." On examination, she had significantly increased tone in the upper and lower extremities bilaterally, visible contraction of the paraspinal muscles, exaggerated lumbar lordosis, and exaggerated startle response. Which of the following statements is incorrect regarding this patient's diagnosis?

   a. Antiglutamic acid decarboxylase antibodies are present in most patients with this disorder

   b. There is an association between this disorder and insulin-dependent diabetes

   c. This disorder can be autoimmune or paraneoplastic, particularly in association with anti-amphiphysin antibodies

d. Levodopa is a useful therapy in patients with this disorder

e. Benzodiazepines and baclofen are useful therapies for patients with this disorder

47. A mother brings her 3-month-old boy to the clinic. She reports that sometimes when he is picked up, he stiffens up for several seconds. When he is put back down, he loosens up again. This happens consistently and is very concerning to her. He also seems to be very "jumpy": even slightly loud or unexpected noises cause him to suddenly jerk. A diagnosis of hyperekplexia is suspected. Which of the following statements is incorrect regarding hyperekplexia?

a. Some patients respond to benzodiazepines or sodium valproate

b. Mutations in the glycine receptor and presynaptic glycine transporter have been identified in familial hyperekplexia

c. Glycine is the inhibitory neurotransmitter at spinal interneurons, including Renshaw cells and Ia inhibitory interneurons

d. Hyperekplexia results from abnormal spinal Ia inhibitory interneuron reciprocal inhibition

e. Hyperekplexia is a startle-evoked epileptic seizure

48. Regarding cerebellar anatomy, which of the following statements is incorrect?

a. Purkinje cells are inhibitory; their neurotransmitter is GABA

b. The superior cerebellar peduncle carries the majority of cerebellar efferents

c. Cerebellar hemisphere lesions lead to contralateral clinical signs

d. Climbing fibers originating from the inferior olive constitute a large component of cerebellar afferents

e. Granule cells are the only cerebellar cell types that are excitatory

49. A 63-year-old man with a history of alcoholism of more than 30 years' duration presents to the clinic complaining of walking difficulties. On examination, he has a wide-based, lurching gait. There is minimal dysmetria on finger-to-nose or heel-to-shin testing. There are no eye movement abnormalities and no nystagmus. MRI of the brain shows cerebellar atrophy, particularly in the midline. Which of the following statements is correct regarding this man's gait disorder?

a. His history of alcoholism is unlikely to be related as only acute alcohol intoxication leads to gait ataxia

b. Chronic alcohol exposure leads to significant cerebellar hemisphere atrophy with relative sparing of midline structures

c. In an alcoholic with ataxia, the cause is most likely a sensory neuropathy because the effects of alcohol on the cerebellum do not lead to clinical signs

d. Chronic alcohol exposure predominantly leads to atrophy of midline cerebellar structures, such as the vermis

e. Thiamine deficiency leads to memory loss and eye movement abnormalities, but not ataxia

50. Which of the following statements is incorrect regarding acquired causes of cerebellar ataxia?

a. Hypothyroidism can lead to gait ataxia, and thyroid-stimulating hormone should be checked in patients with gait ataxia

b. Celiac autoantibodies should be checked in patients with gait ataxia only if there are gastrointestinal symptoms to suggest gluten intolerance

c. The chemotherapeutic agent cytarabine can lead to irreversible cerebellar ataxia

d. Mercury and bismuth both can lead to cerebellar ataxia in toxic amounts

e. Chronic phenytoin can lead to cerebellar atrophy due to Purkinje cell loss

51. A 7-year-old boy is noted to have some clumsiness while walking. Over the subsequent 2 years, his gait becomes significantly ataxic, and he is brought to the clinic. On examination, he has reduced light-touch and vibratory sensation in the lower extremities, with impaired proprioception and hypoactive reflexes, but extensor plantar responses bilaterally. He has high-arched feet and scoliosis. His gait is wide based and lurching. He has dysmetria on finger-to-nose and heel-to-shin testing. Which of the following statements is incorrect regarding this patient's most likely diagnosis?

a. It is autosomal recessive in inheritance

b. It results from an expansion in a CAG trinucleotide repeat in the frataxin gene

c. It result from an expansion in a GAA trinucleotide repeat in the frataxin gene

d. The frataxin protein is a nuclear-encoded mitochondrial protein

e. Cardiac conduction defects and cardiomyopathy occur in patients with this disorder

52. A 9-year-old girl is brought to the clinic for concerns of gait instability. On examination, she has reduced sensation to light-touch and pinprick, reduced vibratory sensation, and impaired proprioception. Deep tendon reflexes are absent in the upper and lower extremities. She is also noted to have truncal and limb ataxia and choreoathetosis. On cranial nerve examination, she cannot move her eyes without thrusting her head in the direction of attempted gaze. Examination also shows multiple dilated tufts of capillary loops in the conjunctiva and oral mucosa. Which of the following statements is correct regarding this patient's most likely diagnosis?

a. It is autosomal dominant in inheritance

b. It results from a trinucleotide repeat expansion

c. It results in impaired DNA repair

d. Patients with this disorder have hypergammaglobulinemia

e. A reduced risk of malignancy is seen with this disorder

53. Which of the following statements is incorrect regarding the spinocerebellar ataxias?

a. They typically present in the third to fifth decades of life

b. They are autosomal dominant in inheritance

c. Cerebellar atrophy is seen on MRI of the brain

d. Neuropathy, upper motor neuron findings, and cognitive decline may occur

e. They all result from a CAG repeat expansion

54. A 63-year-old previously healthy man presents with tremor in both hands as well as gait instability. On examination, he has a bilateral rest and postural tremor, rigidity, bradykinesia, and a wide-based gait. Family history is remarkable only for mental retardation in his grandson. A T2-weighted image from his MRI is shown in Figure 6.3. Which of the following statements is incorrect regarding this patient's disorder?

a. This disorder occurs only in males

b. MRI of the brain may show T2 hyperintensities in the inferior cerebellar peduncle and cerebellum

c. Dysautonomia may occur as part of this syndrome

d. This disorder is X-linked

e. This patient should be checked for a premutation in the fragile X gene

59. The parents of a 7-year-old boy present with him to the clinic, requesting that he be tested for Huntington's disease. A family history of Huntington's disease is present, and the parents would like him to be tested so that they know what to expect for him in the future and to be able to plan accordingly. He has no neuropsychiatric signs or symptoms and no evidence of chorea or other abnormal movements. What is the most appropriate next step?

a. Order genetic testing for the boy, but advise the parents that the family should receive genetic counseling if the test is positive

b. Advise the family that genetic testing will not be ordered until he is 18 years of age and makes the decision himself to be tested

c. Alert social services that the parents are putting their son's autonomy at risk

d. Order genetic testing, but tell the parents that the results would not be revealed until their son is 18 years of age

e. Order genetic testing, but insist that the parents be tested as well

Answer key

1. d	**11.** c	**21.** d	**31.** b	**41.** b	**51.** b
2. c	**12.** a	**22.** b	**32.** d	**42.** c	**52.** c
3. e	**13.** d	**23.** d	**33.** b	**43.** e	**53.** e
4. e	**14.** b	**24.** d	**34.** c	**44.** c	**54.** a
5. d	**15.** b	**25.** a	**35.** e	**45.** b	**55.** d
6. a	**16.** c	**26.** e	**36.** b	**46.** d	**56.** e
7. a	**17.** c	**27.** d	**37.** b	**47.** e	**57.** a
8. c	**18.** b	**28.** c	**38.** c	**48.** c	**58.** d
9. d	**19.** b	**29.** e	**39.** c	**49.** d	**59.** b
10. a	**20.** e	**30.** d	**40.** b	**50.** b	

Answers

1. d, 2. c

The major outflow of the basal ganglia arises in the globus pallidus interna (GPi). Projections from the GPi to the thalamus are inhibitory, as discussed further below.

Projections to the basal ganglia arise from several areas. The majority of cortico-basal ganglia projections target the striatum, which consists of the caudate and putamen. The cortex also projects to the subthalamic nucleus (STN). The striatum also receives projections from the thalamus, substantia nigra, and brainstem (including projections from the norepinephrine-containing neurons in the locus coeruleus and serotonergic raphe nuclei). The lenticular nucleus (also known as the lentiform nucleus) consists of the putamen and globus pallidus. The globus pallidus is divided into globus pallidus externa (GPe) and globus pallidus interna (GPi). The major efferent pathways from the basal ganglia arise from the GPi as well as the substantia nigra pars reticulata (SNr) and project to the ventrolateral and ventroanterior nuclei of the thalamus. This projection of the GPi and SNr is inhibitory. The thalamus then projects to the motor and premotor cortex. The circuitry often referred to in discussion of the basal ganglia can therefore be summarized as cortico-striato-thalamo-cortical. Through various efferent and afferent pathways, the basal ganglia are involved in movement of the trunk and extremities and extraocular muscles, as well as in cognition and emotion.

Basal ganglia circuitry is complex, but certain simplifications allow for a basic understanding of basal ganglia function. The circuits of the basal ganglia can be thought of as consisting of two pathways: the indirect pathway and the direct pathway (Figure 6.5).

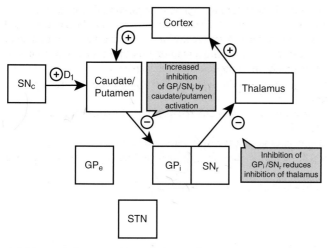

(a) Normal direct pathway schematic

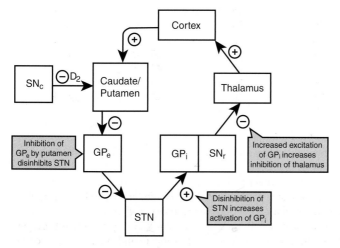

(b) Normal indirect pathway schematic

FIGURE 6.5   Schematic of normal basal ganglia circuitry: (a) direct and (b) indirect pathways (Illustration by David Schumick, BS, CMI. Reprinted with permission of the Cleveland Clinic Center for Medical Art & Photography. ⓒ 2010. All Rights Reserved)

The direct pathway (Figure 6.5a) consists of the caudate/putamen, GPi, SNr, and thalamus. In the direct pathway, the cerebral cortex sends excitatory projections to the caudate/putamen, which send inhibitory projections to the GPi and SNr. The GPi and SNr normally send inhibitory projections to the thalamus, and inhibition of the GPi and SNr therefore disinhibits the thalamus, increasing thalamic outflow to the cortex.

The indirect pathway consists of the caudate/putamen, GPe, STN, GPi, and thalamus (Figure 6.5b). In the indirect pathway, the cortex sends excitatory projections to the caudate/putamen, which sends inhibitory projections to the GPe. The GPe normally has inhibitory projections to the STN, and inhibition of the GPe by striatal projections disinhibits the STN. The STN then sends excitatory projections to the GPi. Recall that the GPi sends inhibitory projections to th thalamus. Therefore, the indirect pathway ultimately inhibits the thalamus, reducing thalamic outflow to the cortex.

The substantia nigra is a structure located between the crus cerebri and the tegmentum of the midbrain. It is a pigmented structure containing a high density of dopaminergic neurons. The substantia nigra pars compacta projects to the striatum, inhibiting the indirect pathway and exciting the direct pathway.

A mnemonic for basal ganglia circuitry is as follows:

Direct pathway: Cinnamon candy great in taste (CCG_iT): Cortex → Caudate/putamen → Globus pallidus interna → Thalamus

Indirect pathway: Cinnamon candy great excitement and supergreat in taste (CCG_eSG_iT): Cortex → Caudate/putamen → Globus pallidus externa → Subthalamic nucleus → Globus pallidus interna → Thalamus

In summary, because projections from the GPi to the thalamus are inhibitory:

– The direct pathway is excitatory: through inhibition of the GPi increases thalamocortical activity.
– The indirect pathway is inhibitory: through excitation of the GPi decreases thalamocortical activity.

These circuits are further discussed in questions 3 and 4.

Bradley WG, Daroff RB, Fenichel GM, et al. Neurology in Clinical Practice, 5th ed. Philadelphia, PA: Elsevier; 2008.

Fahn S, Jankovic J. Principles and Practice of Movement Disorders. Philadelphia, PA: Elsevier; 2007.

3. e,   4. e

Hyperkinetic movement disorders result from reduced activity in the indirect pathway. Thalamic projections to the motor cortex are excitatory; increased activity in thalamocortical projections leads to hyperkinetic movement disorders and decreased activity in hypokinetic movement disorders.

The anatomy of the direct and indirect pathways is described in questions 1 and 2 and Figure 6.5. Because activity in the direct pathway increases activity in thalamic projections to the motor cortex, the direct pathway plays a major role in initiating and maintaining movement. A reduction in activity of the direct pathway therefore reduces movement. Similarly, because the indirect pathway decreases activity in thalamocortical projections, the indirect pathway suppresses movement. Many movement disorders can be explained by reduced or increased activity in the direct or indirect pathway. In general, hyperkinetic movement disorders (those associated with increased and/or extraneous movements) result from reduced activity in the indirect pathway, whereas hypokinetic movement disorders (those marked by a reduction in movement) result from reduced activity in the direct pathway and this will be the premise for the following discussion. (Note however that many movement disorders lead to a combination of hyperkinesia and bradykinesia, with the prototype being Parkinson's disease (PD) (discussed in questions 6 and 7), suggesting that the indirect–direct pathway model is an oversimplification ̀ ̀s not fully explain many movement disorders.)

̀ substantia nigra pars compacta (SNc) inhibits the indirect pathway and excites the direct The SNc degenerates in PD. Reduced SNc activity leads to a reduction in thalamocortical ̀ue to reduced excitation of the direct pathway and reduced inhibition of the indirect ̀Figure 6.6a). Therefore, one hallmark of PD is bradykinesia. Reduced direct pathway ̀viously does not explain the tremor that occurs in PD.

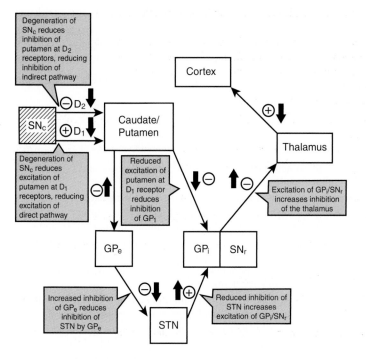

(a) Schematic of basal ganglia circuitry in Parkinson's Disease

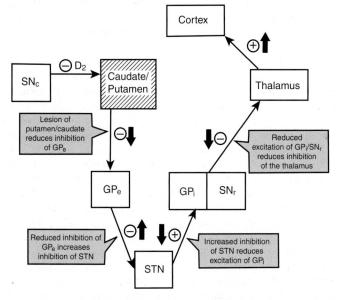

(b) Schematic of basal ganglia circuitry in chorea

FIGURE 6.6   Schematic of basal ganglia circuitry in (a) Parkinson's disease and (b) chorea (Illustration by David Schumick, BS, CMI. Reprinted with permission of the Cleveland Clinic Center for Medical Art & Photography. © 2010. All Rights Reserved)

In disorders in which chorea is the most prominent feature, such as Huntington's disease, a reduction of activity in the indirect pathway disinhibits the thalamus, leading to increased activity (Figure 6.6b). Bradykinesia is also a feature of Huntington's disease, and a reduction in indirect pathway activity does not fully explain the abnormalities of movement seen in this disorder.

Bradley WG, Daroff RB, Fenichel GM, et al. Neurology in Clinical Practice, 5th ed. Philadelphia, PA: Elsevier; 2008.

Fahn S, Jankovic J. Principles and Practice of Movement Disorders. Philadelphia, PA: Elsevier; 2007.

5. d

D_1 receptors are primarily found on neurons involved in the direct pathway, and D_2 receptors on neurons involved in the indirect pathway.

Glutamate is the major excitatory neurotransmitter in the basal ganglia; it is the neurotransmitter released at the majority of excitatory synapses, including cortical projections to the striatum, projections of the subthalamic nucleus to the globus pallidus interna (GPi), and projections of the thalamus to the cortex. GABA is the major inhibitory neurotransmitter of the basal ganglia and is the neurotransmitter released in projections of the striatum to the globus pallidus and the GPi to the thalamus. Various peptides colocalize with these neurotransmitters, including neuropeptide Y, dynorphin, and enkephalin.

Whether or not dopamine acts as an excitatory or inhibitory neurotransmitter depends on the receptor it is acting at. There are two families of dopamine receptors: D_1 and D_2. The D_1 to D_5 subtypes of the D_1 family of dopamine receptors are metabotropic receptors coupled to adenylate cyclase. D_1 receptors are primarily found on neurons involved in the direct pathway, and D_2 receptors on neurons involved in the indirect pathway. The substantia nigra pars compacta inhibits the indirect pathway via activity at D_2 receptors in the striatum and excites the direct pathway via activity at D_1 receptors in the striatum (Figure 6.5). Both D_1 and D_2 receptors are found in neurons of the cortex and the limbic system. D_2 receptors are found in the pituitary gland; activity at D_2 receptors in the pituitary inhibits prolactin release, hence the hyperprolactinemia seen in patients taking antipsychotics (which antagonize D_2 receptors).

Bradley WG, Daroff RB, Fenichel GM, et al. Neurology in Clinical Practice, 5th ed. Philadelphia, PA: Elsevier; 2008.

Fahn S, Jankovic J. Principles and Practice of Movement Disorders. Philadelphia, PA: Elsevier; 2007.

Strange PG. Dopamine receptors in the basal ganglia: Relevance to Parkinson's disease. Mov Disord. 1993; 8(3):263–270.

6. a, 7. a

Both the patients depicted in questions 6 and 7 have histories consistent with idiopathic Parkinson's disease (PD). Parkinsonism is a general term used for patients with tremor, bradykinesia, and/or rigidity. Idiopathic PD is a disorder characterized by tremor, bradykinesia (slowness of movement), and/or rigidity, but in the setting of specific clinical features and a temporal relation of the symptoms, in the absence of other historical and clinical findings that would suggest alternative causes of parkinsonism. The United Kingdom Parkinson's Disease Society Brain Bank's criteria for the diagnosis of PD include the presence of bradykinesia with either rest tremor, rigidity, or postural instability, in addition to at least three of the following features: unilateral onset, rest tremor, progression over time, persistent asymmetry, response to levodopa, levodopa-induced dyskinesias, and/or a clinical course of 10 or more years. As is evident from these criteria, tremor is not necessary for the diagnosis; idiopathic PD can be diagnosed without tremor, as in the case depicted in question 7. Idiopathic PD can be further classified into tremor-predominant and akinetic-rigid forms. Other features of PD are micrographia (small handwriting), hypophonia (reduced voice volume), hypomimia (reduced facial expression), hyposmia or anosmia (reduced or absent sense of smell), and reduced blinking frequency.

The diagnosis of idiopathic PD is purely clinical. Fluorodopa PET studies in patients with idiopathic PD show reduced uptake in the putamen; this and other radiolabeled tracer imaging techniques are predominantly used in the research setting, though in some cases provide an aid in diagnosis.

Several other disorders may be marked by parkinsonism in addition to other clinical and historical features that suggest the diagnosis is not idiopathic PD. DLB is characterized by cognitive dysfunction, hallucinations, and fluctuations in mental status in addition to parkinsonism (discussed in Chapter 12). Absence of these features in the histories provided makes this diagnosis unlikely. Vascular parkinsonism is discussed in question 21, and the history provided makes idiopathic PD more likely. There is no history of exposure to antidopaminergic therapy to suggest drug-induced parkinsonism (discussed in question 21). Corticobasal ganglionic degeneration is discussed in question 20. Absence of a history of falls and no mention of extraocular movement abnormalities makes progressive supranuclear palsy unlikely (discussed in question 17).

Fahn S, Jankovic J. Principles and Practice of Movement Disorders. Philadelphia, PA: Elsevier; 2007.

8. C

Loss of postural reflexes is a feature of idiopathic Parkinson's disease (PD), but typically occurs later in the course of the disease.

The tremor of idiopathic PD is moderate in frequency, 4 to 6 Hz, and is typically more distal than proximal. The tremor has been described as pill rolling, as if the individual is rolling a small pill between the index finger and the thumb. The tremor can involve the legs as well as the head region, most commonly the lips, chin, and jaw, and less often the neck. Although the tremor in idiopathic PD is typically a resting tremor (occurring at rest), postural tremor does occur as well. When a posture (such as outstretched arms) is assumed, there is usually a latency of a few seconds before the tremor appears (this contrasts with the postural tremor of essential tremor, in which the tremor appears immediately on assumption of a posture, as discussed in questions 22–24).

Loss of postural reflexes is usually a feature of more advanced PD, occurring several years after disease onset, often not until after 8 to 10 years. It occurs earlier in other parkinsonian disorders; for example, it occurs within the first 2 years of symptom onset in progressive supranuclear palsy (discussed in question 17) and within the first 5 years of symptom onset in multiple-system atrophy (discussed in questions 18 and 19).

Freezing, or a sudden transient inability to move, is typically a feature of advanced PD. Features of freezing include hesitation in gait initiation, sudden inability to move when walking through a narrow space, such as a door, and when a target is being approached. Rigidity, or increased resistance during passive range of motion, is a feature of idiopathic PD and is often cogwheeling, or ratchety, due to the increased tone being superimposed on a tremor. Rigidity can involve both proximal and distal axial and limb muscles. Chronic rigidity can lead to striatal hand (ulnar deviation at the wrist with flexion at the metacarpophalangeal joints and extension at the interphalangeal joints), striatal toe (extension of the big toe with flexion of the other toes), and camptocormia (extreme flexion of the spine that worsens during walking and improves in the supine position).

Fahn S, Jankovic J. Principles and Practice of Movement Disorders. Philadelphia, PA: Elsevier; 2007.

9. d

Constipation is a prominent symptom in patients with Parkinson's disease (PD). There are many nonmotor symptoms that affect patients with idiopathic PD. In fact, nonmotor features lead to as much, if not more, disability and discomfort as do the motor features. Shoulder pain is a frequent occurrence in PD and can be present years prior to the onset of motor symptoms. Other joints can also be involved. These pains likely result from rigidity and reduced motion at joints; that these pains are due to the underlying disorder rather than arthritis or other orthopedic problems is evidenced by improvement of these pains with dopaminergic therapy. Other types of pain seen in patients with PD include that which is related to dystonia (such as dystonic foot cramping). Nonspecific sensory symptoms (such as paresthesias) in the absence of other physical examination findings indicative of neuropathy also occur.

Urinary frequency, urgency, and nocturia are common in patients with PD, occurring in both sexes and resulting from the more generalized autonomic dysfunction that occurs. In PD, urinary symptoms result in large part from detrusor hyperreflexia. Prostatic enlargement can certainly exacerbate these symptoms. Early neurogenic incontinence in a patient with parkinsonism may suggest the diagnosis of multiple-system atrophy (MSA) instead of PD. As mentioned, patients with idiopathic PD do suffer from autonomic dysfunction, including orthostatic hypotension, and the presence of orthostatic hypotension in patients with parkinsonism does not necessarily imply that their diagnosis is MSA. Unlike MSA, the orthostatic intolerance in PD is usually milder, though it may be severe, and typically occurs later in the course of the disease.

Constipation is a prominent symptom in patients with PD, and may predate the motor symptoms for years. It results from impaired gastrointestinal motility due to involvement of the enteric nervous system with the disease.

REM sleep behavioral disorder (discussed in Chapter 5) can occur in patients with various neurodegenerative disorders, predating other symptoms by years. Its occurrence does not necessarily imply the diagnosis is DLB; it can certainly occur in patients with idiopathic PD.

Fahn S, Jankovic J. Principles and Practice of Movement Disorders. Philadelphia, PA: Elsevier; 2007.

Zesiewicz TA, Sullivan KL, Arnulf I, et al. Practice parameter: treatment of nonmotor symptoms of Parkinson disease. Report of the quality standards subcommittee of the American Academy of Neurology. Neurology. 2010; 74: 924–931.

10. a

Various neuropsychiatric symptoms can occur in patients with idiopathic Parkinson's disease (PD). Depression is common in this patient population, affecting over half of patients at some point during their disease. Depression in PD may in part result from the limitations the disorder imposes on daily life, and as a reaction to having this disease, but is also thought to be secondary to involvement of serotonergic and noradrenergic pathways in the primary disease process. Patients with PD typically have hypomimia (reduced facial expression) and apathy, but in this case, the patient's reported symptoms suggest she is depressed. She should be treated with antidepressant medications; the choice of medications depends on various factors. The majority of antidepressants can be used in patients with PD, except for nonselective monoamine oxidase inhibitors which are contraindicated in patients being treated with concomitant levodopa because of risk of sympathetic overactivation. Anxiety and panic attacks are other common psychiatric disorders seen in patients with PD.

Fahn S, Jankovic J. Principles and Practice of Movement Disorders. Philadelphia, PA: Elsevier; 2007.

Zesiewicz TA, Sullivan KL, Arnulf I, et al. Practice parameter: treatment of nonmotor symptoms of Parkinson disease. Report of the quality standards subcommittee of the American Academy of Neurology. Neurology. 2010; 74:924–931.

11. c

This patient's history is consistent with Parkinson's disease (PD) with dementia. A large number of patients with idiopathic PD develop cognitive dysfunction, and dementia is not uncommon. PD with dementia is a diagnosis made when the patient meets criteria for idiopathic PD for at least 1 year before dementia onset. The dementia in these patients may be accounted for by concurrent Alzheimer's disease in some cases; in others, the pathology relates to the presence of Lewy bodies.

In DLB (discussed further in Chapter 12), cognitive dysfunction and hallucinations antedate the parkinsonism, though they may all occur concurrently. This patient had a near-normal neuropsychologic evaluation 10 years earlier, making DLB unlikely. This patient's history does not suggest normal-pressure hydrocephalus (NPH) (discussed in Chapter 12); NPH can lead to parkinsonism with dementia, but the history suggests this patient had typical idiopathic PD early on, and the dementia occurred years later, without mention of incontinence. Similarly, the description of the patient's disease early on makes corticobasal ganglionic degeneration less likely (discussed in question 20). The history is not consistent with FTD (discussed in Chapter 12), though FTD and idiopathic PD can co-occur.

Jankovic J. Principles and Practice of Movement Disorders. Philadelphia, PA: Elsevier; 2007.

12. a

Parkinson's disease (PD) results from degeneration of dopaminergic neurons in the substantia nigra pars compacta (SNc). The pathologic hallmark of idiopathic PD is the presence of Lewy bodies, which are intracytoplasmic inclusions surrounded by a clear halo (discussed further in Chapter 12). Idiopathic PD is an α-synucleinopathy. The synucleinopathies are a group of neurodegenerative disorders characterized by abnormal deposition of α-synuclein in the brain. Motor manifestations of idiopathic PD result from degeneration of dopaminergic neurons in the SNc. However, widespread pathologic changes occur in PD, including in the olfactory system, dorsal motor nucleus of the vagus nerve, locus coeruleus and raphe nuclei of the brainstem, basal ganglia, and enteric nervous system. Later, the frontal cortex becomes involved, leading to executive dysfunction. These widespread changes are thought to account for the multitude of nonmotor symptoms seen in PD.

In a minority of patients with idiopathic PD, single-gene mutations have been identified. Some of the mutated genes do not necessarily involve Lewy body deposition, pointing to the complexity of the pathophysiology of this disease; the majority of patients with PD do not have an identifiable gene mutation, further suggesting that PD is a complex disorder that is likely the result of both genetic and environmental factors. As of 2010, 15 loci on 11 genes had been implicated in familial PD; these are genotypically and phenotypically heterogeneous, and a full discussion is beyond the scope of this text, but examples include the following:

- α-synuclein (*PARK1* gene), leading to abnormalities in synaptic vesicle trafficking. Autosomal dominant, young onset. Lewy body pathology is seen in this type of familial PD.
- Parkin (*PARK2* gene), a ubiquitin E3 ligase. Autosomal recessive, juvenile onset. Lewy body pathology is not seen in this type of familial PD.
- Leucine-rich repeat kinase 2 (*LRRK2* and *PARK8* gene). The *LRRK2* mutation is one of the most common causes of familial PD. Autosomal dominant. Lewy body pathology is not a prominent feature in this type of familial PD; rather, nigral degeneration is prominent.

Other genes identified in familial PD encode for proteins involved in membrane trafficking, oxidative stress, mitochondrial metabolism, and lysosomal function.

Fahn S, Jankovic J. Principles and Practice of Movement Disorders. Philadelphia, PA: Elsevier; 2007.

Hatano T, Kubo S, Sato S, et al. Pathogenesis of familial Parkinson's disease: new insights based on monogenic forms of Parkinson's disease. J Neurochem. 2009; 11:1075–1093.

13. d

There are several different classes of therapies for the treatment of Parkinson's disease (PD). Entacapone is a catechol-O-methyltransferase (COMT) inhibitor. Dopamine is metabolized by COMT to form 3-O-methyldopa. COMT inhibitors inhibit this conversion, extending the plasma half-life of dopamine, prolonging its duration of action. COMT inhibitors are administered concomitantly with levodopa. They increase the duration of action of levodopa, reducing "off" periods, or periods where the patient is experiencing motor symptoms due to wearing off of the levodopa, and increasing "on" periods.

The first dopaminergic agent available for PD was levodopa, which is a dopamine precursor. After levodopa is ingested, it is converted in the brain and peripherally into dopamine by the enzyme dopa-decarboxylase (also called aromatic amino acid decarboxylase). The peripheral conversion accounts for its side effects such as nausea (discussed in question 14). Carbidopa is a peripheral dopa-decarboxylase inhibitor; it reduces conversion of levodopa into dopamine in the periphery while not inhibiting central conversion. Administration of carbidopa on its own is not of use; it is administered only in combination with levodopa.

The dopamine agonists include pramipexole and ropinirole; older dopamine agonists including bromocriptine, pergolide, and cabergoline are no longer used in the treatment of PD. Ropinirole and pramipexole are agonists predominantly at D_2 and D_3 receptors.

Rasagiline and selegiline are monoamine oxidase type B (MAOB) inhibitors; MAOB is involved in dopamine metabolism. The relatively selective inhibition of MAOB reduces the risk of the "cheese effect" that could be seen with concomitant intake of high levels of tyramine in certain cheeses, resulting in hypertensive crisis (the older MAO inhibitors that inhibited both MAOA and MAOB had a higher risk of this adverse effect).

Trihexyphenidyl is an anticholinergic. Its use in PD is limited to the treatment of tremor, as some of the tremor in PD is thought to result from a relative excess of acetylcholine.

Another therapy used in PD includes amantadine, which has anti-glutamatergic effects, increases presynaptic dopamine release, and inhibits reuptake of synaptic dopamine.

Fahn S, Jankovic J. Principles and Practice of Movement Disorders. Philadelphia, PA: Elsevier; 2007.

14. b

Although patients with premorbid impulse control problems are at higher risk of having worsening with dopamine agonist therapy, the dopamine agonists can cause impulse control disorders even in patients without prior history of such problems. The side effects of dopamine agonists include sedation, lower extremity edema, and impulse control problems, such as hypersexuality, pathologic gambling, and pathologic shopping, in addition to other similar behaviors. The occurrence of such impulse control problems often necessitates discontinuation of dopamine agonists.

Anticholinergic agents such as trihexyphenidyl and benztropine can cause significant cognitive dysfunction, particularly in older adults. Other side effects of these agents include constipation, dry eyes and mouth, and urinary retention.

The main side effect of levodopa is nausea; administration of extra doses of carbidopa (which inhibits peripheral conversion of levodopa into dopamine without affecting its conversion centrally) reduces this side effect. Tolerance develops over time. Dyskinesias, or extraneous choreiform movements, occur with levodopa, with the incidence being related to dosage and duration of therapy. Addition of a catechol-*O*-methyltransferase inhibitor increases the time dopamine is available at the postsynaptic membrane, increasing the occurrence of peak-dose dyskinesias.

Selegiline, a monoamine oxidase type B (MAOB) inhibitor, is metabolized to methamphetamine, which can lead to insomnia. The other MAOB inhibitor, rasagiline, does not have amphetamine-like metabolites.

Fahn S, Jankovic J. Principles and Practice of Movement Disorders. Philadelphia, PA: Elsevier; 2007.

15. b

In younger patients with idiopathic Parkinson's disease (PD), there are several treatment options. In young patients with predominantly tremor, medications such as rasagiline, amantadine, or even an anticholinergic such as trihexyphenidyl can be used. Dopamine agonists can provide significant motor control, and delaying levodopa therapy may reduce risk of levodopa-induced dyskinesias.

In older adults, particularly those with cognitive dysfunction and/or hallucinations, treatment options are more limited. Given this patient's age, and the history of daytime hypersomnolence, a dopamine agonist (such as ropinirole or pramipexole) would not be appropriate given the adverse events discussed in question 14. Bromocriptine is not used in treatment of PD any longer. Trihexyphenidyl would worsen cognitive dysfunction and do little besides perhaps improve the tremor. The most appropriate therapy for this patient would be carbidopa-levodopa.

Fahn S, Jankovic J. Principles and Practice of Movement Disorders. Philadelphia, PA: Elsevier; 2007.

16. c

Deep brain stimulation (DBS) for idiopathic Parkinson's disease (PD) is effective in reducing tremor and bradykinesia, but not gait freezing, falls, or other axial symptoms. In patients with a measurable response to dopaminergic therapy but who over time have less benefits or significant side effects such as dyskinesias, DBS for PD has been proven safe and effective with appropriate case selection.

DBS involves the placement of electrodes into specific target areas, with the assistance of stereotaxis and intraoperative neurophysiologic recording. If symptoms predominantly affect only one side of the body, unilateral DBS to a contralateral brain target is appropriate. In patients with significant symptoms bilaterally, bilateral DBS is done. Target sites have included the subthalamic nucleus, globus pallidus interna, and ventral intermediate (VIM) nucleus of the thalamus. VIM nucleus DBS is particularly effective for tremor and is thus used for the treatment of tremor-predominant PD and essential tremor. Significant cognitive impairment is a contraindication to DBS as significant worsening of cognitive dysfunction can occur postoperatively.

Fahn S, Jankovic J. Principles and Practice of Movement Disorders. Philadelphia, PA: Elsevier; 2007.

17. c

This patient's history and examination is consistent with progressive supranuclear palsy (PSP) (previously known as Steele-Richardson-Olszewski syndrome), a parkinsonism-plus syndrome. PSP typically has onset in the seventh decade of life, later than idiopathic Parkinson's disease

(PD) and multiple-system atrophy (MSA). The most prominent feature of this disorder is gait and balance problems, with frequent falls. Eye abnormalities in PSP include restricted vertical gaze, predominantly downward gaze, making going downstairs difficult, particularly when combined with the involuntary neck hyperextension (retrocollis) that occurs. The downward gaze restriction can be overcome by the oculocephalic maneuver. Examination often reveals square-wave jerks (jerk nystagmus in primary gaze) and impaired optokinetic nystagmus. Other parkinsonian features including bradykinesia, rigidity, micrographia, and gait freezing also occur. MRI of the brain in PSP may show atrophy of the midbrain, leading to the so-called hummingbird sign.

Unlike in idiopathic PD, falling in PSP occurs within 1.5 years of symptom onset, whereas in idiopathic PD, it typically occurs years after symptom onset. Also, the prominent vertical gaze abnormalities help distinguish PSP from idiopathic PD, though eye movement abnormalities can occur in the latter. Also unlike in idiopathic PD, the symptoms in PSP are typically less asymmetric, and response to levodopa is poor. Absence of autonomic features and/or ataxia distinguishes PSP from MSA. In addition, patients with MSA typically have forward neck flexion (antecollis), as opposed to patients with PSP who have retrocollis. PSP is a neurodegenerative disorder, and is a tauopathy, marked by abnormal deposition of the protein tau in various brain regions. In primary autonomic failure (discussed in Chapter 10), parkinsonian features and extraocular movement abnormalities are absent. Corticobasal ganglionic degeneration (discussed in question 20) does not manifest with prominent extraocular movement abnormalities (though eye movement abnormalities can occur) or early frequent falls, and is prominently asymmetric, unlike the case described.

Fahn S, Jankovic J. Principles and Practice of Movement Disorders. Philadelphia, PA: Elsevier; 2007.

18. b, 19. b

Both the patients depicted in questions 18 and 19 have multiple-system atrophy (MSA), a parkinsonism-plus syndrome. MSA has been divided into three types on the basis of the most prominent features: with significant autonomic dysfunction (MSA-A, previously known as Shy-Drager syndrome or Oppenheimer's syndrome, as depicted in question 18), with significant parkinsonism (MSA-P), and with cerebellar ataxia being the most prominent feature (MSA-C, also known as sporadic olivopontocerebellar atrophy (OPCA), depicted in question 19). However, these may occur in combination. All these disorders share in common the presence of parkinsonism that is poorly responsive to levodopa and the neuropathologic finding of glial cytoplasmic inclusions with α-synuclein; they therefore fall under the spectrum of α-synucleinopathies, along with idiopathic Parkinson's disease (PD). MSA has an earlier age of onset as compared to progressive supranuclear palsy (PSP), typically starting in the sixth decade of life. Autonomic dysfunction in MSA manifests with orthostatic hypotension without a compensatory increase in heart rate and urinary incontinence (due to involvement of the group of anterior horn cells in the sacral cord known as Onuf's nucleus) and impotence. A potentially fatal feature that may occur in MSA is laryngeal dystonia.

Imaging features in MSA include hypointensity of the putamen on T2-weighted MRI, a hyperintense slit-like rim around the putamen, and the "hot-cross-buns sign," or cruciform sign: transverse and vertical hyperintensity in the pons, as shown in Figure 6.1, due to loss of pontine neurons and pontocerebellar tracts with intact corticospinal tracts.

Poor response to levodopa, early autonomic dysfunction, and prominent ataxia distinguish the different types of MSA from idiopathic PD. Prominent early falls and restricted downward gaze distinguish PSP from MSA; as mentioned in question 17, patients with PSP have hyperextension of the neck (retrocollis), whereas patients with MSA exhibit involuntary neck flexion (antecollis). In primary autonomic failure (discussed in Chapter 10), parkinsonian features are absent. Corticobasal ganglionic degeneration is discussed in question 20; the prominent dysautonomia in question 18 and ataxia in question 19 make MSA more likely.

Fahn S, Jankovic J. Principles and Practice of Movement Disorders. Philadelphia, PA: Elsevier; 2007.

20. e

This patient's history and examination are consistent with corticobasal ganglionic degeneration (CBGD), a parkinsonism-plus syndrome that is characterized by the presence of focal limb rigidity and/or dystonia, cortical myoclonus, and cortical sensory loss (astereognosis (inability to recognize objects placed in the hand in the absence of primary sensory loss), agraphesthesia (inability to recognize numbers or letters drawn on the hand in the absence of primary sensory loss), and loss of two-point discrimination). Other features include a frontal/subcortical pattern of cognitive dysfunction, apraxia, alien limb phenomena, and parkinsonian features such as rest tremor, rigidity, and bradykinesia. CBGD is pathologically characterized by neuronal degeneration in the pre- and postcentral cortical areas, basal ganglia, and thalamus, as well as the substantia nigra. Achromatic nuclear inclusions are seen in these areas. The presence of myoclonus, higher cortical sensory loss, and dystonic posture with absence of prominent falls makes the other choices less likely.

Fahn S, Jankovic J. Principles and Practice of Movement Disorders. Philadelphia, PA: Elsevier; 2007.

21. d

Manganese toxicity, rather than magnesium toxicity, can lead to parkinsonism. As discussed previously, parkinsonism is the general term applied when bradykinesia, tremor, and/or rigidity are present in a patient, and this term does not imply a specific cause. Many secondary causes of parkinsonism exist.

In the 1920s, during the pandemic of encephalitis lethargica or von Economo encephalitis due to the influenza virus, postencephalitic parkinsonism was seen in several patients after recovery from the acute illness. It has also been seen in more recent years with West Nile virus and Japanese encephalitis virus infection. Parkinsonism may also be a feature of the prion disease CJD.

Vascular parkinsonism results most often from multiple lacunes in the basal ganglia. It classically affects the lower extremities more than the upper extremities, with rigidity, bradykinesia, postural instability, dementia, corticospinal findings, and incontinence occurring. The upper extremities are often relatively spared in this disorder, and tremor is not a prominent feature. Some patients with vascular parkinsonism respond to levodopa therapy.

Drug-induced parkinsonism is most often seen with exposure to antipsychotic agents, with typical antipsychotics such as haloperidol being more likely to cause this adverse effect as compared to atypical antipsychotics such as risperidone. This adverse effect is dose dependent and the risk increases with increasing duration of therapy, but can occur even with low-dose brief exposure.

Manganese toxicity can occur in welders and miners, in chronic liver disease, and in patients on total parenteral nutrition, among other causes. It leads to psychiatric symptoms ("manganese madness"), parkinsonism (but usually without tremor), and a typical gait disorder characterized by toe walking with elbow flexion, the so-called cock walk. On brain MRI, hyperintensity in the basal ganglia on T1-weighted images is seen. Other toxins that can lead to parkinsonism include the neurotoxin abbreviated as MPTP (which is now used to create primate animal models of

Parkinson's disease) and carbon monoxide (which leads to relatively selective toxicity to the globus pallidus interna).

Parkinsonism can be a feature of normal-pressure hydrocephalus (discussed in Chapter 12) and other causes of chronic hydrocephalus. Structural brain lesions affecting the basal ganglia, including strokes, hemorrhages, and tumors, can also lead to parkinsonism, as can paraneoplastic processes.

Bradley WG, Daroff RB, Fenichel GM, et al. Neurology in Clinical Practice, 5th ed. Philadelphia, PA: Elsevier; 2008.

Fahn S, Jankovic J. Principles and Practice of Movement Disorders. Philadelphia, PA: Elsevier; 2007.

22. b, 23. d, 24. d

This patient's history and examination, including her family history, are consistent with essential tremor (ET). ET is characterized by a bilateral (though sometimes asymmetric) postural tremor, typically 4 to 8 Hz with or without a kinetic component (a tremor occurring with action) that may involve the limbs, head, chin, lips, tongue, and even voice. A family history of tremor is present in the majority of patients with ET; ET exhibits an autosomal dominant pattern of inheritance with high penetrance. Although there is this strong familial component, a specific gene causing ET is yet to be identified (as of 2010). The tremor of ET classically improves with alcohol intake. Similar to most movement disorders, it does not continue in sleep (though there are exceptions, discussed in question 41).

Enhanced physiologic tremor is one of the most common causes of postural tremor, but rarely causes enough disability to require treatment. It is faster than ET, 7 to 12 Hz. Both ET and enhanced physiologic tremor increase with anxiety, but in enhanced physiologic tremor, the frequency is variable and can be slowed by mass loading (increasing weight on the arm). The presence of family history also makes ET more likely than enhanced physiologic tremor. There is no mention of abnormal posturing to suggest this patient has a dystonia with a secondary tremor (dystonic tremor). Task-specific tremor is a tremor only occurring, as the name implies, with specific tasks, such as writing or playing of musical instruments. There is no such history presented in the case. Another type of tremor is rubral tremor, also known as Holmes tremor, which is a relatively low-frequency tremor typically present at rest, with posture, and with action. It results from lesions in the dentate nucleus of the cerebellum and/or the superior cerebellar peduncle, and is often seen in patients with multiple sclerosis.

Medications used for the treatment of ET include β-blockers such as propranolol and others, primidone (an anticonvulsant which is converted into phenylethylmalonamide (PEMA) and phenobarbital), antiepileptic agents including topiramate, benzodiazepines including clonazepam, and other agents including gabapentin. Often, combinations of these therapies are necessary. In pharmacotherapy-resistant cases in which the tremor is disabling, deep brain stimulation to the ventral intermediate nucleus of the thalamus can be effective. Although ethanol intake does improve the tremor in ET, it is not an appropriate long-term therapy. Levodopa is not an effective therapy for ET. For the patient depicted in question 22, topiramate is likely the best option, as propranolol will exacerbate her asthma, and given her occupation, a sedating medication such as clonazepam would be relatively contraindicated.

Fahn S, Jankovic J. Principles and Practice of Movement Disorders. Philadelphia, PA: Elsevier; 2007.

Zesiewicz TA, Elble R, Louis ED, et al. Practice parameter: therapies for essential tremor. Report of the quality standards subcommittee of the American Academy of Neurology. Neurology. 2005; 64;2008–2020.

25. a, 26. e, 27. d

This patient's history is consistent with Tourette's syndrome. Tourette's syndrome is a neuropsychiatric disorder diagnosed in the setting of at least one motor and at least one phonic motor tic that occur at some time during the illness (though not necessarily within the same time period) beginning prior to age 18. A tic is a brief and intermittent stereotypic movement (motor tic) or sound (phonic or vocal tic) that is usually preceded by a premonitory sensation. Tourette's syndrome is associated with a variety of behavioral and psychiatric disorders, including attention deficit/hyperactivity disorder (ADHD), obsessive-compulsive disorder, anxiety, depression and other mood disorders, impulse control disorders, and others. The pathophysiology of Tourette's syndrome is complex and not fully understood, but it is thought to involve dopaminergic hyperinnervation of the ventral striatum and limbic system.

An important part of tic management is education of the patient, family, teachers, and peers. Treatment of tics is necessary only when they cause significant social or functional impairment. Nonpharmacologic treatment options include a variety of behavioral therapies, including habit reversal therapy in which the patient is trained to reenact the tics while increasing his/her own awareness of the tics and urges in addition to other components. The mainstay of therapy for Tourette's syndrome and other tic disorders are antidopaminergic agents such as haloperidol, pimozide, and the atypical antipsychotics. Clonidine, an α-2-adrenergic agonist, is useful for the treatment of ADHD and other behavioral aspects of Tourette's syndrome, and improves tics as well. Levodopa would not be the first line of management in Tourette's syndrome, as it may exacerbate tics (though some of the dopamine agonists have been shown in some studies to improve tics, possibly through reduction of endogenous dopamine turnover by action on D_2 autoreceptors).

As mentioned, this patient's constellation of tics and their duration allows for the diagnosis of Tourette's syndrome; when only motor or phonic tics are present and/or their duration is not sufficient enough to make the diagnosis of Tourette's syndrome, the tics are further categorized on the basis of their qualities. Tics that are classified as simple motor consist of a simple isolated movement such as eye blinking or eyebrow raising. Complex motor tics on the other hand consist of coordinated sequenced movements that resemble normal movements such as truncal flexion or head shaking. Simple phonic tics include sniffing, throat clearing, grunting, or coughing. Complex phonic tics include verbalizations such as shouting obscenities (coprolalia), or repeating others (echolalia) or oneself (palilalia). Secondary tourettism is the term given to conditions in which phonic and motor tics are present but an underlying neurologic disorder accounts for the presence of tics; for example, secondary tourettism is seen in autistic spectrum disorders, static encephalopathy, neuroacanthocytosis (discussed in question 33), Huntington's disease (discussed in questions 30 and 31), medications, and other causes. Transient tics have occurred in some patients following infections.

Fahn S, Jankovic J. Principles and Practice of Movement Disorders. Philadelphia, PA: Elsevier; 2007.

Scahill L, Erenberg G, Berlin CM Jr, et al. Contemporary assessment and pharmacotherapy of Tourette syndrome. NeuroRx. 2006; 3(2):192–206.

28. c, 29. e

This patient's history and MRI findings are consistent with Wilson's disease, an autosomal-recessive disorder of copper metabolism resulting from mutations of the gene encoding the copper-transporting P-type ATPase (ATP7B) on chromosome 13. This enzyme normally binds to and transports copper across membranes. A defect in this enzyme leads to inability to excrete copper from the liver into bile, leading to copper accumulation.

The presenting symptoms of the disorder can be neurologic, hepatic, or psychiatric, or a combination of these. Abnormal movements predominate the neurologic presentation, including parkinsonism, dystonia, tremor, ataxia, as well as dysarthria. The tremor may have a variety of features, but classically, it is proximal and of high amplitude, giving the appearance of "wing beating" when the arms are abducted and the elbows flexed. A characteristic grin with drooling also occurs. Psychiatric symptoms include depression, anxiety, and less commonly psychosis. The liver disease may range from mild to fulminant hepatic failure.

Laboratory findings in Wilson's disease include reduced serum levels of the copper-binding protein ceruloplasmin and increased urinary excretion of copper. The presence of Kayser-Fleischer rings, resulting from copper deposits in Descemet's membrane of the cornea, also aids in the diagnosis, and patients suspected of having Wilson's disease should be referred for slit-lamp examination. MRI of the brain shows increased signal on T2-weighted images in the caudate and putamen as seen in Figure 6.2, as well as the midbrain (with sparing of the red nucleus, leading to the so-called "double panda sign" or "face of the giant panda") and thalamus.

The treatment of Wilson's disease includes D-penicillamine or trientine dihydrochloride, in addition to zinc supplementation (which binds copper in the gastrointestinal tract, preventing its absorption), and a low copper diet, including avoidance of nuts, chocolate, and shellfish.

Fahn S, Jankovic J. Principles and Practice of Movement Disorders. Philadelphia, PA: Elsevier; 2007.

30. d, 31. b

This patient's history and examination suggest that she has Huntington's disease, an autosomal dominant disorder due to expansion of the trinucleotide repeat CAG in the Huntington gene on chromosome 4. Age of onset shows anticipation (earlier age of onset in subsequent generations).

The classic clinical features include chorea, gait instability, dystonia, and multiple neuropsychiatric symptoms including depression, psychosis, cognitive dysfunction, executive dysfunction, and personality changes. Other features include motor impersistence, demonstrated by inability of the patient to sustain tongue protrusion and impaired saccades and pursuits, with unsuppressible head movements during eye movements. In some forms, particularly the juvenile form, chorea is absent and the more prominent features are myoclonus and parkinsonism, with significant rigidity (akinetic-rigid syndrome).

In Huntington's disease, neuronal degeneration is seen in the striatum, substantia nigra, globus pallidus, and other areas. MRI of the brain shows caudate and putamen atrophy. The exact role of the Huntington protein in the pathophysiology of Huntington's disease is unclear. Several therapies are under investigation to alter the course of the disease, but until they become available, symptomatic treatment with anti-dopaminergic agents (such as atypical antipsychotics and tetrabenazine) is the mainstay of therapy.

When taking a history and examining a patient with abnormal movements, and in the setting of prior psychiatric history and exposure to anti-dopaminergic therapy, it is important not to attribute the abnormal movements to a tardive phenomenon (discussed in question 35), especially when other features are present that may suggest that there is an underlying disorder leading to the psychiatric symptoms, as is the case in the patient presented in question 30. The prominent chorea, motor impersistence, history of similar illness in the father, and no mention of hepatic dysfunction make Wilson's disease less likely (discussed in question 28). A psychogenic disorder is a diagnosis of exclusion and there are several features in the history to suggest Huntington's disease. Benign hereditary chorea in adulthood is not accompanied by neuropsychiatric changes; it is discussed further in question 32.

Fahn S, Jankovic J. Principles and Practice of Movement Disorders. Philadelphia, PA: Elsevier; 2007.

32. d

Sydenham's disease is best treated with anti-dopaminergic therapies.

Chorea is an involuntary, rapid, and abrupt irregular movement that flows from one body part to another. It may affect any body part, and when affecting the legs and trunks, it leads to a dancing-like gait. There are several causes of chorea.

Sydenham's disease is an autoimmune disorder manifesting with chorea that is usually bilateral but often asymmetric, as well as oculomotor abnormalities and behavioral changes following infection with group A Streptococcus. Unlike other features of rheumatic fever, the chorea can present months after the infection or may be the sole manifestation of rheumatic fever. Patients will have elevated antistreptolysin antibodies and antibasal ganglia antibodies. Treatment of the acute streptococcal infection, as well as subsequent prophylaxis with penicillin in patients who develop rheumatic fever, is essential.

Chorea occurring during pregnancy may signify prior rheumatic fever or an underlying autoimmune disease such as systemic lupus erythematosus (see Chapter 16). It may also reflect an underlying antiphospholipid antibody syndrome.

Benign hereditary chorea is an autosomal dominant nonprogressive syndrome characterized predominantly by chorea, with mild gait ataxia. It results from a mutation in the thyroid transcription factor gene. Mutations in this gene also lead to a more severe childhood syndrome characterized by mental retardation, hypothyroidism, and lung disease (so-called brain-thyroid-lung syndrome).

Fahn S, Jankovic J. Principles and Practice of Movement Disorders. Philadelphia, PA: Elsevier; 2007.

33. b

This patient's history and examination are consistent with neuroacanthocytosis. Age of onset is usually in the third to fourth decades of life. The most prominent clinical features are orolingual dystonias, such as prominent tongue-protrusion dystonia, particularly while eating, self-mutilating behavior, cognitive decline with dementia, dysarthria, ophthalmoplegia, parkinsonism, and behavioral problems. Chorea and athetosis (a slow form of chorea) also occur. Autosomal dominant, X-linked recessive, and sporadic forms have been reported, with genetic heterogeneity. The autosomal recessive form has been associated with a mutation in the chorein gene on chromosome 9. The X-linked form is known as Mcleod's syndrome. The diagnosis of neuroacanthocytosis is made by wet blood smear or Wright-stained blood smear demonstrating acanthocytes.

A form of neuroacanthocytosis associated with abetalipoproteinemia is associated with low serum cholesterol and vitamin E malabsorption, not present in this case. Another syndrome along this spectrum, but with normal vitamin E levels, is hypoprebetalipoproteinemia, acanthocytosis, retinitis pigmentosa, and pallidal degeneration (HARP syndrome).

Dentatorubral-pallidoluysian atrophy is a neurodegenerative autosomal dominant disorder resulting from expansion of the trinucleotide repeat CAG on chromosome 12. It is more common in people of Asian descent. It typically begins in the fourth decade of life, but earlier onset forms exist. Clinical features include myoclonus, choreoathetosis (a combination of chorea and athetosis), epilepsy, dystonia, tremor, parkinsonism, and cognitive dysfunction.

Lesch-Nyhan syndrome is an X-linked recessive disorder resulting from a mutation in hypoxanthine-guanine phosphoribosyltransferase (HGPRT), leading to abnormal purine metabolism. Hyperuricemia with nephrolithiasis, neuropsychiatric symptoms, and abnormal movements including chorea, athetosis, and rigidity occur. Self-mutilation is also a feature of Lesch-Nyhan syndrome, but the normal serum uric acid and prominent tongue-protrusion dystonia make neuroacanthocytosis more likely.

Choreoathetosis is also seen in the disorders of brain iron accumulation, such as pantothenate-kinase–associated neurodegeneration (PKAN), formerly known as Hallervorden-Spatz disease. This is an autosomal recessive disorder of childhood, marked by dystonia, other abnormal movements, and cognitive decline. It results from a mutation in pantothenate kinase 2 gene. The classic MRI appearance is one of hyperintensity in the globus pallidus with a surrounding area of hypointensity, the so-called "eye of the tiger" sign.

Huntington's disease is on the differential diagnosis of patients with a presentation as described above, but the prominent tongue dystonia and self-mutilation make neuroacanthocytosis more likely. A normal uric acid level and the prominent tongue dystonia make Lesch-Nyhan syndrome (discussed in Chapter 14) less likely; self-mutilation is seen in both of these disorders.

Bradley WG, Daroff RB, Fenichel GM, et al. Neurology in Clinical Practice, 5th ed. Philadelphia, PA: Elsevier; 2008.

Fahn S, Jankovic J. Principles and Practice of Movement Disorders. Philadelphia, PA: Elsevier; 2007.

Stevenson VL, Hardie RJ. Acanthocytosis and neurological disorders. J Neurol. 2001; 248:87–94.

34. c

This patient's history is consistent with hemiballism, which can result from an ischemic stroke or other lesions in the contralateral subthalamic nucleus. Ballism is a hyperkinetic movement disorder characterized by forceful, flinging, high-amplitude choreiform movements. Hemiballism, or ballism involving one side of the body, can also occur with contralateral parietal or thalamic lesions. Bilateral ballism may be due to bilateral basal ganglia infarcts. Hemiballism often responds to antidopaminergic therapy.

Fahn S, Jankovic J. Principles and Practice of Movement Disorders. Philadelphia, PA: Elsevier; 2007.

35. e

This patient's history is most consistent with tardive dyskinesia. This disorder is an iatrogenic, typically late (hence the term tardive), adverse effect of dopamine-receptor antagonists, most commonly antipsychotics, but also seen with other therapies such as metoclopramide. It is more likely to occur with typical antipsychotics such as haloperidol and fluphenazine because of their greater antagonism at D_2 receptors, but can also occur with the atypical antipsychotics such as risperidone, with clozapine and quetiapine being least likely to cause tardive dyskinesia. It may occur during therapy with dopamine-receptor antagonists or even years after the medication is discontinued. The manifestations of tardive dyskinesia include oro-bucco-lingual movements (as in this case), akathisia (inner restlessness), dystonia (often of the neck but also other body parts), tremor, parkinsonism, or a combination of these.

Abrupt cessation of a dopamine-receptor antagonist after prolonged use can lead to prominent involuntary dyskinetic movements involving various regions of the body as well as akathisia. A slow taper of the offending agent is therefore recommended when tardive dyskinesia occurs. When psychosis or other indications for dopamine-receptor antagonists persist, switching to an agent with less D_2 antagonism should be attempted when possible. Dopamine-depleting agents such as tetrabenazine or reserpine have been used to treat tardive dyskinesia, with the rationale being that they will reduce dopaminergic synaptic activity without causing dopamine-receptor antagonism. Levodopa, sodium valproate, and clonazepam have also been used successfully. In pharmacotherapy-refractory cases, deep brain stimulation may be effective. Anticholinergics and antihistamines can worsen tardive dyskinesia.

Tardive dyskinesia should be distinguished from an acute dystonic reaction after administration of dopamine-receptor antagonists. This reaction typically occurs within the first few days of exposure to the agent and most often involves the ocular and face muscles, leading to oculogyric crisis (forced eye deviation) and other dystonic manifestations. Treatment involves cessation of the agent and administration of anticholinergics or antihistamines, with resolution of the dystonic reaction within hours.

Fahn S, Jankovic J. Principles and Practice of Movement Disorders. Philadelphia, PA: Elsevier; 2007.

36. b

Dystonia is a sustained contraction of agonist and antagonist muscles, leading to abnormal postures with repetitive twisting movements. Dystonia is classified as focal when it involves a single body part, as in cervical dystonia. If the dystonia spreads to a contiguous body part, it is termed segmental. Generalized dystonia refers to involvement of at least two segmental regions (such as leg plus trunk) with at least one other body part involved. Multifocal dystonia is used to describe the occurrence of dystonia in two noncontiguous body parts, such as foot and hand.

Primary generalized dystonia (also known as Oppenheim's dystonia or dystonia musculorum deformans), depicted in question 36, is an autosomal dominant disorder resulting from a mutation in the torsin A gene on chromosome 9, and referred to as DYT1 dystonia. It is more common in those of Ashkenazi Jewish descent and has relatively low penetrance. Symptoms typically begin in childhood with action-induced limb dystonia that later spreads to involve the trunk and other limbs, with generalization of the dystonia over a few years. In some patients, the dystonia remains focal.

Response to levodopa is typically poor, and a lack of response obviously does not necessarily imply a psychogenic disorder. Treatment of primary generalized dystonia includes anticholinergics, benzodiazepines, and deep brain stimulation of the globus pallidus interna.

Dopa-responsive dystonia (discussed in question 38) shows a good response to levodopa. There are no parkinsonian features to suggest juvenile Parkinson's disease.

Other childhood-onset generalized dystonias including DYT2, DYT4, DYT6, and DYT13 occur because of various mutations. DYT11, or myoclonus-dystonia syndrome, results from a mutation in a sarcoglycan protein (though other mutated genes have been identified) and manifests with tremor, myoclonus, and dystonia typically beginning in the teenage years and associated with various psychiatric symptoms. DYT3 dystonia, or Lubag disease, is X-linked and is seen in males of Filipino descent and manifests with dystonia and parkinsonism.

Fahn S, Jankovic J. Principles and Practice of Movement Disorders. Philadelphia, PA: Elsevier; 2007.

37. b

This patient's history is consistent with primary cervical dystonia, the most common focal dystonia, as well as blepharospasm. Cervical dystonia typically begins in adulthood and manifests with involuntary head posture, neck pain, and in some cases a tremor (dystonic tremor; essential tremor can also lead to head tremor, but the presence of dystonia in her case makes dystonic tremor the likely diagnosis). A sensory trick (geste antagoniste), such as touching the face or head or positioning the head in a specific manner against an object, may partially relieve symptoms. In a proportion of patients with focal dystonia, blepharospasm, or dystonic eyelid movements manifesting as involuntary blinking often followed later by more forceful involuntary eyelid closure occur, often worsened with driving or light exposure. Other forms of dystonia such as oromandibular dystonia (involving the mouth and lips) may occur as well. Therapies including anticholinergics, benzodiazepines, and baclofen may be helpful, but botulinum toxin therapy is the mainstay of treatment. Blepharospasm may be seen as part of Meige's syndrome, in which oromandibular dystonia occurs as well.

Bradley WG, Daroff RB, Fenichel GM, et al. Neurology in Clinical Practice, 5th ed. Philadelphia, PA: Elsevier; 2008.

Fahn S, Jankovic J. Principles and Practice of Movement Disorders. Philadelphia, PA: Elsevier; 2007.

38. c

This patient's history is consistent with dopa-responsive dystonia, or Segawa's syndrome. This disorder is more common in females and the occurrence of dystonia frequently shows a diurnal variation, being worse in the afternoon and evening. Parkinsonism is a common associated finding on examination. It typically presents in childhood, but adult-onset forms exist as well. Response to low-dose levodopa is typically present, without risk of significant dyskinesias.

Dopa-responsive dystonia, or DYT5, is autosomal dominant and most commonly results from a mutation in the enzyme GTP cyclohydrolase I (GCH1) on chromosome 14. GCH1 is the rate-limiting enzyme in tetrahydrobiopterin synthesis, which is a cofactor for tyrosine hydroxylase, the enzyme that catalyzes the rate-limiting step of dopamine synthesis.

Tyrosine hydroxylase deficiency can lead to a phenotype of dopa-responsive dystonia, but is a more severe childhood dystonia syndrome. Mutations in other genes encoding other enzymes involved in dopamine synthesis or metabolism can also lead to dystonia and other abnormal movements. Mutations in the enzyme aromatic acid decarboxylase lead to a syndrome of dystonia, parkinsonism, oculogyric crisis, dysautonomia, and other manifestations.

Bradley WG, Daroff RB, Fenichel GM, et al. Neurology in Clinical Practice, 5th ed. Philadelphia, PA: Elsevier; 2008.

Fahn S, Jankovic J. Principles and Practice of Movement Disorders. Philadelphia, PA: Elsevier; 2007.

39. c

This patient has a primary, focal, task-specific dystonia. Although the dystonia may overflow to involve more proximal areas over time during specific activities, it is unlikely that she will develop a generalized dystonia given her age.

The most common task-specific dystonia is writer's cramp, a dystonia occurring during writing. This type of dystonia, occurring only with specific activities, is most often primary, without an underlying secondary cause. It most often occurs after the activity is performed for some time. This type of dystonia can occur during playing of various musical instruments; in horn or woodwind players, embouchure dystonia, or dystonia of the lips, jaw, or tongue can be seen. Treatment may include focal injections of botulinum toxin in a manner that minimizes the dystonia, but also minimizes impact on musical performance.

Fahn S, Jankovic J. Principles and Practice of Movement Disorders. Philadelphia, PA: Elsevier; 2007.

40. b

The following discussion of myoclonus is limited to nonepileptic myoclonus (see Chapter 5 for discussion of epileptic myoclonus). Myoclonus is a brief, sudden, jerky movement that may be either generalized (involving the whole body at once in a single jerk), multifocal (involving different body parts, not necessarily all at once), segmental or focal (involving only one region of the body).

Cortical myoclonus is the term given to myoclonus resulting from abnormal activity in the sensorimotor cortex. A cortical discharge preceding this type of myoclonus can be detected by electrophysiologic techniques that involve back-averaging. Lance-Adams syndrome, depicted in question 40, manifests after hypoxic–ischemic brain injury, and may not be evident for months or even years after the insult. The most prominent feature is an action myoclonus, and when the myoclonus involves the legs, gait is prominently affected. Treatment includes benzodiazepines such as clonazepam, piracetam, levetiracetam, as well as sodium valproate.

Myoclonus may also have brainstem origin, as well as spinal cord origin, the latter resulting in either segmental myoclonus (restricted to a specific limb or area of the trunk) or propriospinal myoclonus (involving axial muscles). Nerve root or peripheral nerve lesions can rarely result in segmental myoclonus as well. Multifocal myoclonus is often seen in the context of a variety of metabolic disorders such as uremia and liver failure; in the latter, negative myoclonus or asterixis is seen (discussed in Chapter 16). Not all myoclonus is pathologic; physiologic myoclonus includes hypnic jerks, which are hypnagogic lower extremity jerks (occurring in the early stages of sleep) and hiccups.

Bradley WG, Daroff RB, Fenichel GM, et al. Neurology in Clinical Practice, 5th ed. Philadelphia, PA: Elsevier; 2008.

Fahn S, Jankovic J. Principles and Practice of Movement Disorders. Philadelphia, PA: Elsevier; 2007.

41. b

Palatal myoclonus or tremor, depicted in question 41, is characterized by rhythmic palatal movements that may lead to audible clicks due to eustachian tube contraction (these are not hallucinations). The contractions may also involve other head regions. Palatal myoclonus may be essential (without a discernible cause) or symptomatic, due to a brainstem lesion such as stroke or tumor. The symptomatic form is one of the few movement disorders that persist during sleep. Palatal myoclonus results from dysfunction in pathways connecting the dentate nucleus of the cerebellum, the inferior olive, and the red nucleus, all of which make up the Guillain-Mollaret triangle. Hypertrophy of the inferior olive on MRI of the brain may be seen.

Bradley WG, Daroff RB, Fenichel GM, et al. Neurology in Clinical Practice, 5th ed. Philadelphia, PA: Elsevier; 2008.

Fahn S, Jankovic J. Principles and Practice of Movement Disorders. Philadelphia, PA: Elsevier; 2007.

42. c

Blepharospasm typically involves both eyes and does not involve the cheek and mouth (discussed in question 37).

This patient's history is consistent with hemifacial spasm, in which there are synchronous contractions of one side of the face. In the majority of cases, an identifiable structural lesion is not present, but some cases can occur after facial nerve paresis or due to identifiable compressive lesions of cranial nerve VII such as a tumor or a vascular loop. Contractions most often begin around the eye and spread to ipsilateral face muscles; bilateral involvement is rare but can occur, though contractions on each side of the face are asynchronous. Treatment may involve nerve decompression if there is a clear compressive lesion, but botulinum toxin therapy is otherwise the mainstay of treatment.

Although an identifiable structural cause is usually not seen on imaging, this disorder is hypothesized to occur due to a demyelinating lesion in the facial nerve that leads to abnormal spontaneous discharges, with ephaptic transmission or spread of electrical discharges between adjacent fibers of a demyelinated nerve. Because the blink reflex test (the electrophysiologic equivalent of the corneal reflex) is abnormal in patients with hemifacial spasm, another theory is that this disorder results from hyperexcitability in the facial nerve nucleus.

Fahn S, Jankovic J. Principles and Practice of Movement Disorders. Philadelphia, PA: Elsevier; 2007.

Simpson DM, Blitzer B, Brashear A, et al. Assessment: Botulinum neurotoxin for the treatment of movement disorders (an evidence-based review): Report of the therapeutics and technology subcommittee of the American Academy of Neurology. Neurology. 2008; 70;1699–1706.

43. e

Given this patient's history, the episodes of arm flapping are likely stereotypies. Stereotypies are patterned, repetitive, stereotyped movements, or vocalizations that occur in response to an external or internal stimulus. Common stereotypies are head nodding, arm flapping, body rocking, head banging, grunting, humming, or moaning. They may occur in otherwise normal children during times of excitement or boredom, but more often occur in children with developmental delay and autism. When associated with the latter, self-injurious stereotypies may be present, as in the case described above. In Rett's syndrome (discussed in Chapter 14), several stereotypies are often seen, including hand wringing, body rocking, and others.

Stereotypies are distinguished from complex motor tics in that they are not associated with an urge with relief after executing the movement or vocalization. This patient's history is not consistent with Tourette's syndrome (discussed in questions 25-27) or paroxysmal dyskinesias (discussed in question 44).

Fahn S, Jankovic J. Principles and Practice of Movement Disorders. Philadelphia, PA: Elsevier; 2007.

44. c

This patient's history is consistent with paroxysmal kinesigenic dyskinesias (PKDs). There are several categories of paroxysmal dyskinesias, all sharing in common episodes of hyperkinetic abnormal movements with intervening normalcy. The abnormal movements may include dystonia, chorea or choreoathetosis, ballism, or dysarthria. These disorders differ in the length of the paroxysm, triggers for the episodes, pharmacologic therapy, and genetics.

PKD is characterized by episodes that last seconds to at most 5 minutes, precipitated by sudden movement as well as by startle and hyperventilation. PKD may be either familial or sporadic, and secondary forms occur in multiple sclerosis, following trauma, in patients with a history of perinatal hypoxic encephalopathy, and in the setting of other underlying neurologic disorders. The primary form responds well to anticonvulsants such as carbamazepine.

In paroxysmal nonkinesigenic dyskinesia (PNKD), attacks last 2 minutes to several hours, and there are sometimes no clear precipitants, although episodes can be aggravated by alcohol, caffeine, and fatigue. Episodes are less frequent than in PKD. PNKD does not typically respond to anticonvulsants.

A third form of paroxysmal dyskinesias is referred to as paroxysmal exertional dyskinesias, in which episodes are triggered by prolonged exercise and last typically 5 to 30 minutes but sometimes up to 2 hours.

Paroxysmal hypnogenic dyskinesias were previously thought to be nonepileptic dyskinesias but are now known to be frontal lobe seizures as part of the syndrome autosomal dominant nocturnal frontal lobe epilepsy, which results from mutations in the nicotinic acetylcholine receptor, among other genetic mutations. The paroxysmal dyskinesias are not epileptic, but there is an association between PKD or PNKD and epilepsy; families have been reported that have both PNKD and infantile convulsions with choreoathetosis, and a mutation in the gene encoding a sodium/glucose transporter on chromosome 16 has been identified.

Fahn S, Jankovic J. Principles and Practice of Movement Disorders. Philadelphia, PA: Elsevier; 2007.

45. b

This patient's history is consistent with episodic ataxia type II (EAII). The episodic ataxias are a group of disorders that are categorized on the basis of clinical and genetic differences. They may be familial or sporadic.

Episodic ataxia type I (EAI) is marked by episodes of ataxia in association with facial twitching that may be myokymia (rippling muscle movements) or neuromyotonia. These attacks occur up to several times per day, last seconds to minutes, and may be triggered by startle, movement, or exercise. This disorder is due to a mutation in the voltage-gated potassium channel gene *KCNA1* on chromosome 12. These episodes may respond to anticonvulsants, such as carbamazepine, in some cases.

In EAII, the episodes of ataxia may be associated with brainstem symptoms such as nystagmus and dysarthria; facial twitching does not occur. The episodes last minutes to hours, can occur daily to monthly, and may be triggered by stress and alcohol intake. EAII results from a mutation in the calcium channel *CACN1A4*, the same gene mutated in familial hemiplegic migraine, and many patients with EAII have migraines during or outside of the ataxia attacks. EAII episodes may respond to the carbonic anhydrase inhibitor acetazolamide.

Episodic ataxia type III is an autosomal dominant disorder in which the attacks of ataxia are associated with tinnitus and vertigo, and in between attacks myokymia occurs. These attacks respond to acetazolamide. In episodic ataxia type IV, episodes of ataxia are associated with ocular motion abnormalities, and the attacks may be triggered by sudden head movement. The genes for these two types of episodic ataxia have yet to be identified (as of 2010).

Fahn S, Jankovic J. Principles and Practice of Movement Disorders. Philadelphia, PA: Elsevier; 2007.

46. d

This patient's history and examination are consistent with stiff person syndrome. Levodopa is not useful for the treatment of this disorder.

Stiff person syndrome is a syndrome that typically begins in the fourth and fifth decades. It is characterized by increased tone affecting predominantly the axial muscles, including the paraspinal muscles, leading to exaggerated lumbar lordosis, in addition to abdominal muscles, leading to a "board-like" abdomen. The limbs later become involved. Superimposed spasms in response to anxiety or excitement occur, as does an exaggerated startle response. This disorder may be autoimmune, in association with glutamic acid decarboxylase (GAD) antibodies. GAD catalyzes the synthesis of the inhibitory neurotransmitter GABA. In patients with anti-GAD antibodies, insulin-dependent diabetes and other endocrinopathies may occur as well. More focal forms of the disorder, as in stiff leg syndrome, also occur. Stiff person syndrome may also be paraneoplastic in association with anti-amphiphysin antibodies. The mainstays of therapy for stiff person syndrome are benzodiazepines and baclofen for their GABA effect.

Fahn S, Jankovic J. Principles and Practice of Movement Disorders. Philadelphia, PA: Elsevier; 2007.

47. e

Hyperekplexia is not epileptic, but it must be distinguished from startle-evoked seizures.

Hyperekplexia, or exaggerated startle, can manifest with sudden brief exaggerated startle reactions (blinking, flexion of the neck and trunk, abduction and flexion of the arms) or more prolonged tonic startle spasms. These sometimes occur secondary to minor stimuli and do not habituate.

There are primary familial forms of hyperekplexia in which mutations in the glycine receptor and presynaptic glycine transporter have been identified. Glycine is the inhibitory neurotransmitter at spinal interneurons including Renshaw cells and Ia inhibitory interneurons, and abnormal spinal Ia inhibitory interneuron reciprocal inhibition is thought to be the cause of startle in these cases. Secondary forms of exaggerated startle occur in a variety of brainstem disorders as well as in Creutzfeldt–Jakob disease (discussed in Chapter 15) and stiff person syndrome (discussed in question 46).

Fahn S, Jankovic J. Principles and Practice of Movement Disorders. Philadelphia, PA: Elsevier; 2007.

48. c

Cerebellar hemisphere lesions lead to ipsilateral clinical signs.

The cerebellum consists of two cerebellar hemispheres, a midline vermis, and several deep gray nuclei interspersed among the cerebellar white matter. The cerebellar cortex consists of three layers. The molecular layer is outermost and consists of inhibitory neurons known as stellate and basket cells. Purkinje cells lie in a layer under these neurons, and are the main output of the cerebellum to the deep cerebellar and vestibular nuclei. The main neurotransmitter of Purkinje cells is GABA, an inhibitory neurotransmitter. The innermost layer is the granular layer, and consists of granule cells and Golgi interneurons. Parallel fibers, axons of the granule cells, travel to synapse with Purkinje cells. Granule cells are the only cerebellar cell types that are excitatory.

Inhibitory fibers arise from the Purkinje cells of the cerebellum and project to the deep cerebellar nuclei. Fibers arising from the deep cerebellar nuclei, including the dentate, emboliform, and globose nuclei, are excitatory and are carried through the superior cerebellar peduncle, decussate, and then synapse in the thalamus. The thalamus in turn projects to the cortex, which in turn projects back to the brainstem through the corticobulbar, corticospinal, and other descending pathways. Because the fibers from the cerebellum to the thalamus cross, and motor fibers from the cortex ultimately cross (in the decussation of the corticospinal tract in the pyramids), lesions to one cerebellar hemisphere lead to ipsilateral cerebellar signs and symptoms.

Afferents into the cerebellum are carried through the inferior, middle, and superior cerebellar peduncle (note that the superior cerebellar peduncle carries predominantly cerebellar efferents, though it carries afferents to the cerebellum as well). These afferents include axons of the spinocerebellar tract, which are termed mossy fibers, as well as projections from the pons, vestibular nuclei, and reticular nuclei. Another main afferent pathway to the cerebellum arises from the inferior olivary nucleus and travels in the form of climbing fibers around Purkinje cells.

The clinical features of cerebellar dysfunction include ataxia, dysmetria (uncoordinated movement with under- or overshooting of target), dysdiadochokinesia (impaired rapid alternating movements), hypometric or hypermetric saccades (under- or overshooting of eye movements to a target, respectively), hypotonia, and rebound (inability to control the extent of movement particularly when resistance is released).

Ropper AH, Samuels MA. Adams and Victor's Principles of Neurology, 9th ed. New York: McGraw-Hill; 2009.

49. d

Chronic alcoholism can lead to a variety of neurologic signs and symptoms through several mechanisms. Malnourishment can lead to thiamine and vitamin B_{12} deficiency, which can lead to a variety of neurologic manifestations (discussed in Chapter 17). However, alcohol itself is toxic to the cerebellum. It predominantly affects midline structures such as the vermis, and this accounts for the prominent truncal ataxia, though cerebellar hemisphere atrophy leading to limb ataxia can also be seen.

Bradley WG, Daroff RB, Fenichel GM, et al. Neurology in Clinical Practice, 5th ed. Philadelphia, PA: Elsevier; 2008.

50. b

Celiac disease can lead to isolated cerebellar dysfunction in the absence of gastrointestinal symptoms. In a patient with ataxia of unclear etiology, celiac antibodies should be checked as gluten-free diet can improve the ataxia (discussed also in Chapter 16).

There are several causes of acquired cerebellar ataxia. Hypothyroidism can lead to gait ataxia, and checking serum thyroid-stimulating hormone is indicated in an adult presenting with ataxia. Supplementation with thyroid hormone can lead to improvement of the gait disorder. Chemotherapeutic agents including 5-fluorouracil and cytarabine can lead to significant cerebellar toxicity. In cytarabine toxicity, Purkinje cell loss and gliosis occur, and there is loss of dentate neurons as well; the cerebellar dysfunction is typically irreversible. Metals such as mercury can lead to cerebellar toxicity as well as visual cortex toxicity, leading to a syndrome of ataxia, visual field deficits, and paresthesias. Bismuth salicylate can also lead to cerebellar toxicity if ingested in high amounts. Other cerebellar toxins include the solvent toluene.

Chronic intake of phenytoin can lead to cerebellar atrophy due to damage to Purkinje cells. Acute phenytoin toxicity can lead to a reversible cerebellar ataxia. Other causes of acquired cerebellar ataxia include infection (as in HIV infection, Creutzfeldt–Jakob disease, and Whipple's disease; see Chapter 15) or postinfection (such as is seen after varicella zoster infection in children). The Miller–Fisher variant of Guillain–Barre (discussed in Chapter 9) leads to ataxia in addition to areflexia, ophthalmoplegia, and involvement of other cranial nerves.

Bradley WG, Daroff RB, Fenichel GM, et al. Neurology in Clinical Practice, 5th ed. Philadelphia, PA: Elsevier; 2008.

Ropper AH, Samuels MA. Adams and Victor's Principles of Neurology, 9th ed. New York: McGraw-Hill; 2009.

51. b

Friedreich's ataxia (FA) is an autosomal recessive hereditary ataxia characterized by cerebellar dysfunction, neuropathy, and upper motor neuron findings. High-arched feet and spinal deformities occur. Cardiac involvement is common, including cardiac conduction abnormalities and hypertrophic cardiomyopathy. It most often presents in young adulthood, but presentation in early childhood or even late adulthood may occur. FA results from an expansion of the trinucleotide repeat GAA in the frataxin gene on chromosome 9. The exact role of frataxin is unclear, but it is thought to be a nuclear-encoded mitochondrial protein. Idebenone, a synthetic coenzyme Q10 analogue, improves the cardiomyopathy in FA.

Bradley WG, Daroff RB, Fenichel GM, et al. Neurology in Clinical Practice, 5th ed. Philadelphia, PA: Elsevier; 2008.

Trujillo-Martín MM, Serrano-Aguilar P, Monton-Alvarez F, et al. Effectiveness and safety of treatments for degenerative ataxias: a systematic review. Mov Disord. 2009; 24(8):1111–1124.

52. c

Ataxia–telangiectasia (AT) is an autosomal recessive disorder that typically presents in childhood with neuropathy, ataxia, and extraocular movement abnormalities, characteristically marked by inability to move the eyes without head thrusting. Telangiectasias are present in the conjunctiva and other areas. These patients are at increased risk of hematologic and other malignancies, and are prone to infections due to immunodeficiency, including hypogammaglobulinemia. This disorder results from a mutation in the *ATM* gene on chromosome 11. Mutations in this gene result in impaired DNA repair. A high-serum α-fetoprotein is seen in AT as well as in ataxia with oculomotor apraxia type 2, a disorder clinically similar to AT.

Bradley WG, Daroff RB, Fenichel GM, et al. Neurology in Clinical Practice, 5th ed. Philadelphia, PA: Elsevier; 2008.

53. e

The spinocerebellar ataxias (SCAs) are a group of autosomal dominant ataxias that are clinically and genetically heterogeneous. Repeat expansions are common to many of them, with the CAG repeat most often expanded, but other repeats of different lengths have been identified on different chromosomes, as have been point mutations and other genetic abnormalities. The pathophysiology of the SCAs resulting from repeat expansion is thought to relate to a toxic gain of function, leading to a protein product that is misfolded and abnormally aggregates.

The spinocerebellar ataxias (SCAs) typically present in the third to fifth decades of life, but can present at any age, with each of the SCAs having a different mean age of onset. Although clinically heterogeneous, they share in common the occurrence of a progressive truncal and limb ataxia, often with associated spasticity and other upper motor neuron findings. Other abnormalities depending on the subtype include impaired saccades and smooth pursuits, cranial nerve abnormalities, and in some cases neuropathy. In some of the SCAs, epilepsy and cognitive decline occur. In SCA7, there is retinopathy with vision loss. MRI of the brain shows cerebellar atrophy and in some cases, atrophy of the brainstem and cervical spinal cord.

The most common spinocerebellar ataxia (SCA) is SCA3, also known as Machado–Joseph disease. Like SCA1 and SCA2, age of onset is typically in the third to fourth decades of life, though wide variability again occurs. In addition to ataxia and other cerebellar signs, facial and tongue atrophy and fasciculations occur, and bulbar symptoms such as dysphagia are common. Levodopa-responsive parkinsonism may occur. Neuropathy is a late feature. SCA3 results from expansion of the CAG repeat in the gene ataxin 3 on chromosome 14.

Bradley WG, Daroff RB, Fenichel GM, et al. Neurology in Clinical Practice, 5th ed. Philadelphia, PA: Elsevier; 2008.

Ropper AH, Samuels MA. Adams and Victor's Principles of Neurology, 9th ed. New York: McGraw-Hill; 2009.

54. a

This disorder may present clinically in females, though uncommon. This patient likely has fragile X tremor–ataxia syndrome, an X-linked ataxia. Fragile X syndrome results from expansion of CGG repeat in the *FMR1* gene on chromosome X to more than 200 repeats. In the grandparents of patients with fragile X syndrome, a repeat number of 55 to 200, in the premutation range, may result in clinical manifestations, including tremor, ataxia, parkinsonism, dysautonomia, and cognitive decline. Although the clinical presentation resembles the cerebellar type of multiple-system atrophy (discussed in questions 18 and 19), a family history of mental retardation should prompt consideration of this disorder. Woman may be affected as well, though less commonly and typically with less prominent features. MRI of the brain may show hyperintensities in the cerebellum and inferior cerebellar peduncle on T2-weighted images, as seen in Figure 6.3.

Bradley WG, Daroff RB, Fenichel GM, et al. Neurology in Clinical Practice, 5th ed. Philadelphia, PA: Elsevier; 2008.

55. d

Cerebrotendinous xanthomatosis is the most likely diagnosis in this patient. This is an autosomal recessive disorder caused by a defect in the enzyme 27-sterol hydroxylase on chromosome 2, which results in deposition of cholesterol and cholestanol in a variety of tissues, including the brain, lungs, lens of the eye, and tendons. This results in a variety of clinical manifestations in multiple organ systems, including neuropsychiatric symptoms (cognitive decline, personality changes, and psychiatric symptoms), ataxia (in the limbs and trunk), parkinsonism, neuropathy, tendon xanthomas particularly in the Achilles tendon, diarrhea, and cataracts. Diagnosis is made by measurement of serum cholestanol; serum cholesterol is often not elevated and not helpful in making the diagnosis. MRI of the brain shows cortical and cerebellar atrophy and white matter abnormalities. Treatment includes chenodeoxycholic acid as a means of lowering serum cholestanol; long-term therapy may lead to improvement in neurologic signs and symptoms.

Although the tests listed would help evaluate for other disorders that can lead to ataxia and neuropsychiatric symptoms, the constellation of signs and symptoms including ataxia, cataracts, and tendon xanthomas make cerebrotendinous xanthomatosis the most likely diagnosis. Machado–Joseph disease (SCA3, discussed in question 53) is diagnosed by analysis of CAG repeat number on chromosome 14. Copper and ceruloplasmin are tested for diagnosis of Wilson's disease (discussed in questions 28 and 29).

Bradley WG, Daroff RB, Fenichel GM, et al. Neurology in Clinical Practice, 5th ed. Philadelphia, PA: Elsevier; 2008.

56. e

This patient's history and examination are consistent with orthostatic tremor. This type of tremor affects the trunk and thighs. It is characteristically high frequency: surface EMG electrodes on the thighs would show a tremor frequency of 14 to 16 Hz. Symptoms include unsteadiness or shakiness on standing, with improvement when given physical support or with ambulation.

The gait disorder is not described as magnetic or apraxic, and there is no history of incontinence or cognitive decline to suggest normal-pressure hydrocephalus (discussed in Chapter 12). Unfortunately, patients with orthostatic tremor may be misdiagnosed with psychogenic gait disorder because the tremor may not be visible on examination, though it is most often detectable by surface EMG. There are no features of parkinsonism on examination to suggest vascular parkinsonism. Essential tremor can affect the legs, but it would not lead to the symptoms described in the case.

Bradley WG, Daroff RB, Fenichel GM, et al. Neurology in Clinical Practice, 5th ed. Philadelphia, PA: Elsevier; 2008.

57. a

This patient's CT scan, shown in Figure 6.4, shows bilateral calcification of the basal ganglia and cerebellum, or striopallidodentate calcinosis, also known as Fahr's disease. The differential diagnosis of hyperdense lesions on CT scan does include hemorrhage, but given the time course of this patient's symptoms as well as the symmetry and density of the lesions on CT scan (being comparable to that of the bone), calcium deposition is more likely. Although small basal ganglia calcifications are an incidental imaging finding of little clinical significance in most patients, the extent of calcification seen on this patient's CT scan combined with the history and examination findings suggest that this is clinically relevant and likely contributing to his parkinsonism. The distribution of calcium deposition includes most often the caudate, but also putamen, thalamus, and cerebellum, among other areas. Striopallidodentate calcinosis can be idiopathic, but can also be seen in both autosomal dominant and recessive familial forms, and a variety of metabolic disorders including secondary hyperparathyroidism as is seen in end-stage renal disease, primary hyperparathyroidism, as well as hypoparathyroidism.

Bradley WG, Daroff RB, Fenichel GM, et al. Neurology in Clinical Practice, 5th ed. Philadelphia, PA: Elsevier; 2008.

Manyam BV. What is and what is not "Fahr's disease." Parkinsonism Relat Disord. 2005; 11: 73–80.

58. d, 59. b

Patients should receive genetic counseling prior to obtaining a genetic test in order to allow them to make an informed decision regarding whether or not to have the test. During counseling, the positive and negative predictive value of the test, meaning of false positives and false negatives, and implications of testing should be discussed. Potential consequences including insurance concerns should be addressed, but testing should not be denied by the physician because of potential problems with insurance. Rather, the patient should be provided with information regarding potential consequences and be allowed to make an informed decision. It is the physician's obligation to maintain strict confidentiality, and the patient should be supported regardless of when he or she is going to disclose the information to family members. Although all patients with progressive neurodegenerative disorders should be encouraged to draft advanced directives early on, this should not be a prerequisite to diagnostic testing.

On the other hand, testing of asymptomatic minors should be avoided regardless of family history; genetic testing of asymptomatic children at their parents' request should not occur, regardless of the parents' intentions, particularly when the disorder is not treatable and there is no intervention that can be taken to prevent the disease. Testing should occur only after the age of 18, after an informed decision has been made by the patient (after genetic counseling).

Kodish E. Testing children for cancer genes: The rule of earliest onset. J Pediatr. 1999; 135(3): 390–395.

Statement of the Practice Committee Genetics Testing Task Force of the American Academy of Neurology. Practice parameter: genetic testing alert statement of the Practice Committee genetics testing Task Force of the American Academy of Neurology. Neurology. 1996;47: 1343–134.

Buzz Phrases	Key Points
Direct pathway: inhibitory or excitatory to cortex?	Excitatory (increases thalamic excitation of cortex)
Indirect pathway: inhibitory or excitatory to cortex?	Inhibitory (decreases thalamic excitation of cortex)
Hyperkinetic movement disorders (direct or indirect pathway dysfunction)?	Reduced activity of indirect pathway
Hypokinetic movement disorders (direct or indirect pathway dysfunction)?	Reduced activity of direct pathway
Sites involved in indirect pathway (name 5)	Caudate/putamen, globus pallidus externa (GPe), subthalamic nucleus (STN), globus pallidus interna (GPi), and thalamus
Sites involved in direct pathway (name 4)	Caudate/putamen, globus pallidus interna (GPi), substantia nigra reticulate (SNr), and thalamus
Mechanism of action: ropinirole and pramipexole	Dopamine agonists at D_2 and D_3 receptors
Mechanism of action: entacapone	Catechol-O-methyltransferase (COMT) inhibitor
Mechanism of action: levodopa	Dopamine precursor, converted into dopamine by action of dopa-decarboxylase
Mechanism of action: carbidopa	Peripheral dopa-decarboxylase inhibitor
Parkinson's disease therapy that causes impulse control problems	Dopamine agonists
Most common gene mutated in hereditary Parkinson's disease	Leucine-rich repeat kinase 2 (LRRK2)
Tongue-protrusion dystonia, chorea, acanthocytes on wet mount peripheral smear	Neuroacanthocytosis
Huntington's disease: chromosome, mode of inheritance, protein, genetic abnormality	Chromosome 4, autosomal dominant, Huntington, CAG trinucleotide repeat expansion
Torsin A mutation	Primary generalized dystonia, autosomal dominant, chromosome 9, DYT1 dystonia
Filipino with dystonia and parkinsonism	DYT3, Lubag, X-linked dystonia-parkinsonism
Dystonia in a young girl with diurnal variation and parkinsonism on examination	Dopa-responsive dystonia, autosomal dominant, GTP cyclohydrolase I (GCH1) on chromosome 14
Episodes of ataxia with facial twitching: diagnosis, gene, triggers, treatment	Episodic ataxia type I. Gene: KCN1A. Triggers: exercise, startle. Treatment: anticonvulsants such as carbamazepine
Episodes of ataxia with nystagmus and dysarthria: diagnosis, gene, triggers, treatment	Episodic ataxia type II. Gene: CACN1A4. Triggers: alcohol, fatigue, stress. Treatment: acetazolamide
Neurotransmitter implicated in familial hyperekplexia (exaggerated startle syndrome)	Glycine
Antibodies in stiff person syndrome	Autoimmune: anti-glutamic acid decarboxylase (GAD). Paraneoplastic: anti-amphiphysin

(*continued*)

Buzz Phrases	Key Points
High-arched feet, scoliosis, neuropathy, ataxia, cardiomyopathy. Diagnosis, gene	Friedreich's ataxia, trinucleotide repeat GAA expansion in frataxin gene on chromosome 9, autosomal recessive
Telangiectasia, ataxia, oculomotor abnormalities, immunodeficiency, hematologic malignancy	Ataxia–telangiectasia, autosomal recessive, ATM gene on chromosome 11, results in impaired DNA repair
Ataxia with high serum α-fetoprotein	Ataxia–telangiectasia and ataxia with oculomotor apraxia type 2
Cause and mode of inheritance of spinocerebellar ataxia type 3 (Machado–Joseph disease), clinical presentation	CAG repeat expansion, autosomal dominant. Ataxia, spasticity, neuropathy
Ataxia, parkinsonism in the grandfather of a boy with fragile X syndrome. Disorder, gene, imaging findings	Fragile X tremor–ataxia syndrome (FXTAS), from premutation (55-200 repeats) in CGG in FMR1 gene on chromosome X. T2 hyperintensities in cerebellum and inferior cerebellar peduncle
Ataxia, cataracts, tendon xanthomas. Disorder, diagnosis	Cerebrotendinous xanthomatosis, serum cholestanol
"Eye of the tiger"	Hyperintensity surrounded by hypointensity in the basal ganglia, seen in pantothenate-kinase–associated neurodegeneration (PKAN)
Medication that improves outcome of cardiomyopathy in Friedreich's ataxia	Idebenone, a coenzyme Q10 analogue

Chapter 7

Neuroimmunology

Questions

Questions 1–3

1. A 24-year-old right-handed Caucasian woman comes to your clinic for the first time. One year ago she had one episode of a tingling sensation ascending to the mid-chest region lasting 2 weeks. One month ago she lost vision in her right eye and had pain behind the eye, worse with movement, that resolved incompletely after 2 weeks. Her MRI of the brain and cervical spine are shown in Figures 7.1 and 7.2. This presentation and MRI are consistent with:

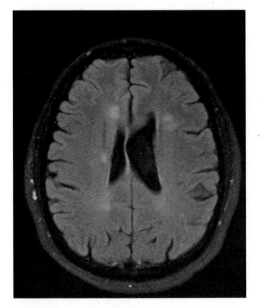

FIGURE 7.1   Axial FLAIR MRI

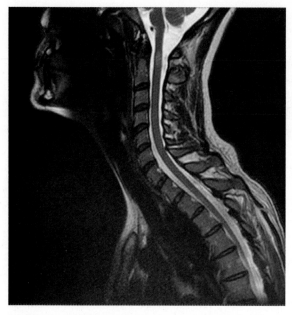

FIGURE 7.2 Sagittal T2-weighted MRI

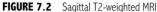

    a. A clinically isolated syndrome of demyelination
    b. Primary progressive multiple sclerosis
    c. Acute disseminated encephalomyelitis
    d. Fulminant multiple sclerosis because of two episodes in a year
    e. Relapsing-remitting multiple sclerosis

2. Other tests that may be useful diagnostically for this problem include:
    a. Laboratory testing to exclude a vitamin B_{12} deficiency and lupus erythematosus
    b. Skin biopsy for small-fiber neuropathy
    c. Brainstem auditory-evoked potentials
    d. CSF analysis for cells, protein, glucose, and oligoclonal bands
    e. a and d

3. What is correct regarding the prognosis?
    a. Will progress to using a wheelchair within 5 years
    b. Has benign multiple sclerosis and will not progress
    c. Will likely be unable to walk after 15 years
    d. Should avoid pregnancy due to worsening of her disease
    e. Will likely have measurable disability on neurologic examination after 10 years

Questions 4–6

4. A 32-year-old Caucasian woman developed left retro-orbital pain, worse with eye movement, 1 week ago. Over the past 2 days she has lost central vision, has reduced perception of light brightness, and colors seem "washed out." You examine her and find a normal fundus, a left relative afferent pupillary defect (RAPD), and visual acuity of 20/200 in the left eye. The following are correct, except:

a. This condition usually improves over about 6 weeks
b. Oral steroids are appropriate treatment
c. This condition is sometimes associated with the emergence of multiple sclerosis
d. Intravenous steroids with an oral steroid taper are the treatment of choice
e. For visual acuity of 20/50 or better, steroid treatment has not been shown to be beneficial

5. The presence of a relative afferent pupillary defect implies:
   a. An imminent early third nerve palsy
   b. Dampened efferent arm of the pupillary light reflex
   c. A particularly good prognosis
   d. A meningeal inflammatory component
   e. Involvement proximal to the Edinger-Westphal nucleus

6. Testing that is valuable in such a patient includes:
   a. Syphilis serology
   b. Angiotensin-converting enzyme
   c. MRI of the brain and orbits with gadolinium
   d. Brainstem auditory-evoked potentials
   e. Retinal angiography

7. A 45-year-old woman with relapsing-remitting multiple sclerosis of 5 years' duration develops new right leg weakness, with trouble walking more than 10 feet unsupported. She has no recent fever or infection and has not recently started a new medication. You examine her in the office and note increased reflexes in the right leg compared with prior examination, a Babinski sign on the right, and a right crossed adductor. Which of the following answers is correct?
   a. A Babinski sign is consistent with a spinothalamic tract demyelinating plaque
   b. Her weakness is due to a lower motor neuron disorder
   c. Intravenous methylprednisolone is the treatment of choice
   d. She should immediately begin working out harder
   e. A crossed adductor is a clear sign of cervical spinal cord disease

8. Your patient with newly diagnosed multiple sclerosis comes to you and wants to know a few things about this disease. The only statement that is correct in multiple sclerosis is that:
   a. Multiple sclerosis is more common further from the equator
   b. Drinking milk definitely prevents multiple sclerosis
   c. Her identical twin has a 100% chance of getting multiple sclerosis too
   d. Multiple sclerosis is definitely due to mononucleosis
   e. Multiple sclerosis is environmentally transmitted

9. The pathology of active multiple sclerosis can consist of all of the following, except:
   a. Involvement of cortical gray matter
   b. Involvement of white matter
   c. Loss of myelin from axons
   d. Axonal transections
   e. Profuse basophilic infiltration in the meninges

10. Typical symptoms of multiple sclerosis may include all of the following, except:
    a. Tingling, burning, aching, or "numb" sensations
    b. Weakness of the legs

c. Double vision
> d. Distal limb atrophy *(Lupper ard N disorder. dess & cames atrophy)*
e. Ataxia

11. Your 34-year-old African-American female patient with relapsing neurologic symptoms has spinal fluid testing. Which of the following findings would prompt you to consider diagnoses other than multiple sclerosis?
    a. Elevated kappa chains
    b. WBC count of 22 (normal 0 to 5 cells/mm^3)
  ^ c. Neutrophilic pleocytosis
    d. Elevated immunoglobulin G synthesis rate
    e. Normal CSF immunologic parameters

12. You see a 21-year-old male college student of Asian-American descent. He has had three episodes of neurologic symptoms, including an episode of hemiparesis lasting 3 weeks, one episode of optic neuritis in the left eye lasting 2 weeks, and one episode of paresthesias of both legs and lower abdomen with reduced bladder sensation with residual symptoms. His MRI of the brain is shown in Figures 7.3 and 7.4. The only statement that is true is:

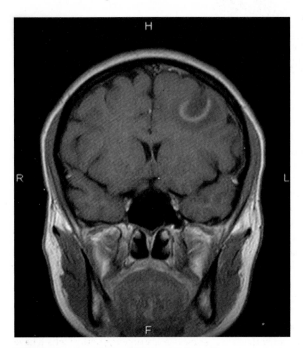

FIGURE 7.3   Coronal T1-weighted postcontrast MRI

    a. This is multifocal glioma and he should have a brain biopsy
  ^ b. This may respond to intravenous steroids or may require other immunosuppression
    c. The open-ring sign indicates abscess formation
    d. Prognosis is dismal with this MRI finding
    e. *Chlamydia pneumoniae* has been proven to cause this picture

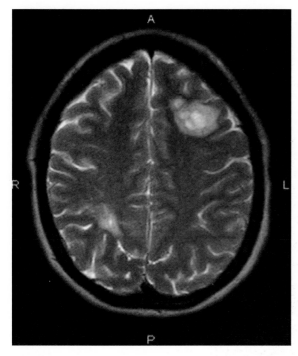

FIGURE 7.4   Axial T2-weighted MRI

13. Your patient with relapsing multiple sclerosis has an MRI with gadolinium. The following statements are incorrect, except:
    a. Typical lesions of multiple sclerosis have decreased T2 signal and increased T1 signal
    b. Spinal cord multiple sclerosis lesions usually extend over more than three segments
    c. Spinal cord lesions in multiple sclerosis never show mass effect
    d. Typical multiple sclerosis lesions are periventricular and oval shaped
    e. Multiple sclerosis lesions are always well defined on FLAIR imaging
    f. Higher-field-strength MRI magnets are less likely to show multiple sclerosis lesions

Questions 14–18

14. You see a 45-year-old Caucasian man in your office. Two months ago he developed a nearly complete loss of vision in the left eye, which has not resolved despite intravenous steroids and a tapering course of oral steroids. Two weeks ago he developed visual loss in the right eye, which has persisted. He has burning paresthesias of both feet and some urinary urgency, both of which have been present for 1 year. His MRI of the cervical cord is seen in Figure 7.5. His spinal fluid shows 50 WBCs/mm^3, with 45% neutrophils and 55% lymphocytes, protein of 75 mg/dL, and negative oligoclonal banding. CSF VDRL is negative, HIV is negative, HTLV I and II are negative, and vitamin B$_{12}$ level is normal. ANA is moderately elevated at a titer of 1:128. Which of the following is the most likely diagnosis?
    a. Lupus myelitis
    b. Fulminant multiple sclerosis

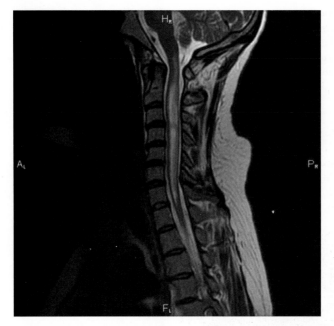

FIGURE 7.5 Sagittal T2-weighted MRI

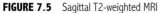
c. Neuromyelitis optica
d. Subacute combined degeneration
e. Neurosarcoidosis

15. In terms of the most recent episode of neurologic symptoms:
a. Treatment is nonurgent as most of these events resolve
b. Intravenous steroids are ineffective and counterproductive
c. Interferon β-1b is the drug of choice
d. Recovery is often incomplete
e. Natalizumab is indicated due to its higher efficacy profile

16. Long-term treatment could consist of all of the following, except:
a. Oral steroids
b. Azathioprine
c. Cyclosporine pulse therapy
d. Rituximab therapy
e. Weekly intramuscular interferon β-1a

17. The disease course in this condition can be all of the following, except:
a. Gradual worsening over time
b. Relapsing
c. Monophasic
d. Severe
e. Isolated spinal cord involvement

18. In this condition, all of the following are true about the brain MRI findings, except:

    a. The brain is always normal in this condition
    b. The brain is often normal in this condition
    c. Involvement of the spinal cord extending into the brainstem can occur
    d. Posterior reversible encephalopathy syndrome can occur
    e. Lesions atypical for multiple sclerosis can occur

Questions 19–21

19. A 12-year-old right-handed Caucasian girl comes to the hospital. She had a mild upper respiratory tract infection 2 weeks ago and then over the past 4 days developed headache, fever, visual blurring, trouble walking, and paresthesias of her limbs. Her MRI is shown in Figures 7.6 and 7.7. Her examination shows bilateral papillitis, brisk reflexes with some limb ataxia, and upgoing toes. She is moderately confused and febrile. CSF shows a mild lymphocytic pleocytosis and negative oligoclonal banding. This syndrome is most consistent with:

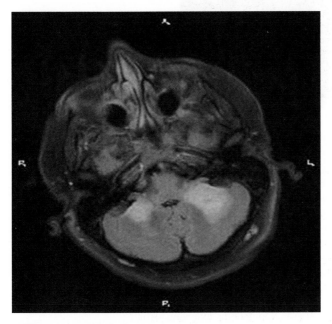

FIGURE 7.6   Axial FLAIR MRI

    a. Relapsing-remitting multiple sclerosis
    b. Acute disseminated encephalomyelitis
    c. Hemorrhagic leukoencephalopathy of Weston Hurst
    d. Balo's concentric sclerosis
    e. Viral meningitis

20. In terms of how this is related to multiple sclerosis:

    a. It appears to be a separate neuroimmunologic disorder
    b. It usually transitions into multiple sclerosis
    c. It never transitions into multiple sclerosis

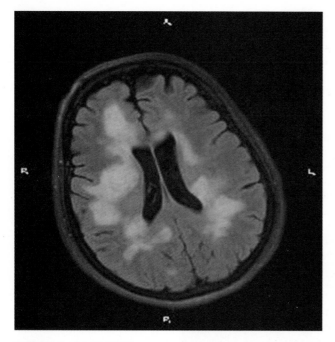

FIGURE 7.7   Axial FLAIR MRI

   d. It is the pediatric equivalent of multiple sclerosis
   e. It is the same as multiple sclerosis

21. You decide to treat the patient with the following:
   a. Intravenous diphenhydramine
   b. Intravenous ceftriaxone
   c. Intravenous acyclovir
   d. Intravenous gentamicin
   e. Intravenous methylprednisolone

22. Regarding fatigue in multiple sclerosis, which of the following is true?
   a. Is always due to depression
   b. Is due to sleep disorders in most cases
   c. Is a frequent symptom in patients with multiple sclerosis
   d. Has a precisely defined pathophysiology
   e. Is untreatable

23. You see a patient with multiple sclerosis who wants to become pregnant. You tell her that:
   a. She should never get pregnant because it will worsen her multiple sclerosis
   b. She will need to have a Cesarean section
   c. She should start prenatal vitamins
   d. She cannot receive steroids during pregnancy
   e. She can continue her interferon β-1b during pregnancy

24. Your 37-year-old African-American female patient with early relapsing multiple sclerosis wants to consider a disease-modifying agent. You tell her that:
    a. She should start nothing as these agents only work in 30% of patients
    b. The agents reduce relapse rate and reduce MRI activity in relapsing-remitting multiple sclerosis
    c. There is one best choice in terms of medicines
    d. Antibodies that neutralize medicine form in all patients on these medications
    e. She should expect to feel better after 6 months on medicine

Questions 25–27

25. Your 42-year-old right-handed Caucasian female patient has been on an interferon and then glatiramer acetate, but has continued to have exacerbations with weakness of the left leg and diplopia. Her MRI shows two enhancing lesions. You start her on monthly natalizumab 300 mg intravenously. Your initial counseling to her includes all the following, except:
    a. This medicine reduces exacerbations by 60% to 70% in relapsing forms of MS
    b. It requires participation in a monitoring program
    c. It has a 1 in 1000 risk of causing progressive multifocal leukoencephalopathy
    d. Natalizumab is more risky than using mitoxantrone for multiple sclerosis
    e. There is a 1 in 50 risk of anaphylaxis during natalizumab use

26. During the third infusion of natalizumab, the patient develops shortness of breath, tachycardia, and a pruritic erythematous rash on her chest and abdomen. You recommend:
    a. A trial of diphenhydramine prophylaxis
    b. Referral to an allergist for desensitization
    c. Retrial with 150 mg of natalizumab for the next dose
    d. Evaluation for immunoglobulin A deficiency
    e. Terminating the infusion, treating for anaphylaxis, and avoiding future doses

27. After 2 years on treatment, the patient develops headaches, mild right hemiparesis, and word-finding difficulty. There is a new subcortical lesion on MRI. You recommend all of the following, except:
    a. Stopping natalizumab during evaluation
    b. Double the natalizumab dose in future treatments
    c. CSF for JC virus PCR
    d. Considering plasmapheresis depending on evaluation
    e. Careful clinical monitoring

28. Your 54-year-old male patient with multiple sclerosis has painful spasms of both legs, which are worse at bedtime, increased when he has to have a bowel movement, and worse with stress. His examination shows a spastic paraparesis. The following statement about spasticity is true:
    a. Spasticity is the same as weakness
    b. Treatment with baclofen or tizanidine is usually not beneficial
    c. If he works out hard, it will go away
    d. Stretching may be helpful
    e. Botulinum toxin injections are not indicated in focal spasticity

29. You are called to the emergency department to see a 23-year-old female Caucasian patient. She has been previously well, but about a week ago without prodromal illness, she developed ascending paresthesias of the legs and trunk. She had progressive unsteadiness and leg weakness

and now cannot walk. Her examination shows mildly reduced reflexes in the legs, upgoing toes, and a sensory level. Her MRI of the spine is shown in Figure 7.8. CSF shows a mild lymphocytic pleocytosis, negative studies for syphilis, herpes zoster, *Mycoplasma*, and HIV. Which of the following is the most likely diagnosis?

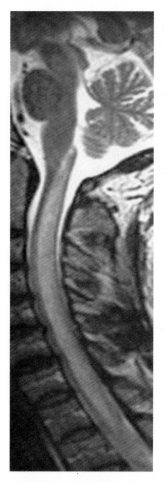

FIGURE 7.8   Sagittal T2-weighted MRI

  a. Ascending myelitis
  b. Transverse myelitis
  c. Lupoid myelitis
  d. Guillain-Barre syndrome
  e. Early multiple sclerosis

30. Fingolimod is an oral agent used in relapsing multiple sclerosis. Its mechanism of action is best described by:

  a. Interferon-based therapy that alters cytokine trafficking
  b. Polymer that simulates the antigenicity of myelin basic protein
  c. DNA polymerase inhibitor

d. Modulator of sphingosine-1 phosphate receptors
e. Selectively inhibits B-cell maturation

31. Dalfampridine is a medication that:
a. Reduces pseudobulbar affect in patients with neurologic injury
b. Reduces relapses in patients with relapsing-remitting multiple sclerosis
c. Is FDA approved to improve visual contrast sensitivity in multiple sclerosis
d. Is FDA approved to improve the speed of walking in multiple sclerosis
e. Is not indicated for patients with multiple sclerosis

32. A patient comes to you asking about new oral agents for multiple sclerosis in research studies. She is specifically interested in oral cladribine. All the following statements about this medicine are incorrect, except:
a. Oral cladribine is a chemotherapeutic agent and therefore cannot be used in multiple sclerosis
b. Oral cladribine is a purine nucleoside analogue
c. Oral cladribine is a nonspecific inhibitor of T-cell adhesion to endothelial cells
d. Oral cladribine has an unknown mechanism, but reduces immunoglobulin production
e. Oral cladribine has no hematologic side effects

33. Your patient with secondary progressive multiple sclerosis comes to her appointment asking about her low vitamin D. She wants to know what the relationship with multiple sclerosis is and exactly how much vitamin D she should be taking to prevent a worsening of her multiple sclerosis. You tell her all of the following, except:
a. The exact relationship between vitamin D and multiple sclerosis is not known
b. Low vitamin D is the reason why multiple sclerosis is more common further from the equator
c. In a large prospective cohort nursing study, nurses who used vitamin D supplementation were less likely to get multiple sclerosis
d. Vitamin D can be an immunomodulator in animal models of multiple sclerosis
e. Vitamin D is often lower in African-Americans who also tend to have more severe clinical multiple sclerosis

Answer key

1. e	7. c	13. d	19. b	25. d	31. d
2. e	8. a	14. c	20. a	26. e	32. b
3. e	9. e	15. d	21. e	27. b	33. b
4. b	10. d	16. e	22. c	28. d	
5. e	11. c	17. a	23. c	29. b	
6. c	12. b	18. a	24. b	30. d	

Answers

1. e, 2. e, 3. e

This patient has relapsing-remitting multiple sclerosis (RRMS). Most patients with this disorder have onset between age 20 and 40, though age of onset ranges from early childhood to late adulthood. Females are affected more than males in a 3:2 ratio. It is more common further north and south of the equator, and more common in Caucasians. RRMS is defined by relapses consistent with demyelination, with or without clinical improvement, but with episodes of clinical stability in between relapses. The term "remitting" is confusing as these patients may not return to clinical normalcy after a relapse. In addition, on MRI, they may have new lesion formation while remaining clinically stable five to ten times as often as they have new clinical episodes. A "relapse" is defined as an episode of new or worsened neurologic symptoms, lasting more than 24 hours, not due to fever or infection. Other synonyms for this are an attack, bout, or exacerbation. The diagnosis is based on two relapses separated in time with clinical evidence of multiple lesions in the central nervous system. The diagnosis can also be made on the basis of multiple lesions on the MRI in combination with an appropriate history and examination, new lesion formation on MRI over time, and new clinical activity over time.

A clinically isolated syndrome of demyelination is a single clinical episode consistent with demyelination, but no "second episode" to make a clinical diagnosis of multiple sclerosis. Primary progressive multiple sclerosis usually occurs in older patients. These patients have a gradually progressive course from onset and do not have relapses. They may have a lower burden of MRI lesions than do patients with RRMS. Acute demyelinating encephalomyelitis is an acute disorder, more common in childhood, and often occurring soon after an infection or vaccination. Patients develop a subacute severe disorder with multifocal demyelination in the brain and spinal cord (see discussion to questions 19 to 21). Fulminant multiple sclerosis indicates a rapidly progressive course with repeated relapses that are refractory to standard treatment.

There are no laboratory tests that are presently useful in the diagnosis of multiple sclerosis. On occasion, other disorders can mimic multiple sclerosis. Diseases commonly tested for in early evaluation of multiple sclerosis include vitamin B_{12} deficiency, lupus, Lyme disease in endemic areas, and other inflammatory disorders depending on clinical suspicion. Skin biopsy for small-fiber neuropathy may be useful for patients with paresthesias that affect the limbs and face, that are persistent, and in whom there is no evidence to suggest central demyelination. Brainstem auditory-evoked potentials can be abnormal in the population with multiple sclerosis, but generally are not helpful diagnostically (insensitive in early multiple sclerosis for subclinical brainstem lesions). Somatosensory-evoked, or visual-evoked, potentials may be useful in selected patients to ascertain a second lesion or show slowing, suggestive of central demyelination. CSF may show mild elevation in WBCs, predominantly lymphocytes. Measures of immune activity are sometimes but not always abnormal, including immunoglobulin G synthesis rate and the presence of oligoclonal bands (indicating antibody formation in the spinal fluid compartment).

The prognosis for RRMS is better than most people expect. Various studies have shown a good prognosis over 10 years in a representative population without treatment. However, neurologic examination shows abnormalities after 10 years of disease in most patients. The diagnosis of benign multiple sclerosis is a retrospective one after 15 to 20 years of disease without measurable disability. This occurs in approximately 10% to 20% of patients with multiple sclerosis.

Fox R, Bethoux F, Goldman MD, et al. Multiple sclerosis: Advances in understanding, diagnosing, and treating the underlying disease. Cleve Clin J Med. 2006; 73:91–102.

4. b, 5. e, 6. c

This patient has optic neuritis. The results of a large randomized double-blind treatment trial for acute optic neuritis compared intravenous methylprednisolone with prednisone taper, oral prednisone taper, and placebo. This study showed that recovery was hastened by intravenous methylprednisolone with oral prednisone taper but that visual outcome at 1 year was not significantly affected. Oral steroids were at best no better than placebo, and possibly worse.

In about 80% of patients with acute optic neuritis, recovery occurs over weeks. This may be incomplete. Over a 15-year period after an episode of optic neuritis, multiple sclerosis occurs in about 50% of cases. Factors that increase the risk of multiple sclerosis developing include the presence of brain MRI lesions consistent with demyelination and abnormal CSF findings. In the Optic Neuropathy Treatment Trial, patients with visual acuity of 20/50 or better did not measurably benefit from intravenous steroids treatment.

Relative afferent pupillary defect is a sign seen in optic neuritis. In this condition, there is involvement of the optic nerve with impaired response to light stimulation. The afferent arm of the pupillary light reflex is affected, in the side of the optic neuritis as compared to the normal eye. This leads to a relative reduction in signal traveling to the Edinger Westphal nucleus in the midbrain from the affected eye. Thus light shone into the affected eye causes a normal consensual light reflex. (Both the pupils constrict.) When the stimulus is shifted to the "good" eye, pupils remain constricted, and then when shifted back to the affected eye, there is relatively less "light," so the pupils dilate (see also Chapter 1). This is not an indication of an effect on the third nerve, which is the efferent arm of the pupillary light reflex. This does not suggest a particular prognosis. This does not imply a meningeal component.

MRI of the brain is ordered primarily to assess evidence and risk of progression to multiple sclerosis. On occasion, imaging of the optic nerve can confirm optic nerve involvement, but it is not critical for the diagnosis of optic neuritis. Rarely, retro-orbital or meningeal processes can cause sudden visual loss, simulating optic neuritis. On occasion, sinus cystic disease can cause impingement on or inflammation in the optic nerve. If there are one or more well-defined demyelinating lesions on MRI, the risk of multiple sclerosis goes from about 20% in 5 years to approximately 80% over 5 years. Multiple treatment trials in patients with a single episode of demyelination and MRI brain lesions have shown benefit from starting medicines that are FDA approved for multiple sclerosis treatment in such patients. In general, when the MRI does not show such lesions, treatment is not indicated beyond steroid therapy acutely.

Unless the patient has a history suggestive of syphilis, syphilis serology is not useful. Angiotensin-converting enzyme testing is not useful in this situation unless there are other indications to suggest sarcoidosis. Brainstem auditory-evoked potentials are of low yield in this situation. There is no indication for retinal angiography in typical optic neuritis. It may be useful if there are atypical features such as a horizontal scotoma or very sudden painless onset suggesting a vascular etiology.

Balcer LJ. Optic neuritis. N Engl J Med. 2006; 354:1273–1280.

Beck RW, Cleary PA, Anderson MM Jr, et al. A randomized, controlled trial of corticosteroids in the treatment of acute optic neuritis. The Optic Neuritis Study Group. N Engl J Med. 1992; 326:581–588.

7. C

The patient is having an acute relapse. In this case there is a functional deficit interfering with walking, which is an indication for treatment rather than conservative management. Intravenous methylprednisolone usually given as a dose of 1000 mg daily for 3 to 5 days, with an oral steroid taper, is presently the treatment of choice for acute relapses. Other options include other forms of steroids, different dosing or duration of taper, not using a tapering dose, and high-dose steroids. The goal of treatment is to reduce the functional deficit and increase the speedy recovery of function.

The Babinski sign is elicited by stroking the lateral border of the sole of the foot with a moderately sharp object. A normal response is that the great toe goes down (plantar flexion). A positive Babinski sign is when the great toe goes up, often with fanning of the other toes. A full "triple flexion" response is when the ankle dorsiflexes, the knee flexes, and the hip flexes in addition to the Babinski sign. The presence of a Babinski sign implies dysfunction in the corticospinal (pyramidal) tract between the cortex and the lumbar spinal cord. A positive Babinski sign is an indication of an upper motor neuron disorder (corticospinal tract) and not a lower motor neuron disorder (problem affecting the lower motor neuron from the anterior horn of the spinal cord to the neuromuscular junction).

Increased exercise during an acute exacerbation has not been shown to be beneficial. However regular exercise in multiple sclerosis has been shown to improve quality-of-life measures and reduce fatigue and depression scales. A crossed adductor sign is seen when performing the patellar reflex. The opposite (crossed) leg adducts (moves medially from the hip). This implies a spread of reflex above the L4 level into L2 and L3 segments of the cord, indicating disinhibition of the reflex arc. This is another upper motor neuron sign.

Frohman EM, Shah A, Eggenberger E, et al. Corticosteroids for multiple sclerosis: I. application for treating exacerbations. Neurotherapeutics. 2007; 4(4):618–626.

8. a

Multiple sclerosis is more prevalent the further north or south of the equator one lives. The cause for this has not been established. Moving after the age of 12 does not seem to alter this risk. There is no evidence that drinking milk or other dietary measures affect the development of multiple sclerosis. However various epidemiologic studies suggest a link between vitamin D levels and multiple sclerosis, with lower vitamin D levels being correlated with higher risk of multiple sclerosis. Whether this is related to the cause of multiple sclerosis or common factors is unclear. Monozygotic (identical) female twins have a 33% chance of both being affected by multiple sclerosis if one develops multiple sclerosis. This indicates a mixture of genetic and nongenetic factors in the disease causation. Although mononucleosis has been linked to multiple sclerosis at times, the relationship is unclear and no definitive pathogenic relationship can be shown at present. The best evidence against environmental transmission of multiple sclerosis comes from adoption studies that do not show an increase in multiple sclerosis in children adopted into multiple sclerosis-affected families. Multiple sclerosis exacerbations are more likely to occur after infections, but are not related to any specific infection. Motor vehicle accidents and surgical procedures have not been linked to the onset or exacerbation of multiple sclerosis.

Fox RJ, Bethoux F, Goldman MD, et al. Advances in understanding, diagnosing and treating the underlying disease. Cleve Clin J Med. 2006; 73:91–102.

9. e

Multiple sclerosis is not associated with basophilic or eosinophilic infiltration of the meninges. Lymphocytes enter the CNS from the periphery. There are focal areas of demyelination (plaques) with glial cell infiltration and inflammatory cell accumulation. Macrophages are present in the core of the plaques. Areas of remyelination can be seen ("shadow plaques"). Oligodendroglial cells are reduced in the plaque core and increased at the periphery. Normal-appearing white matter may show loss of axons and some gliosis. Cortical gray matter is affected in multiple sclerosis, but this is poorly visualized with present imaging techniques and is thus under-recorded during life. White matter is typically affected in multiple sclerosis; myelin is removed from around axons, and early in lesion formation, axons are also injured and measurably transected.

Lucchinetti CF, Parisi J, Bruck W. The pathology of multiple sclerosis. Neurol Clin. 2006; 23:77–105.

10. d

Multiple sclerosis is typically an upper motor neuron or CNS disorder and does not cause muscle atrophy. However there are reported cases of some peripheral involvement and muscle atrophy in late multiple sclerosis, but these would be atypical features and suggest other diagnoses. Paresthesias of various types including the above as well as focal areas of pruritus or a sensation of wetness are common in multiple sclerosis. These can occur anywhere on the body. Weakness and gait difficulties are key common symptoms in multiple sclerosis, but do not occur in every patient. Double vision can occur and is usually due to brainstem involvement. Gait or limb ataxia occurs commonly and can be due to cerebellar, cerebellar connection, or sensory tract involvement in multiple sclerosis.

Noseworthy JH, Lucchinetti C, Rodriguez M, et al. Multiple sclerosis. N Engl J Med. 2000; 343:938–952.

11. c

White cells can be elevated in the CSF in multiple sclerosis. Usually there is a predominance of lymphocytes and no more than 50 cells/mm^3. A neutrophilic pleocytosis would be unusual and might suggest another diagnosis. For example this can be seen in Devic's disease at times (neuromyelitis optica; see discussion to questions 14 to 18). Elevated kappa chains are an indication of antibody formation in the CNS compartment and can be seen in multiple sclerosis. Immunoglobulin G synthesis rate elevation is one measure of increased intrathecal elaboration of antibody and can be seen in multiple sclerosis. Some patients with multiple sclerosis can have normal CSF. The frequency of this finding varies, but a normal CSF does not "rule out" multiple sclerosis.

Noseworthy JH, Lucchinetti C, Rodriguez M, et al. Multiple sclerosis. N Engl J Med. 2000; 343:938–952.

12. b

This picture is consistent with tumefactive multiple sclerosis. Although the diagnosis of multifocal glioma is in the differential of multicentric lesions in the brain, the relapsing pattern and the presence of an open-ring sign with limited mass effect on the MRI in Figure 7.3 would all argue against this diagnosis. Tumefactive multiple sclerosis appears to be a subform of relapsing multiple sclerosis with large, mass-like lesions. These often have incomplete peripheral enhancement, showing the "open-ring sign," which is suggestive of this pathology. Patients may improve with intravenous steroids but, on occasion, may require other immunologic treatment such as plasmapheresis or intravenous immunoglobulin. The open-ring sign is consistent with tumefactive multiple sclerosis and does not suggest abscess. The prognosis is similar to that seen in relapsing and remitting multiple sclerosis and is not "dismal." There is no specific evidence that *Chlamydia pneumoniae* is causative for tumefactive multiple sclerosis. There is some evidence that may suggest that *Chlamydia pneumoniae* may be related to multiple sclerosis, but this has not been corroborated.

Lucchinetti CF, Gavrilova RH, Metz I, et al. Clinical and radiographic spectrum of pathologically confirmed tumefactive multiple sclerosis. Brain. 2008; 131:1759–1775.

13. d

Typical multiple sclerosis lesions are periventricular and oval shaped. They have increased T2 signal. Characteristically, they are oval shaped and periventricular, but may be irregular, small or large, sharply defined or ill-defined, and may involve subcortical and juxtacortical brain. They may be seen in the infratentorial compartment typically around the fourth ventricle and in the brainstem white matter. They may show T1-reduced signal (so-called black holes). This appears to suggest more significant axonal loss or an older plaque. With gadolinium, some, but not all lesions can enhance. Enhancement of all lesions or persistent enhancement for weeks would be atypical for an multiple sclerosis plaque. Spinal cord lesions in multiple sclerosis usually extend only one to two vertebral segments and tend to involve a segment of the cord. A longitudinally extensive lesion over three or more segments suggests other disorders such as Devic's disease (see discussion to questions 14 to 18), transverse myelitis, sarcoidosis, lupus, or an intraspinal mass. Spinal cord lesions may show mass effect acutely, with gradual reduction in mass effect over time and eventual focal atrophy. Some multiple sclerosis lesions can be ill-defined. Some patients have a poorly defined change in brain MRI signal on FLAIR and T2, known as "dirty white matter," in which cloudy-appearing changes without sharply defined borders are seen.

There is an increased detection of focal lesions with increased field strength. This can be very useful for infratentorial lesions that may not be evident with lower-field-strength magnets.

Pretorius PM, Quaghebeur G. The role of MRI in the diagnosis of MS. Clin Radiol. 2003; 58:434–448.

14. c, **15.** d, **16.** e, **17.** a, **18.** a

Neuromyelitis optica (Devic's disease) is a neuroinflammatory condition with a distinct pathology and clinical course. Histologically, focal areas of demyelination are seen with significant leukocyte infiltration and some areas of frank necrosis and cavitation. There may be nearly complete axon loss within lesions. There are antibodies, neuromyelitis optica immunoglobulin G (NMO-IgG), that bind selectively to the aquaporin-4 water channel. This is a component of the dystroglycan-protein complex located in astrocytic foot processes at the blood-brain barrier.

Lupus myelitis can be acute as well, but patients have other markers of lupus, such as skin rash, arthritis, and renal involvement. Relapsing optic neuritis and myelitis together would be unusual in lupus myelitis. Fulminant multiple sclerosis could cause this syndrome, but the presence of severe optic neuritis bilaterally should suggest the diagnosis of Devic's disease first. Laboratory testing for NMO-IgG is positive in 70% of such cases. Subacute combined degeneration could cause paresthesias of the feet but does not cause a relapsing optic neuritis. Neurosarcoidosis can mimic most neurologic disorders but is usually a diagnosis of exclusion or diagnosed when systemic markers of this disease are present (e.g., skin, lung, and other organ involvement; see Chapter 16).

Devic's disease progresses with relapses, but does not tend to progress in between relapses. It can have a monophasic or relapsing course. It can be severe. It can exhibit a spinal form. Relapses are frequently severe and may not recover completely. Treatment is urgent in relapses of Devic's disease and many of the deficits do not resolve completely. Interferon β does not seem to be effective in Devic's disease. There are no data on the use of natalizumab in Devic's disease. Medicines that have been used anecdotally include steroids, azathioprine, Cytoxan, rituximab, and other immunosuppressants. For acute exacerbations, IV steroids or plasmapheresis can be used.

Early in Devic's disease the brain tends to be spared. However, later in the course it may have some atypical features, with brainstem disease extending up from the spinal cord, lesions atypical for multiple sclerosis in the brain, and imaging findings consistent with posterior reversible encephalopathy syndrome.

Lennon VA, Kryzer TJ, Pittock SJ. IgG marker of optic-spinal multiple sclerosis binds to the aquaporin-4 water channel. N Engl J Med. 2005; 202:473–477.

Pittock SJ, Lennon VA, Krecke K, et al. Brain abnormalities in neuromyelitis optica. Arch Neurol. 2006; 63:390–396.

19. b, **20.** a, **21.** e

This syndrome is most consistent with acute disseminated encephalomyelitis (ADEM). ADEM is usually a monophasic syndrome often occurring after an infection or vaccination. It is a multifocal demyelinating syndrome with large lesions that can be peripheral and may involve the basal ganglia. CSF may show a pleocytosis, but usually does not show oligoclonal bands. Patients are often febrile and encephalopathic. It may leave residual deficits.

First-line treatment for ADEM is intravenous methylprednisolone. All treatment recommendations are anecdotal. Treatment consists of initial intravenous methylprednisolone and if this fails, trial of plasmapheresis. There is no indication for antibacterial or antiviral agents.

The hemorrhagic leukoencephalopathy of Weston Hurst is a severe immune-mediated encephalopathy with areas of hemorrhage often in the temporal lobes. It may be a subform of ADEM. Balo's concentric sclerosis refers to a progressive demyelinating disorder in which concentric rings of demyelination are seen either pathologically or on MRI. This is not consistent with viral meningitis as the patient has CNS parenchymal findings on MRI.

ADEM appears to be a separate neuroimmunologic disorder from multiple sclerosis. However, some patients diagnosed with ADEM later develop a relapsing pattern consistent with multiple sclerosis. This may be due to a tendency in the pediatric population to diagnose ADEM rather than a first episode of multiple sclerosis.

Tenembaum S, Chitnis T, Ness J, et al. ADEM. Neurology. 2007; 68:S23–S36.

22. c

Approximately 95% of patients with multiple sclerosis have fatigue as a symptom at some time during their course. This may be part of the biology of the disease, but its pathogenesis has not been fully defined. It is not usually due to depression or sleep disorders, but both of these are worth inquiring about. In addition, some medicines used for multiple sclerosis can cause fatigue. Fatigue in multiple sclerosis can be treated with good sleep hygiene, naps during the day, regular exercise, and sometimes medicines such as amantadine or modafinil.

Fox RJ, Bethoux F, Goldman MD, et al. Advances in understanding, diagnosing and treating the underlying disease. Cleve Clin J Med. 2006; 73:91–102.

23. c

Pregnancy does not change the course of multiple sclerosis appreciably. Like other women contemplating pregnancy, patients should be on prenatal vitamins with folic acid. There are no specific issues in the conduct of pregnancy and patients can have an epidural anesthetic and can have a regular delivery or Cesarean section as needed obstetrically. Steroids can be used during pregnancy though should be limited as much as possible and preferably should not be given in the first trimester. Interferons (category C in pregnancy) should be stopped at least 1 month before conception. Glatiramer acetate is category B in pregnancy, but it is usually stopped before conception. Women with multiple sclerosis tend to have fewer exacerbations during pregnancy and more in the first 6 months after delivery (see Chapter 16). Breast-feeding may be protective against exacerbations. Children of women with multiple sclerosis have a 3% to 5% lifetime chance of developing multiple sclerosis.

Ferrero S, Pretta S, Ragna N. Multiple sclerosis: Management issues during pregnancy. Eur J Obstet Gynecol Reprod Biol. 2004; 115:3–9.

24. b

All the standard disease-modifying agents for early relapsing-remitting multiple sclerosis (interferon β-1b, interferon β-1a intramuscularly or subcutaneously, and glatiramer acetate) reduce relapse rate, reduce new lesion formation on MRI, and tend to slow progression of measurable disability on neurologic examination. They are similar in effect profile. They vary in side effects, route of administration, and frequency of administration. The interferons as a class cause flu-like symptoms after injections and may cause injection site reactions. They require laboratory monitoring for liver function changes and hematologic change. Glatiramer acetate causes local injection site reactions and occasional idiosyncratic chest pain. Although all agents reduce attack frequency 30% on average, this varies widely in individuals. None of the agents promote neural repair or cause "improvement" as an outcome. There is no one best choice for treatment. Higher dose interferons tend to cause neutralizing antibodies in one-third of cases that may not interfere with the efficacy of these medicines.

Fox RJ, Bethoux F, Goldman MD, et al. Advances in understanding, diagnosing and treating the underlying disease. Cleve Clin J Med. 2006; 73:91–102.

25. d, 26. e, 27. b

Natalizumab is a humanized monoclonal antibody against the cellular adhesion molecule α4-integrin. It binds to lymphocytes and prevents adherence at the endothelial surface of blood vessels in the brain and gut. It therefore reduces the entry of immunologically active cells into the CNS compartment. Trials have shown a 60% to 70% reduction in exacerbation rate, reduced activity on MRI, and slowed progression with the use of this medicine in relapsing forms of multiple sclerosis. In the United States, it is indicated for relapsing forms of multiple sclerosis usually when patients have failed other forms of disease-modifying therapy. Use of natalizumab requires an FDA-approved monitoring program.

There is an approximately 1 in 1000 risk of developing progressive multifocal leukoencephalopathy (PML) in patients on natalizumab. The risk appears to be higher with prior or additional immunosuppressing medicines and after 2 years of continuous use. There are no comparative studies of natalizumab and mitoxantrone in multiple sclerosis. Mitoxantrone has been associated with treatment-related acute leukemia and dose-dependent cardiomyopathy.

Anaphylaxis occurs in about 1 in 50 patients often by the second to fourth dose of natalizumab. Symptoms include shortness of breath, wheezing, hypotension, rash, and tachycardia. The infusion should be stopped immediately if this occurs and procedures for anaphylaxis instituted. This is an absolute contraindication to restarting natalizumab. There is no desensitization procedure, nor should the medicine be retried with premedication or at a lower dose. This is not related to immunoglobulin A deficiency. PML occurs in about 1 in 1000 patients treated with natalizumab. Symptoms include aphasia, visual field deficits, headache, hemiparesis, and cognitive dysfunction progressing over weeks. Patients develop focal subcortical lesions in multiple brain areas that can at times be difficult to discriminate from multiple sclerosis lesions. CSF may be positive for JC virus PCR. JC virus is the causative agent for PML. Treatment for PML in this population includes stopping natalizumab and beginning plasmapheresis to clear residual natalizumab more rapidly from the system.

Carson KR, Focosi D, O'Major E, et al. Monoclonal antibody-associated progressive multifocal leukoencephalopathy in patients treated with rituximab, natalizumab, and efalizumab. Lancet Oncol. 2009; 10:816–824.

Polman CH, O'Connor PW, Havrdova E, et al. A randomized, placebo-controlled trial of natalizumab for relapsing multiple sclerosis. N Engl J Med. 2006; 354:899–910.

28. d

Spasticity is defined as a velocity-dependent increase in stretch reflexes. There are both tonic (stiffening in place) and phasic (movement of a limb with spasm) spasms. Spasticity can occur with or without concurrent weakness. It indicates disinhibition of the upper motor neuron pathway.

Both baclofen and tizanidine are indicated for multiple sclerosis-related spasticity. They have similar efficacy. Side effects of baclofen include fatigue, dizziness, and dose-related leg weakness at higher doses. Sudden cessation of baclofen may cause withdrawal seizures. Side effects of tizanidine include light-headedness and hypotension, fatigue, and rarely liver function changes. There is no evidence that exercise "takes away" spasticity. Judicious stretching and a regular exercise program both are part of spasticity management. For patients in whom medications are ineffective or cause too many side effects, selective botulinum injections may improve symptoms. For some patients, implantation of a subcutaneous pump that delivers baclofen at the spinal cord level through a catheter may be beneficial.

Goldman MD, Cohen JA, Fox RJ, et al. Multiple sclerosis: Treating symptoms, and other general medical issues. Cleve Clin J Med. 2006; 73(2):177–186.

29. b

Figure 7.8 demonstrates an extensive lesion in the cervical spinal cord consistent with transverse myelitis. Transverse myelitis is a term used for patients with a subacute onset of myelopathy, which appears to be on an immunologic basis. It may occur after a viral illness, *Mycoplasma* infection, or vaccination, but is often not preceded by an illness. Symptoms include paresthesias and sensory deficit often ascending to a specific level, weakness, back pain, and bowel and bladder dysfunction.

Ascending myelitis does not exist. Myelitis can occur in systemic lupus erythematosus but is usually acute and in the setting of active lupus symptomatology. This would be in the differential diagnosis of this condition along with other inflammatory disorders of the spinal cord or a lesion impinging on or compressing the spinal cord. Vascular disorders of the spinal cord are usually acute in onset. Guillain-Barre syndrome is a lower motor neuron disorder and toes would not be upgoing. It rarely causes a sensory level and does not cause a longitudinally extensive lesion, such as shown in the figure.

Kerr D, Ayetey H. Immunopathogenesis of acute transverse myelitis. Curr Opin Neurol. 2002; 15:339–347.

30. d

Fingolimod is an orally active modulator of four of the five sphingosine-1 phosphate (S1P$_1$) receptors. It acts as a superagonist at the S1P$_1$ receptor on thymocytes and lymphocytes. It induces an uncoupling and internalization of that receptor. This makes these cells unresponsive to such signaling. They therefore lack the signal necessary for egress from the lymph nodes and secondary lymphoid tissues. In clinical trials it reduces relapses of multiple sclerosis in patients with relapsing-remitting multiple sclerosis (RRMS), as well as reduces MRI measures of clinical activity. In addition, there appear to be direct effects on neurons and glial cells, which also express S1P$_1$ receptors. It is unclear if this effect is active in vivo, but may indicate some potential for neuroprotection.

Kappos L, Radue EW, O'Connor P, et al. A placebo-controlled trial of oral fingolimod in relapsing multiple sclerosis. N Engl J Med. 2010; 362:387–401.

31. d

Dalfampridine was FDA approved as an oral medication to improve walking in patients with multiple sclerosis. Dalfampridine is a symptomatic therapy, and can be used in combination with disease-modifying agents. It is an extended-release form of 4-aminopyridine (previously known as fampridine). Dalfampridine is a broad-spectrum inhibitor of voltage-sensitive potassium channels. In laboratory studies, dalfampridine has been found to improve impulse conduction in demyelinated nerve fibers and to increase synaptic transmitter release at nerve endings. Dalfampridine is administered as a 10-mg timed-release pill every 12 hours. In two phase III trials in patients with multiple sclerosis randomized to dalfampridine versus placebo, a significantly greater percentage of patients were "responders" on dalfampridine than on placebo. A responder was defined as a patient who showed faster walking speed while on therapy than while not on therapy. About one-third patients responded to dalfampridine in these studies. The increased response rate in the dalfampridine group was observed across all four major types of multiple sclerosis (relapsing-remitting, secondary progressive, progressive relapsing, and primary progressive).

Goodman AD, Brown TR, Krupp LB, et al. Sustained-release oral fampridine in multiple sclerosis: A randomized, double-blind, controlled trial. Lancet. 2009; 373:732–738.

32. b

Cladribine is a purine nucleoside analogue that interferes with the behavior and proliferation of certain WBCs, particularly lymphocytes, which are involved in the pathological process of multiple sclerosis. In phase III trials, oral cladribine reduced measures of multiple sclerosis disease activity, such as relapse rate and new lesion formation on MRI. Major adverse events in phase III trials included lymphocytopenia and herpes zoster.

Giovannoni G, Comi G, Cook S, et al. A placebo-controlled trial of oral cladribine for relapsing multiple sclerosis. N Engl J Med. 2010; 362:416–426.

33. b

It is not a definite causation that low vitamin D is the reason why multiple sclerosis is more common further from the equator. Although vitamin D levels may be lower further from the equator, the exact relationship between vitamin D levels and multiple sclerosis is not yet known. There are a number of interesting epidemiologic observations that suggest there may be a link, but no definite causative association has been proven. Low vitamin D levels are more common further away from the equator, as is the prevalence and incidence of multiple sclerosis. In a large nursing health cohort study, multiple sclerosis was less common in nurses who took vitamin D supplements. African-Americans with multiple sclerosis have both lower vitamin D levels than Caucasians and a more severe clinical course. There is no well-defined dose of vitamin D for multiple sclerosis at present. Some trials are under way to further understand this link.

Smoldersa J, Damoiseauxb J, Menheerec P, et al. Vitamin D as an immune modulator in multiple sclerosis, a review. J Neuroimmunol. 2008; 194:7–17.

Buzz Phrases	Key Points
Multiple sclerosis relapse	Episode of neurologic worsening or new symptoms in multiple sclerosis not due to fever or infection lasting >24 hours
Dawson's fingers	Finger-like extensions of demyelination and inflammation extending rostrally from the corpus callosum in multiple sclerosis
Lhermitte's sign	Electrical sensations down the neck, back or limbs with neck flexion. Often related to demyelination in cervical spine
Uhthoff's phenomenon	Visual blurring with exercise in patients with heat-sensitive multiple sclerosis
Internuclear ophthalmoplegia	Due to disorder in MLF common in multiple sclerosis. With a right internuclear ophthalmoplegia on left gaze, cannot adduct right eye, with left eye abduction nystagmus. May be bilateral
Balo's concentric sclerosis	Form of demyelination with concentric sclerosis, may appears as onion skin lesion on MRI
Devic's disease	Also known as neuromyelitis optica, neuromyelitis optic immunoglobulin G to aquaporin-4
Useless hand of Oppenheim	Because of sensory deafferentation where the hand feels useless with otherwise-normal motor function

Chapter 8

Neuro-oncology

Questions

Question 1

1. A 5-year-old boy is brought in for evaluation of abnormal jerks and chaotic REM in all directions. He is also ataxic when attempting to walk and has sudden brief truncal and limb jerks. Which of the following is incorrect regarding this condition?
   a. This paraneoplastic syndrome is most commonly associated with medulloblastoma
   b. In adults, this condition may be associated with breast and small cell lung carcinoma
   c. The neurologic manifestations respond to ACTH
   d. Resection of the primary tumor will lead to resolution of this syndrome
   e. In adults, it may be associated with Anti-Ri antibodies

Questions 2–3

2. Which of the following is a variant of diffuse astrocytomas?
   a. Gemistocytic
   b. Protoplasmic
   c. Pleomorphic xanthoastrocytoma
   d. a and b
   e. All of the above

3. Which of the following is a variant of diffuse astrocytoma?
   a. Pleomorphic xanthoastrocytoma
   b. Subependymal giant cell astrocytoma
   c. Pilocytic astrocytoma
   d. Fibrillary astrocytoma
   e. None of the above

4. A 47-year-old woman with breast cancer presents with headache and multiple cranial neuropathies. Her MRI shows leptomeningeal enhancement, and CSF shows abnormal cells on cytologic examination. Which of the following is correct?

277

a. This patient has brain stem infiltration by the breast cancer causing multiple cranial neuropathies
b. CSF examination is very sensitive for this condition, with few false negatives
c. Some cases are treated with a combination of whole-brain radiation and intraventricular methotrexate
d. γ knife is the treatment of choice
e. Melanomas infiltrating the meninges have a better prognosis than lymphomas

5. Which of the following risk factors is clearly associated with the development of gliomas?
   a. Use of cell phones
   b. Infections
   c. Immunosuppression
   d. Tobacco use
   e. Radiation exposure

Questions 6–8

6. A 60-year-old man with a history of headaches and recent personality change presents with altered mental status. An MRI of the brain is obtained and shown in Figure 8.1. Which of the following is the most likely diagnosis?

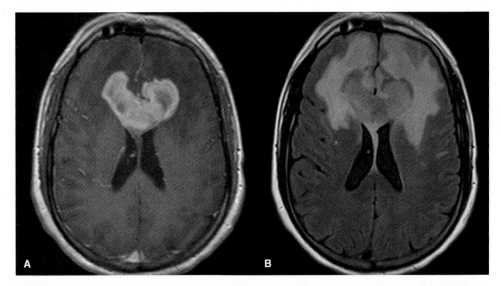

FIGURE 8.1 **(A)** Axial T1-weighted post-contrast MRI; **(B)** axial FLAIR MRI

a. Meningioma
b. Astrocytoma WHO grade II
c. Astrocytoma WHO grade IV
d. Ependymoma
e. Oligodendroglioma

7. Which of the following histopathologic findings do you expect to find in a biopsy of the lesion shown in Figure 8.1?
   a. Cells with "fried egg" appearance
   b. Nuclear pseudopalisading
   c. Perivascular pseudorosettes
   d. Homer-Wright rosettes
   e. Rosenthal fibers

8. Which is the most likely survival time for the patient depicted in question 6?
   a. 15 years
   b. 10 years
   c. 5 years
   d. 3 years
   e. 15 months or less

9. Which of the following tumors does not typically present with seizures?
   a. Ganglioglioma
   b. Dysembryoplastic neuroepithelial tumor
   c. Oligodendroglioma
   d. Ependymoma
   e. Astrocytoma

10. A 49-year-old woman presents with 3 weeks of gradually progressive dysarthria, unsteadiness, and frequent falls. On examination she is found to have prominent nystagmus in all directions, with marked dysarthria. She also has truncal ataxia and dysmetria, which is more prominent in the upper than lower extremities. The patient has also been losing weight for the past 4 months. An MRI shows diffuse cerebellar atrophy, but no evidence of intracranial mass. Complete work-up detects a pelvic mass originating in the ovary. Which of the following is correct regarding this condition?
   a. A leptomeningeal biopsy will certainly demonstrate an infiltrative neoplasm
   b. CSF cytology and flow cytometry are very specific for the diagnosis of this condition
   c. Anti-Tr antibodies are most likely to be positive in this patient
   d. Anti-Hu antibodies are the most common cause of this condition especially in the setting of breast carcinomas
   e. Anti-Yo antibodies are likely to be positive in this patient

11. A patient presents with an MRI that is shown in Figure 8.2, and the histopathology shows a glial neoplasm with necrosis and endothelial hyperplasia. What treatment options will be potentially beneficial?
   a. Surgical resection
   b. Radiation therapy
   c. Temozolomide
   d. a and c
   e. a, b, and c

12. Regarding gliomas, which of the following is not a poor prognostic factor?
   a. Older age
   b. Mixed oligoastrocytoma as compared to pure astrocytic type

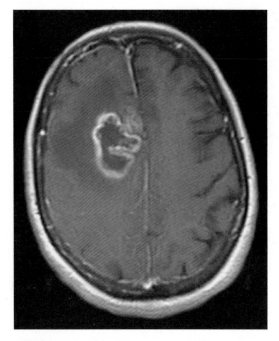

FIGURE 8.2 Axial T1-weighted postcontrast MRI

    c. Ring enhancing with gadolinium
    d. Poor performance status
    e. Necrotic center with pseudopalisading nuclei

13. Which of the following paraneoplastic syndromes is associated with the wrong antibody and neoplasm?
    a. Retinal degeneration—anti-recoverin—small cell lung carcinoma
    b. Optic neuropathy—anti-Hu—breast cancer
    c. Paraneoplastic sensory neuropathy—anti-Hu—small cell lung cancer
    d. Sensory neuronopathy—anti-Hu—small cell lung cancer
    e. Lambert-Eaton myasthenic syndrome—anti-voltage-gated calcium channel (P/Q type)—small cell lung cancer

14. A 59-year-old woman presents with headaches and is found to have a brain mass. A biopsy is obtained, which is shown in Figure 8.3. Which of the following is the most likely diagnosis?
    a. Fibrillary astrocytoma
    b. Oligodendroglioma
    c. Glioblastoma
    d. Meningioma
    e. Ependymoma

15. Which of the following is correct regarding anaplastic astrocytoma?
    a. It is a WHO grade II tumor
    b. It is well circumscribed, with no infiltration seen microscopically

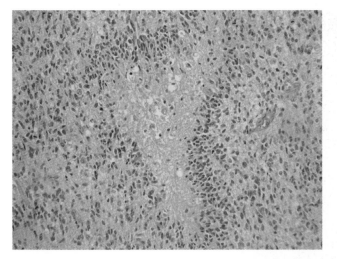

FIGURE 8.3   Brain specimen (Courtesy of Dr. Richard A. Prayson). Shown also in color plates

  c. Median survival is 10 to 15 years
  d. p53 mutations are seen in these type of tumors
  e. 1p19q deletion is common in this tumor and carries a better prognosis

16. A 5-year-old patient presents with 2 weeks of gradually worsening headaches, now with nausea and vomiting. An MRI is obtained, which is shown in Figure 8.4. Which is the most likely diagnosis?
  a. Glioblastoma multiforme
  b. Oligodendroglioma
  c. Diffuse fibrillary astrocytoma
  d. Pilocytic astrocytoma
  e. Acoustic schwannoma

17. A 17-year-old boy with focal epilepsy undergoes surgical resection of a right temporal lobe lesion, and the biopsy is consistent with a pleomorphic xanthoastrocytoma. Which of the following is correct regarding this lesion?
  a. It is a deeply seated and infiltrating lesion
  b. Eosinophilic granular bodies are not typically seen
  c. Intercellular reticulin deposition is common
  d. Prognosis is generally poor with more than 50% undergoing malignant transformation
  e. Can be seen in the temporal lobe, but is more common in the frontal lobes

18. A 12-year-old boy is found to have a subependymal giant cell astrocytoma. Which of the following is correct regarding this lesion?
  a. It is commonly sporadic and rarely associated with tuberous sclerosis
  b. It is infiltrative
  c. The presence of "candle gutterings" suggests an alternative diagnosis
  d. It is benign (WHO grade I)
  e. Even though it can be seen in young patients, it is most commonly encountered in the elderly

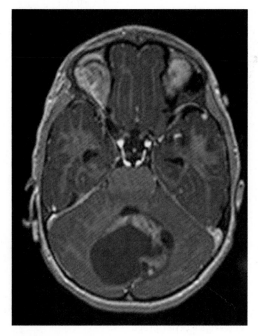

FIGURE 8.4 Axial T1-weighted postcontrast MRI

19. Which of the following is incorrect regarding oligodendroglioma?
    a. WHO grade II oligodendrogliomas are usually nonenhancing
    b. They are usually found superficially and involve the cortex
    c. They occur more frequently in the frontal lobes
    d. Borders are ill-defined as the tumor is infiltrating
    e. In the classic type of this tumor, glial fibrillary acidic protein is positive

20. A 7-year-old patient presents with a posterior fossa tumor. A biopsy is obtained, which is shown in Figure 8.5. Which is the most likely diagnosis?
    a. Cerebellar hemangioblastoma
    b. Pilocytic astrocytoma
    c. Glioblastoma multiforme
    d. Oligodendroglioma
    e. Meningioma

21. A 42-year-old patient presents with a seizure and is found to have a brain mass. A biopsy is obtained, which is shown in Figure 8.6. Which of the following is the most likely diagnosis?
    a. Pilocytic astrocytoma
    b. Glioblastoma
    c. Oligodendroglioma
    d. Ependymoma
    e. Hemangioblastoma

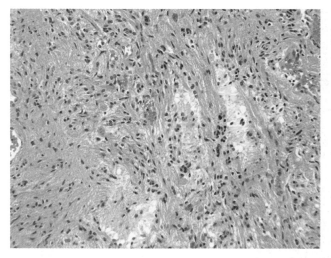

FIGURE 8.5   Brain specimen (Courtesy of Dr. Richard A. Prayson). Shown also in color plates

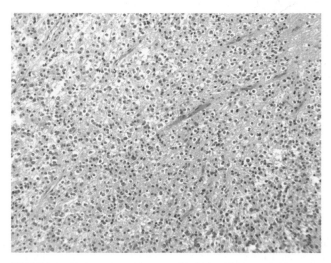

FIGURE 8.6   Brain specimen (Courtesy of Dr. Richard A. Prayson). Shown also in color plates

Questions 22–23

22. A 5-year-old boy presents with headaches, nausea, and vomiting. A posterior fossa tumor is found on imaging and a biopsy is obtained, shown in Figure 8.7. Which of the following is correct regarding this tumor?

   a. In children, this tumor more commonly occurs in the spinal cord as compared to the intracranial region

   b. When intracranial, this tumor is more commonly supratentorial than infratentorial

   c. Homer-Wright rosettes are common in this type of tumor

   d. It is highly infiltrative

   e. Patients younger than 3 years of age have a worse prognosis

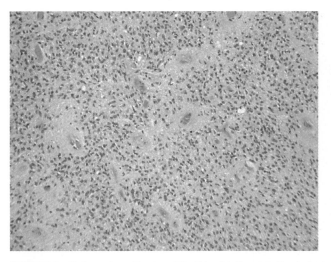

FIGURE 8.7 Brain specimen (Courtesy of Dr. Richard A. Prayson). Shown also in color plates

23. Which of the following is incorrect regarding this type of tumor?
   a. There are perivascular pseudorosettes
   b. The myxopapillary variant arises from the filum terminale
   c. Surgical resection may be curative, and prognosis depends on the extent of resection
   d. It may produce drop metastases
   e. It may be associated with neurofibromatosis type 1 (NF1)

24. A patient with epilepsy is found to have an abnormality on an MRI of the brain. The biopsy was consistent with a diagnosis of ganglioglioma. Which of the following is correct regarding this abnormality?
   a. These tumors are composed only of glia
   b. These tumors are composed only of neurons
   c. Eosinophilic granular bodies are commonly encountered
   d. They are highly infiltrative
   e. Treatment requires a combination of surgical resection, radiation, and chemotherapy

25. A 29-year-old man undergoes an MRI for evaluation of headaches. A lateral ventricular mass is found, and after surgical resection, the pathology is consistent with a neurocytoma. Which of the following is correct regarding this tumor?
   a. Positive for synaptophysin
   b. Highly infiltrative tumor
   c. WHO grade III
   d. Most commonly located in the fourth ventricle
   e. Glial fibrillary acidic protein positive

Questions 26–27

26. A 50-year-old man presents with a seizure and is found to have an intracranial tumor on MRI, which is shown in Figure 8.8. Which of the following is correct?
   a. This tumor arises from glia
   b. The origin is glioneuronal

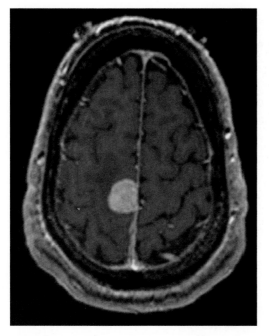

FIGURE 8.8   Axial T1-weighted postcontrast MRI

   c. This tumor originates from arachnoid cap cells
   d. This is a metastatic tumor
   e. This tumor frequently infiltrates the brain parenchyma

27. Which of the following is correct regarding this tumor?
   a. This tumor is more common in men
   b. It may be associated with neurofibromatosis type 2
   c. These are rapidly growing, infiltrative tumors
   d. A dural tail on MRI is not likely to be seen with these type of tumors
   e. Previous radiation is not associated with this type of tumor

28. A 29-year-old man undergoes surgical resection of a cerebellar mass. The histopathologic specimen is shown in Figure 8.9. Which of the following is correct?
   a. The MRI of this type of lesion shows a cyst with an enhancing mural nodule
   b. Is a highly infiltrative lesion
   c. This tumor is classified as WHO grade III
   d. Is more common in children
   e. More than 90% of the cases are associated with von Hippel-Lindau

29. A biopsy of a cerebellar mass is obtained from a 7-year-old patient, shown in Figure 8.10. Which of the following is the most likely diagnosis?
   a. Medulloblastoma
   b. Oligodendroglioma
   c. Pilocytic astrocytoma

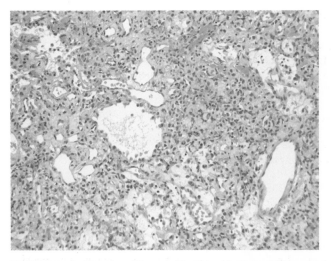

FIGURE 8.9 Brain specimen (Courtesy of Dr. Richard A. Prayson). Shown also in color plates

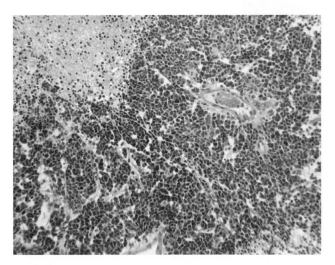

FIGURE 8.10 Brain specimen (Courtesy of Dr. Richard A. Prayson). Shown also in color plates

    d. Meningioma
    e. Glioblastoma

30. Which of the following is correct regarding pineal tumors?
    a. Pineocytomas are more common in children
    b. Pineoblastomas are more common in the elderly
    c. Pineoblastomas may spread via the craniospinal axis or metastasize
    d. Pineoblastoma cells may resemble mature pineocytes
    e. Pineocytomas have very high mitotic activity

31. Which of the following options is incorrect regarding the various types of cysts that can be found in the CNS?

a. Colloid cysts can be associated with acute hydrocephalus and sudden death

b. Dermoid cysts contain hair follicles, sebaceous glands, and sweat glands

c. Epidermoid cysts are most commonly located in the cerebellopontine angle

d. An MRI of epidermoid cysts shows hyperintensity on T1 and T2 with no restriction on DWI

e. Arachnoid cysts are lined by arachnoid cap cells

32. Which of the following is incorrect regarding medulloblastoma?

a. It is associated with genetic defects in chromosome 17

b. It originates from pluripotential cells

c. *N-myc* amplification is associated with poorer prognosis

d. Patients with younger age at diagnosis have better prognosis

e. It is more common in males

33. A 9-year-old boy with intractable epilepsy undergoes temporal lobectomy. The histopathologic specimen is shown in Figure 8.11. Which of the following is incorrect regarding this tumor?

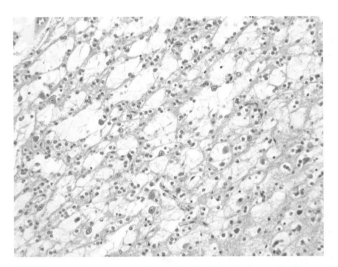

FIGURE 8.11   Brain specimen (Courtesy of Dr. Richard A. Prayson). Shown also in color plates

a. Most common location is the temporal lobe

b. This lesion often has a cortical or juxtacortical location

c. Floating neurons are characteristic of this lesion

d. It is a WHO grade I tumor

e. On MRI, it has a heterogeneous contrast-enhancing pattern

Questions 34–35

34. A 35-year-old man with HIV presents with headaches and altered mental status, and is found to have an intracranial mass. A biopsy is obtained, which is shown in Figure 8.12. Which of the following is the most likely diagnosis?

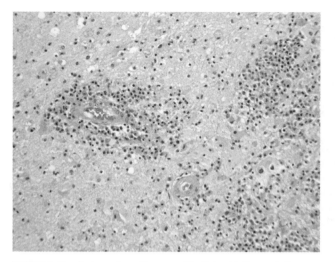

FIGURE 8.12   Brain specimen (Courtesy of Dr. Richard A. Prayson). Shown also in color plates

    a. Glioblastoma
    b. Lymphoma
    c. Oligodendroglioma
    d. Meningioma
    e. Ependymoma

35. Which of the following is incorrect regarding this condition?
    a. It is most commonly a diffuse, large B-cell tumor
    b. Primary tumors of this type usually involve the parenchyma rather than the leptomeninges
    c. Steroid use should be avoided prior to biopsy if this neoplasm is suspected
    d. It is associated with Epstein-Barr virus, especially in immunocompromised patients
    e. Surgical resection is the cornerstone of treatment

36. A 12-year-old boy with a bitemporal hemianopia is found to have a suprasellar mass. The lesion is resected, and a biopsy specimen is shown in Figure 8.13. Which of the following is incorrect regarding this tumor?
    a. It can be associated with diabetes insipidus
    b. It is seen only in children
    c. The cysts contain material that resembles machine-oil fluid
    d. The fluid in the cysts may elicit a xanthogranulomatous inflammatory process
    e. It originates from remnants of Rathke's pouch

37. A 4-year-old boy is found to have an intraventricular mass, which is biopsied. The histopathologic specimen is shown in Figure 8.14. Which of the following is incorrect regarding this lesion?
    a. Most common location is in the lateral ventricles
    b. CSF production may be increased
    c. It may present with hydrocephalus and features of increased intracranial pressure
    d. It is a WHO grade II tumor
    e. It is more common in children

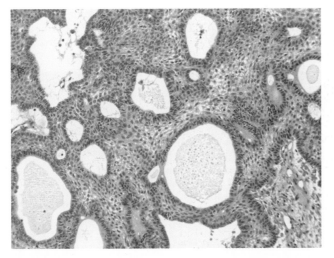

FIGURE 8.13   Suprasellar mass specimen (Courtesy of Dr. Richard A. Prayson). Shown also in color plates

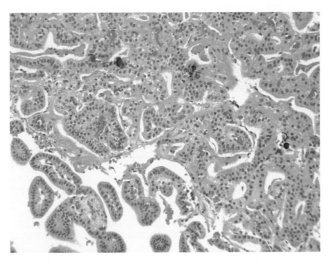

FIGURE 8.14   Intraventricular mass specimen (Courtesy of Dr. Richard A. Prayson). Shown also in color plates

38. A 41-year-old man presents with multiple cranial neuropathies. An intracranial tumor is found compressing the brain stem, and given the radiologic appearance, there is suspicion for a chordoma. Which of the following is incorrect regarding this tumor?

 a. The clivus and sacrococcygeal regions are the most common locations
 b. It originates from the notochord
 c. It is infiltrative and lobulated
 d. It consists of physaliphorous cells
 e. It invades nervous tissue but spares the bone

39. A 36-year-old woman presents with gradually progressive unsteadiness and hearing loss in the left ear. An MRI is obtained, which is shown in Figure 8.15. Which of the following is the most likely diagnosis?

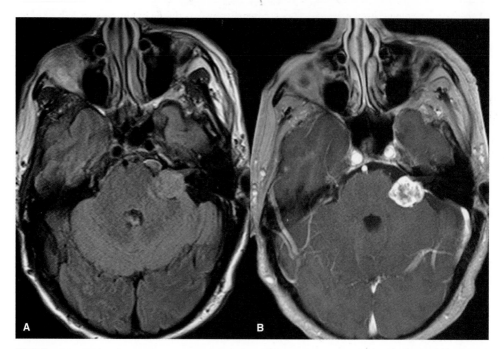

FIGURE 8.15 **(A)** Axial T1-weighted postcontrast MRI; **(B)** axial FLAIR MRI

    a. Vestibular schwannoma
    b. Oligodendroglioma
    c. Cerebellar hemangioblastoma
    d. Ependymoma
    e. Metastatic lesion

Questions 40–41

40. Which of the following is the order of frequency from most common to least common origin of brain metastases:
    a. Lung, melanoma, prostate, breast
    b. Lung, breast, melanoma, colon
    c. Breast, lung, melanoma, kidney
    d. Lung, melanoma, thyroid, breast
    e. Colon, breast, lung, melanoma

41. Which of the following is incorrect regarding brain metastases?
    a. They are more common than primary brain tumors
    b. Hemorrhagic metastasis can be seen with melanomas, non–small cell carcinomas, and renal cell carcinomas

c. The majority are infratentorial

d. Multiple metastatic lesions can be seen with small cell carcinomas and melanomas

e. Steroids are used to treat surrounding edema in brain metastasis

42. A histopathologic specimen from a pontocerebellar mass is shown in Figure 8.16. Which of the following is correct regarding this tumor?

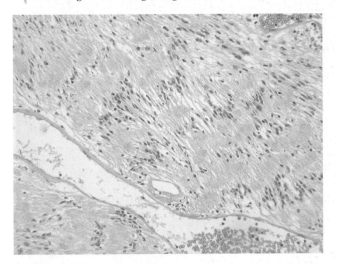

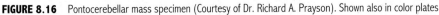

FIGURE 8.16 Pontocerebellar mass specimen (Courtesy of Dr. Richard A. Prayson). Shown also in color plates

a. Most common location is the facial nerve

b. Antoni A pattern has a loose appearance

c. Verocay bodies are seen in this picture and are characterized by a palisading arrangement of the cells

d. This is a malignant tumor, categorized as WHO grade III

e. This tumor is diffusely infiltrating

43. A 72-year-old man with diabetes is undergoing visual assessment for renewal of his driver's license and he fails the vision examination. On evaluation by his ophthalmologist he is found to have bitemporal hemianopia. An MRI of the brain is done, which is shown in Figure 8.17; the lesion measures 1.9 by 1.3 by 2.3 cm. The mass is resected, and pathological analysis reveals the findings shown in Figure 8.18. What is the most likely diagnosis in this patient?

a. Craniopharyngioma

b. Pituitary microadenoma

c. Pituitary macroadenoma

d. Rathke's cleft cyst

e. Pituitary apoplexy

44. A patient presents with a seizure, and the MRI obtained is shown in Figure 8.19. Which of the following is the most likely diagnosis?

a. Metastasis

b. Meningioma

c. Low-grade diffuse fibrillary astrocytoma

47. A 21-year-old man presented initially with depression 3 months ago, treatment was started, however, since then the patient has significant personality changes, with visual hallucinations and confusion. He also has prominent anterograde amnesia. The progression has been very gradual. His MRI and PET scan are shown in Figure 8.20. Which of the following is incorrect regarding this syndrome?

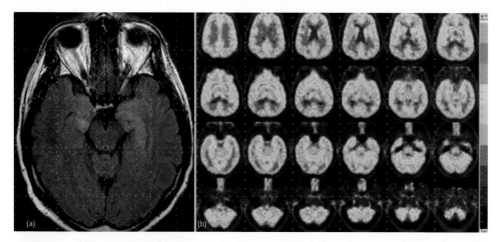

FIGURE 8.20   **(A)** Axial FLAIR MRI; **(B)** FDG-PET scan. Shown also in color plates

   a. This patient has limbic encephalitis
   b. This patient most likely has a testicular mass with anti-Hu antibodies in the serum
   c. Seizures may occur
   d. Can occur in older patients, in which case it is associated with small cell lung cancer and ANNA-1 antibodies
   e. The testicular tumor most often associated with this syndrome is a germ cell tumor

48. Regarding the prognosis of oligodendrogliomas, which of the following is correct?
   a. Chromosome 1p and 19q deletions confer a worse prognosis
   b. Younger patients have better survival
   c. p16 gene deletion is associated with better outcomes
   d. p53 mutations occur in more than 50% of the cases
   e. The prognosis in oligodendrogliomas is worse than in astrocytomas

49. A 52-year-old man presents with headaches and is diagnosed with a glioblastoma multiforme of the right frontal lobe. He is offered treatment with surgery, radiation, and chemotherapy, but decides not to be treated at all, except with medications that might symptomatically help his headache. He states to his neuro-oncologist that he understands that lack of any treatment could shorten his survival by several months, but says he would rather spend what time he has left traveling with his family and seeing friends. His family supports his decision. The neuro-oncologist feels that the patient could gain a few months with relatively good quality of life with the right treatment plan, and is surprised at the patient's decision. Which of the following statements would be an appropriate reaction from the neuro-oncologist on the basis of the principle of autonomy?

a. "I would like to obtain a psychiatric evaluation because I don't think you understand the implications of your decision and I want to get a court-order to treat you with surgery, radiation, and chemotherapy"

b. "It's a free world, if you don't want therapy that's fine, but if you're not going to listen to my opinion, then I can't give you prescriptions for corticosteroids or any other treatment for your headaches, maybe you should see your primary doctor about that"

c. "I respect your decision, even though I feel there are some benefits of therapy, and therapy will always be an option for you if you change your mind down the line. There are some options to treat your headache that I will prescribe to you"

d. "You are in denial right now, you clearly don't understand the implications of your decisions, let's talk about this again in a few days, I'm sure you'll change your mind, you'd be crazy not to"

e. "I wouldn't be recommending all these treatment options if I wasn't sure that's the best thing for you, this is my area of expertise, and I think you should strongly re-consider, and take the treatment I am offering"

Answer key

1. a	10. e	19. e	28. a	37. d	46. b
2. d	11. e	20. b	29. a	38. e	47. b
3. d	12. b	21. c	30. c	39. a	48. b
4. c	13. b	22. e	31. d	40. b	49. c
5. e	14. c	23. e	32. d	41. c	
6. c	15. d	24. c	33. e	42. c	
7. b	16. d	25. a	34. b	43. c	
8. e	17. c	26. c	35. e	44. a	
9. d	18. d	27. b	36. b	45. a	

Answers

1. a

This patient has opsoclonus myoclonus syndrome. This syndrome can present in adults with breast, ovarian, and small cell lung cancer, as well as in children with neuroblastoma (not medulloblastoma).

Clinically, these patients have spontaneous rapid, irregular, and high-amplitude conjugate eye movements that occur in any direction, as well as diffuse myoclonic jerks, and frequent ataxia.

CSF may be normal or show a mild pleocytosis, and MRI is typically normal.

Anti-Ri (also known as ANNA-2) antibodies are seen in this syndrome and especially associated with breast cancer, but can also be seen in a small percentage of small cell lung cancer. Anti-Hu (or ANNA-1) antibodies have been reported in adults with small cell lung cancer and children with neuroblastoma. There is no specific neuropathologic finding.

Characteristically, children with neuroblastoma respond to treatment with ACTH, and may have resolution of the neurologic manifestations when the neuroblastoma is treated. The prognosis is worse in adults.

Ropper AH, Samuels MA. Adams and Victor's Principles of Neurology, 9th ed. New York: McGraw-Hill; 2009.

2. d, 3. d

Diffuse astrocytomas can be classified according to the histopathologic cell type into fibrillary, gemistocytic, and protoplasmic. Diffuse astrocytomas are infiltrating neoplasms, categorized as WHO grade II. These are slow-growing tumors that may evolve to an anaplastic astrocytoma or glioblastoma. In general, the MRI shows a T2-hyperintense lesion with no enhancement with gadolinium.

Fibrillary astrocytomas are prototypical and more common, with elongated hyperchromatic nuclei, scant cytoplasm, and the presence of a fibrillary background. Gemistocytic astrocytomas are characterized by a round prominent eosinophilic cytoplasm. Protoplasmic astrocytomas are composed of cells with oval-shaped nuclei with scant cytoplasm and a microcystic background.

Pleomorphic xanthoastrocytoma is not a diffuse astrocytoma and is rather a different type of astrocytoma, which is localized superficially, more commonly in the temporal lobe, with well-demarcated borders, and frequently associated with seizures.

Subependymal giant cell astrocytoma and pilocytic astrocytomas are also well-circumscribed neoplasms and not categorized under the diffuse astrocytomas.

Prayson RA, Goldblum JR. Neuropathology, 1st ed. Philadelphia, PA: Elsevier; 2005.

Ropper AH, Samuels MA. Adams and Victor's Principles of Neurology, 9th ed. New York: McGraw-Hill; 2009.

4. c

This patient has meningeal carcinomatosis, and these cases are sometimes treated with whole-brain radiation plus intraventricular methotrexate.

Certain cancers can spread to the meninges producing a carcinomatous meningitis. This can be seen with adenocarcinoma of the breast, lung and gastrointestinal tract, melanoma, childhood leukemia, and systemic lymphoma. Prostate cancer has been described to spread to the leptomeninges, and this is thought to occur through dissemination via the Batson's plexus, which is a network of valveless veins that connect pelvic veins with internal vertebral veins.

The clinical manifestations of leptomeningeal disease are varied, but frequently, these patients present with headache and backache. Polyradiculopathies, multiple cranial neuropathies, and altered mental status are frequently seen. Some patients have features of increased intracranial pressure and hydrocephalus. The MRI shows leptomeningeal enhancement. The diagnosis can be established with CSF studies using cytologic evaluation and flow cytometry. CSF also will show a pleocytosis with increased protein and sometimes reduced glucose. However, CSF cytologic analysis is not sensitive, and many times repeated testing may be needed. In some cases, leptomeningeal biopsy may be required.

The treatment consists of radiation therapy to symptomatic areas, sometimes requiring whole-brain radiation. Some cases are treated with intrathecal chemotherapy and, preferably, intraventricular chemotherapy with methotrexate via an Ommaya reservoir. Unfortunately, the combination of brain radiation and chemotherapy carries a significant risk of leukoencephalopathy. Patients with meningeal carcinomatosis have a poor prognosis, usually with survivals of less than 6 months. In general, best response occurs in lymphomas, breast cancer, and small cell lung cancers. Worse prognosis is seen with other types of lung cancer and melanomas.

In this case, the leptomeningeal disease explains the multiple cranial neuropathies, and there is no indication to think about a brain stem infiltrative disease.

γ knife targets focal lesions, and is not useful in diffuse meningeal disease.

Cone LA, Koochek K, Henager HA, et al. Leptomeningeal carcinomatosis in a patient with metastatic prostate cancer: Case report and literature review. Surg Neurol. 2006; 65:372–376.

Prayson RA, Goldblum JR. Neuropathology, 1st ed. Philadelphia, PA: Elsevier; 2005.

Ropper AH, Samuels MA. Adams and Victor's Principles of Neurology, 9th ed. New York: McGraw-Hill; 2009.

5. e

Radiation exposure is a well-established risk factor known to be associated with the development of gliomas. Radiation for previous neoplasia of the CNS may increase the risk of developing a glioma, frequently a malignant one.

Gliomas are the most common primary brain tumor, and incidence increases with age. There are no other clearly associated risk factors. There is no clear link between these tumors and cell phone use. Immunosuppression and tobacco use have not been associated with these neoplasms.

Rowland LP, Pedley TA. Merritt's Neurology, 12th ed. Philadelphia, PA: Lippincott Williams & Wilkins; 2010.

6. c

This patient has an astrocytoma WHO grade IV, or glioblastoma. The MRI demonstrates a neoplasm crossing the corpus callosum, with strong gadolinium enhancement. There are hypointense areas that may correlate with necrosis, and there is also significant edema as seen on the FLAIR image. The typical tumor that crosses the corpus callosum is glioblastoma, and this appearance is called a "butterfly lesion." Lymphomas have also been reported to cross the corpus callosum; however, this is less common.

Glioblastoma is the most common primary brain tumor, accounting for close to 50% of all gliomas. They typically present in adult patients usually above 50 years of age, manifesting with focal neurologic deficits, headaches, and other features of increased intracranial pressure and seizures.

Meningioma is an extra-axial tumor that arises from the meninges rather than from within the brain parenchyma, though orbitofrontal and falcine meningiomas can often present with symptoms related to frontal lobe dysfunction. The MRI shown in Figure 8.1 clearly demonstrates an intra-axial tumor, within the brain parenchyma, which is not consistent with meningiomas.

Astrocytoma WHO grade II typically shows T2 hyperintensity, but no contrast enhancement. Ependymomas originate from the ependyma and are typically localized in the ventricles. Oligodendrogliomas are hemispheric masses usually arising superficially and with cortical involvement.

Prayson RA, Goldblum JR. Neuropathology, 1st ed. Philadelphia, PA: Elsevier; 2005.

Rowland LP, Pedley TA. Merritt's Neurology, 12th ed. Philadelphia, PA: Lippincott Williams & Wilkins; 2010.

7. b

The patient depicted in question 6 has a glioblastoma, in which nuclear pseudopalisading, or arrangement of nuclei in a palisading pattern around areas of necrosis, can be found. Glioblastoma (astrocytoma WHO grade IV) is the most common primary brain tumor, and is a highly infiltrating and invasive tumor. Other histopathologic features of glioblastoma include nuclear atypia, mitoses, endothelial hyperplasia, and necrosis.

Cells with "fried egg" appearance are seen in oligodendrogliomas. Perivascular pseudorosettes are seen in ependymomas, and Homer-Wright rosettes are seen in medulloblastoma. Rosenthal fibers can be seen in Alexander's disease, pilocytic astrocytoma, pleomorphic xanthoastrocytoma, and chronic reactive gliosis.

Prayson RA, Goldblum JR. Neuropathology, 1st ed. Philadelphia, PA: Elsevier; 2005.

Rowland LP, Pedley TA. Merritt's Neurology, 12th ed. Philadelphia, PA: Lippincott Williams & Wilkins; 2010.

8. e

This patient most likely has a survival time of about 15 months or less. Patients with astrocytomas will have different prognoses depending on the histologic grade, being approximately 5 to 10 years for grade II, 2 to 3 years for grade III, and 1 year or less for grade IV.

The prognosis depends on other factors as well. Age is a very important factor, and younger patients do better than older ones. Performance status is also very important, and patients with poor baseline condition and significant neurologic deficits have a worse prognosis.

Prayson RA, Goldblum JR. Neuropathology, 1st ed. Philadelphia, PA: Elsevier; 2005.

Rowland LP, Pedley TA. Merritt's Neurology, 12th ed. Philadelphia, PA: Lippincott Williams & Wilkins; 2010.

9. d

Ependymoma does not typically present with seizures. This type of tumor is the third most common CNS tumor in children, and 90% occur intracranially, most commonly in the infratentorial region, typically in the fourth ventricle. Given the location, these tumors tend to obstruct CSF flow, and features of increased intracranial pressure and hydrocephalus are the most common manifestations. Ependymomas in the supratentorial region occur in the periventricular region, but they may uncommonly be more superficial. Ependymomas can also occur in the spinal cord, more commonly in adults.

Ganglioglioma, dysembryoplastic neuroepithelial tumors, oligodendrogliomas, and astrocytomas frequently present with seizures.

Bradley WG, Daroff RB, Fenichel GM, et al. Neurology in Clinical Practice, 5th ed. Philadelphia, PA: Elsevier; 2008.

Prayson RA, Goldblum JR. Neuropathology, 1st ed. Philadelphia, PA: Elsevier; 2005.

10. e

This patient has a paraneoplastic syndrome consistent with paraneoplastic cerebellar degeneration. It has a prominent association with ovarian and breast carcinoma, but can also be seen in Hodgkin's lymphoma, small cell carcinoma of the lung, and other visceral tumors.

The patient presents with cerebellar symptoms with a subacute, gradual course over a period of weeks to months. Typically, patients have ataxia that affects the trunk and limbs. They also have nystagmus and prominent dysarthria. Other neurologic manifestations may occur, including diplopia, vertigo, and sensorineural hearing loss.

CSF studies may be completely normal but in some cases, may show slight increase in the white cell count and protein. CT and MRI may be normal at the onset, but there may be evidence of increased signal in the cerebellar white matter and eventually atrophy of the cerebellum. Pathologically, there are diffuse degenerative changes of the cerebellar cortex and deep nuclei, and loss of Purkinje cells.

Anti-Yo antibodies (also known as anti–Purkinje cell antibodies) are seen in the serum of about 50% of patients with this syndrome, especially in those with ovarian cancer, but in smaller percentages of patients with breast carcinoma. Some patients may have anti-Hu antibody (also known as ANNA-1), especially in the setting of small cell carcinoma of the lung. Anti-Tr antibody is associated with lymphomas.

In many cases, the paraneoplastic syndrome develops in a patient with advanced malignancy; however, in some patients the paraneoplastic neurologic manifestations precede the malignancy and ongoing work-up for malignancy is required.

There is little evidence to guide therapy of paraneoplastic cerebellar degeneration. The progression may subside with removal of the underlying neoplasm, if possible, and there have been reports of some improvement with plasmapheresis, intravenous corticosteroids, and intravenous immunoglobulin, though the prognosis is generally poor.

Ropper AH, Samuels MA. Adams and Victor's Principles of Neurology, 9th ed. New York: McGraw-Hill; 2009.

11. e

Surgical resection, radiation therapy, and chemotherapy with temozolomide are potentially beneficial for patients with glioblastoma, the most likely tumor type in this patient, based on the imaging and histopathologic findings.

Complete removal of the tumor is not possible given that astrocytomas (especially glioblastoma) are infiltrating tumors with no clear margins. However, if the tumor characteristics permit, surgery with near-complete resection or debulking improves neurologic function, reduces mass effect, and prolongs survival. Unfortunately, this may not be possible with very large tumors or with those crossing the corpus callosum.

Radiotherapy with focal radiation is an important treatment option, and it is given with a target total dose of 60 Gy for high-grade gliomas, divided in several fractions over 6 to 7 weeks.

Adjuvant chemotherapy has been shown to prolong survival in meta-analyses in which older nitrosourea agents such as carmustine were used. Temozolomide is an alkylating agent that has replaced nitrosoureas and is currently widely used as an adjuvant therapy. The addition of temozolomide to radiotherapy for newly diagnosed glioblastoma results in significant survival benefit with minimal additional toxicity to the patient.

Prayson RA, Goldblum JR. Neuropathology, 1st ed. Philadelphia, PA: Elsevier; 2005.

Rowland LP, Pedley TA. Merritt's Neurology, 12th ed. Philadelphia, PA: Lippincott Williams & Wilkins; 2010.

Stupp R, Mason WP, Van Den Bent MJ, et al. Radiotherapy plus concomitant and adjuvant temozolomide for glioblastoma. N Engl J Med. 2005; 352:987–996.

12. b

Histologic type and grade are very important prognostic factors in patients with astrocytomas. The histologic type influences prognosis, and mixed variants, such as oligoastrocytomas, have a better prognosis than pure astrocytomas but worse than oligodendrogliomas. Regarding the histologic grade, a patient with a grade II astrocytoma has an average survival of 5 to 10 years, grade III has an average survival of 2 to 3 years, and grade IV has an average survival of 15 months or less. The presence of gadolinium enhancement on MRI represents a disruption of the blood-brain barrier and correlates with the WHO grade. Usually grade II tumors have no enhancement, grade III tumors have some degree of enhancement, and grade IV tumors characteristically demonstrate ring enhancement, therefore correlating with a poorer prognosis. However, it is important to note that lower grade tumors may ring-enhance and higher grade tumors may heterogeneously enhance and rarely minimally enhance.

The age of the patient is also very important, and elderly patients usually have a worse prognosis than younger patients with the same diagnosis. Performance status is also important in prognostication and when deciding the treatment options, because those with worse baseline pretreatment condition and neurologic impairment will do worse.

Pathologic findings with the presence of a necrotic center with pseudopalisading nuclei are characteristic of glioblastoma (astrocytoma WHO grade IV), and these tumors have the worst prognosis among the astrocytomas.

Prayson RA, Goldblum JR. Neuropathology, 1st ed. Philadelphia, PA: Elsevier; 2005.

Ropper AH, Samuels MA. Adams and Victor's Principles of Neurology, 9th ed. New York: McGraw-Hill; 2009.

13. b

The predominant antibody in paraneoplastic optic neuropathy is anti-CRMP-5, which is associated with lung cancer. These patients present with vision loss.

The predominant antibody in paraneoplastic retinal degeneration is anti-recoverin or anti-CAR, and is associated with small cell lung cancer, thymoma, renal cell carcinoma, and melanoma. These patients present with scotomas, vision loss, predominantly nocturnal, and disc swelling.

Paraneoplastic subacute sensory neuropathy and neuronopathy are associated with anti-Hu (ANNA-1) antibodies and linked to small cell lung cancer.

Lambert-Eaton myasthenic syndrome is a paraneoplastic syndrome presenting in the setting of small cell lung carcinoma and associated with anti-voltage-gated calcium channels of the P/Q type (see Chapter 10).

Paraneoplastic chorea, presenting with bilateral choreoathetosis and in the setting of lung cancer, is associated with anti-Hu and anti-CRMP-5 antibodies.

Ropper AH, Samuels MA. Adams and Victor's Principles of Neurology, 9th ed. New York: McGraw-Hill; 2009.

14. c

The findings in Figure 8.3 are consistent with glioblastoma. The histopathologic specimen shows a glial neoplasm with hypercellularity, nuclear pleomorphism, necrosis, and pseudopalisading nuclei around the area of necrosis. Glioblastoma is a WHO grade IV astrocytoma, which is the most common primary brain tumor in adults and accounts for 50% of all gliomas. Grossly, it is a heterogeneous mass with necrosis and hemorrhage. Microscopically, it is very hypercellular, with nuclear atypia and abundant mitoses. Endothelial hyperplasia, necrosis, and pseudopalisading nuclei differentiate glioblastoma from other neoplasms, and from astrocytomas of lower grades.

Fibrillary astrocytoma is a diffuse astrocytoma, but it does not have necrosis or pseudopalisading. Oligodendrogliomas are hypercellular tumors with uniformly rounded nuclei and clear perinuclear haloes, giving it a "fried egg" appearance, which is not seen in this picture. Meningiomas are dural-based tumors originating from meningothelial or arachnoid cap cells, and are histologically composed of monomorphic cells with oval nuclei, sometimes with the presence of psammoma bodies, without pseudopalisading necrosis. Ependymomas are microscopically arranged in sheets of cells with round nuclei, with the presence of perivascular pseudorosettes and true ependymal rosettes.

Prayson RA, Goldblum JR. Neuropathology, 1st ed. Philadelphia, PA: Elsevier; 2005.

15. d

With anaplastic astrocytomas, p53 mutations may be seen in nearly half of these tumors. Anaplastic astrocytoma is a WHO grade III tumor, characterized by the presence of nuclear atypia, significant cellular proliferation, and mitotic activity, but without necrosis, pseudopalisading nuclei, or endothelial hyperplasia. These tumors are highly infiltrating.

Genetic mutations are seen in these tumors, such as p53 mutation in almost half, and loss of p16 and other genes of the retinoblastoma regulatory pathway. 1p19q deletion is common in oligodendrogliomas and rare in anaplastic astrocytomas. Patients with astrocytomas WHO grade III have an average survival of 2 to 3 years.

Prayson RA, Goldblum JR. Neuropathology, 1st ed. Philadelphia, PA: Elsevier; 2005.

16. d

This patient has a pilocytic astrocytoma, which is a WHO grade I astrocytoma and the most common glioma in children, occurring usually in the first or second decade of life. These tumors are well circumscribed, frequently located in the cerebellum, but can also be seen in the hypothalamus, third ventricle, optic nerve, spinal cord, and dorsal brain stem. In the cerebellum, they are characteristically cystic with a gadolinium-enhancing mural nodule, as depicted in Figure 8.4. In the hypothalamus and optic nerves these tumors are solid.

Most pilocytic astrocytomas are sporadic; however, neurofibromatosis type 1 is associated with these tumors, especially in the optic nerve.

Given the well-demarcated lesion, these tumors tend to be surgically curable with a good prognosis. If the tumor cannot be completely resected, radiation therapy or chemotherapy may be required.

This MRI showing a cyst with an enhancing nodule localized in the cerebellum in the age group of this patient is characteristic of pilocytic astrocytoma. The other gliomas are more common in older patients and in the supratentorial region. Acoustic schwannoma typically occurs in the cerebellopontine angle.

Bradley WG, Daroff RB, Fenichel GM, et al. Neurology in Clinical Practice, 5th ed. Philadelphia, PA: Elsevier; 2008.

Prayson RA, Goldblum JR. Neuropathology, 1st ed. Philadelphia, PA: Elsevier; 2005.

17. c

Pleomorphic xanthoastrocytoma (PXA) is a well-demarcated tumor, typically superficial and affecting the cortex, and most commonly encountered in the temporal lobes. It is more common in children and young adults, and manifests clinically as focal epilepsy.

On MRI, it is seen as a cyst with an enhancing mural nodule. Macroscopically, it is cystic, sometimes with calcifications. Microscopically, it is composed of pleomorphic astrocytes arranged in fascicles, with intercellular reticulin deposition. There are lipidized astrocytes in about 25% of the cases. Eosinophilic granular bodies are typically seen, and Rosenthal fibers may be seen in the periphery of the lesion.

These tumors are often surgically resectable, and the prognosis is favorable. In about 15% to 20% of the cases, PXA undergoes malignant transformation. PXA is classified as WHO grade II, unless there are foci of anaplasia, in which case it is considered grade III.

Bradley WG, Daroff RB, Fenichel GM, et al. Neurology in Clinical Practice, 5th ed. Philadelphia, PA: Elsevier; 2008.

Prayson RA, Goldblum JR. Neuropathology, 1st ed. Philadelphia, PA: Elsevier; 2005.

18. d

Subependymal giant cell astrocytoma (SEGA) is a benign hamartomatous tumor, WHO grade I, located in the intraventricular region, commonly in the third or lateral ventricles. It is seen in tuberous sclerosis almost exclusively, and it occurs in children and young adults, but not in elderly patients. Macroscopically, it is solid, well demarcated, noninfiltrative, and sometimes has calcifications. SEGA is surgically resectable. Microscopically, there is a glioneuronal appearance, and the cells are packed in fascicles and around blood vessels, giving the appearance of perivascular pseudorosettes. "Candle gutterings" are masses along the ventricular surface, similar histologically to SEGA, and seen in this condition.

Bradley WG, Daroff RB, Fenichel GM, et al. Neurology in Clinical Practice, 5th ed. Philadelphia, PA: Elsevier; 2008.

Prayson RA, Goldblum JR. Neuropathology. Philadelphia, PA: Elsevier; 2005.

19. e

Oligodendroglioma of the classic type is usually negative for glial fibrillary acidic protein (GFAP).

Oligodendrogliomas are diffuse gliomas that are infiltrating with ill-defined borders. They occur at any age, but more commonly occur in middle-aged adults (40 to 50 years of age), and are slightly more common in males (3:2). These tumors arise superficially and involve the cortex, with the most frequent location being in the frontal lobes. Given their cortical location, a common initial presenting manifestation is seizures.

WHO grade II oligodendrogliomas typically grow slowly, are seen as T2-hyperintense lesions on MRI, and are typically nonenhancing, whereas WHO grade III or anaplastic oligodendrogliomas progress more rapidly and are enhancing. Anaplastic oligodendrogliomas are hypercellular, with numerous mitoses and microvascular proliferation.

These tumors are usually negative for GFAP, except when minigemistocytic or gliofibrillary oligodendrocytes are present.

Bradley WG, Daroff RB, Fenichel GM, et al. Neurology in Clinical Practice, 5th ed. Philadelphia, PA: Elsevier; 2008.

Prayson RA, Goldblum JR. Neuropathology, 1st ed. Philadelphia, PA: Elsevier; 2005.

20. b

Given the age of the patient, tumor location, and pathologic features, this patient's diagnosis is pilocytic astrocytoma.

The histopathologic specimen shown in Figure 8.5 is consistent with pilocytic astrocytoma, showing a glial neoplasm that demonstrates a biphasic pattern of compact regions along with microcystic components. There are piloid or hair-like astrocytic processes, which give the name to this tumor. In addition, Rosenthal fibers and a few eosinophilic granular bodies are seen, both of which are not pathognomonic, but are typically seen in these tumors. Eosinophilic granular bodies are also seen in pleomorphic xanthoastrocytomas and gangliogliomas. Rosenthal fibers are also seen in gliosis and in Alexander's disease.

The clinical and histopathologic features are not consistent with the other options provided. Cerebellar hemangioblastoma are prominently vascular tumors with abundant capillaries and stromal vacuolated cells. Histopathologic features of glioblastoma multiforme include necrosis, pseudopalisading, and endothelial hyperplasia. Oligodendrogliomas are hypercellular tumors with uniformly rounded nuclei and clear perinuclear haloes, giving it a "fried egg" appearance. Meningiomas are dural-based tumors originating from meningothelial or arachnoid cap cells, and are histologically composed of monomorphic cells with oval nuclei, sometimes with the presence of psammoma bodies.

Bradley WG, Daroff RB, Fenichel GM, et al. Neurology in Clinical Practice, 5th ed. Philadelphia, PA: Elsevier; 2008.

Prayson RA, Goldblum JR. Neuropathology, 1st ed. Philadelphia, PA: Elsevier; 2005.

21. c

The histopathologic specimen in Figure 8.6 shows a hypercellular tumor with uniformly rounded nuclei and clear perinuclear haloes, giving it a "fried egg" appearance. There are also capillaries with a "chicken wire" appearance. These features are characteristic of oligodendrogliomas. The clear haloes are helpful in making the diagnosis; however, this appearance is caused by a delayed fixation artifact, is not pathognomonic, and may not be present in rapidly fixed specimens and frozen sections.

The histopathologic features are not consistent with the other options provided. Pilocytic astrocytoma is a glial neoplasm with piloid or hair-like astrocytic processes, which demonstrates a biphasic pattern of compact regions along with microcystic components. Histopathologic features of glioblastoma multiforme include necrosis, pseudopalisading, and endothelial hyperplasia. Ependymomas are microscopically arranged in sheets of cells with round nuclei, with the presence of perivascular pseudorosettes and true ependymal rosettes. Cerebellar hemangioblastomas are prominently vascular tumors with abundant capillaries and stromal vacuolated cells.

Bradley WG, Daroff RB, Fenichel GM, et al. Neurology in Clinical Practice, 5th ed. Philadelphia, PA: Elsevier; 2008.

Prayson RA, Goldblum JR. Neuropathology, 1st ed. Philadelphia, PA: Elsevier; 2005.

22. e, 23. e

This patient has an ependymoma. These types of tumors are associated with neurofibromatosis type 2 (NF2) (not NF1; see Chapter 14).

As seen in Figure 8.7, there are sheets of cells with the presence of perivascular pseudorosettes, which is characteristic of this type of tumor. Ependymomas are the third most common CNS tumor in children, more common intracranially and especially in the infratentorial region. When supratentorial, these tumors tend to occur in the periventricular region; however, they can also be present more superficially. About 10% of these tumors occur in the spinal cord, more frequently in adults.

Macroscopically, these tumors are well demarcated with a tendency to compress rather than infiltrate the parenchyma. Some cases are cystic, especially the supratentorial ones. Microscopically, they are arranged in sheets of spindled cells with round nuclei and small nucleoli. There are perivascular pseudorosettes, in which the cells surround blood vessels (as in Figure 8.7). There are also true ependymal rosettes, in which the cells are arranged around a clear space. Homer-Wright rosettes are not seen in these types of tumors (but rather in medulloblastoma).

Most ependymomas are WHO grade II. Anaplastic ependymomas are graded as WHO III, and are characterized by the presence of increased mitotic activity, hypercellularity, and microvascular proliferation. WHO grade II ependymomas may be surgically curable with a good prognosis, being the extent of resection an important prognostic factor. Radiation therapy may be used for residual disease. Prognosis is worse in patients younger than 3 years of age at presentation. Ependymomas in contact with the CSF may produce drop metastases conferring a worse prognosis.

Myxopapillary ependymoma is a WHO grade I variant that occurs almost exclusively in the filum terminale. It is more common in adults, has a red appearance grossly, and a thin collagenous capsule. These tumors have a better prognosis.

Genetically, ependymomas may be associated with chromosome 22q deletions, and spinal ependymomas may be related to NF2 mutations.

Bradley WG, Daroff RB, Fenichel GM, et al. Neurology in Clinical Practice, 5th ed. Philadelphia, PA: Elsevier; 2008.

Prayson RA, Goldblum JR. Neuropathology, 1st ed. Philadelphia, PA: Elsevier; 2005.

24. c

Ganglioglioma is a CNS tumor with glial and neuronal components. These tumors occur most commonly in children and young adults, arising from the temporal lobe, extending superficially, and presenting with seizures. Radiologically, the MRI may show a cyst with an enhancing mural nodule. Macroscopically, gangliogliomas are partially cystic, with solid components that may be calcified. Microscopically, there is a fibrillary background with dysmorphic ganglion cells showing nuclear pleomorphism, multinucleation, or cytoplasmic vacuolation. Other features include the presence of eosinophilic granular bodies, perivascular lymphocytic cuffing, microcystic spaces, and collagen deposition. The glial component shows glial fibrillary acidic protein positivity, whereas the neuronal component reacts with synaptophysin, chromogranin, and neurofilament.

Gangliogliomas are WHO grade I, they have a good prognosis, and the treatment is surgical resection.

Bradley WG, Daroff RB, Fenichel GM, et al. Neurology in Clinical Practice, 5th ed. Philadelphia, PA: Elsevier; 2008.

Prayson RA, Goldblum JR. Neuropathology, 1st ed. Philadelphia, PA: Elsevier; 2005.

25. a

Neurocytoma is a tumor that is reactive with synaptophysin, a marker of neuronal differentiation and which detects neuronal vesicle proteins.

Neurocytomas are encountered more frequently between the third and fifth decades of life. The location is intraventricular, more commonly in the lateral ventricles and in the third ventricle near the foramen of Monro. Macroscopically, they are well demarcated, gray, and friable. Microscopically, this neoplasm has round cells in a fibrillary background with prominent capillary vasculature. This tumor resembles oligodendroglioma; however, neurocytomas are immunoreactive for neuronal differentiation, but not for glial markers, being positive for synaptophysin but negative for glial fibrillary acidic protein. Ultrastructurally (on electron microscopy), neurocytoma shows neurotubules, neurofilaments, and neurosecretory granules.

These tumors are WHO grade II, with good prognosis. The treatment is surgical resection.

Bradley WG, Daroff RB, Fenichel GM, et al. Neurology in Clinical Practice, 5th ed. Philadelphia, PA: Elsevier; 2008.

Prayson RA, Goldblum JR. Neuropathology, 1st ed. Philadelphia, PA: Elsevier; 2005.

26. c, 27. b

The imaging findings in Figure 8.8 are consistent with a meningioma, which originates from meningothelial or arachnoid cap cells. These tumors account for 13% to 26% of primary intracranial tumors, and are more common in women, with a peak in the sixth or seventh decades of life. The most common sites include the cerebral convexities, parasagittal region, sphenoid wing, parasellar region, and spinal canal. Clinically, patients may be asymptomatic and the tumor may be found incidentally; however, depending on their location and size, meningiomas may produce focal neurologic manifestations, seizures, or headaches.

Meningiomas are dural-based tumors, often with a dural tail seen on imaging and sometimes with mass effect on the adjacent parenchyma. Calcifications may occur. These tumors are generally benign, slow growing, firm, rubbery, and well demarcated, compressing brain tissue rather than infiltrating it. However, in malignant meningiomas, there may be tissue infiltration.

Microscopically, these tumors are composed of monomorphic cells with oval nuclei, and the presence of psammoma bodies is common. However, meningiomas are very heterogeneous, with multiple histologic variants ranging in the spectrum of histologic WHO grade I, II, and III. The majority of meningiomas are syncytial, fibrous, or transitional types, which are benign variants.

Radiologically, on MRI meningiomas are isointense to gray matter on T1 and T2, with homogeneous enhancement. A dural tail may be appreciated as mentioned.

In general, most meningiomas are benign and surgically resectable, with the extent of the resection being the major predictor of recurrence. WHO grade III tumors and a high proliferative index predict a higher recurrence rate. Radiotherapy may be used for aggressive tumors.

More than half of meningiomas are associated with loss of chromosome 22, and there are associations of meningiomas with neurofibromatosis type 2, previous radiation, and breast carcinoma.

Bradley WG, Daroff RB, Fenichel GM, et al. Neurology in Clinical Practice, 5th ed. Philadelphia, PA: Elsevier; 2008.

Prayson RA, Goldblum JR. Neuropathology, 1st ed. Philadelphia, PA: Elsevier; 2005.

28. a

Figure 8.9 shows a tumor characterized by prominent capillary vasculature and stromal cells showing a vacuolated cytoplasm. This is consistent with hemangioblastoma.

Hemangioblastomas are benign, vascular tumors, and the most common primary cerebellar neoplasm in adults. They can occur at any age, with a peak incidence between 25 and 40 years, being slightly more common in males. Macroscopically, they are well demarcated and cystic. Histopathologically, there are abundant capillaries and stromal vacuolated cells. They may present with mass effect and CSF obstruction, leading to increased intracranial pressure. About 10% of these tumors secrete an erythropoietin-like substance leading to secondary polycythemia. MRI demonstrates a cyst with an enhancing mural nodule.

This tumor is WHO grade I, and can be resected surgically. Hemangioblastomas are associated with von Hippel-Lindau (VHL) in about 25% of the cases, related to mutations in the *VHL* gene on chromosome 3p25–26.

Bradley WG, Daroff RB, Fenichel GM, et al. Neurology in Clinical Practice, 5th ed. Philadelphia, PA: Elsevier; 2008.

Prayson RA, Goldblum JR. Neuropathology, 1st ed. Philadelphia, PA: Elsevier; 2005.

29. a

Figure 8.10 shows a hypercellular neoplasm, with a sheet-like proliferation of small blue cells and a high nuclear-to-cytoplasm ratio, characteristic of medulloblastoma. Homer-Wright pseudorosettes, even though not appreciated in this picture, are seen in about a third of cases. Macroscopically, medulloblastomas are soft tumors, with necrosis and hemorrhage.

Medulloblastoma is a rapidly growing and invasive tumor, which arises from the cerebellum. It is seen in children, and accounts for 20% of childhood brain tumors.

The histopathologic features are not consistent with the other options provided. Oligo-dendrogliomas are hypercellular tumors with uniformly rounded nuclei and clear perinuclear haloes, giving it a "fried egg" appearance. Pilocytic astrocytoma is a glial neoplasm with piloid or hair-like astrocytic processes, and demonstrates a biphasic pattern of compact regions along with microcystic components. Meningiomas are dural-based tumors originating from meningothe-lial or arachnoid cap cells, histologically composed of monomorphic cells with oval nuclei, sometimes with the presence of psammoma bodies. Histopathologic features of glioblastoma multiforme include necrosis, pseudopalisading nuclei, and endothelial hyperplasia.

Prayson RA, Goldblum JR. Neuropathology, 1st ed. Philadelphia, PA: Elsevier; 2005.

Ropper AH, Samuels MA. Adams and Victor's Principles of Neurology, 9th ed. New York: McGraw-Hill; 2009.

30. c

Pineocytomas and pineoblastomas are tumors arising from the pineal gland parenchyma, pre-senting with various manifestations, including ophthalmologic findings such as Parinaud syn-drome, brain stem and cerebellar manifestations, features of increased intracranial pressure, and hypothalamic dysfunction.

Pineocytomas are more frequent in young adults. These tumors are well demarcated and homogeneous. Histopathologically, this tumor is composed of small uniform cells that resemble pineocytes, with low mitotic activity. There may be rosette formations.

Pineoblastomas are more frequent in children and macroscopically are soft and poorly demarcated, with areas of necrosis and hemorrhage. The cells may resemble those of other embryonal tumors, such as medulloblastomas, and there is significant proliferation of small round cells with high nuclear-to-cytoplasmic ratio, and prominent mitotic activity. These cells lack differentiation and resemble primitive neuroectodermal tumors, and not mature pineocytes. Pineoblastomas are associated with a deletion on chromosome 11q, and may spread via the craniospinal axis or may metastasize. The prognosis of pineocytomas is better than that of pineoblastomas.

Prayson RA, Goldblum JR. Neuropathology, 1st ed. Philadelphia, PA: Elsevier; 2005.

Ropper AH, Samuels MA. Adams and Victor's Principles of Neurology, 9th ed. New York: McGraw-Hill; 2009.

31. d

Several types of benign cysts arise in the neuroaxis. These cysts can be resected if symptomatic, and do not undergo malignant degeneration.

Colloid cysts arise near the foramen of Monro, and may produce several manifestations including headache and mental status changes, and if there is obstruction of the foramen of Monro, patients may present with drop attacks, acute hydrocephalus, and even sudden death. Symptoms may be intermittent, and syncope and other symptoms may be positional, occurring when the patient bends forward or with Valsalva. Radiologically, these cysts have increased signal on T1, with no enhancement. Colloid cysts have a thin-walled lining and contain thick and cloudy gelatinous fluid. Microscopically, there is a single layer of columnar ciliated or goblet cells. The treatment is surgical resection, and sometimes shunt placement is required for management of hydrocephalus.

Epidermoid and dermoid cysts arise from ectopic ectodermal tissue. Epidermoid cysts occur in young adults and arise from the cerebellopontine angle. On MRI, epidermoid cysts have CSF intensity on T2, being slightly hyperintense to CSF fluid on FLAIR. They have a characteristic restricted diffusion appearance on DWI, which helps to distinguish these cyst from arachnoid cysts. Epidermoid cysts are microscopically lined by squamous-type epithelium filled with keratinaceous material.

Dermoid cysts arise in children, and tend to occur in the cerebellar vermis, parasellar, or parapontine region and in the lumbosacral region in the spinal canal. They are a "pearly" white structure, with a content similar to epidermoid cysts, and lined by squamous epithelium; however, dermoid cysts also contain hair follicles, sebaceous glands, and sweat glands. Dermoid cysts can rupture, and the content can incite a chemical meningitis characterized by a granulomatous inflammation.

Arachnoid cysts are basically a cystic space bound by arachnoid membranes, with a location associated with the meninges, predominantly in the temporal lobe region. They are lined by arachnoid cap cells.

Rathke's cleft cysts occur in between the anterior and posterior hypophysis. They have a thin-walled lining containing a cloudy fluid, and are lined by columnar epithelium with ciliated and goblet cells.

Bradley WG, Daroff RB, Fenichel GM, et al. Neurology in Clinical Practice, 5th ed. Philadelphia, PA: Elsevier; 2008.

Prayson RA, Goldblum JR. Neuropathology, 1st ed. Philadelphia, PA: Elsevier; 2005.

32. d

In medulloblastomas, a diagnosis at a younger age (usually younger than 3 years of age) confers a poorer prognosis.

Medulloblastomas are embryonal tumors that arise from pluripotential cells and are encountered in children, more commonly in males, and located in the posterior fossa, more specifically in the cerebellum. The clinical presentation includes manifestations of increased intracranial pressure, hydrocephalus, and cerebellar findings. The most common genetic defect is on chromosome 17. This tumor can metastasize or spread via CSF, and therefore, MRI of the entire neuroaxis should be obtained.

Treatment involves maximal surgical resection, in addition to chemotherapy and radiation therapy, with survival rates up to 80% at 5 years.

A desmoplastic variant confers a better prognosis. Features of poor prognosis include early age at the onset (younger than 3 years of age), incomplete resection, presence of brain stem invasion, metastasis, large cell variants, glial differentiation, and N-myc transcription factor amplification.

Prayson RA, Goldblum JR. Neuropathology, 1st ed. Philadelphia, PA: Elsevier; 2005.

Ropper AH, Samuels MA. Adams and Victor's Principles of Neurology, 9th ed. New York: McGraw-Hill; 2009.

33. e

The pathologic features in Figure 8.11 are typical of a dysembryoplastic neuroepithelial tumor (DNET), demonstrating prominent clear spaces that seem to contain ganglion cells. In between these clear spaces, there are multiple cells and a glial component that resembles an oligodendroglioma.

DNET is a benign superficial tumor that is an important cause of refractory seizures in children. These tumors are located in the cortical or juxtacortical region, most commonly in the temporal lobe. The MRI shows a nodular or cystic lesion that is hyperintense on T2-weighted images and does not enhance with contrast. It grows very slowly, and macroscopically, it has a multinodular architecture, with mucinous cysts. Histologically, it is seen as multiple areas in which ganglion cells appear to float within mucin-filled spaces ("floating neurons"). In between these nodules, there is a component with more glial characteristics, sometimes resembling an oligodendroglioma. At the edges of these lesions, there may be cortical dysplasia.

DNET is a WHO grade I tumor, and surgical resection is helpful for the cure or control of the seizures.

Prayson RA, Goldblum JR. Neuropathology, 1st ed. Philadelphia, PA: Elsevier; 2005.

Ropper AH, Samuels MA. Adams and Victor's Principles of Neurology. 9th ed. New York: McGraw-Hill; 2009.

34. b, 35. e

This patient has a lymphoma, likely primary CNS lymphoma (PCNSL) given the parenchymal invasion of lymphocytes with an angiocentric pattern. Surgical resection does not play a role in the treatment of lymphomas.

PCNSL occur predominantly in immunocompromised patients, such as patients with AIDS and posttransplant patients. In these cases they are frequently associated with Epstein-Barr virus (EBV). PCNSL can also occur in immunocompetent hosts; however, this is rare, and there is a lower association with EBV.

PCNSL is usually a diffuse, large B-cell lymphoma, and rarely caused by T-cell proliferation. In contrast to secondary invasion by lymphomas from other primary sites, PCNSL invades the parenchyma more than the leptomeninges, and histologically, it is characterized by proliferation and diffuse infiltration of atypical lymphocytes with an angiocentric pattern as seen in Figure 8.12. These neoplasms can be single or multicentric, and can involve the corpus callosum. PCNSL can also involve the eye, and therefore, an ophthalmology evaluation is warranted to examine the vitreous for lymphoma cells.

Clinically, the presentation is variable, manifesting with headaches, signs of increased intracranial pressure, seizures, focal neurologic deficits, or alteration in the mental status. MRI shows a lesion with T2 hyperintensity, edema, and contrast enhancement.

The prognosis is poor, with 5-year survival rates of 25% to 45%, being much worse in immunocompromised patients.

This neoplasm is steroid responsive, and steroids should be avoided before biopsy because they may reduce the yield of this diagnostic test. However in cases of emergency, especially in the presence of significant mass effect and herniation, steroid use may be required.

Surgery is not indicated because this neoplasm is often deep and multicentric. The treatment includes radiation therapy and chemotherapy, with agents such as cytosine arabinoside and intrathecal methotrexate. This combination prolongs survival; however, it is associated with leukoencephalopathy and systemic side effects. In patients with HIV-related PCNSL, highly active antiretroviral therapy is the treatment of choice.

Given the clinical and histopathologic features shown, this is not a glioblastoma, oligodendroglioma, meningioma, or ependymoma.

Prayson RA, Goldblum JR. Neuropathology, 1st ed. Philadelphia, PA: Elsevier; 2005.

Ropper AH, Samuels MA. Adams and Victor's Principles of Neurology, 9th ed. New York: McGraw-Hill; 2009.

36. b

This is a craniopharyngioma, which is most common in children, but has a bimodal age distribution and is also seen in adults.

Figure 8.13 shows a tumor with multicystic components, characterized by proliferation of cords of epithelial-appearing cells, with a palisade of basaloid cells toward the lumen of the cysts. This is consistent with a craniopharyngioma. Craniopharyngiomas are benign epithelioid tumors that originate from remnants of the Rathke's pouch and arise in the sellar region, where they grow to produce manifestations from mass effect on adjacent structures, such as the optic chiasm, pituitary, hypothalamus, bony structures, and ventricular system, even to the point of being able to obstruct CSF flow. Common manifestations are therefore visual disturbances, endocrine deficiencies, diabetes insipidus, and findings of increased intracranial pressure. Craniopharyngiomas occur in a bimodal distribution, seen with a peak incidence in childhood and middle-aged adults. Macroscopically, these tumors are partially solid with a cystic component, frequently filled with lipid- and cholesterol-rich brown fluid, also called "machine-oil–like fluid," which if spilled, may cause a xanthogranulomatous inflammation. Microscopic calcifications, keratin, and xanthogranulomatous inflammation are seen more commonly in the adamantinomatous variant. In the papillary variant, the sheets of cells form pseudopapillae.

These tumors are in general surgically resectable. They have a benign behavior, but may recur if there is incomplete resection.

Prayson RA, Goldblum JR. Neuropathology, 1st ed. Philadelphia, PA: Elsevier; 2005.

Ropper AH, Samuels MA. Adams and Victor's Principles of Neurology, 9th ed. New York: McGraw-Hill; 2009.

37. d

Figure 8.14 shows a proliferation of epithelial cells in a papillary pattern lining fibrovascular cores, consistent with choroid plexus papilloma, which is a WHO grade I tumor.

Choroid plexus papillomas are tumors of childhood, and most commonly arise from the lateral ventricles, followed by the fourth ventricle and then the third ventricle. Clinically, they may be asymptomatic, or present with hydrocephalus and manifestations of increased intracranial pressure, sometimes due to a combination of obstructed flow and increased CSF production.

Choroid plexus papillomas are circumscribed masses composed of epithelium lining fibrovascular cores, resembling normal choroid plexus. In contrast to papillomas, choroid plexus carcinomas are invasive, with nuclear pleomorphism, demonstrating atypia, mitosis, and necrosis.

Choroid plexus papillomas are surgically resectable and considered low grade or WHO grade I. Choroid plexus carcinomas are higher grade (WHO grade III), and after surgical resection, radiotherapy and chemotherapy may be needed.

Prayson RA, Goldblum JR. Neuropathology, 1st ed. Philadelphia, PA: Elsevier; 2005.

Ropper AH, Samuels MA. Adams and Victor's Principles of Neurology, 9th ed. New York: McGraw-Hill; 2009.

38. e

Chordomas are invasive osseo-destructive tumors encountered in adults, more commonly in males, and arise from remnants of the primitive notochord. They are located most commonly in the clivus and sacrococcygeal region. If in the clivus, they may present clinically with headaches, neck pain, and multiple cranial neuropathies due to brain stem compression. If in the sacrococcygeal region, they may present with sphincter dysfunction and pain.

These tumors are locally invasive and tend to destroy the bone, which is appreciated on radiologic studies such as CT and MRI. Grossly, this tumor is infiltrative and lobulated. Microscopically, there is a lobulated pattern with fibrovascular septa and cords of epithelioid cells. Vacuolated cells are present and are called physaliphorous cells.

The treatment is surgical excision and sometimes radiotherapy for residual disease. There may be recurrences from residual tumor.

Prayson RA, Goldblum JR. Neuropathology, 1st ed. Philadelphia, PA: Elsevier; 2005.

Ropper AH, Samuels MA. Adams and Victor's Principles of Neurology, 9th ed. New York: McGraw-Hill; 2009.

39. a

This patient has a vestibular schwannoma. These are tumors that occur more commonly in the fourth and fifth decades, and most commonly arise from the vestibular portion of cranial nerve VIII. They grow in the cerebellopontine angle, and may compress the brain stem and erode into the internal auditory meatus. Clinically, they grow slowly and may be asymptomatic, or present with hearing loss, tinnitus, and in some cases cerebellar findings given that the cerebellar peduncles are compressed. Radiologically, they are seen as circumscribed isointense tumors with contrast enhancement as seen in Figure 8.15. The location and radiologic appearance of the tumor as shown in Figure 8.15 distinguish it from the other choices. It is extra-axial (not within the brain parenchyma) and is not within the ventricular system. This is not a location typical for metastatic lesions. Given the clinical and radiologic findings, this patient does not have an oligodendroglioma, cerebellar hemangioblastoma, ependymoma, or metastatic tumor.

Bradley WG, Daroff RB, Fenichel GM, et al. Neurology in Clinical Practice, 5th ed. Philadelphia, PA: Elsevier; 2008.

Prayson RA, Goldblum JR. Neuropathology, 1st ed. Philadelphia, PA: Elsevier; 2005.

40. b, 41. c

Metastatic lesions are more common than primary brain tumors. Eighty percent of brain metastases are supratentorial and 20% intratentorial. Intracranial metastatic lesion can affect the skull and dura and brain parenchyma or produce a meningeal carcinomatosis.

The most common source of metastasis to the brain is the lung, followed by breast and then melanoma. Other tumors that may produce brain metastasis include gastrointestinal tumors especially from the colon and rectum—also, kidney cancer and tumors originating from the gallbladder, liver, thyroid, testicle, uterus, ovary, and pancreas. It is very rare to have parenchymal brain metastases originating from the prostate, esophagus, oropharynx, and skin (other than melanoma). Colon and pelvic cancers have a tendency to spread to the posterior fossa.

Metastatic lesions can be multiple or single. Multiple metastases are seen with small cell carcinomas and melanomas. Those that are frequently found as single metastasis originate from the kidney, breast, thyroid, or adenocarcinoma of the lung. Hemorrhagic metastases are seen with melanoma, choriocarcinomas, non–small cell carcinomas, thyroid carcinomas, and renal cell carcinomas.

Patients harboring metastasis typically present with a seizure, focal neurologic findings, headaches, and sometimes with increased intracranial pressure. Symptom onset is typically relatively rapid and abrupt rather than gradual.

The treatment of brain metastasis includes brain irradiation, surgical intervention for solitary metastasis in some cases, and chemotherapy. Steroids play a significant role in the treatment of surrounding edema.

Prayson RA, Goldblum JR. Neuropathology, 1st ed. Philadelphia, PA: Elsevier; 2005.

Ropper AH, Samuels MA. Adams and Victor's Principles of Neurology, 9th ed. New York: McGraw-Hill; 2009.

42. C

The histopathologic findings in Figure 8.16 are consistent with a vestibular schwannoma.

Schwannomas most commonly arise from the vestibular portion of CN VIII and grow in the cerebellopontine angle. Grossly, they have a yellowish color and are well demarcated. Histologically, there is a biphasic pattern with a more compact phase (or Antoni A area) and a looser pattern (or Antoni B area). The cells and nuclei tend to be elongated, sometimes with an arrangement in a palisade configuration, which is called Verocay body, as seen in Figure 8.16. This figure shows an Antoni A pattern. Immunohistochemically, these tumors are S-100 positive.

Vestibular schwannomas are associated with neurofibromatosis type 2, and the presence of bilateral tumors is diagnostic for this latter condition.

These tumors are benign, categorized as WHO grade I, and surgically resectable. Gamma knife may also be a therapeutic option.

Bradley WG, Daroff RB, Fenichel GM, et al. Neurology in Clinical Practice, 5th ed. Philadelphia, PA: Elsevier; 2008.

Prayson RA, Goldblum JR. Neuropathology, 1st ed. Philadelphia, PA: Elsevier; 2005.

43. C

The imaging findings in Figure 8.17 and appearance of the lesion in Figure 8.18 are consistent with a pituitary adenoma. Pituitary adenomas greater than 1 cm in size are classified as macroadenomas, whereas those less than 1 cm in size are classified as microadenomas. Most pituitary adenomas are nonsecretory; of the secretory ones, prolactin-secreting adenomas, so-called prolactinomas, are most common, though those secreting growth hormone, ACTH, and thyroid-stimulating hormone also occur. Follicle-stimulating hormone–secreting adenomas may occur; luteinizing hormone–secreting adenomas are rare. Patients may be asymptomatic, as in this patient's case in which the visual field deficit was detected incidentally. In women, symptoms including galactorrhea and amenorrhea lead to earlier diagnosis, particularly in the case of prolactinomas. In men, prolactinomas may present with impotence. Endocrine disturbances may occur with nonsecretory adenomas when the lesion is large enough to compromise normal pituitary tissue function. Other symptoms include headache, ophthalmoparesis, and vision loss. Pressure on or invasion into the cavernous sinus may lead to cranial neuropathies.

Pituitary adenomas are the most common masses in the sellar region. The lesion is isointense on T1, and enhances almost homogeneously with contrast, as seen in Figure 8.17. Figure 8.18 shows evidence of monomorphic eosinophilic cells. Besides tumors of pituitary origin, other tumors that may occur in the sellar region include gliomas, meningiomas, chordomas, metastases, and others. Pituitary apoplexy, or hemorrhage into, most commonly, a pituitary macroadenoma, presents with sudden severe headache, ophthalmoparesis, and in some cases evidence of increased intracranial pressure.

The histopathologic findings are not consistent with a craniopharyngioma or Rathke's cleft cyst. Craniopharyngiomas are benign epithelioid tumors that originate from remnants of the Rathke's pouch and arise in the sellar region, where they grow to produce manifestations from mass effect on adjacent structures. Craniopharyngiomas are multicystic, with squamous epithelial cells and sometimes calcifications.

Rathke's cleft cysts occur in between the anterior and posterior hypophysis. They have a thin-walled lining containing a cloudy fluid, and they are lined by columnar epithelium with ciliated and goblet cells.

Aminoff MJ. Neurology and General Medicine, 4th ed. Philadelphia, PA: Elsevier; 2008.

Bradley WG, Daroff RB, Fenichel GM, et al. Neurology in Clinical Practice, 5th ed. Philadelphia, PA: Elsevier; 2008.

44. a

Figure 8.19 shows a lesion with typical characteristics of metastasis. Metastases are round and demarcated, located in the gray-white junction, and hyperintense on T2-weighted images, with significant enhancement with gadolinium, and prominent surrounding vasogenic edema, which is appreciated on the FLAIR image in Figure 8.19 as hyperintensity around the main lesion.

Meningiomas are dural-based tumors, which is not the case in Figure 8.19. Low-grade diffuse fibrillary astrocytomas will not show this degree of edema. Glioblastoma is an aggressive lesion that demonstrates surrounding edema; however, it usually will have a more heterogeneous enhancement pattern with areas of necrosis. This is not a location for an ependymoma, which will have a closer relationship with the ventricular surface.

Bradley WG, Daroff RB, Fenichel GM, et al. Neurology in Clinical Practice, 5th ed. Philadelphia, PA: Elsevier; 2008.

45. a

Various immunohistochemical markers are utilized to help in the diagnosis and typification of certain neoplasms. Glial fibrillary acidic protein (GFAP) is positive with glial intermediate filaments, cytokeratin is positive with epithelial intermediate filaments, Melan-A and HMB-45 are positive with melanocytic cells, CD45 is a marker of lymphocytes, CD3 for T cells, and CD20 for B cells. Ki-67 is a marker of nuclear proliferation.

In this case, with positive GFAP and very high percentage of Ki-67, the most likely diagnosis is an astrocytoma. Given that GFAP can be positive in gliosis, Ki-67 helps distinguish between the two. A carcinoma will likely be cytokeratin positive. Melanoma will likely show Melan-A and HMB-45 positivity. Absence of positive markers for lymphocytes makes lymphoma unlikely.

Prayson RA, Goldblum JR. Neuropathology, 1st ed. Philadelphia, PA: Elsevier; 2005.

46. b

Pilocytic astrocytoma is a WHO grade I, not grade II, tumor. Astrocytomas are neoplasms that originate from the neuroglia. These may arise from different regions of the CNS, including the brain, cerebellum, hypothalamus, optic nerve, optic chiasm, brain stem, and spinal cord. The location is influenced by age, and in adults, they are most frequently encountered in the cerebral hemispheres. The clinical presentation may be variable, with headaches, focal neurologic manifestations, and frequently seizures.

The WHO grades these tumors on the basis of the St. Anne–Mayo grading system, using extent of atypia, mitoses, endothelial hyperplasia, and necrosis as criteria. Astrocytomas are classified as at least WHO grade II in the presence of atypia. Anaplastic astrocytomas are classified as WHO grade III on the basis of the presence of atypia and mitotic activity. Glioblastoma multiforme are WHO grade IV, having endothelial hyperplasia and necrosis. Pilocytic astrocytoma is a WHO grade I well-circumscribed tumor, frequently located in the cerebellum, but can also be seen in the hypothalamus, third ventricle, optic nerve, spinal cord, and dorsal brain stem.

Astrocytomas can also be classified as diffuse astrocytomas, pilocytic astrocytomas, pleomorphic xanthoastrocytomas, and subependymal giant cell astrocytomas. Diffuse astrocytomas can be subdivided according to the predominant histologic cell type (see questions 2 and 3).

Prayson RA, Goldblum JR. Neuropathology, 1st ed. Philadelphia, PA: Elsevier; 2005.

Ropper AH, Samuels MA. Adams and Victor's Principles of Neurology, 9th ed. New York: McGraw-Hill; 2009.

47. b

Figure 8.20 shows signal hyperintensity in both mesial temporal lobes, as well as a PET scan demonstrating increased fluorodeoxyglucose uptake in the mesial temporal lobes bilaterally. These findings are consistent with limbic encephalitis. In young patients with paraneoplastic limbic encephalitis, a testicular germ cell tumor may be the cause, and most often associated with anti-Ma antibodies, not anti-Hu.

Paraneoplastic encephalomyelitis may affect various parts of the CNS. Paraneoplastic limbic encephalitis is a subset of this syndrome, in which bilateral temporal lobes and other limbic structures are involved. These patients present with a neuropsychiatric syndrome characterized by personality changes, depression, agitation, hallucinations, psychosis, and a confusional state. Typically, these patients have amnesia, with prominent short-term anterograde component. Sometimes seizures occur as well. The onset is usually gradual and progressive over weeks to months, but there are cases of more rapid evolution. CSF may show mild pleocytosis and increased protein. The MRI demonstrates a characteristic hyperintensity in bilateral mesial temporal lobes, as shown in Figure 8.20. Histopathologically, there is inflammation with perivascular lymphocytes and monocytes, microglial proliferation, neuron loss, and foci of necrosis.

This syndrome presents in patients with small cell lung cancer associated with anti-Hu (ANNA-1) antibodies. In young males, it may also be seen associated with testicular germ cell tumors, in which case the most common antibody encountered is anti-Ma. An autoimmune, nonparaneoplastic limbic encephalitis associated with voltage-gated potassium channel antibodies (anti-VGKC antibodies) may lead to a similar presentation.

Treatment involves addressing the primary neoplasm. Some cases are responsive to steroids or other immunomodulatory therapies such as plasmapheresis or intravenous immunoglobulins.

A paraneoplastic encephalitis has been reported in patients with ovarian teratomas associated with antibodies to NMDA receptors. This type of encephalitis manifests with psychiatric symptoms, amnesia, seizures, dyskinesias, autonomic dysfunction, and decreased level of consciousness. In these patients, tumor resection and immunotherapy lead to improvement, and in some cases, to full recovery.

Bradley WG, Daroff RB, Fenichel GM, et al. Neurology in Clinical Practice, 5th ed. Philadelphia, PA: Elsevier; 2008.

Dalmau J, Tuzun E, Wu HY, et al. Paraneoplastic anti-N-methyl-D-aspartate receptor encephalitis associated with ovarian teratoma. Ann Neurol. 2007; 61:25–36.

Ropper AH, Samuels MA. Adams and Victor's Principles of Neurology, 9th ed. New York: McGraw-Hill; 2009.

48. b

The prognosis in oligodendrogliomas is better than in astrocytomas. Other factors that influence prognosis include age of the patient (better survival with younger patients), presurgical performance status (worse prognosis with poorer baseline functional and neurologic status), bulk of resection (the greater the extent of resection the better), and genetic alterations. Important genetic alterations are chromosome 1p and 19q codeletions, which occur in 50% to 80% of the cases, and are associated with a better prognosis, enhanced survival, and better response to chemotherapy, radiation therapy, or both. Mutation of p53 is not typically seen in oligodendrogliomas, and its presence suggests the possibility of an astrocytic neoplasm. Deletion of the chromosomal region p16 is more commonly seen in anaplastic astrocytomas and glioblastomas, and is associated with progression.

Treatment of oligodendrogliomas involves surgical resection, chemotherapy, and radiation therapy. The chemotherapy used includes temozolomide, which has replaced PCV (procarbazine, lomustine, and vincristine).

Bradley WG, Daroff RB, Fenichel GM, et al. Neurology in Clinical Practice, 5th ed. Philadelphia, PA: Elsevier; 2008.

Prayson RA, Goldblum JR. Neuropathology, 1st ed. Philadelphia, PA: Elsevier; 2005.

49. c

The principle of autonomy is based on the premise that patients are their own ultimate decision makers. Autonomy contrasts with physician paternalism, which dominated the physician-patient relationship in the past, in which the physician was viewed, and viewed him- or herself, as the authoritative decision maker that would simply tell the patient what was best for him or her. The modern-day physician-patient relationship is built around patient autonomy, creating room for shared decision making, in which the physician presents treatment options to the patient and provides the education necessary for the patient to make a decision with the help and support of the physician.

In the case presented, the physician has offered all treatment options to the patient, and the patient has made an informed decision to have only symptomatic treatment. The patient clearly understands the implications of his decision, and although the physician does not agree with it, he or she will still support the patient and care for him. Assessment of the patient's capacity to make decisions for himself is not indicated in this case as the patient clearly demonstrates understanding of the consequences of his or her decision. Denying the patient further care because of the decision the patient has made is clearly the incorrect answer. Making sure to frequently reassess the patient's understanding and discussing treatment options at later encounters is important, but use of derogatory remarks to coerce the patient into a specific treatment option is clearly not in line with respecting patient autonomy. Option e is a demonstration of paternalism; while physicians should clearly state their medical opinion on the basis of best evidence as to what they feel the best course of action would be, shared decision making, taking into account the patient's values and wishes, is the basis of respecting patient autonomy.

Jonsen A, Siegler M, Winslade W. Clinical Ethics: A Practical Approach to Ethical Decisions in Clinical Medicine, 6th ed. New York: McGraw-Hill; 2006.

Buzz Phrase	Key Points
Glial neoplasm with necrosis and pseudopalisading nuclei	Glioblastoma multiforme
"Fried egg" appearance	Oligodendrogliomas (fixation artifact)
Perivascular pseudorosettes	Ependymomas
True rosettes	Ependymomas
Homer-Wright rosettes	Medulloblastoma
Ki-67	Marker of nuclear proliferation
Glial fibrillary acidic protein	Glial fibrillary acidic protein. Marker of glial intermediate filaments
Cytokeratin	Marker of epithelial intermediate filaments
Melan-A and HMB-45	Positive in melanocytic cells
CD3	T cells
CD20	B cells
Rosenthal fibers	Pilocytic astrocytoma, pleomorphic xanthoastrocytoma, Alexander's disease, chronic reactive gliosis
Chromosome 1p and 19q deletion	Good prognostic factor in oligodendrogliomas
Subependymal giant cell astrocytomas	Tuberous sclerosis
Tumors typically presenting with seizures	Oligodendrogliomas, gangliogliomas, dysembryoplastic neuroepithelial tumors
von Hippel-Lindau	Cerebellar hemangioblastoma, chromosome 3, autosomal dominant
"Zellballen" arrangement of nests of cells	Paraganglioma
Common origin of brain metastasis	Lung > breast > melanoma
Paraneoplastic cerebellar degeneration associated with ovarian carcinoma or breast carcinoma	Anti-Yo antibodies
Small cell lung carcinoma. Associated with sensory neuropathy and neuronopathy, but may be associated with other paraneoplastic syndromes	Anti-Hu (ANNA-1) antibodies
Opsoclonus myoclonus associated with breast cancer and ovarian cancer	Anti-Ri (ANNA-2) antibodies
Opsoclonus myoclonus in children	Neuroblastoma
Paraneoplastic retinal degeneration, small cell lung carcinoma	Anti-recoverin antibodies
Lambert-Eaton myasthenic syndrome	Anti-voltage-gated calcium channel P/Q type antibodies
Limbic encephalitis and testicular germ cell tumor	Anti-Ma antibodies
Paraneoplastic encephalitis associated with ovarian teratoma	Anti-NMDA receptor antibodies

Chapter 9

Neuromuscular I

(Neurophysiology, Plexopathy, and Neuropathy)

Questions

Questions 1–2

1. A 3-year-old boy is seen by a pediatric neurologist for multiple concerns including cognitive and motor developmental delay. The parents reported that the patient did not walk like his siblings, but rather seemed to walk on the insides of his feet. Unlike his siblings, he also had tightly curled hair. Examination revealed nystagmus, bilateral weakness of the legs, and brisk reflexes with ankle clonus. One year later, the patient requires insertion of a peg tube, has developed significant spasticity in his arms and legs, and has had significant vision loss. He has significant language delay as well. Two years later, the patient passes away from complications of aspiration pneumonia, and on autopsy, pathologic analysis of nerve fibers demonstrates large focal axonal swellings filled with neurofilaments. What is the most likely diagnosis in this patient?
   a. Dejerine-Sottas syndrome
   b. Charcot-Marie-Tooth (CMT) type 2A
   c. CMT type 4
   d. Giant axonal neuropathy
   e. Metachromatic leukodystrophy

2. A 25-year-old man is referred to the clinic by his ophthalmologist. In early childhood, he was noted to have a retinal disorder, and in his teenage years, he was denied a driver's license due to night blindness and visual field deficits. In recent years, he had begun to complain of tingling in his legs and later, of clumsiness and weakness. Examination revealed evidence of bilateral symmetric sensory loss and distal bilateral lower extremity weakness. A serum phytanic acid level is obtained and is elevated. What is the most likely diagnosis in this patient?
   a. Myoneurogastrointestinal encephalopathy
   b. Kearns-Sayre syndrome
   c. Neurogenic muscle weakness, ataxia, and retinitis pigmentosa syndrome
   d. Abetalipoproteinemia
   e. Refsum's disease

Questions 3–4

3. Which of the following is incorrect regarding electrophysiologic studies of the peripheral nervous system?

a. SNAP amplitude is a measure of the number of axons that conduct between the stimulation and recording sites

b. Sensory distal latency is the time it takes for the action potential to travel between the nerve stimulation site and the recording site

c. Axon loss lesions result in reduced conduction velocities

d. CMAP amplitude depends on the status of the motor axons, neuromuscular junctions, and muscle fibers

e. The F-wave and H-reflex are late responses

4. Which of the following is incorrect regarding electrophysiologic studies of the peripheral nervous system?

a. CMAP amplitudes may be reduced in axon loss lesions

b. Prolonged distal latency is seen in demyelinating lesions

c. The H-reflex is the electrophysiologic equivalent of the ankle reflex

d. The H-reflex is obtained by stimulating the tibial nerve

e. The F-wave is obtained after submaximal stimulation of a motor nerve

5. Regarding needle EMG, which of the following is incorrect?

a. Insertional activity is increased in denervated muscles

b. Fibrillation and fasciculation potentials are examples of spontaneous activity

c. Short-duration motor unit potentials (MUPs) are seen more frequently in myopathic processes

d. Large polyphasic MUPs are seen in acute neuropathic lesions

e. Reduced recruitment is seen in axon loss lesions

6. Which of the following is incorrect regarding the evaluation of a radiculopathy associated with an axon loss intraspinal canal lesion?

a. Fibrillation potentials can be seen in a segmental myotome 3 weeks after the onset

b. There are abnormal sensory SNAPs in a segmental dermatome

c. Reinnervation or collateral innervation occurs in a proximal to distal gradient

d. The H-reflex tests the S1 reflex arc, and is helpful in the diagnosis of S1 radiculopathy

e. Large polyphasic motor unit potentials can be detected in chronic radiculopathies

Questions 7–8

7. A patient presents for evaluation of weakness in the upper extremities that had been occurring for the prior few months. NCS and EMG were unremarkable. With rapid repetitive stimulation and evaluation after exercise, there was no increase in CMAP amplitude. Slow repetitive nerve stimulation was obtained, and is shown in Figure 9.1. Which of the following is the most likely diagnosis?

a. A myopathy

b. A demyelinating neuropathy

c. An axon loss neuropathy

d. Myasthenia gravis

e. Botulism

Resp (#)	NPamp (mV)	NPamp (%chg)	NParea (mVms)	NParea (%chg)
1	1.1	0.0	6.6	0.0
2	0.9	−15.9	5.5	−16.7
3	0.8	−29.9	4.5	−31.5

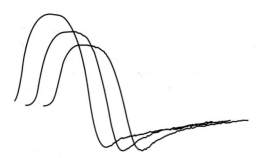

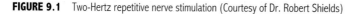

0.5 mV

2 ms   Train 1

FIGURE 9.1 Two-Hertz repetitive nerve stimulation (Courtesy of Dr. Robert Shields)

8. A patient is referred for an EMG/NCS for a possible diagnosis of a neuromuscular junction disorder. Which of the following is correct?
   a. CMAP increment after rapid repetitive stimulation is a feature of myasthenia gravis (MG)
   b. CMAP increment after brief exercise is a feature of MG
   c. A decrement in the CMAP after 2- to 3-Hz repetitive stimulation is consistent with MG
   d. Abnormal jitter on single-fiber EMG is a very specific finding for the diagnosis of MG
   e. Sensory NCS are typically abnormal in MG

9. A patient with lung cancer is being referred for evaluation of Lambert-Eaton myasthenic syndrome (LEMS). Which of the following is incorrect?
   a. Needle EMG is usually normal in LEMS
   b. Low to borderline-low CMAP amplitudes at rest are common in LEMS
   c. Slow repetitive stimulation (2 to 3 Hz) results in a decremental response of the CMAP amplitudes
   d. Rapid repetitive stimulation (20 to 50 Hz) results in an incremental response of the CMAP amplitudes
   e. Voluntary single-fiber jitter analysis helps to distinguish myasthenia gravis from LEMS

10. Regarding the types of skeletal muscle fibers, which of the following is correct?

a. Type I fibers have low oxygen consumption
⌐ b. Type IIa fibers are fast with large glycolytic capacity
c. Type I fibers are large in size
d. Type IIb fibers are fast with high oxidative capacity
e. Type IIb fibers are slow

Questions 11–12

11. A 55-year-old man presents with weakness, which initially developed in the lower extremities. He undergoes evaluation and treatment and is eventually admitted to a rehabilitation facility. He returns 9 weeks later with worsening of his weakness, which is affecting upper extremities distally and lower extremities proximally and distally. He also has distal paresthesias, and his examination demonstrates diffuse areflexia. CSF shows 3 WBCs/mm^3 (normal up to 5 lymphocytes/mm^3) and protein is 100 mg/dL (normal up to 45 mg/dL). An EMG/NCS is obtained and right median nerve NCS is shown in Figure 9.2. Which of the following is the most likely diagnosis?

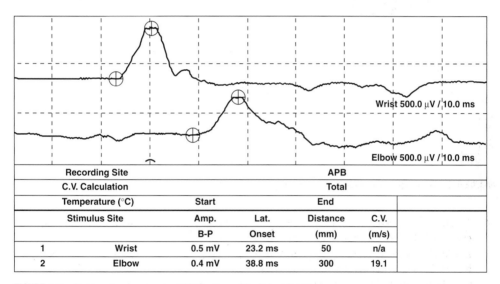

Recording Site			APB		
C.V. Calculation			Total		
Temperature (°C)	Start		End		
Stimulus Site	Amp.	Lat.	Distance	C.V.	
	B-P	Onset	(mm)	(m/s)	
1	Wrist	0.5 mV	23.2 ms	50	n/a
2	Elbow	0.4 mV	38.8 ms	300	19.1

FIGURE 9.2 Right median nerve motor NCS (Courtesy of Dr. Robert Shields)

a. Guillain-Barre syndrome
, b. Chronic inflammatory demyelinating polyneuropathy
c. Multifocal motor neuropathy
d. Lambert-Eaton myasthenic syndrome
e. Myasthenia gravis

12. Which of the following is incorrect regarding this condition?
! a. Sensory NCS are required to establish the diagnosis
b. There may be prolongation of distal motor latencies
c. CSF albuminocytologic dissociation can be seen in this condition
d. Sural nerve biopsy shows evidence of inflammation, demyelination, and remyelination
e. Conduction block is a common finding

13. Which of the following is incorrect regarding an axon loss peripheral nerve injury?
   a. Fibrillation potentials appear by the third week of the injury
   b. Conduction block 10 days after the injury suggests segmental demyelination
   c. The presence of conduction block can help localize the site of segmental demyelination
   d. NCS 3 weeks after the injury are useful to localize a focal axon loss lesion
   e. Axon loss leads to wallerian degeneration

14. A 62-year-old retired secretary presents to the clinic complaining of painful tingling sensations and numbness in her left thumb, index, and middle finger that wake her up at night. On examination, motor power in her left arm, forearm, and hand is normal. There is subtle loss of pinprick and light touch on the distal first to third digits (at the finger tips). Biceps and brachioradialis deep tendon reflexes are normal. A tracing from her median nerve sensory NCS is shown in Figure 9.3 (normal median nerve SNAP latency is 4.0 ms); motor NCS and EMG are normal. What is the most likely diagnosis?

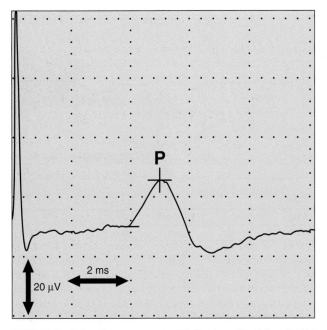

FIGURE 9.3   Left median nerve sensory NCS (Courtesy of Dr. Robert Shields)

   a. C6 radiculopathy
   b. C7 radiculopathy
   c. Carpal tunnel syndrome
   d. Median neuropathy at the elbow
   e. Brachial plexopathy

Questions 15–16

15. A 28-year-old woman presents with numbness and tingling in her feet. She was seen in the emergency department, and after no neurologic abnormalities were found, she was reassured and discharged home. Four days later she returns, unable to walk. She complains of numbness and tingling from her toes up to just above her knees, and also affecting her hands. On examination, she has distal more than proximal weakness in the lower extremities and subtle weakness in her hands. Ankle and patellar reflexes are absent. She recalls having a viral illness a couple of weeks ago. Which of the following is the most likely diagnosis?

- a. Guillain-Barre syndrome
- b. Multiple sclerosis
- c. Stroke
- d. Myelopathy
- e. Myasthenia gravis

16. The patient is admitted to the hospital, and continues to worsen. Which of the following tests should be obtained to ensure adequate care, and may affect the subsequent management of this patient?

- a. MRI of the lumbar spine
- b. Evaluation of respiratory parameters, including negative inspiratory force and vital capacity
- c. MRI of the brain
- d. CSF studies for various antibodies, oligoclonal bands, and myelin basic protein
- e. EMG/NCS as soon as possible

17. Regarding innervation of the upper extremity, which of the following is incorrect?

- a. The brachial plexus is formed from the anterior rami of the C5 to T1 nerve roots
- b. The middle trunk is formed from the C7 root
- c. The lower (inferior) trunk is formed from the C8 and T1 roots
- d. The dorsal scapular nerve is the only nerve that branches directly off the nerve roots
- e. The cords of the brachial plexus are named according to their anatomic relationship to the axillary artery

Questions 18–19

18. A 40-year-old man presents to the clinic complaining of bilateral lower extremity sharp burning pains. Examination reveals bilateral symmetric loss of sensation to temperature and pinprick, with mild reduction in vibratory sense and fine touch, and normal proprioception. Review of systems reveals dyspnea on exertion, early satiety, erectile dysfunction, and constipation. Routine laboratory testing and monoclonal protein analysis are negative. His father suffered from similar symptoms in middle age, and was in a wheelchair prior to his death at the age of 65 from heart and renal failure. What is the most likely diagnosis in this patient?

- a. Familial amyloid polyneuropathy type 1
- b. Familial amyloid polyneuropathy type 2
- c. Familial amyloid polyneuropathy type 3
- d. Primary amyloidosis
- e. Secondary amyloidosis

19. A 55-year-old woman presents with complaints of tingling and sensory loss over the right thumb, second digit, and third digit that wake her up at night. She has a history of left carpal tunnel syndrome, requiring surgery 3 years earlier. Examination reveals bilateral symmetric distal loss of pinprick sensation in the feet, but it is otherwise normal. Her mother and sister both have had bilateral carpal tunnel release. Review of systems is otherwise negative. What is the most likely diagnosis in this patient?

a. Familial amyloid polyneuropathy type 1
b. Familial amyloid polyneuropathy type 2
c. Familial amyloid polyneuropathy type 3
d. Primary amyloidosis
e. Secondary amyloidosis

20. A patient with long-standing diabetes has autonomic dysfunction. Which of the following is least likely to occur with diabetic autonomic neuropathy?

a. Impotence
b. Silent myocardial infarction
c. Resting tachycardia and loss of respiratory influence on the heart rate
d. Diarrhea that occurs typically during the daytime
e. Delayed gastric emptying

Questions 21–22

21. A 13-year-old girl is brought to the clinic by her mother for bilateral foot drop. As an infant and young child, she had always been clumsy and seemed to trip on her own feet, and could not participate in ballet classes. Over more recent years, her feet became noticeably weak. On examination, she had bilateral symmetric weakness of foot dorsiflexion and plantarflexion. She had hammertoes and high-arched feet. Ankle and knee deep tendon reflexes were absent. Examination of the mother also revealed hammertoes and high-arched feet. Conduction velocities of approximately 30 cm/second were revealed in all NCS of the legs, with no identifiable conduction block. What is the most likely diagnosis in this patient?

a. Charcot-Marie-Tooth (CMT) 1
b. CMT2
c. A muscular dystrophy
d. CMT3
e. CMT4

22. Regarding the various manifestations of the different subtypes of Charcot-Marie-Tooth (CMT), which of the following statements is incorrect?

a. Hammertoes and spine deformities are more prominent in CMT1 than CMT2
b. CMT2 typically has a later age of onset as compared to CMT1
c. CMT3, or Dejerine-Sottas syndrome, presents in infancy and typically leads to disabling weakness
d. Respiratory muscle involvement is common in the most common type of CMT
e. In some subtypes of CMT4, one of the axonal CMTs, vision or hearing loss occurs

23. Which of the following is correct regarding the median nerve?

a. The median nerve arises solely as a continuation of the medial cord
b. The median nerve carries C6 to T1 fibers
c. The median nerve innervates all forearm flexors
d. The median nerve innervates all intrinsic hand muscles
e. The median nerve innervates only forearm and hand muscles; it does not innervate any upper arm muscles

24. Which of the following treatment options has evidence to support its use for Guillain-Barre syndrome?

    a. Intravenous immunoglobulins (IVIGs) combined with steroids

    b. Steroids alone

    c. Plamapheresis combined with steroids

    d. Pyridostigmine

    e. IVIGs or plasmapheresis

Questions 25–26

25. Which of the following is incorrect regarding the lumbosacral plexus?

    a. The femoral nerve forms from posterior divisions of L2, L3, and L4

    b. The obturator nerve forms from anterior divisions of L2, L3, and L4

    c. Iliohypogastric, ilioinguinal, and genitofemoral nerves arise from the lumbosacral trunk

    d. The lumbosacral trunk joins the sacral plexus

    e. The lateral femoral cutaneous nerve arises from L2 and L3

26. Which of the following is incorrect regarding the lumbosacral plexus?

    a. The lumbosacral trunk originates from L4 and L5

    b. The posterior femoral cutaneous nerve provides sensory innervation to the lower buttock and posterior thigh

    c. The pudendal nerve arises from S2, S3, and S4 and provides sensory innervation to the perineal region

    d. The tensor fascia latae abducts the thigh when the hip is extended

    e. The largest nerve of the lumbosacral plexus is the sciatic nerve

27. A 22-year-old woman presents to the neuromuscular clinic with painless right foot drop. NCS show a conduction block at the fibular head. She admits to frequently crossing her legs. She is prescribed an ankle-foot orthosis, undergoes physical therapy, and does well, eventually regaining back all of the strength of her right foot. Six years later, she presents with weakness of her intrinsic hand muscles, and NCS show conduction block of the ulnar nerve at the elbow. She does recall hitting her "funny bone" several times a few days prior to evaluation. Her family history reveals that her father and brother had a history of similar episodes of weakness in the foot or arm since they were young adults. Which of the following is incorrect regarding the diagnosis of this patient?

    a. The peroneal nerve is most often affected, followed by the ulnar nerve

    b. It is caused by a deletion in peripheral myelin protein 22 (*PMP22*) gene

    c. It is autosomal dominant in inheritance with incomplete penetrance

    d. This patient has hereditary neuralgic amyotrophy

    e. Neuropathologic analysis of a nerve biopsy from this patient would show sausage-like thickening of the myelin, known as tomacula

28. Which of the following is correct regarding lower extremity innervation?

    a. Gluteus medius and tensor fascia latae receive innervation from the superior gluteal nerve

    b. Gluteus minimus receives innervation from the inferior gluteal nerve

    c. The long head of the biceps femoris is innervated by the peroneal division of the sciatic nerve

    d. Tibialis anterior is innervated by a branch of the tibial nerve

    e. A patient with inability to dorsiflex and evert the foot most likely has a lesion in the deep peroneal nerve

a. HIV testing
b. Monoclonal protein analysis
c. Hepatitis C antibody
d. Acetylcholine receptor antibodies
e. EMG/NCS

39. Which of the following inherited neuropathies are not autosomal dominant?
  a. Charcot-Marie-Tooth type (CMT) 1
  b. Hereditary sensory and autonomic neuropathy type 1
  c. CMT4
  d. Familial amyloid polyneuropathies
  e. Hereditary neuropathy with liability to pressure palsy

40. A 40-year-old man presents with pain in the right lower extremity radiating from the buttock down to his foot. He has pain and sensory deficit along the posterior thigh, leg, and lateral aspect of the foot. There is weakness on plantarflexion. Patellar reflex is normal, but the ankle reflex is depressed on the right side. Which of the following is the most likely diagnosis?
  a. L2 and L3 radiculopathy
  b. L4 radiculopathy
  c. L5 radiculopathy
  d. S1 radiculopathy
  e. Peroneal neuropathy

41. A 40-year-old man presents to the clinic complaining of left-hand weakness. He complains of significant loss of fine motor coordination in the left hand. On examination, he has atrophy of the intrinsic hand muscles, weakness of wrist flexion in an ulnar direction, flexion at the distal interphalangeal joint of fourth and fifth digits, and abduction and adduction of all the fingers. There is loss of sensation over the hypothenar eminence and the fourth and fifth digits, but not more proximally. Proximal arm muscle strength, forearm flexion and pronation, and flexion of the second and third digits at both the proximal and distal interphalangeal joints are of normal strength. Thumb abduction is mildly weak. On attempt to make a fist, there is hyperextension at the metacarpophalangeal joint of the fourth and fifth digits and flexion at the proximal but not distal interphalangeal joints. Ulnar nerve CMAPs are shown in Figure 9.4. What is the most likely diagnosis in this patient?
  a. A C8 radiculopathy
  b. Ulnar neuropathy at the wrist
  c. Medial cord lesion
  d. A C7 radiculopathy
  e. Ulnar neuropathy at or above the elbow

42. A 65-year-old man with type 2 diabetes mellitus presents with right lower extremity pain and weakness. He reports that symptoms began with severe low back pain radiating down his right hip and thigh. He then noticed difficulty flexing his hip and extending his knee. On examination, he has atrophy of the right thigh muscles and severe weakness of the hip flexors, adductors, quadriceps, and hamstring muscles on the right side. There are sensory deficits in the antero-medial thigh. His patellar reflex is absent on the same side. Which of the following is the most likely diagnosis?
  a. Small-fiber diabetic neuropathy
  b. Large-fiber diabetic neuropathy

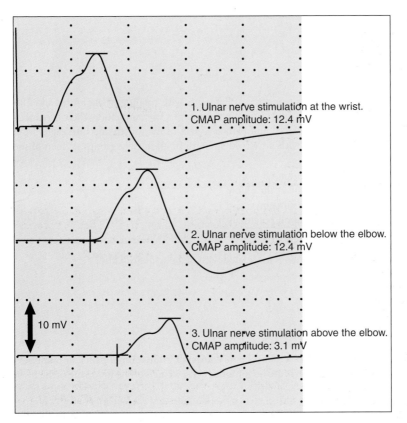

1. Ulnar nerve stimulation at the wrist.
CMAP amplitude: 12.4 mV

2. Ulnar nerve stimulation below the elbow.
CMAP amplitude: 12.4 mV

10 mV

3. Ulnar nerve stimulation above the elbow.
CMAP amplitude: 3.1 mV

FIGURE 9.4 Ulnar nerve motor NCS (Courtesy of Dr. Robert Shields)

   c. Diabetic autonomic neuropathy
   d. Diabetic mononeuropathy
   e. Diabetic amyotrophy

43. Which of the following is incorrect regarding the radial nerve?
   a. It is a continuation of the posterior cord
   b. It carries C5, C6, C7, and C8 fibers
   c. It innervates all three heads of the triceps muscle
   d. It provides sensory innervation to most of the posterolateral arm and forearm
   e. All of the forearm muscles innervated by the radial nerve are forearm extensors

44. A 50-year-old woman is admitted for asthma exacerbation, and suffers multiple medical complications during her hospitalization. She is bedridden for more than 4 weeks and is found to have a right foot drop. On neurologic evaluation, there is weakness in dorsiflexion and eversion of the foot. An NCS is performed and demonstrates reduced CMAP amplitude of the tibialis anterior and extensor digitorum brevis, as well as reduced SNAP amplitude of the superficial peroneal. EMG shows fibrillations in the tibialis anterior, extensor hallucis, extensor digitorum brevis, and peroneus longus. Short head of the biceps femoris is normal. Other muscles tested demonstrated no abnormalities. Which of the following is the most likely diagnosis?

a. Common peroneal nerve
b. Deep peroneal nerve
c. L5 nerve root
d. Sciatic nerve
e. Tibial nerve

45. A 52-year-old truck driver since his teenage years presents with tingling in the fourth and fifth digits of his left hand. The tingling is mild but annoying to him. On examination, there is reduced sensation to all modalities on the dorsal and palmar aspect of the fourth and fifth digits from the wrist crease to the finger tips, with preserved strength in all muscle groups. Which of the following statements is correct?
a. This man has carpal tunnel syndrome
b. This man has an ulnar neuropathy at the elbow
c. This man should be referred to a surgeon
d. EMG is expected to show fibrillation potentials in the C6 and C7 myotomes
e. Conservative management frequently fails in this type of disorder

46. Which of the following complications is associated with diabetic neuropathy?
a. Foot ulcers
b. Arthropathy affecting the ankles
c. Sensory ataxia
d. Acute third nerve palsy
e. All of the above

47. A 30-year-old obese man who works as a mechanic comes for evaluation of pain and numbness in the lateral aspect of his thigh. There are no motor deficits. Which of the following is the most likely structure involved?
a. Lateral femoral cutaneous nerve
b. Femoral nerve
c. Saphenous nerve
d. Obturator nerve
e. Lumbosacral plexus

48. A 50-year-old man undergoes coronary artery stenting performed through a femoral artery puncture. After the procedure, he becomes hypotensive and requires admission to the ICU. His hematocrit drops and he needs blood transfusion. He later notices pain with hip flexion and numbness in the anterior and medial thigh. He also has difficulty flexing the hip and extending the knee, and his patellar reflex is absent. Three weeks later, NCS show a reduced saphenous SNAP. On needle EMG, fibrillation potentials are seen in the iliacus and quadriceps muscles. Thigh adductors and muscles below the knee show no abnormalities. Which of the following is correct?
a. This is consistent with a femoral nerve injury at the inguinal region
b. This is consistent with a femoral nerve injury in the intrapelvic region
c. This patient has a lumbar plexopathy
d. This patient has an obturator nerve injury
e. This patient has involvement of the nerve arising from the anterior divisions of L2, L3, and L4 spinal roots

49. A 50-year-old woman with a 10-year history of type 2 diabetes mellitus presents with burning pain in both feet. Sensation to vibration and proprioception is preserved, as are the deep tendon reflexes. Which of the following most likely explains her symptoms?

a. Small fiber diabetic neuropathy
b. Large fiber diabetic neuropathy
c. Diabetic polyradiculoneuropathy
d. Diabetic mononeuropathy
e. Diabetic amyotrophy

50. A 73-year-old man with poorly controlled diabetes presents with complaints of painless weakness of extension of the fingers in the left hand. On examination, forearm extension and wrist extension and abduction (wrist extension in a radial direction) are normal in strength, but wrist extension and adduction (wrist extension in an ulnar direction) are weak. Forearm supination is weak, particularly when tested with the forearm extended, but there is no pain with active supination. Finger extension at the metacarpophalangeal joints is also weak, as is thumb abduction in the plane of the palm, and thumb extension at the interphalangeal and metacarpophalangeal joint. Sensory examination is normal. On NCS, the superficial sensory radial nerve is normal. Triceps deep tendon reflex is normal. What is the most likely diagnosis?
    a. Radial neuropathy at the spiral groove
    b. C7 radiculopathy
    c. Posterior interosseus nerve palsy
    d. Radial neuropathy at the elbow
    e. Supinator syndrome

51. A 38-year-old man presents with pain in the left lower extremity. The pain and sensory deficits are localized to the anterior thigh and medial leg. There is weakness on hip flexion, knee extension, and ankle dorsiflexion. The patellar reflex on the left is depressed and the ankle reflex is normal. Saphenous SNAP is normal. On EMG, fibrillation potentials are seen in the iliacus, vastus lateralis and medialis, rectus femoris and tibialis anterior muscles. Paraspinal fibrillations are also appreciated. Which of the following is the most likely diagnosis?
    a. Lumbar plexopathy
    b. L2, L3 and L4 radiculopathy
    c. L5 radiculopathy
    d. S1 radiculopathy
    e. Femoral neuropathy

52. A 24-year-old man undergoes minimally invasive mitral valve repair. He does well with normal arm strength until 3 days postoperatively when he begins experiencing severe shoulder and arm pain. The pain resolves 7 days later, but his arm becomes weak over ensuing days. He has weakness of shoulder abductors, arm external rotators, forearm flexors, forearm pronators, and finger flexors. What is the most likely diagnosis in this patient?
    a. Cervical-brachial-pharyngeal variant of Guillian-Barre syndrome
    b. Acute brachial plexitis (Parsonage-Turner syndrome)
    c. Post-sternotomy brachial plexus lesion
    d. Infectious polyradiculitis
    e. An axillary neuropathy due to positioning during the operation

Questions 53–54

53. A 32-year-old man sustains a knife stab wound to the left antecubital fossa. He is brought to the emergency department where he is treated for brachial artery hemorrhage and is otherwise stabilized. On follow-up 8 weeks later, he denies any pain in his limb. He has Medical Research

Council grade 2/5 strength in forearm pronation, thumb opposition, flexion, and abduction, flexion at the distal interphalangeal joint of the second digit, and flexion at the proximal interphalangeal joint of the second to fifth digits. Wrist flexion is 4/5, but the hand deviates in an ulnar direction during flexion. Flexion at the distal interphalangeal joint of the fourth and fifth digits is normal. Sensation is markedly reduced on the distal dorsal aspect of the first three digits and on the lateral (radial) aspect of the palm and first three digits, as well as the lateral (radial) aspect of the fourth digit. When asked to make a fist, the patient can barely flex the thumb, can partially flex the second digit, and has normal flexion of the fourth and fifth digits. What is the most likely diagnosis in this patient?

  a. Complete median nerve palsy at the level of the antecubital fossa
  b. Ischemic monomelia
  c. Anterior interosseus nerve syndrome
  d. A medial cord lesion
  e. A C7 radiculopathy

54. A 52-year-old woman presents to the neuromuscular clinic complaining of finger weakness in the right hand. She reports difficulty holding a teacup with the right hand using a pincer grasp. She denies any sensory symptoms. On examination of the right upper limb, there is weakness of flexion at the distal interphalangeal joint of the second and third digits, weakness of thumb flexion, and weakness of forearm pronation when the forearm is fully flexed. Otherwise, all other muscles groups are of normal strength, and there is no evidence of sensory loss. What is the most likely diagnosis in this patient?

  a. Complete median nerve palsy at the level of the antecubital fossa
  b. Ischemic monomelia
  c. Anterior interosseus nerve syndrome
  d. A medial cord lesion
  e. A C7 radiculopathy

Questions 55–56

55. An lumbar puncture is obtained on a patient with suspected Guillain-Barre syndrome. Which of the following findings do you expect?

  a. Increased lymphocytes with normal protein
  b. Increased neutrophils with normal protein
  c. Increased protein with normal cell count
  d. Abnormal CSF production of immunoglobulins, with the presence of oligoclonal bands and myelin basic protein
  e. Increased RBCs

56. Which of the following findings does not occur in Guillain-Barre syndrome?

  a. MRI showing gadolinium enhancement in the cauda equina
  b. Abnormal or prolonged F-responses on NCS
  c. Persistently normal distal latencies on NCS
  d. Conduction block
  e. Abnormal H-reflex

57. A 62-year-old woman presents to the neuromuscular clinic with complaints of painless right upper extremity weakness and sensory loss. She has a history of cancer of the right breast for which she had undergone surgery, chemotherapy, and radiation 3 years earlier. On examination, she has weakness in arm abduction and adduction, forearm flexion and extension, wrist flexion and extension, and sensory loss over the entire arm. EMG confirms involvement of all muscles examined, and myokymic discharges are evident on the EMG. Her left arm and lower extremities are normal. What is the most likely diagnosis in this patient?

a. Carcinomatous invasion of the brachial plexus
b. Chemotherapy-induced neuropathy
c. Radiation-induced brachial plexopathy
d. Paraneoplastic sensorimotor neuropathy
e. Cervical spine stenosis

58. A 56-year-old man with a history of diarrhea 2 weeks prior, presents with 4 days of difficulty walking and diplopia. On examination, he is very unsteady, and cannot walk straight. The motor examination shows full strength; however, the ankle and patellar reflexes are absent. Which of the following antibodies may be involved?

a. GM1
b. GD1a
c. GD1b
d. GQ1b
e. GalNac-GD1a

59. A 19-year-old man is hired as a packager on an assembly line. His main job is to take heavy objects off the conveyer belt and place them in a box that immediately follows the object on the belt. He does this hundreds of times a day using his right arm. He presents to the company physician 3 months after he starts his job complaining of a deep aching pain in the proximal right forearm that worsens with forearm pronation against resistance. On examination, motor testing is limited due to pain, but weakness of wrist flexion, thumb abduction, and flexion of the second digit is apparent. Strength of forearm pronation appears normal. What is the most likely diagnosis?

a. Complete median nerve palsy at the elbow
b. Pronator teres syndrome
c. Anterior interosseus nerve syndrome
d. A medial cord lesion
e. A C7 radiculopathy

60. Which of the following is incorrect regarding the management of patients with carpal tunnel syndrome?

a. In patients without known risk factors for carpal tunnel, and in the appropriate clinical setting, testing for hypothyroidism and diabetes is indicated
b. Acromegaly can be a cause of carpal tunnel syndrome
c. Amyloidosis can be a cause of carpal tunnel syndrome
d. Surgical therapy is indicated in asymptomatic carpal tunnel syndrome
e. Surgical release for carpal tunnel syndrome is indicated in severe cases

Questions 61–62

61. A 34-year-old woman fractures her left tibia. Because of several complications, she requires the use of crutches over several months. She later presents to the neuromuscular clinic with complaints of weakness in her right arm. On examination, she has weakness in forearm extension, wrist extension, and finger extension, as well as sensory loss along the posterolateral arm, forearm, and dorsolateral hand. The triceps deep tendon reflex is absent. Arm adduction and abduction, forearm pronation, and wrist flexion are normal in strength. What is the most likely diagnosis in this patient?

a. Radial neuropathy at the spiral groove

b. Radial neuropathy at the axilla

c. Radial neuropathy at the elbow

d. C7 radiculopathy

e. Posterior cord lesion

62. A 37-year-old man is involved in a motor vehicle accident and fractures his right humerus. He later presents to a clinic with complaints of weakness in wrist and finger extension. On examination, forearm extension is strong. Wrist extension in both the radial and ulnar direction and finger extension are weak, and there is loss of sensation on the lower lateral arm and posterior forearm. What is the most likely diagnosis in this patient?

a. C7 radiculopathy

b. Radial neuropathy at the axilla

c. Radial neuropathy at the elbow

d. Radial neuropathy at the spiral groove

e. Posterior cord lesion

63. A 52-year-old man is diagnosed with a neck mass, and undergoes excision of the mass, with intraoperative frozen sections showing adenocarcinoma with positive margins. The surgeon elects to pursue a radical neck dissection with extensive excision. Following initial recovery, the patient reports weakness in raising his right arm above his head. On examination, his right shoulder is noted to be hanging at a lower level as compared to the left. Right arm abduction to 90 degrees is normal, but there is weakness of arm abduction above that level. Shoulder shrug is Medical Research Council 4/5 in strength. There is weakness in head turning to the left. Otherwise, upper extremity examination is normal, and there is no sensory loss in the head, neck, or arm region. Cranial nerve examination and gag reflex are otherwise normal as well. What is the most likely diagnosis in this patient?

a. Lesser occipital nerve injury

b. Jugular foramen syndrome

c. Cervical plexus injury

d. Spinal accessory nerve injury

e. Greater occipital nerve injury

64. Which of the following presentations of nervous system involvement can occur with diabetes?

a. Small-fiber neuropathy

b. Large-fiber neuropathy

c. Autonomic neuropathy

d. Only a and c

e. All of the above

65. A 48-year-old man presents with numbness, tingling, and weakness. He initially experienced weakness in the right hand and later developed weakness in the left hand and left foot. He also has painful paresthesias in the right hand and left foot. Deep tendon reflexes are normal in the right lower limb, but decreased everywhere else. His CSF shows a protein level of 75 mg/dL (normal up to 45 mg/dL) and cell count of 3/mm^3 (normal up to 5 lymphocytes/mm^3). There is

evidence of conduction block in many peripheral nerves and abnormal sensory NCS. Which of the following is the most likely diagnosis?

a. Chronic inflammatory demyelinating polyneuropathy
b. Acute inflammatory demyelinating polyeneuropathy
c. Multifocal motor neuropathy
d. Multifocal acquired demyelinating sensory and motor neuropathy
e. Subacute inflammatory demyelinating polyneuropathy

66. A 19-year-old man is arrested during attempted robbery. While he is transported to the jail, he is agitated, and keeps pulling on the handcuffs. The prison physician is later called to see him for numbness of his right hand, because there was concern that he was having a stroke. On examination, he had decreased sensation over the dorsolateral aspect of the right hand, with normal motor strength and normal sensation in other areas. What is the most likely diagnosis?

a. Acute ischemic stroke in the hand area of the postcentral sulcus
b. Carpal tunnel syndrome
c. The symptoms are not consistent with any particular neurologic disorder; this man is malingering
d. Superficial sensory radial neuropathy
e. C8 radiculopathy

67. A 32-year-old man is involved in a motorcycle accident and sustains an anterior shoulder dislocation. Six weeks later, he presents to the clinic complaining of weakness in flexion of his right forearm at the elbow. On examination, right forearm flexion strength is Medical Research Council grade 2/5, and there is minimal palpable contraction of arm muscles during attempted forearm flexion. Forearm supination is 2/5 in strength with the forearm flexed, and 4/5 in strength with the forearm extended. The biceps deep tendon reflex is absent. Arm adduction is normal in strength. Forearm pronation, and distal motor strength, such as wrist flexion, is normal. There is diminished sensation over the lateral aspect of the forearm, but sensation over the thumb and second digit is normal. What is the most likely diagnosis in this patient?

a. Biceps tendon rupture
b. C6 radiculopathy
c. Median neuropathy at the elbow
d. Lateral cord lesion
e. Musculocutaneous neuropathy

68. A 62-year-old woman presents for evaluation of severe pain and paresthesias in her feet. Sensory examination shows impairments to pinprick and temperature below the ankles. Motor examination and reflexes are preserved. A small-fiber neuropathy is considered. Which of the following is incorrect regarding this condition?

a. Diabetes is a common cause of this condition
b. Quantitative sudomotor axon reflex test can be used for diagnosis
c. Skin biopsy and intraepidermal nerve fiber density can be used for diagnosis
d. Thermoregulatory sweat test can be used for diagnosis
e. EMG/NCS are usually abnormal

69. A 10-year-old girl falls off a ledge and fractures the proximal humerus. After her cast is removed, she is noted to have weakness of the arm, and neurologic consultation is requested. On examination, she is able to abduct the arm up to around 30 degrees, but not beyond that. Arm flexion

is Medical Research Council grade 2/5. Sensory examination reveals a small area of hypoesthesia on the lateral aspect of the upper arm, but is otherwise normal. Arm adduction, forearm pronation, and forearm, wrist, and finger extension, are of normal strength. What is the most likely diagnosis in this patient?

a. Axillary neuropathy
b. Radial neuropathy
c. Posterior cord lesion
d. C5 radiculopathy
e. Middle trunk lesion

70. A 39-year-old man is admitted to the ICU with an acute pontine infarct. Work-up shows a dolichoectatic basilar artery with a partially thrombosed aneurysm. Echocardiogram reveals a dilated cardiomyopathy. On questioning of family members, it is revealed that since adolescence, he had complained of severe burning pains in his hands and feet with heat exposure or exercise, but his pediatrician had attributed them to growing pains and they had not been fully investigated. On examination, he has several dark-purplish punctuate lesions on his trunk and scrotum. His father suffered from burning hands and feet and in middle age required dialysis for renal failure of unclear etiology. Which of the following is correct regarding the disorder depicted in this case?

a. It is due to a deficiency of the enzyme arylsulfatase A
b. It is due to a deficiency in the enzyme α-galactosidase A
c. It is autosomal dominant in inheritance
d. The stroke in this patient is likely unrelated to his underlying condition
e. It is a glycogen storage disease

71. A 38-year-old athlete sustains an injury while playing football. Eight weeks later, he presents to a neuromuscular clinic with right arm weakness. He has Medical Research Council motor power of 4/5 in external rotation of the arm, forearm flexion, and shoulder abduction. There is sensory loss over the lateral aspect of the arm and forearm. The biceps deep tendon reflex is absent. On EMG, there are fibrillation potentials in the biceps, brachialis, deltoid, brachioradialis, supraspinatus, and rhomboid muscles. EMG examination of the triceps, pronator teres, brachioradialis, and intrinsic hand muscles is normal. Which of the following best explains this patient's weakness?

a. An upper brachial plexus trunk lesion
b. An axillary nerve lesion
c. A C5 and C6 root lesion
d. A lesion to the musculocutaneous nerve
e. A lesion to the lateral cord of the brachial plexus

72. A 45-year-old athlete who spends several hours a day weight lifting presents with deep, aching shoulder pain and arm weakness. On examination, he has weakness of shoulder abduction and external rotation with the forearm flexed while the elbow is stabilized against the patient's side. Sensory examination is normal, and arm adduction is normal. Winging of the scapula is not evident. Forearm flexion is normal, and the biceps deep tendon reflex is normal. This is most consistent with

a. Injury to the thoracodorsal nerve
b. Suprascapular nerve entrapment
c. Long thoracic nerve injury
d. C5 radiculopathy
e. An upper trunk lesion

73. A 55-year-old man with mild truncal obesity, hyperlipidemia, and long-standing diabetes comes referred from gastroenterology. Four months ago, he developed bulging in the right lower abdomen with a patch of numbness and a sensation of burning to touch in this area. You examine him and find that he has an absent superficial abdominal reflex in the right lower quadrant of the abdomen, as well as patchy reduction to pinprick and light touch on both sides of the abdominal wall at approximately T10 to T12. You feel his history is most consistent with the following:

a. Spinal cord ischemia
b. Stretch neuropathy due to obesity
c. Femoral nerve injury
d. Thoracoabdominal polyradiculopathy
e. Malingering

74. An 18-year-old woman presents to the clinic complaining of right-hand weakness. She reports that for many months while cheerleading, with her arms abducted and externally rotated and forearms flexed (holding up her pom-poms) she feels a dull ache and tingling in her hand, mainly in the fourth and fifth digits. More recently, the aching has become more continuous and she has noted some numbness of the medial forearm. Examination shows weakness of thumb abduction away from the plane of the palm, and weakness of finger abduction and adduction, with subtle atrophy of the hand muscles. There is sensory loss over the medial aspect of the hand and forearm. What is the most likely diagnosis in this patient?

a. Ulnar neuropathy at the elbow
b. Carpal tunnel syndrome
c. Neurogenic thoracic outlet syndrome
d. C8 radiculopathy
e. Median neuropathy at the elbow

Questions 75–77

75. A 20-year-old woman presents to the clinic with debilitating shooting pains in the feet and legs. Examination shows loss of sensation to pinprick and temperature, with mildly reduced sensation to vibration and fine touch. Proprioception is intact in the fingers and toes. She is fearful that she is developing the condition that her father and paternal grandfather suffered from; they both are deceased, and she does not recall details, but remembers that as far back as she could remember, they had problems with foot ulcerations and odd deformities in their toes and ankles, and her father had required a below-the-knee amputation. On directed questioning, she admits to heat intolerance and feels she does not sweat the way other people normally would. What is the most likely diagnosis in this patient?

a. Hereditary sensory and autonomic neuropathy (HSAN) type 1
b. Charcot-Marie-Tooth 1A
c. HSAN type 2
d. HSAN type 3
e. HSAN type 4

76. The parents of a 1-year-old boy bring him to the clinic with multiple concerns. In the first month of life he was noted to have trouble swallowing and suffered from aspiration pneumonia, and a percutaneous gastrostomy tube was placed. During that admission, his blood pressure was noted to be "all over the place." His parents noticed that when he cried, he would not produce tears, but would become very flushed and sweat dramatically. What is the most likely diagnosis in this patient?

 a. Hereditary sensory and autonomic neuropathy (HSAN) type 1
 b. Charcot-Marie-Tooth 1A
 c. HSAN type 2
 d. HSAN type 3
 e. HSAN type 4

77. A 2-year-old girl is brought to the pediatric neurologist by her parents. She had suffered from recurrent fevers since childhood, but no matter what fluctuations occurred in her body temperature, she would never sweat. An infectious cause to her fevers could not be identified. They noticed that she did not cry when she received her vaccinations, and since she had started walking, if she bumped into an object or fell, she did not seem to feel pain, even when she sustained a significant abrasion or bruise. What is the most likely diagnosis in this patient?
 a. Hereditary sensory and autonomic neuropathy (HSAN) type 1
 b. Charcot-Marie-Tooth 1A
 c. HSAN type 2
 d. HSAN type 3
 e. HSAN type 4

78. Which of the following conditions does not present as mononeuritis multiplex?
 a. Vasculitic neuropathy
 b. Diabetes
 c. Guillain-Barre syndrome
 d. Cryoglobulinemic vasculitis
 e. Neuropathy associated with HIV

79. A 37-year-old man presents with right wrist drop and left foot drop, associated with painful paresthesias, rash, and arthralgias. A blood sample is sent for evaluation, detecting precipitation of protein when exposed to cold temperature. Which of the following is incorrect?
 a. Commonly associated with hepatitis C
 b. This patient has multiple mononeuropathies associated with cryoglobulinemia
 c. Complement levels are elevated
 d. May be associated with HIV
 e. Multiple myeloma may be associated

80. A 22-year-old man presents to the clinic with complaints of severe pain and redness of the limbs with exercise or whenever the weather is warm. When these episodes occur, he goes home and sits in a tub of ice water until he cools down. These episodes have become so severe that he minimizes physical exertion despite having a love for sports, and is actually thinking of moving north to prevent heat exposure. He is otherwise healthy, and physical examination is normal. His father suffers from similar symptoms. Routine laboratory testing, including complete blood count and fasting glucose, are normal. What is the most likely diagnosis in this patient?
 a. Hereditary sensory and autonomic neuropathy type 1
 b. Primary erythromelalgia
 c. Secondary erythromelalgia
 d. Fabry's disease
 e. Small fiber neuropathy associated with glucose intolerance

81. A 57-year-old man presents with 3 months of gradually progressive neurologic symptoms that began with numbness and dysesthesias in his hands and feet, which have worsened. More recently, he has been having difficulty walking, especially when it is dark, and reports that he feels unsteady when he closes his eyes. On examination, he has ataxia in all four limbs when he closes his eyes, patchy sensory deficits in various parts of his body without a distal-to-proximal gradient, and areflexia. His strength is normal. NCS demonstrate bilateral asymmetric reduction of SNAPs in various sensory nerves, more in the upper than lower extremities, with normal CMAPs. Which of the following is incorrect regarding this condition?
    a. SSA and SSB antibodies should be obtained
    b. Anti-Hu antibodies should be obtained
    c. Lung cancer should be ruled out
    d. The dorsal root ganglia are likely involved
    e. Pyridoxine should be supplemented at high doses

82. A 36-year-old man is standing on the ledge of the balcony of his fourth-floor apartment and is putting up Christmas lights. He starts to fall, but luckily grabs onto the railing of the balcony with his left hand, and is left barely hanging from the railing with his finger tips. His brother hears him crying for help and assists him. He experiences severe pain in his arm, but is relieved to have not fallen to the ground. Over the next several days, he notices difficulty with fine motor movements of his left hand. On examination, he has weakness of finger flexion at the proximal and distal interphalangeal joint of the second to fifth digits, weakness of finger abduction and adduction, weakness of thumb abduction away from the plane of the palm, and weakness of wrist flexion in an ulnar (medial) direction. There is sensory loss over the medial forearm and fourth and fifth digits, but sensation is otherwise intact. Arm and forearm flexors and extensors as well as wrist and finger extensors are strong. What is the most likely diagnosis in this patient?
    a. Ulnar neuropathy at the wrist
    b. Median neuropathy at the elbow
    c. Radial neuropathy
    d. Lower trunk lesion
    e. Lateral cord lesion

83. A 14-year-old girl presents to the emergency department with severe abdominal pain, nausea, and vomiting. Routine laboratory testing including liver enzymes is normal. She is admitted to the hospital and treated with intravenous fluids. Two days later, she is witnessed to have a generalized tonic-clonic seizure. She subsequently begins experiencing hallucinations and delusions. MRI of the brain with contrast and CSF analysis are normal. Four days after admission, she is noted to have mild weakness of wrist extension; one week later, examination shows bilateral wrist drop. What is the most likely diagnosis in this patient?
    a. Wilson's disease
    b. Systemic lupus erythematosuis
    c. Acute inflammatory demyelinating polyneuropathy
    d. Acute disseminated encephalomyelitis
    e. Acute intermittent porphyria

84. A 32-year-old man is being evaluated by a company physician prior to employment. The physician notices the patient's arm is weak; on further questioning, the patient states, "I've been like this since I was born, my mom said that's just how I was made." On examination, he holds his right arm close to his body, internally rotated, with his wrist and fingers flexed. Arm abduction and flexion are weak. Arm extension is normal in strength. Biceps deep tendon reflex is absent,

but triceps deep tendon reflex is normal. There is sensory loss along the lateral half of the arm and forearm and the thumb and index finger. EMG shows no evidence of denervation in the rhomboids. What is the most likely diagnosis in this patient?

a. An axillary neuropathy
b. An upper trunk lesion
c. A C7 root lesion
d. A middle trunk lesion
e. A C5 and C6 root lesion

85. A 39-year-old woman with type 1 diabetes mellitus presents for evaluation. She has numbness in a glove and stocking distribution affecting hands and feet. She has no pain. There is loss of sensation to vibration and proprioception, and she is hyporeflexic distally. Which of the following most likely explains her symptoms?

a. Small fiber diabetic neuropathy
b. Large fiber diabetic neuropathy
c. Diabetic polyradiculoneuropathy
d. Diabetic mononeuropathy
e. Diabetic amyotrophy

86. A 60-year-old woman presents with 2 months of pain radiating from her buttock down to her right leg. She has foot drop on the right, with severe foot dorsiflexion weakness. There is sensory deficit in the right lateral leg and dorsum of the foot. NCS show reduced peroneal CMAPs recording from the tibialis anterior and extensor digitor brevis muscles and normal superficial peroneal SNAP. Needle EMG shows fibrillations and reduced recruitment in the tibialis anterior, extensor digitorum brevis, extensor hallucis, peroneous longus, tibialis posterior, and flexor digitorum longus. Which of the following is the most likely diagnosis?

a. L5 radiculopathy
b. S1 radiculopathy
c. Common peroneal neuropathy
d. Deep peroneal injury
e. Sciatic nerve injury

Answer key

1. d	16. b	31. e	46. e	61. b	76. d
2. e	17. d	32. d	47. a	62. d	77. e
3. c	18. a	33. d	48. b	63. d	78. c
4. e	19. b	34. e	49. a	64. e	79. c
5. d	20. d	35. c	50. c	65. d	80. b
6. b	21. a	36. d	51. b	66. d	81. e
7. d	22. d	37. b	52. b	67. e	82. d
8. c	23. e	38. d	53. a	68. e	83. e
9. e	24. e	39. c	54. c	69. a	84. b
10. b	25. c	40. d	55. c	70. b	85. b
11. b	26. d	41. e	56. c	71. c	86. a
12. a	27. d	42. e	57. c	72. b	
13. d	28. a	43. e	58. d	73. d	
14. c	29. a	44. a	59. b	74. c	
15. a	30. d	45. b	60. d	75. a	

Answers

1. d

The history and examination of the patient in question 1 are consistent with giant axonal neuropathy (GAN). This is a rare autosomal recessive disorder that manifests in early childhood. It affects intermediate filaments of both the central and peripheral nervous system, leading to a sensorimotor neuropathy, corticospinal tract involvement with upper motor neuron signs, and optic atrophy leading to vision loss. The characteristic gait includes walking on the inner edges of the feet. The integument is also involved, and patients often have tightly curled hair. The neuropathy is predominantly axonal, and neuropathologic analysis of nerves from patients with this disorder reveal pathognomonic findings of large focal axonal swelling that contain tightly packed disorganized neurofilaments. This disorder is due to mutations in the *GAN* gene that encodes for gigaxonin, which is involved in cross-linking of intermediate filaments. It is progressive, and death typically occurs by adolescence.

The clinical history, particularly the hair findings, characteristic gait, evidence of CNS involvement, and neuropathologic findings distinguish GAN from Dejerine-Sottas syndrome, or Charcot-Marie-Tooth type (CMT) type 3 (discussed in questions 21 and 22), CMT4 (discussed in question 39), and CMT2A (discussed in questions 21 and 22), which also manifest in childhood and can be quite severe. Metachromatic leukodystrophy (MCL) (discussed in Chapter 14) is also a severe neurodegenerative disorder that manifests in early life; clinical manifestations include both central and peripheral nervous system manifestations. MCL is distinguished from GAN on the basis of the neuropathologic and imaging features, as well as biochemical studies, including elevated urine sulfatides in MCL (see Chapter 14).

Bradley WG, Daroff RB, Fenichel GM, et al. Neurology in Clinical Practice, 5th ed. Philadelphia, PA: Elsevier; 2008.

2. e

This patient's history, examination, and laboratory testing are consistent with Refsum's disease (RD). RD is an autosomal dominant peroxisomal disorder that results from a defect in an enzyme involved in fatty acid metabolism, leading to accumulation of an intermediate in this pathway, phytanic acid. Clinical manifestations include retinitis pigmentosa (with night blindness and visual field constriction), cardiomyopathy, and skin changes. Neurologic manifestations include neuropathy, hearing loss, anosmia, ataxia, and cerebellar signs. The neuropathy is a large-fiber sensorimotor neuropathy. The presence of overriding toes due to a shortened fourth metatarsal may aid in the diagnosis. Treatment includes dietary modification to reduce dietary intake of phytanic acid.

Clinical features of the other disorders listed also include retinitis pigmentosa and neuropathy, but elevated phytanic acid levels are diagnostic of Refsum's disease. In myoneurogastrointestinal encephalopathy (MNGIE), intestinal pseudo-obstruction is a prominent feature; other features include ophthalmoparesis and a demyelinating neuropathy. MNGIE is due to a mutation in the thymidine phosphorylase gene.

Abetalipoproteinemia, also known as Bassen-Kornzweig syndrome, is an autosomal recessive disorder that results in defective triglyceride transport, leading to abnormal very low density lipoprotein secretion. Fat malabsorption results in deficiencies in vitamins A, E, D, and K. Low levels of serum β-lipoprotein and vitamin E in the serum suggest the diagnosis. Peripheral smear shows acanthocytes. Clinical manifestations include retinitis pigmentosa, neuropathy, and ataxia.

Neurogenic muscle weakness, ataxia, and retinitis pigmentosa syndrome is a mitochondrial cytopathy that results from a mutation in the adenosine triphosphate 6 gene. Patients may present with a predominantly sensory axonal neuropathy. Other mitochondrial cytopathies including mitochondrial encephalopathy with lactic acidosis and stroke-like symptoms and disorders due to polymerase γ mutations can also lead to neuropathy.

Kearns-Sayre syndrome (KSS) is a mitochondrial disorder resulting from a mutation in mitochondrial DNA. It manifests before the age of 20 with retinitis pigmentosa, progressive opthalmoplegia, cardiac conduction defects, ataxia, myopathy, and hearing loss; neuropathy is not a prominent feature of KSS.

Bradley WG, Daroff RB, Fenichel GM, et al. Neurology in Clinical Practice, 5th ed. Philadelphia, PA: Elsevier; 2008.

Ropper AH, Samuels MA. Adams and Victor's Principles of Neurology, 9th ed. New York: McGraw-Hill; 2009.

3. c, 4. e

Significant axon loss lesions produce reductions in action potential amplitudes and tend to have preserved or mildly reduced conduction velocities. The F-wave is obtained after supramaximal stimulation of a motor nerve.

NCS are classified into sensory and motor conduction studies. Sensory NCS are obtained by stimulating a sensory nerve while recording the transmitted potential at a different site along the same nerve. Three main measures can be obtained: SNAP amplitude, sensory distal latency, and conduction velocity. The SNAP amplitude (in microvolts) represents a measure of the number of axons conducting between the stimulation site and the recording site. Sensory distal latency (in ms) is the time that it takes for the action potential to travel between the stimulation site and the recording site of the nerve. The conduction velocity is measured in meters per second and is obtained dividing the distance between two sites of stimulation by the differences of the latencies between these two sites: Conduction velocity = Distance/(Proximal latency − Distal latency).

Motor NCS are obtained by stimulating a motor nerve and recording at the belly of a muscle innervated by that nerve. The CMAP is the resulting response, and depends on the motor axons transmitting the action potential, status of the neuromuscular junction, and muscle fibers. The CMAP amplitudes, motor latencies, and conduction velocities are routinely assessed and analyzed.

In general, for sensory and motor responses, a decrease in the amplitudes correlates with axon loss lesions. On the other hand, prolonged latencies and slow conduction velocities correlate with demyelination. Low amplitudes can result from demyelinating conduction block when the nerve stimulation is proximal to the block.

The F-wave and the H-reflex are late responses. The F-wave is obtained after supramaximal stimulation of a motor nerve while recording from a muscle. The electrical impulse travels antidromically (conduction along the axon opposite to the normal direction of impulses) along the motor axons toward the motor neuron, backfiring and traveling orthodromically (conduction along the motor axon in the normal direction) down the nerve to be recorded at the muscle. The H-reflex is the electrophysiologic equivalent of the ankle reflex (S1 reflex arc) and is obtained by stimulating the tibial nerve at the popliteal fossa while recording at the soleus. The electrical impulse travels orthodromically through a sensory afferent, enters the spinal cord, and synapses with the anterior horn cell, traveling down the motor nerve to be recorded at the muscle.

Katirji B. Electromyography in Clinical Practice: A Case Study Approach, 1st ed. St. Louis: Mosby; 1998.

Preston DC, Schapiro BE. Electromyography and Neuromuscular Disorders, 2nd ed. Philadelphia, PA: Elsevier; 2005.

5. d

Large polyphasic motor unit potentials (MUPs) are not seen in acute neuropathic lesions, but rather in chronic ones.

When performing needle EMG examination, insertional and spontaneous activity as well as voluntary MUP activity should be characterized. Insertional activity is recorded as the needle is inserted into a relaxed muscle. It is increased in denervated muscles and myotonic disorders, and is decreased when the muscle is replaced by fat or connective tissue and during episodes of periodic paralysis. Spontaneous activity is assessed with the muscle at rest, and examples include fibrillation potentials, fasciculation potentials, and myokymia and myotonic potentials. All spontaneous activity is abnormal.

MUPs are obtained while the needle is inserted into the muscle during voluntary contraction. Various characteristics are of consideration, including recruitment pattern and MUP parameters, such as duration, amplitude, and configuration. Recruitment is a measure of the number of MUPs firing during increased force of voluntary muscle contraction. In axon loss lesions, reduced recruitment is characterized by a less-than-expected number of MUPs firing rapidly. Early or rapid recruitment occurs in myopathic processes with loss of muscle fibers, in which an excessive number of short-duration and small-amplitude MUPs fire during the muscle contraction. With poor voluntary effort or with CNS disorders causing weakness, recruitment is reduced with normal MUPs firing at slow or moderate rates, sometimes in a variable fashion. In neuropathic disorders with denervation and reinnervation, MUPs disclose increased duration and amplitude, and may be polyphasic. In myopathic disorders, MUPs are of reduced duration and amplitude, and may also be polyphasic.

Katirji B. Electromyography in Clinical Practice: A Case Study Approach, 1st ed. St. Louis: Mosby; 1998.

Preston DC, Schapiro BE. Electromyography and Neuromuscular Disorders, 2nd ed. Philadelphia, PA: Elsevier; 2005.

6. b

In a radiculopathy, there are normal SNAPs despite sensory symptoms.

The dorsal root ganglion is located just outside the spinal canal within the intervertebral foramen. It has sensory unipolar neurons with preganglionic fibers that extend proximally and enter the spinal cord through the dorsal horns, projecting rostrally in the spinal cord. The postganglionic fibers project distally through the spinal nerves and peripheral nerves, carrying information from a dermatome. On the other hand, the motor fibers originate from the anterior horn cells within the spinal cord, projecting distally through spinal nerves and peripheral nerves, carrying motor innervation to a myotome.

A radiculopathy occurs from an intraspinal canal lesion resulting in damage of the preganglionic fibers, leaving unaffected the cell body in the dorsal root ganglia and the postganglionic fibers, and therefore, even though sensory symptoms are prominent, the SNAPs are normal.

An axon loss radiculopathy will also injure motor fibers in the intraspinal canal region, affecting the respective myotome. This leads to denervation, with fibrillation potentials seen 3 weeks after the onset of motor axon loss, decreased recruitment, and 3 to 6 months later, large and polyphasic motor unit potentials (MUPs). The presence of these large and polyphasic MUPs is dependent on reinnervation and collateral innervation, typically occurring in a proximal-to-distal fashion, with proximal muscles more successfully reinnervated as compared to distal muscles.

The H-reflex is the electrophysiologic equivalent of the ankle reflex, which is an S1 reflex, and this test is helpful in the evaluation of S1 radiculopathies.

Katirji B. Electromyography in Clinical Practice: A Case Study Approach. 1st ed. St. Louis: Mosby; 1998.

Preston DC, Schapiro BE. Electromyography and Neuromuscular Disorders, 2nd ed. Philadelphia, PA: Elsevier; 2005.

7. d, 8. c

The 2-Hz repetitive nerve stimulation shown in Figure 9.1 demonstrates a more than 10% decremental response of the CMAP amplitude, which is consistent with a diagnosis of myasthenia gravis (MG).

MG is a disorder of the neuromuscular junction, due to an antibody-mediated destruction of postsynaptic nicotinic acetylcholine receptors (discussed further in Chapter 10). Electrodiagnostic studies are important to diagnose this condition and to help differentiate it from other neuromuscular junction disorders. Sensory NCS are normal in MG, and motor NCS are usually normal as well. Whenever CMAPs are found to be low in amplitude, a presynaptic disorder such as Lambert-Eaton syndrome or botulism should be suspected. An increment in the CMAP amplitudes after exercise or rapid repetitive stimulation is a feature of a presynaptic disorder, and not of MG.

Repetitive stimulation is a helpful test in the diagnosis of MG, in which there is a decrement of CMAP amplitudes with slow repetitive nerve stimulation (2 to 3 Hz), with a decrement of greater than 10% being consistent with MG. The decremental responses occur due to a normal reduction in the release of acetylcholine after subsequent stimulation and the reduced availability of receptors from the disease, leading to a loss of end-plate potentials and reduction of the motor action potentials. In presynaptic neuromuscular junction disorders, rapid stimulation with frequencies of 20 to 50 Hz produces an incremental response by overcoming the efflux of calcium (which occurs within 100 to 200 ms); this is not seen in postsynaptic disorders where the limiting factor is at the postsynaptic membrane.

Jitter analysis by single-fiber EMG (SFEMG) is performed by recording with a single-fiber needle electrode positioned to detect potentials from two muscle fibers of the same motor unit. The variability of the interpotential interval between these two potentials is the jitter, and it is abnormal in MG due to delayed neuromuscular transmission. Neuromuscular blocking can also be detected, and is measured by the percentage of discharges in which one of the potentials is missing. SFEMG is highly sensitive but not specific for MG, being frequently abnormal in other neuromuscular junction disorders.

Moment-to-moment variation of the motor unit potentials (MUPs) may be present in MG, meaning that the MUPs vary in amplitude and configuration with successive discharges, due to blocking at some of the neuromuscular junctions of the muscle fibers composing the MUP.

Given the abnormal slow repetitive stimulation, as well as the normal NCS and needle examination on this patient, the diagnoses of myopathy and neuropathy are unlikely. The time frame of the presentation is not consistent with botulism.

Katirji B. Electromyography in Clinical Practice: A Case Study Approach, 1st ed. St. Louis: Mosby; 1998.

Preston DC, Schapiro BE. Electromyography and Neuromuscular Disorders, 2nd ed. Philadelphia, PA: Elsevier; 2005.

9. e

Jitter on single-fiber EMG is an indication of a neuromuscular junction abnormality, but it is not specific and cannot distinguish between myasthenia gravis and Lambert-Eaton myasthenic syndrome (LEMS).

LEMS is a disorder of neuromuscular transmission characterized by a reduced release of acetylcholine, and antibodies to presynaptic voltage-gated calcium channels. LEMS is frequently detected as a paraneoplastic syndrome associated with small cell lung carcinoma (discussed in Chapter 10). Electrodiagnostic studies are helpful in diagnosing this condition. Sensory NCS are normal, but CMAP amplitudes are usually low to borderline low at rest because many fibers fail to reach threshold after a stimulus, given inadequate release of acetylcholine vesicles. Brief exercise facilitates a release of acetylcholine and results in an increment in the CMAP amplitudes.

Patients with LEMS have a decremental response with slow repetitive stimulation, given that there is a decline in acetylcholine release with each stimulus, leading to loss of end-plate potentials and reduction of the motor action potential. However, these patients have an incremental response with rapid repetitive stimulation, given that the calcium availability in the presynaptic terminal is enhanced with repetitive stimulation, resulting in a larger release of quanta and larger end-plate potentials. This occurs with rapid stimulation because the frequency of stimulation is faster than the time it takes for calcium to leave the presynaptic terminal (100 to 200 ms), leading to higher levels of calcium influx and larger end-plate potentials. The incremental response has to be more than 50% to be considered diagnostic.

Needle EMG is usually normal in LEMS.

Katirji B. Electromyography in Clinical Practice: A Case Study Approach, 1st ed. St. Louis: Mosby; 1998.

Preston DC, Schapiro BE. Electromyography and Neuromuscular Disorders, 2nd ed. Philadelphia, PA: Elsevier; 2005.

10. b

There are different types of skeletal muscle fibers, which vary in their contractile speed, ATPase activity, and source of energy, among other characteristics. Muscle fibers type I are also called slow-oxidative, have slow ATPase activity and large oxidative capacity, with large numbers of mitochondria. They are red in color and small in diameter. Type IIa fibers are also called fast-oxidative-glycolytic, and these fibers have fast ATPase activity, with high glycolytic capacity and moderate oxidative capacity. These fibers are fast and resistant to fatigue. They are red in color and large in diameter. Type IIb fibers are also called fast-glycolytic, and these fibers have fast ATPase activity, with high glycolytic capacity but low oxidative capacity. These fibers are fast and fatigable. Their color is pale and diameter is large.

Barret KE, Barman SM, Boitano S, et al. Ganong's Review of Medical Physiology, 23rd ed. New York: McGraw-Hill; 2010.

11. b, 12. a

This patient has chronic inflammatory demyelinating polyneuropathy (CIDP), which is a symmetric demyelinating polyneuropathy presenting with proximal and distal weakness with or without sensory loss and hypo- or areflexia. Autonomic involvement may occur, but it is less common than in Guillain-Barre syndrome (GBS). CIDP usually presents in adult patients between 40 and 60 years of age, and it is progressive and/or relapsing, with a time course of at least 8 weeks necessary for the diagnosis to be made.

In CIDP, CSF may demonstrate albuminocytologic dissociation. If the CSF cell count is elevated more than $10/mm^3$ (normal up to 5 lymphocytes/mm^3), an alternative cause should be investigated.

In CIDP, electrophysiologic studies demonstrate features of a demyelinating neuropathy. Figure 9.2 shows right median motor NCS with stimulation at the wrist and at the elbow, with findings consistent with a demyelinating neuropathy. On NCS, demyelination is associated with marked slowing of conduction velocity (slower than 75% of the lower limit of normal), marked prolongation of distal latency (longer than 130% of the upper limit of normal), or both. In this case, the peak latency is prolonged (normal is <4 ms) and the conduction velocity is reduced (normal >50 m/s), with the presence of CMAP amplitude dispersion. All these features are consistent with demyelination. Although not present in this case, conduction block is common in CIDP. Sensory NCS do not play a major role in the diagnosis of CIDP.

Sural nerve biopsy should be considered when the CSF or electrophysiologic studies are not supportive of the diagnosis. In CIDP the biopsy will typically show evidence of demyelination and remyelination with onion bulb formation, and sometimes evidence of inflammation. Nerve biopsy may be helpful to exclude other conditions.

When the clinical symptoms do not progress beyond 4 weeks, GBS is the likely diagnosis. When symptoms relapse after treatment and/or symptom progression extends beyond 4 weeks (but <8 weeks), the diagnosis is controversial. Some authors suggest the term subacute inflammatory demyelinating polyradiculoneuropathy to describe patients in this time frame, with manifestations similar to both acute inflammatory demyelinating polyneuropathy and CIDP. CIDP is the diagnosis when symptoms progress or relapse beyond 8 weeks.

GBS is discussed in questions 15, 16, 24, 55, and 56. Multifocal motor neuropathy is discussed in questions 35 and 36. This patient does not have a disorder of the neuromuscular junction, and therefore this is not myasthenia gravis or Lambert-Eaton myasthenic syndrome (discussed in Chapter 10).

Saperstein DS. Chronic acquired demyelinating polyneuropathies. Semin Neurol. 2008; 28:168–184.

13. d

After 3 weeks from an injury, NCS cannot localize a focal axon loss lesion.

Peripheral nerve injury severity can range from focal demyelination to axonal injury and finally nerve transection with discontinuity of the nerve. Electrophysiologic studies can help determine the degree of injury.

A focal nerve injury can cause segmental demyelination, which is characterized by the presence of slowing at a specific site or the presence of a conduction block, which is a decrease in the CMAP amplitude with proximal stimulation as compared to distal stimulation, without significant temporal dispersion. The presence of conduction block therefore suggests segmental demyelination and helps localize the site of injury. A conduction block is reversible, given that the lesion is demyelinating.

If the injury is severe, an axon loss lesion may occur, eventually leading to wallerian degeneration, which is typically completed in 7 to 10 days from the injury. During this time, a conduction block may be observed due to axon loss. After 10 days, the distal axon degenerates and can no longer conduct. Therefore the conduction block due to axonal interruption resolves.

Once denervation occurs, spontaneous muscle activity appears on EMG, manifested by fibrillation potentials, which usually appear after the third week from the injury.

Katirji B. Electromyography in Clinical Practice: A Case Study Approach, 1st ed. St. Louis: Mosby; 1998.

Preston DC, Schapiro BE. Electromyography and Neuromuscular Disorders, 2nd ed. Philadelphia, PA: Elsevier; 2005.

14. C

This patient's history is consistent with carpal tunnel syndrome, the most common entrapment neuropathy. The carpal tunnel is bounded dorsally and laterally by the carpal bones, and the transverse carpal ligament forms the palmar border. The structures that pass through the carpal tunnel include the median nerve most superficially (on the palmar aspect), flexor pollicis longus tendon, four tendons of the flexor digitorum superficialis, and four tendons of the flexor digitorum profundus.

Carpal tunnel syndrome may be unilateral or bilateral. Symptoms of carpal tunnel include pain and paresthesias in the medial half of the palm and first three digits and lateral half of the fourth digit that classically awaken the patient at night, with patients shaking their hand to relieve symptoms. Shooting pains may radiate up the forearm or even the upper arm; therefore, presence of forearm or upper arm symptoms should not exclude the diagnosis of carpal tunnel syndrome. Sensation is spared over the thenar eminence because the palmar sensory branch that innervates the thenar eminence travels outside the carpal tunnel. Physical examination may show provocation of symptoms with repetitive tapping on the median nerve at the wrist (Tinel's sign) and with hyperflexion of the wrists for a period of time (Phalen's maneuver). The only motor branch of the median nerve distal to the carpal tunnel is the thenar (or recurrent) motor branch; in advanced carpal tunnel, the thenar muscles are therefore weak and atrophied and show evidence of denervation on EMG. In such cases, there is weakness of thumb abduction and opposition, with weakness in activities requiring fine motor coordination of the first three digits such as buttoning.

Figure 9.3 shows prolonged distal median nerve SNAP latency. Motor NCS and EMG are normal, indicating mild carpal tunnel. With more advanced demyelination, evidence of conduction block at the wrist may be found, but it requires more distal stimulation near or at the palm for confirmation. With more severe carpal tunnel, with axon loss, prolonged distal motor latencies and reduced amplitudes of the CMAP and SNAP are seen. When severe, there is also evidence of denervation in median nerve–innervated thenar muscles on EMG.

Absence of neck pain makes radiculopathy less likely. In addition, the brachioradialis deep tendon reflex is intact. Although a C6 radiculopathy would lead to sensory loss over the lateral thumb, it would also lead to sensory loss over the lateral forearm, in addition to weakness in forearm flexion and supination, which are not evident in this case. A C7 radiculopathy leads to sensory loss over the third digit, but both a C6 and C7 radiculopathy are less likely on the basis of the abnormal median nerve sensory NCS, and absence of weakness or fibrillation potentials in C6- and C7-innervated muscles. In radiculopathy, because the dorsal root ganglion lies distal to the lesion, sensory NCS remain normal, despite sensory complaints the patient may have. A brachial plexopathy would usually not lead to the limited distribution of sensory symptoms without motor symptoms as well. Absence of weakness in more proximal median nerve–innervated muscles, and the presence of conduction block at the wrist, supports the lesion being at the level of the wrist rather than the elbow.

Guillain-Barre syndrome is discussed in questions 15, 16, 24, 55, and 56.

Preston DC, Shapiro BE. Electromyography and Neuromuscular Disorders. 2nd ed. Philadelphia, PA: Elsevier; 2005.

Russell SM. Examination of Peripheral Nerve Injuries, New York: Thieme; 2006.

15. a, 16. b

This patient has Guillain-Barre syndrome (GBS). This is an acute inflammatory demyelinating polyradiculoneuropathy and a common cause of ascending paralysis. It affects any age group and any gender in all parts of the world. In about 60% of cases, there is a preceding respiratory or gastrointestinal illness 1 to 3 weeks prior. *Campylobacter jejuni* is an identifiable etiology of the preceding gastrointestinal illness; however, it is the cause in only a limited number of cases and predominantly associated with the axonal variant.

GBS is considered to be caused by an immunologic reaction to the peripheral nerves. It is not clear what triggers the immunologic reaction, but it is thought that an infectious or environmental process may contribute to the process in susceptible individuals. The main mechanism is a T-cell-mediated response against myelin proteins that occurs after encountering a cross-reactive antigen, leading to the release of cytokines and activation of macrophages that will damage peripheral myelin. During the process, there is mononuclear infiltration into the peripheral nerves, T-lymphocyte activation, and antibody binding to Schwann cells and myelin components, with macrophages targeting the myelin components. Axonal variants of GBS exist, and are less responsive to treatment with protracted course and worse prognosis.

The typical clinical presentation begins with sensory symptoms, especially numbness and paresthesias beginning distally, usually in the toes and feet, ascending through the lower extremities, and later the upper extremities. Some patients complain of burning pain, with cramps or muscle discomfort. Lower extremity weakness begins later, and is usually symmetric and ascending from distal to proximal, evolving over days. There is subsequent involvement of the hands and upper limbs, and weakness of the respiratory and bulbar muscles may occur later. Reduced or absent reflexes are evident on examination.

Involvement of the autonomic nervous system and respiratory muscles may occur in patients with GBS, and there may be rapid progression with life-threatening complications, such as arrhythmias, bradycardia, tachycardia, hemodynamic instability, and respiratory failure. A patient who is rapidly worsening should be observed with cardiac monitoring and frequent vital signs, as well as frequent evaluation of respiratory parameters, including negative inspiratory force and vital capacity. A negative inspiratory force of less than -30 cc H_2O or vital capacity of less than 15 to 20 mL/kg support elective endotracheal intubation.

The diagnosis of GBS is based on clinical history and examination, and monitoring respiratory function in a rapidly deteriorating patient with a characteristic history and examination is paramount. Other supporting tests are sometimes helpful to make the diagnosis and exclude other potential causes. Identifying cytoalbuminologic dissociation (i.e., high CSF protein and few WBCs) supports the diagnosis. EMG/NCS may be normal in the acute setting and will not likely affect the acute care of the patient. MRI of the lumbar spine may show gadolinium enhancement of the cauda equina, but this will not affect the treatment. MRI of the brain is not indicated.

Hughes RAC, Cornblath DR. Guillain-Barre syndrome. Lancet. 2005; 366:1653–1666.

Ropper AH, Samuels MA. Adams and Victor's Principles of Neurology, 9th ed. New York: McGraw-Hill; 2009.

17. d

As discussed further below and shown in Figure 9.5, both the dorsal scapular nerve and the long thoracic nerve arise directly from the ventral (anterior) rami of the nerve roots.

The upper extremity receives innervation from the C5 to T1 nerve roots. In the intervertebral foramina, the motor and sensory roots join to form a spinal nerve, which then branches into

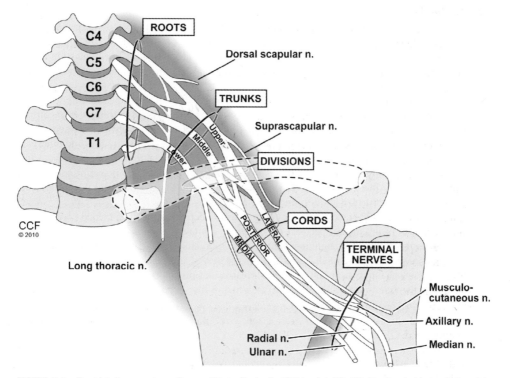

FIGURE 9.5   Brachial plexus anatomy diagram (Illustration by David Schumick, BS, CMI. Reprinted with permission of the Cleveland Clinic Center for Medical Art & Photography. © 2010. All Rights Reserved)

ventral and dorsal rami before exiting the foramina. The ventral (anterior) rami of these nerve roots join to form a plexus of nerves known as the brachial plexus (Figure 9.5). The innervation of the upper extremities is discussed below.

-Roots

Two nerves that innervate the upper extremity branch off the nerve roots themselves. The dorsal scapular nerve, which innervates the rhomboids and levator scapulae, arises from the C5 nerve root. The long thoracic nerve, which innervates the serratus anterior, arises from the C5 to C7 roots.

-Trunks

The ventral rami of the C5 to T1 nerve roots join to form the trunks of the brachial plexus.

The upper (or superior) trunk, formed from the C5 and C6 nerve roots, gives off two branches: the suprascapular nerve, which innervates the supraspinatus and infraspinatus, and the nerve to subclavius. The point where the C5 and C6 nerve roots meet is called Erb's point.

The middle trunk is formed from the C7 root. There are no branches from the middle trunk.

The lower (inferior trunk) is formed from the C8 and T1 roots. There are no branches from the inferior trunk.

The trunks then divide into anterior and posterior divisions.

-Cords and nerves

The cords are named according to their relationship to the axillary artery.

The lateral cord is formed from the anterior divisions of the superior and middle trunk, and therefore carries fibers from C5 to C7. The lateral cord gives rise to the lateral pectoral nerve, which innervates the pectoralis major. The lateral cord ends as two nerves, the median nerve (which also receives a contribution from the medial cord), discussed further in question 23, and the musculocutaneous nerve, which contains the lateral antebrachial cutaneous nerve and is further discussed in question 67.

The posterior cord is formed from the posterior divisions of the upper, middle, and lower trunk, and therefore carries fibers from C5 and C8. Three nerves arise from the posterior cord: (1) the upper subscapular nerve, which contains predominantly C7 and C8 fibers and innervates the subscapularis; (2) the lower subscapular nerve, which contains C5 and C6 fibers and innervates the teres major and the lower part of the subscapularis; and (3) the thoracodorsal nerve, which contains C6, C7, and C8 fibers and innervates the latissimus dorsi. The posterior cord ends as two nerves, the axillary nerve, which is discussed further in question 69, and the radial nerve, which is discussed further in question 43.

The medial cord is a continuation of the lower (inferior) trunk. The medial cord gives off three nerves: (1) the medial pectoral nerve, which contains predominantly C8 and T1 fibers and innervates the pectoralis minor; (2) the medial brachial cutaneous nerve, which provides sensory innervation to the medial arm; and (3) the medial antebrachial cutaneous nerve, which provides sensory innervation to the medial forearm. The medial cord gives fibers to the median nerve and then continues as the ulnar nerve, which is discussed further in question 37.

Russell SM. Examination of Peripheral Nerve Injuries. New York: Thieme; 2006.

18. a, 19. b

The patient in question 18 has familial amyloid polyneuropathy (FAP) type 1, as evidenced by an examination suggestive of a polyneuropathy, autonomic features, and a family history. The patient in question 19 has FAP2, as evidence by the presence of carpal tunnel, a family history of carpal tunnel, mild predominantly sensory polyneuropathy, and absence of prominent autonomic features.

The familial FAPs are a group of autosomal dominant multisystem disorders that result from deposition of amyloid proteins in the peripheral nerves and other organs including the heart and kidney.

The most common FAPs, types 1 and 2, result from various mutations in transthyretin, a plasma protein that is synthesized predominantly in the liver and transports thyroxine and other proteins.

FAP1 is characterized by onset of symptoms in the third to fourth decades of life. Both small and large nerve fibers are affected, but loss of pain and temperature sensation is most pronounced, with relative sparing of posterior column modalities. Symptoms include lancinating pains and dysesthesias, and autonomic dysfunction, including sexual dysfunction, orthostatic hypotension, urinary symptoms, gastrointestinal symptoms, anhidrosis, and pupillary abnormalities. Cardiac and renal involvement may occur from amyloid deposition in these organs. Nerve, rectal, or fat pad biopsy with congo red staining demonstrates amyloid, which exhibits an apple-green birefringence on polarized light; transthyretin molecular gene testing is also available for diagnosis. Liver transplant may be helpful for FAPs resulting from transthyretin mutations.

FAP2, as depicted in question 19, manifests later than FAP1, in the fourth and fifth decades, and its main features are carpal tunnel syndrome and a slowly progressive polyneuropathy, with absence of autonomic features.

FAP3 and -4 are rare and not related to abnormalities in transthyretin. FAP3 is similar to FAP1 in clinical manifestations, but with earlier renal involvement and more gastrointestinal involvement, with a higher incidence of duodenal ulcers. Other features may include hypothyroidism, adrenal insufficiency, and sexual dysfunction. It results from abnormalities in the apolipoprotein *A1* gene. FAP4 manifests in the third decade of life, with corneal dystrophy being a prominent early feature. In later life, cranial neuropathies and skin changes occur; cranial nerves VII, VIII, and XII are commonly affected. Other features include a peripheral sensorimotor neuropathy and carpal tunnel syndrome, without autonomic signs or symptoms. FAP4 results from abnormalities in the amyloid protein gelsolin.

The FAPs are distinguished on the basis of family history and laboratory testing from primary systemic amyloidosis (which results from deposition of AL amyloid, and is associated with monoclonal protein), and secondary amyloidosis (which results from deposition of AA amyloid, and occurs in the setting of systemic inflammatory diseases).

Bradley WG, Daroff RB, Fenichel GM, et al. Neurology in Clinical Practice, 5th ed. Philadelphia, PA: Elsevier; 2008.

Ropper AH, Samuels MA. Adams and Victor's Principles of Neurology, 9th ed. New York: McGraw-Hill; 2009.

20. d

The diarrhea that occurs from diabetic autonomic neuropathy typically occurs at night.

Autonomic dysfunction resulting from diabetic neuropathy can involve multiple organ systems. In the cardiovascular system, manifestations include resting tachycardia or bradycardia, loss of the respiratory variability of the heart rate, loss of the normal tachycardic response, orthostatic hypotension, and increased risk of silent myocardial infarction. Gastrointestinal abnormalities may occur, ranging from delayed gastric emptying, constipation from colonic atony, bacterial overgrowth, and diarrhea, which is typically nocturnal. Neurogenic bladder may occur, as well as sexual dysfunction caused by impotence, erectile dysfunction, and retrograde ejaculation. Abnormalities in sudomotor function also occur, with areas of anhidrosis and hyperhydrosis.

Bradley WG, Daroff RB, Fenichel GM, et al. Neurology in Clinical Practice, 5th ed. Philadelphia, PA: Elsevier; 2008.

Ropper AH, Samuels MA. Adams and Victor's Principles of Neurology, 9th ed. New York: McGraw-Hill; 2009.

21. a, 22. d

This patient's history and examination are consistent with Charcot-Marie-Tooth (CMT) 1. The clinical manifestations are discussed further below, but respiratory compromise is not usually seen in the most common forms of CMT, but occurs in some cases of CMT2C.

The CMTs, also known as hereditary sensorimotor neuropathies or peroneal muscular atrophy, are a large, heterogeneous group of inherited peripheral neuropathies. The CMTs can be divided into demyelinating, axonal, and combined demyelinating and axonal forms. They are genetically heterogeneous.

The demyelinating CMTs include CMT1 and CMTX. CMT4, discussed in question 39, involves both demyelination and axon loss. In the demyelinating CMTs, NCS generally show diffuse, uniformly slow conduction velocities without conduction blocks or temporal dispersion, indicating a hereditary as opposed to acquired demyelinating process (discussed in question 12). There may be evidence of axon loss in the demyelinating forms as well, particularly in patients with long-standing disease; this is secondary axon loss, and conduction velocities as well as CMAP and SNAP amplitudes will be reduced. In contrast, with the axonal forms, motor and sensory potential amplitudes will be reduced, but conduction velocities will be normal or minimally reduced (discussed in question 3, 4, and 13).

At the time of this publication, there were seven subtypes of CMT1; they are all inherited in an autosomal dominant fashion. CMT1A is the most common inherited demyelinating neuropathy. Clinical manifestations typically begin in the first two decades of life and include slowly progressive weakness, muscle atrophy, kyphosis, and mild (often asymptomatic) sensory loss. Other signs include hammertoes, high-arched feet, palpably enlarged nerves due to peripheral nerve hypertrophy (which more commonly occurs in the CMT1 group compared to the other CMTs), and pes cavus. Involvement of the upper extremities typically occurs later in life. There is often a family history of neuropathy, though due to variable expression, some affected family members may only have mild features such as hammertoes and may remain undiagnosed for a large part of their life; sporadic cases without a clear family history also exist. Other forms of CMT may be congenital and severe. In the CMT1 group, many of the genes involved are related to myelin synthesis. CMT1A is due to a duplication in the peripheral myelin protein 22 (*PMP22*) gene on chromosome 17, whereas CMT1B is due to a mutation in the myelin protein 0 gene. CMT1B is more severe in terms of clinical manifestations as compared to CMT1A. In patients with CMT1, CSF shows elevated protein levels in some cases. Roussy-Levy syndrome is phenotypically similar to CMT1A but is associated with the presence of a static tremor and gait ataxia. It has been associated with mutations in both the *PMP22* and myelin protein 0 genes.

On nerve biopsy, pathologic features of the demyelinating inherited polyneuropathies include demyelination and an onion-bulb appearance due to Schwann cell proliferation. Onion bulbs are not specific for CMT, and also occur with chronic inflammatory demyelinating polyneuropathy (discussed in questions 11, 12, and 38).

CMTX is the second most common type of CMT. It is demyelinating and is clinically similar to CMT1, but it is X-linked in inheritance; males therefore tend to be more severely affected compared to females. It is due to a mutation in the connexin 32 gene.

CMT2 accounts for approximately one-third of the autosomal dominant inherited neuropathies. The CMT2 group are axonal neuropathies; NCS show normal conduction velocities, and nerve biopsy shows axon loss without evidence of significant demyelination. Compared to CMT1, in CMT2, symptoms and signs typically appear later and foot and spine deformities are less severe. Clinical manifestations do not always help distinguish the different CMTs, but some clinical features occur more frequently in the different subtypes. Optic atrophy occurs more in CMT2A2, foot ulcerations in CMT2B, and vocal cord paralysis, intercostal, and diaphragmatic weakness in CMT2C. In CMT2D, unlike in the other CMTs, the hands are involved more than the feet. Peripheral nerve hypertrophy does not occur. They are all autosomal dominant in inheritance, except for a subtype of CMT2A. The genes implicated in the CMT2 group are involved in axonal transport and membrane trafficking. CMT2A2 is one of the most common of this group and is due to mutations in mitofusin 2.

CMT3, also known as Dejerine-Sottas syndrome or hypertrophic neuropathy of infancy, is one of the more severe forms of the demyelinating CMTs. It presents in infancy with proximal weakness, absent deep tendon reflexes, and hypertrophy of the peripheral nerves. Prominent sensory symptoms including pain and dysesthesias occur. Patients typically have extensive disability early in life. Both autosomal recessive and dominant forms exist. CSF protein is usually elevated. Congenital hypomyelination is seen along the spectrum of this disorder. CMT3 is genetically heterogeneous; mutations in several genes including *PMP22*, protein myelin 0, and other genes implicated in defective demyelination are associated with CMT3. CMT4 is discussed in question 39.

The CMTs can be misdiagnosed as muscular dystrophy; NCS findings, as well as the presence of hammertoes and high-arched foot, distinguish between the two.

Bradley WG, Daroff RB, Fenichel GM, et al. Neurology in Clinical Practice, 5th ed. Philadelphia, PA: Elsevier; 2008.

Ropper AH, Samuels MA. Adams and Victor's Principles of Neurology, 9th ed. New York: McGraw-Hill; 2009.

23. e

If the upper extremity were to be divided into upper arm (above the elbow), forearm (elbow to wrist), and hand (below the wrist), the median nerve does not innervate any muscles in the upper arm.

The median nerve is derived from the lateral and medial cords. The median nerve runs down the midline of the arm and crosses over the brachial artery to lie just medial to it as it passes under the bicipital aponeurosis in the antecubital fossa. In the forearm, the median nerve innervates pronator teres, flexor carpi radialis, and flexor digitorum superficialis (see Table 9.1 for root innervations and action of the muscles innervated by the median nerve).

TABLE 9.1 Upper extremity muscles innervated by the median nerve, their root innervation, and action

Muscle	Nerve Innervation	Root Innervation	Action
Pronator teres	Median nerve	C6, C7	Forearm pronation
Flexor carpi radialis	Median nerve	C6, C7	Wrist flexion in a radial direction
Flexor digitorum superficialis	Median nerve	C8, T1	Flexion of second to fifth proximal interphalangeal joint
Flexor digitorum profundus	Median nerve, anterior interosseus branch	C8, T1	Flexion of distal interphalangeal joint of second and part of third digit
Flexor pollicis longus	Median nerve, anterior interosseus branch	C8, T1	Flexion of distal phalanx of thumb
Pronator quadratus	Median nerve, anterior interosseus branch	C7, C8	Forearm pronation (best tested with forearm fully flexed to reduce action of pronator teres)
Abductor pollicis brevis	Median nerve	C8, T1	Thumb abduction (palmar abduction away from the plane of palm)
Flexor pollicis brevis	Median nerve (along with ulnar nerve)	C8, T1	Thumb flexion at metacarpophalangeal joint
Opponens pollicis	Median nerve	C8, T1	Thumb opposition
First and second lumbricals	Median nerve	C8, T1	Extension of the proximal interphalangeal joint of the second and third digits

In the forearm, the median nerve gives off the anterior interosseus nerve that innervates flexor digitorum profundus to the second and third digits, flexor pollicis longus, and pronator quadratus. Before entering the carpal tunnel, the median nerve gives off the palmar cutaneous sensory nerve, a pure sensory nerve. The median nerve then passes through the carpal tunnel (discussed in question 14) and gives off the thenar motor branch, which innervates abductor pollicis brevis and opponens pollicis. The median nerve also innervates the first and second lumbricals.

The median nerve provides sensory innervations to the lateral (radial) two-thirds of the palm and the distal dorsal aspect of the first to third digits and the distal lateral (radial) half of the fourth digit through the palmar cutaneous nerve and through digital branches.

The median nerve is prone to injury with supracondylar fractures. Median nerve palsy can also occur due to entrapment in ligaments or between muscles (discussed in question 59).

Russell SM. Examination of Peripheral Nerve Injuries. New York: Thieme; 2006.

24. e

Intravenous immunoglobulins (IVIG) and plamapheresis both are used for the treatment of Guillain-Barre syndrome (GBS). Plasmapheresis (plasma exchange) has been evaluated in clinical trials, demonstrating benefit within the first 4 weeks from symptom onset and a trend toward additional benefit when administered earlier. Benefits include reduction of the duration of hospitalization, need for mechanical ventilation, more improvement on disability scales, and shortened time to walking unaided. Plasmapheresis is used in four to six treatments of 200 to 250 mL/kg. IVIG has been tested as well, and its use has shown similar efficacy to plasmapheresis. Its dose is 400 mg/kg/day for 5 days. The combination of plasmapheresis and IVIG has failed to show additional improvement when compared to either therapy alone. The use of steroids is not beneficial and not recommended. Pyridostigmine is used for symptomatic treatment of myasthenia gravis (discussed in Chapter 10), and not for GBS.

Hughes RAC, Cornblath DR. Guillain-Barre syndrome. Lancet. 2005; 366:1653–1666.

Hughes RAC, Widjicks EFM, Barohn R, et al. Practice parameter: Immunotherapy for Guillain-Barre syndrome: Report of the Quality Standards Subcommittee of the American Academy of Neurology. Neurology. 2003; 61:736–740.

Ropper AH, Samuels MA. Adams and Victor's Principles of Neurology, 9th ed. New York: McGraw-Hill; 2009.

25. c, 26. d

The iliohypogastric, ilioinguinal, and genitofemoral nerves do not arise from the lumbosacral trunk, but rather from the lumbar plexus. The tensor fascia latae abducts the thigh when the hip is flexed, not extended.

The lumbosacral plexus consists of the lumbar and sacral plexus, connected via the lumbosacral trunk (Figure 9.6).

The lumbar plexus is formed by contributions from T12 to L4 and gives rise to three major and three minor nerves. The three minor nerves are the iliohypogastric, ilioinguinal, and genitofemoral. The first two arise from a common trunk originating from L1 with some contributions from T12. The genitofemoral nerve arises from L1 and L2. The three major nerves are the femoral, obturator, and lateral femoral cutaneous. The lateral femoral cutaneous nerve originates from L2 and L3 (discussed in question 47). The femoral nerve originates from the posterior divisions of L2, L3, and L4 (see question 29 and Figure 9.7). The obturator nerve originates from the anterior divisions of L2, L3, and L4 and divides into an anterior and a posterior division. The anterior division gives innervation to the adductor brevis, adductor longus, and gracilis muscles. The posterior division gives innervation to the obturator externus and a portion of the adductor magnus, which is also innervated by the sciatic nerve.

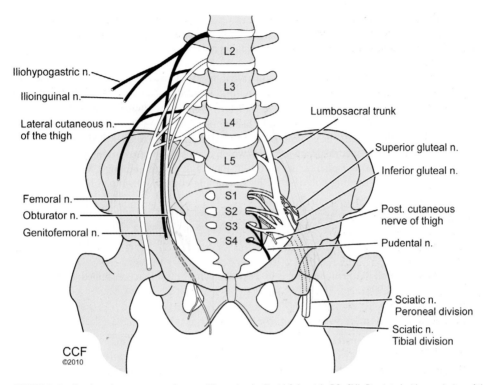

FIGURE 9.6 Lumbar plexus anatomy diagram (Illustration by David Schumick, BS, CMI. Reprinted with permission of the Cleveland Clinic Center for Medical Art & Photography. © 2010. All Rights Reserved)

The lumbosacral trunk is a structure that originates from L4 and L5 and joins the sacral plexus to form the sciatic nerve, which is not only the largest nerve of the lumbosacral plexus, but the largest nerve in the body.

The sacral plexus originates from the L4, L5, S1, S2, S3, and S4 nerve roots, with L4 and L5 provided by the lumbosacral trunk as already described. The anterior divisions of L4 through S3 contribute to form the tibial division of the sciatic nerve. The posterior divisions from L4 through S2 contribute to the common peroneal division of the sciatic nerve.

The superior gluteal nerve originates from L4, L5, and S1 and innervates the gluteus medius, gluteus minimus, and tensor fascia latae. These muscles contribute to thigh abduction, with the tensor fascia latae acting as the main abductor when the hip is flexed, and the gluteus medius and minimus acting as the main abductors when the hip is extended. The inferior gluteal nerve originates from L5, S1, and S2 and innervates the gluteus maximus, which is an extensor of the thigh. The posterior cutaneous nerve of the thigh originates from S1, S2, and S3 and gives sensory cutaneous innervation to the lower buttock and posterior thigh. The pudendal nerve originates from S2, S3, and S4 and provides sensory innervation to the perineal region and perianal region through the inferior rectal nerve, perineal nerve, and dorsal nerve of the penis or clitoris (discussed in Chapter 10).

Katirji B. Electromyography in Clinical Practice: A Case Study Approach, 1st ed. St. Louis: Mosby; 1998.

Russell SM. Examination of Peripheral Nerve Injuries. New York: Thieme; 2006.

27. d

This patient has hereditary neuropathy with liability to pressure palsies (HNPP). It is an autosomal dominant predominantly demyelinating hereditary neuropathy with incomplete penetrance and is caused by a deletion in the peripheral myelin protein 22 gene. Duplications in this same gene are the cause of Charcot-Marie-Tooth type (CMT) 1A. Patients with HNPPs classically present with recurrent episodes of focal mononeuropathies or plexopathies of the upper or lower limbs; the peroneal nerve is most commonly affected, followed by the ulnar nerve. The presentation is typically in young adulthood, and a history of compression or traction on the involved nerve can often be elicited. The weakness is not preceded or accompanied by pain, distinguishing HNPP from hereditary neuralgic amyotrophy, which can also lead to recurrent upper extremity mononeuropathies. Other phenotypes of HNPP, including one resembling CMT or a chronic sensorimotor demyelinating polyneuropathy resembling chronic inflammatory demyelinating polyneuropathy, also exist.

NCS show prolonged distal latencies, focal slowing at sites of compression, and in some cases diffuse reductions in SNAP amplitudes. Nerve biopsy shows a characteristic pattern of focal, sausage-like areas of thickening in the myelin called tomacula, as well as evidence of segmental demyelination and axon loss.

Bradley WG, Daroff RB, Fenichel GM, et al. Neurology in Clinical Practice, 5th ed. Philadelphia, PA: Elsevier; 2008.

28. a

The sciatic nerve originates from the L4, L5, S1, S2, and S3 roots. This nerve is the largest nerve in the body, and gives off two initial branches: the superior and inferior gluteal nerves. The superior gluteal nerve innervates the gluteus medius, minimus, and tensor fascia latae. The inferior gluteal nerve innervates the gluteus maximus (see Table 9.2).

TABLE 9.2 Lower extremity muscles innervated by superior and inferior gluteal nerves, their root innervation, and action

Muscle	Nerve Innervation	Root Innervation	Action
Tensor fascia lata	Superior gluteal	L4, L5, S1	Thigh abduction with the hip flexed
Gluteus medius and minimus	Superior gluteal	L4, L5, S1	Thigh abduction with the hip extended
Gluteus maximus	Inferior gluteal	L5, S1, S2	Thigh extension

The sciatic nerve is composed of two different nerves running together: the tibial nerve medially and the common peroneal nerve laterally. In the thigh, the tibial division innervates the adductor magnus, semimembranosus, semitendinosus, and long head of the biceps femoris. The short head of the biceps femoris is supplied by the common peroneal division. The tibial nerve then continues in the posterior aspect of the leg and gives innervation to the gastrocnemius, soleus, and tibialis posterior. The peroneal nerve continues, and after the popliteal fossa, it passes behind the fibular head and divides into the superficial and deep peroneal nerves. The superficial peroneal nerve gives off branches to the peroneus longus and brevis, which permit foot eversion. The deep peroneal nerve supplies the tibialis anterior, extensor hallucis, extensor digitorum longus and brevis, and peroneus tertius. A lesion in the deep peroneal nerve produces foot drop with inability to dorsiflex the foot without impairing eversion of the foot. Preservation of foot inversion distinguishes peroneal neuropathy from L5 radiculopathy, in which the tibialis posterior muscle (innervated by the tibial nerve) is involved, impairing foot inversion.

Katirji B. Electromyography in Clinical Practice: A Case Study Approach, 1st ed. St. Louis: Mosby; 1998.

Russell SM. Examination of Peripheral Nerve Injuries. New York: Thieme; 2006.

29. a

The femoral nerve (Figure 9.7) is a large nerve that originates from the posterior divisions of L2, L3, and L4, traveling through the psoas major muscle which it innervates, then passing through the iliacus muscle which it also innervates. After this course, the femoral nerve passes under

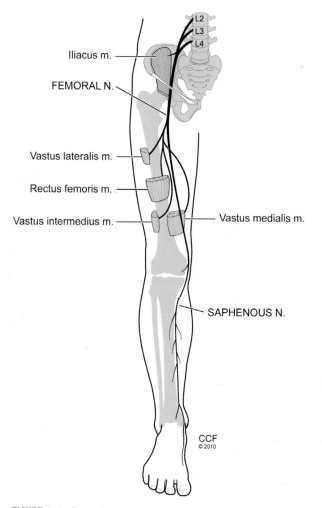

FIGURE 9.7   Femoral nerve anatomy diagram (Illustration by David Schumick, BS, CMI. Reprinted with permission of the Cleveland Clinic Center for Medical Art & Photography. © 2010. All Rights Reserved)

the inguinal canal into the femoral triangle, located lateral to the femoral artery. It then divides into several terminal branches. There are three cutaneous branches: (1) the medial femoral cutaneous, (2) intermediate femoral cutaneous, and (3) saphenous nerve.

These branches carry sensory information from the anteromedial thigh, medial leg, medial malleolus, and arch of the foot. The motor branches provide innervation to the quadriceps (rectus femoris, vastus lateralis, medialis, and intermedius), sartorius, and pectineus (see Table 9.3). The patellar reflex is carried through the femoral nerve.

TABLE 9.3	Lower extremity muscles innervated by the femoral and obturator nerves, their root innervation, and action		
Muscle	**Nerve Innervation**	**Root Innervation**	**Action**
Iliacus	Femoral	L2, L3	Hip flexion
Psoas major	Femoral	L2, L3, L4	Hip flexion
Quadriceps	Femoral	L3, L4	Knee extension
Sartorius	Femoral	L2, L3, L4	Thigh abduction, flexion and external rotation
Adductor brevis	Obturator	L2, L3, L4	Thigh adduction
Adductor longus	Obturator	L2, L3, L4	Thigh adduction
Adductor magnus	Obturator, tibial	L4	Thigh adduction

Femoral nerve injury will manifest as weakness in hip flexion and knee extension, loss of the patellar reflex and sensory findings in the anteromedial thigh and medial leg. The femoral nerve can be injured in the retroperitoneal or intrapelvic space, or at the inguinal ligament. Clinically, the distinction between injury at these sites can be made by detection of weakness on hip flexion that will represent psoas compromise and electrophysiologically by the presence of fibrillations in the iliacus muscle. Both these muscles are innervated before the inguinal ligament, and their compromise will suggest an intrapelvic injury rather than an inguinal injury.

At the inguinal region, the femoral nerve can be damaged by inguinal masses or hematomas, during hip surgery or perineal surgeries, especially associated with prolonged lithotomy position, such as in this case.

It is important to distinguish femoral nerve injury from L2-L3-L4 radiculopathy and lumbar plexopathy. The presence of impairment of other nerves will suggest these possible diagnoses. For example, adductor weakness suggests involvement of the obturator nerve, which can occur in L2-L3-L4 radiculopathy or a lumbar plexopathy. Also, the presence of weakness in the distal lower extremity muscles will imply injury to other nerves, excluding a selective femoral nerve injury. Abnormal SNAPs do not correlate with a radiculopathy from an intraspinal canal lesion, because SNAPs will be normal in these lesions (discussed in questions 3, 4, and 6).

Katirji B. Electromyography in Clinical Practice: A Case Study Approach, 1st ed. St. Louis: Mosby; 1998.

Russell SM. Examination of Peripheral Nerve Injuries. New York: Thieme; 2006.

30. d

This patient's history and examination are consistent with Tangier's disease. Tangier's disease is a very rare autosomal recessive disorder. Neurologic manifestations include a symmetric predominantly sensory neuropathy with dissociated sensory loss (loss of pain and temperature with relative preservation of posterior column modalities), mimicking syringomyelia. In other patients, relapsing multifocal mononeuropathies may occur. It results from mutations in an adenosine triphosphate transporter protein that results in low-serum cholesterol levels and elevated triglyceride levels. Deposition of triglycerides occurs in the reticuloendothelial system, and bone marrow biopsy may show fat-laden macrophages; deposition of triglycerides in the tonsils accounts for the orange appearance of the tonsils in these cases.

Bradley WG, Daroff RB, Fenichel GM, et al. Neurology in Clinical Practice, 5th ed. Philadelphia, PA: Elsevier; 2008.

Ropper AH, Samuels MA. Adams and Victor's Principles of Neurology, 9th ed. New York: McGraw-Hill; 2009.

31. e

This patient has a sensory neuronopathy and possibly a peripheral neuropathy in the setting of small cell lung cancer, and most likely this is a paraneoplastic syndrome. Paraneoplastic syndromes are manifestations of malignancy, and commonly manifest with neurologic involvement. Small cell lung cancer is the most common neoplasm associated with neurologic paraneoplastic syndromes; however, other malignancies can also present this way, including breast, ovarian, kidney, and prostate cancers, thymomas, and lymphomas.

Certain antibodies have been found to correlate with characteristic clinical presentations, and it is thought that these antibodies are directed against the nervous system, either peripheral or central. Anti-Hu (also known as ANNA-1) antibody is typically associated with peripheral neuropathy and sensory neuronopathy in the setting of small cell lung cancer, and will most likely be positive in this case, though anti-Hu antibody has been associated with a variety of other neurologic manifestations as well. Anti-voltage-gated calcium channel is present in Lambert-Eaton myasthenic syndrome in association with small cell lung cancer (discussed in Chapter 10). Anti-Yo is present in ovarian carcinoma and other malignancies, and manifests with cerebellar degeneration. Anti-Ri is associated with opsoclonus-myoclonus with or without ataxia in the setting of neoplasms of the lung or breast. Anti-MAG antibodies are antibodies against myelin-associated glycoprotein and are associated with demyelinating neuropathy in the setting of monoclonal gammopathy of unknown significance (discussed in Chapter 16).

Bradley WG, Daroff RB, Fenichel GM, et al. Neurology in Clinical Practice, 5th ed. Philadelphia, PA: Elsevier; 2008.

Darnell RB, Poster JB. Paraneoplastic syndromes involving the nervous system. N Engl J Med. 2003; 349:1543–1554.

Ropper AH, Samuels MA. Adams and Victor's Principles of Neurology, 9th ed. New York: McGraw-Hill; 2009.

32. d

The sciatic nerve (Figure 9.8) arises from the L4, L5, S1, S2, and S3 nerve roots. It is composed of two nerves: (1) the tibial nerve located medially and (2) the common peroneal nerve located laterally (Figure 9.9). Both are in the same sheath, but remain separated throughout their course with no intercrossing fibers. The common peroneal nerve is more prone to injuries, because it is smaller, more lateral, and has less supportive tissue.

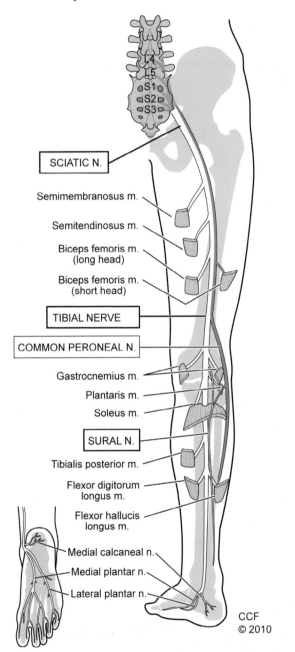

FIGURE 9.8 Sciatic nerve anatomy diagram (Illustration by David Schumick, BS, CMI. Reprinted with permission of the Cleveland Clinic Center for Medical Art & Photography. © 2010. All Rights Reserved)

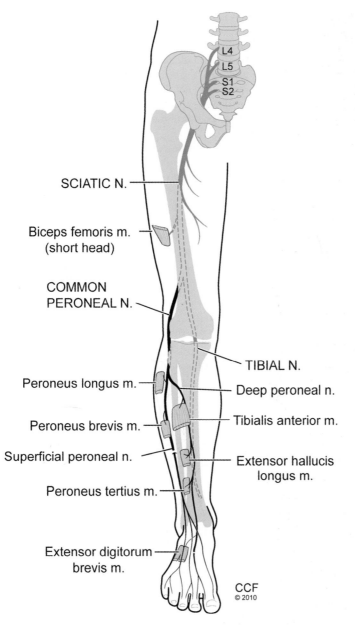

SCIATIC N.

Biceps femoris m.
(short head)

COMMON
PERONEAL N.

TIBIAL N.

Peroneus longus m.

Deep peroneal n.

Peroneus brevis m.

Tibialis anterior m.

Superficial peroneal n.

Extensor hallucis
longus m.

Peroneus tertius m.

Extensor digitorum
brevis m.

L4
L5
S1
S2

CCF
© 2010

FIGURE 9.9 Peroneal nerve anatomy diagram (Illustration by David Schumick, BS, CMI. Reprinted with permission of the Cleveland Clinic Center for Medical Art & Photography. © 2010. All Rights Reserved)

The sciatic nerve exits the pelvis through the sciatic notch, gives off the superior gluteal nerve, and then passes under the piriformis muscle, after which it gives off the inferior gluteal nerve. In the thigh, the tibial division of the sciatic nerve gives innervation to the semitendinosus, semimembranosus, long head of the biceps femoris, and adductor magnus. The peroneal division of the sciatic nerve gives a branch to the short head of the biceps femoris in the thigh. Proximal to the popliteal fossa, the sciatic nerve bifurcates into the tibial and common peroneal nerves. Abnormalities in the short head of the biceps femoris help distinguish a sciatic nerve lesion from a common peroneal lesion at the fibular head, as the short head of the biceps femoris is spared in the latter.

The tibial nerve gives off the sural nerve that provides sensory innervation to the lateral aspect of the leg and foot. The tibial nerve then continues down the leg, innervating the gastrocnemius, soleus, tibialis posterior, flexor digitorum longus, and flexor hallucis longus. At the medial ankle, the tibial nerve passes through the tarsal tunnel and gives three terminal branches: (1) the calcaneal, (2) medial plantar, and (3) lateral plantar nerves.

The common peroneal nerve runs around the fibular head from posterior to anterior and divides into the superficial and deep peroneal nerves. The superficial peroneal innervates the peroneus longus and brevis, as well as the skin in the lower two-thirds of the lateral aspect of the leg and dorsum of the foot. The deep peroneal innervates the tibialis anterior, extensor hallucis, extensor digitorum longus and brevis, and peroneus tertius (see Table 9.4). The sensory territory of the deep peroneal nerve is the web space between the first and second toes.

TABLE 9.4	Lower extremity muscles innervated by the tibial and peroneal nerves, their root innervation, and action		
Muscle	**Nerve Innervation**	**Root Innervation**	**Action**
Tibialis anterior	Deep peroneal	L4, L5	Foot dorsiflexion
Extensor hallucis	Deep peroneal	L5, L4	First toe extension
Peroneus longus and brevis	Superficial peroneal	L5, S1	Foot eversion
Extensor digitorum brevis	Peroneal	L5, S1	Toe extension at the metatarsophalangeal joint
Adductor magnus	Tibial, obturator	L4	Thigh adduction
Semitendinosus, Semimembranosus	Tibial	L5	Knee flexion
Biceps femoris, long head	Tibial	S1, S2	Knee flexion
Biceps femoris, short head	Peroneal	S1, S2	Knee flexion
Tibialis posterior	Tibial	L5, S1	Foot inversion
Flexor digitorum longus	Tibial	L5, S1	Toe flexion
Gastrocnemius	Tibial	S1, S2	Plantarflexion with the knee straight
Soleus	Tibial	S1, S2	Plantarflexion with the knee straight or bent

In this patient, both tibial and peroneal nerve–innervated muscles are affected, including the short head of the biceps femoris, suggesting a sciatic nerve lesion, rather than individual tibial or peroneal nerve involvement. The fact that the sural and superficial peroneal SNAPs are affected excludes the possibility of a radiculopathy. Finally, the conspicuous absence of gluteal nerve–innervated muscles makes the diagnosis of a lumbosacral plexopathy unlikely. The final diagnosis is thus a sciatic mononeuropathy.

Common and deep peroneal neuropathies are discussed in question 44. L5 radiculopathy is discussed in question 86. Tibial nerve injury is discussed in question 34.

Katirji B. Electromyography in Clinical Practice: A Case Study Approach, 1st ed. St. Louis: Mosby; 1998.

Russell SM. Examination of Peripheral Nerve Injuries. New York: Thieme; 2006.

33. d

There is evidence supporting the efficacy of steroids, plasmapheresis, and/or intravenous immunoglobulin (IVIG) for chronic inflammatory demyelinating polyneuropathy (CIDP, discussed in questions 11, 12, and 38). Natalizumab is used for the treatment of multiple sclerosis, not CIDP.

Prednisone can be used for initial therapy from doses of 1 mg/kg/day up to 100 mg/day. Once improvement is noticed, the dose can be slowly tapered to a maintenance dose. A steroid-sparing agent may be required, such as azathioprine, cyclosporine, methotrexate, or mycophenolate mofetil. IVIG can be used with a dose of 2 g/kg over 2 to 5 days and repeated every 4 to 6 weeks according to the response. Plasmapheresis can be used with two to three treatments per week for a total of five to ten treatments. The benefits, however, are transient, and may last from 3 to 8 weeks, requiring repeated treatments. Plasmapheresis may be effective in patients who have significant weakness and those who relapse on steroids, in which case the dose of steroids should be increased along with the frequency and number of plasmapheresis treatments.

Ropper AH, Samuels MA. Adams and Victor's Principles of Neurology, 9th ed. New York: McGraw-Hill; 2009.

Saperstein DS. Chronic acquired demyelinating polyneuropathies. Semin Neurol. 2008; 28:168–184.

34. e

The tibial nerve is a division of the sciatic nerve, and at the level of the thigh, it provides innervation to the semimembranosus, semitendinosus, and long head of the biceps femoris (see Figure 9.8). Proximal to the popliteal fossa, the tibial division of the sciatic nerve separates from the peroneal division and gives off the sural nerve, which provides sensory innervation to the lateral aspect of the leg and foot. The tibial nerve then continues down the leg innervating the gastrocnemius, soleus, tibialis posterior, flexor digitorum longus, and flexor hallucis longus. The tibialis anterior is an L5 deep peroneal nerve–innervated muscle.

At the medial ankle, the tibial nerve passes under the flexor retinaculum through the tarsal tunnel and gives three terminal branches: (1) calcaneal, (2) medial plantar, and (3) lateral plantar. The calcaneal branch is purely sensory and innervates the heel. The medial plantar branch innervates the abductor hallucis, flexor digitorum brevis, and flexor hallucis brevis, as well as the skin of the medial sole. The lateral plantar branch innervates the abductor digiti quinti pedis, flexor digiti quinti pedis, adductor hallucis, and interossei, as well as the skin of the lateral sole.

An entrapment neuropathy of the tibial nerve at the level of the tarsal tunnel will not produce weakness on plantarflexion. This entrapment neuropathy may manifest with burning pain in the plantar region, worse with standing and walking, with sensory deficits in the sole and sometimes atrophy in this area. Sensation in the dorsum of the foot is normal, as well as the ankle reflex.

Katirji B. Electromyography in Clinical Practice: A Case Study Approach, 1st ed. St. Louis: Mosby; 1998.

Russell SM. Examination of Peripheral Nerve Injuries. New York: Thieme; 2006.

35. c, 36. d

This patient has multifocal motor neuropathy (MMN), also known as multifocal motor neuropathy with conduction block. This condition is a purely motor demyelinating neuropathy that presents with asymmetric weakness from involvement of individual peripheral nerves, hypo- or areflexia in the distribution of affected nerves, and no sensory manifestations. CSF studies show normal protein levels, in contrast to acute and chronic demyelinating polyneuropathies. Anti-GM1 antibodies have been detected in this condition, but the presence of these antibodies is not required to make the diagnosis, and does not predict response to therapy. Electrophysiologic testing demonstrates typical conduction block in various nerve distributions. The presence of conduction block is not however required to make the diagnosis if there are other features of demyelination, and the response to treatment is not different between patients with or without conduction block. Sensory NCS are normal.

Patients with MMN do not have a good response to steroids or plasmapheresis, and some may worsen with these therapies. The use of intravenous immunoglobulin has shown to be of benefit and is associated with clinical improvement. Other therapies that have been reported to be beneficial are rituximab and cyclophosphamide.

Chronic inflammatory demyelinating polyneuropathy (CIDP) is discussed in questions 11, 12, and 38. Acute inflammatory demyelinating polyneuropathy (AIDP) is discussed in questions 15, 16, 24, 55, and 56. Subacute inflammatory demyelinating polyneuropathy is a controversial diagnosis that is not generally accepted, but some authors have used this term to define patients with manifestations similar to AIDP and CIDP, with a time evolution between 4 and 8 weeks. Multifocal acquired demyelinating sensory and motor neuropathy is discussed in question 65.

Saperstein DS. Chronic acquired demyelinating polyneuropathies. Semin Neurol. 2008; 28:168–184.

37. b

The ulnar nerve is a continuation of the medial cord. The medial cord gives a contribution to the median nerve and then gives off two branches: (1) the medial brachial cutaneous nerve and (2) medial antebrachial cutaneous nerve, which provide sensory innervation to the medial half of the arm and forearm, respectively. It then continues as the ulnar nerve. The ulnar nerve predominantly carries C8 and T1 fibers. If the upper extremity were to be divided into upper arm (above the elbow), forearm (elbow to wrist), and hand (below the wrist), the ulnar nerve does not innervate any muscles in the arm.

At the elbow, it emerges from the triceps and enters the post-condylar groove, a bony canal between the medial epicondyle and the olecranon of the ulna. This is where the ulnar nerve is most susceptible to injury (see questions 41 and 45). The ulnar nerve then travels down the forearm, where it gives branches to flexor carpi ulnaris and then flexor digitorum profundus to the fourth and fifth digits (see Table 9.5 for root innervations and action of the muscles innervated by the ulnar nerve). It gives off two sensory branches: (1) the dorsal ulnar cutaneous nerve and (2) palmar ulnar cutaneous nerve. Proximal to the wrist it is joined by the ulnar artery.

| TABLE 9.5 | Upper extremity muscles innervated by the ulnar nerve, their root innervation, and action |

Muscle	Nerve Innervation	Root Innervation	Action
Flexor carpi ulnaris	Ulnar nerve	C7, C8, T1	Wrist flexion in an ulnar direction
Flexor digitorum profundus	Ulnar nerve	C8, T1	Flexion at distal interphalangeal joint of fourth and fifth digits
Palmaris brevis	Ulnar nerve	C8, T1	Corrugates hypothenar skin, aiding in grasp
Abductor digiti minimi	Ulnar nerve	C8, T1	Abduction of the fifth digit
Flexor digiti minimi	Ulnar nerve	C8, T1	Flexion at metacarpophalangeal joint of the fifth digit
Opponens digiti minimi	Ulnar nerve	C8, T1	Opposition of fifth digit
Third and fourth lumbricals	Ulnar nerve	C8, T1	Extension at proximal interphalangeal joints of fourth and fifth digits
Dorsal interossei	Ulnar nerve	C8, T1	Finger abduction
Palmar interossei	Ulnar nerve	C8, T1	Finger adduction
Adductor pollicis	Ulnar nerve	C8, T1	Thumb adduction (in plane parallel to palm)
Flexor pollicis brevis	Ulnar nerve (along with median nerve)	C8, T1	Thumb flexion at metacarpophalangeal joint

The ulnar nerve then enters the hand via Guyon's canal, which is bounded by the carpal bones dorsally and laterally, the transverse carpal ligament medially, and the palmar carpal ligament ventrally. The ulnar nerve then bifurcates into a deep motor branch and a superficial sensory branch distal to Guyon's tunnel. The deep motor branch innervates hypothenar eminence muscles: abductor digiti minimi, flexor digiti minimi, and opponens digiti minimi. The ulnar nerve provides motor innervation to many of the intrinsic hand muscles, which are largely involved in fine finger movements: the fourth and fifth lumbricals, and the dorsal and palmar interossei. It also innervates two thenar muscles: (1) adductor pollicis and (2) flexor pollicis brevis.

The ulnar nerve provides sensory innervation to the hypothenar eminence, the palmar and dorsal medial portion of the hand, fifth digit, and half of the fourth digit.

Russell SM. Examination of Peripheral Nerve Injuries. New York: Thieme; 2006.

38. d

This patient is not suspected of having a neuromuscular junction disorder such as myasthenia gravis, and therefore acetylcholine receptor antibodies are not helpful. This patient has clinical features to suggest a chronic inflammatory demyelinating polyneuropathy (CIDP). In cases of CIDP in which the CSF shows a WBC count of more than $10/mm^3$, an underlying cause should be ruled out and tests should be obtained to investigate other etiologies, including HIV, hepatitis C, lymphoproliferative or myeloproliferative disorders, Lyme disease, and neurosarcoidosis.

Monoclonal protein analysis should be obtained to evaluate for a serum paraprotein. EMG and NCS are part of the work-up of CIDP, and will show features of demyelination with conduction block.

Saperstein DS. Chronic acquired demyelinating polyneuropathies. Semin Neurol. 2008; 28:168–184.

39. c

By convention, recessive forms of Charcot-Marie-Tooth (CMT) are classified as CMT4. The CMT4 group consists of eight subtypes, which include both demyelinating and axon loss forms. These disorders are rare. They have a young age of onset, in early childhood, with significant disability. Clinical features of some of these subtypes include vision loss, severe scoliosis, and hearing loss.

The hereditary sensory and autonomic neuropathies are also autosomal dominant and discussed in questions 75 to 77. Hereditary neuropathy with liability to pressure palsy is discussed in question 27, and the familial amyloid polyneuropathies are discussed in questions 18 and 19.

Preston DC, Shapiro BE. Electromyography and Neuromuscular Disorders, 2nd ed. Philadelphia, PA: Elsevier; 2005.

40. d

Lumbosacral radiculopathy is commonly caused by disc herniation or degenerative spine changes. S1 radiculopathy commonly manifests as pain radiating from the buttock down the posterior thigh, posterior leg, and lateral foot, with sensory impairment in this dermatomal region, especially the lateral foot and fifth toe. The most prominent weakness is plantarflexion and toe flexion, and the ankle deep tendon reflex will be reduced or absent. Muscles involved in S1 radiculopathies include the abductor hallucis, abductor digiti quinti pedis, soleus, medial and lateral gastrocnemius, extensor digitorum brevis, biceps femoris (long and short head), and gluteus maximus. Muscles partially innervated by S1 that may also be affected are the tibialis posterior, flexor digitorum brevis, gluteus medius, and tensor fascia latae. Although the SNAPs should be normal in S1 radiculopathies, the H-reflex is commonly reduced or absent.

L2-L3-L4 radiculopathy is discussed in question 51. L5 radiculopathy is discussed in question 86. Peroneal neuropathy is discussed in question 44.

Katirji B. Electromyography in Clinical Practice: A Case Study Approach, 1st ed. St. Louis: Mosby; 1998.

Russell SM. Examination of Peripheral Nerve Injuries. New York: Thieme; 2006.

41. e

This patient's history and examination are consistent with an ulnar neuropathy at or above the elbow. This can occur with trauma, lacerations, or blunt injury. There is significant loss of fine motor coordination due to weakness of the third and fourth lumbricals and the palmar and dorsal interossei. Flexor pollicis brevis is innervated by both the median and ulnar nerve, so even with complete ulnar palsy, some thumb abduction can still be achieved by the part of the muscle innervated by the median nerve. When asked to make a fist, the hand assumes the appearance of a claw, with the fourth and fifth digits hyperextended at the metacarpophalangeal joint and partially flexed at the interphalangeal joint. This occurs because the third and fourth lumbricals as well as the interossei and flexor digiti minimi are weak, and there is unopposed action of the radial nerve–innervated muscles (see Table 9.6), causing hyperextension at the metacarpophalangeal joints. Other signs seen with ulnar nerve palsy include (1) Wartenberg's sign, or fifth digit abduction at rest due to paralysis of the third palmar interossei with unopposed action of extensor digiti minimi and extensor digitorum communis (radial nerve–innervated muscles), and (2) Froment's sign, whereby during attempted forceful adduction of the thumb, as with an attempt to hold a piece of paper between the thumb and the index finger, thumb flexion occurs. This occurs because the adductor pollicis is weak, and thumb flexion (by the intact flexor pollicis longus) substitutes with thumb flexion. In the case described, reduction in CMAP amplitude of more than 50% with stimulation above as compared to below the elbow (Figure 9.4) further supports the diagnosis.

In patients with ulnar nerve compression at the wrist, at Guyon's canal (as occurs in bicycle riders or others who frequently place pressure at the medial wrist area), claw hand, Wartenberg's sign, and Froment's sign can be seen. Involvement of flexor carpi ulnaris and flexor digitorum profundus (which receive motor branches from the ulnar nerve in the forearm) indicate that the lesion is proximal to the wrist. In addition, with lesions at or distal to the wrist, sensation over the hypothenar eminence is spared because the palmar cutaneous branch arises proximal to Guyon's canal. With a lesion at the wrist, CMAP amplitudes would be abnormally low with stimulation at the wrist, and a reduction in CMAP amplitude would not occur with more proximal stimulation.

Other C8-innervated muscles such as the flexor digitorum profundus to the second digit are of normal strength, and forearm pronation is normal, providing evidence that this is not a C7 or C8 radiculopathy. Intact sensation proximal to the wrist excludes a proximal medial cord lesion; when sensory loss extends 2 cm or more proximal to the wrist, the territory innervated by the medial antebrachial cutaneous nerve (which branches directly off the medial cord), involvement of the medial cord should be suspected. Another feature distinguishing an ulnar nerve palsy from a medial cord lesion is intact strength of median nerve-innervated C8 and T1 muscles, such as flexor pollicis brevis, abductor pollicis brevis, opponens pollicis, and the median nerve–innervated lumbricals (see Table 9.1).

Russell SM. Examination of Peripheral Nerve Injuries. New York: Thieme; 2006.

42. e

This patient has diabetic amyotrophy, which is a polyradiculoneuropathy. These patients are usually older, and the beginning of symptoms may occur in the setting of mild diabetes; however, the onset is frequently associated with a period of transition, such as during the initiation or adjustment of insulin treatment, or associated with episodes of hypo- or hyperglycemia. The presentation begins with pain starting in the low back or hip and radiating down to the lower limb. Deep pain with superimposed lancinating sensation is described, and commonly more severe at night. The sensory deficit may involve the L2, L3, and L4 distributions. Days to weeks later, these patients develop weakness and eventually atrophy, which involve the pelvic girdle and thigh muscles. Muscles most frequently involved are the iliopsoas, glutei, thigh adductors, quadriceps, hamstrings, and sometimes the anterior tibial muscles. Patellar reflex is absent. The EMG shows evidence of denervation in the involved myotomes.

The progression is gradual and may continue for months. The pain often resolves spontaneously, and subsequently, there may be recovery of strength, but this may take many months and sometimes years. Contralateral involvement may occur in some cases, appearing months or years later.

This is not a diabetic mononeuropathy. Small-fiber diabetic neuropathy is discussed in question 49. Large-fiber diabetic neuropathy is discussed in question 85. Diabetic autonomic neuropathy is discussed in question 20.

Bradley WG, Daroff RB, Fenichel GM, et al. Neurology in Clinical Practice, 5th ed. Philadelphia, PA: Elsevier; 2008.

Ropper AH, Samuels MA. Adams and Victor's Principles of Neurology, 9th ed. New York: McGraw-Hill; 2009.

43. e

One of the forearm muscles innervated by the radial nerve, the brachioradialis, is a forearm flexor.

The radial nerve is a continuation of the posterior cord. It carries C5, C6, C7, and C8 fibers. The first branch of the radial nerve is the posterior cutaneous nerve to the arm. In the arm, the radial nerve gives branches to long, medial, and lateral heads of the triceps muscle and then travels along the spiral groove (see Table 9.6 for root innervations and action of the muscles innervated by the radial nerve). It then gives off the posterior cutaneous nerve, which runs with the radial nerve in the spiral groove of the humerus. In the spiral groove, the radial nerve gives off the lateral

TABLE 9.6	Upper extremity muscles innervated by the radial nerve, their root innervation, and action		
Muscle	**Nerve Innervation**	**Root Innervation**	**Action**
Triceps	Radial nerve	C6, C7, C8	Forearm extension
Brachioradialis	Radial nerve	C5, C6	Forearm flexion in mid-supination
Extensor carpi radialis longus	Radial nerve	C5, C6	Wrist extension and abduction (radial extension)
Extensor carpi radialis brevis	Radial nerve	C5, C6	Wrist extension and abduction (radial extension)
Supinator	Radial nerve, posterior interosseus nerve	C6, C7	Forearm supination (best tested with forearm extended to reduce action of biceps brachii)
Extensor carpi ulnaris	Radial nerve, posterior interosseus nerve	C7, C8	Wrist extension and adduction (ulnar extension)
Extensor digitorum communis	Radial nerve, posterior interosseus nerve	C7, C8	Extension at metacarpophalangeal joints of second to fifth digits
Extensor digiti minimi	Radial nerve, posterior interosseus nerve	C7, C8	Extension at metacarpophalangeal joint of fifth digit
Abductor pollicis longus	Radial nerve, posterior interosseus nerve	C7, C8	Thumb abduction (radial abduction in plane of palm)
Extensor pollicis longus	Radial nerve, posterior interosseus nerve	C7, C8	Thumb extension at interphalangeal joint
Extensor pollicis brevis	Radial nerve, posterior interosseus nerve	C7, C8	Thumb extension at metacarpophalangeal joint
Extensor indices	Radial nerve, posterior interosseus nerve	C7, C8	Extension at metacarpophalangeal joints of second digit

cutaneous nerve to the arm. Distal to the spiral groove, it gives branches to the brachioradialis, and extensor carpi radialis longus and brevis. Distal to the elbow, it bifurcates into the posterior interosseus and superficial sensory radial nerves. The posterior interosseus nerve innervates extensor carpi ulnaris, extensor digitorum communis, extensor digiti minimi, abductor pollicis longus, extensor pollicis longus and brevis, and extensor indices.

The radial nerve provides sensory innervation to the posterior arm through the posterior cutaneous nerve to the arm, to the lateral arm via the lateral cutaneous nerve to the arm, and to the posterior forearm through the posterior cutaneous nerve to the forearm. The superficial sensory radial nerve provides sensory innervation to the dorsolateral half of the hand, the proximal two-thirds of the thumb (including the lateral thumb, over the anatomic snuffbox), and the second and third digits (discussed in question 66). Remember that the distal dorsal aspects of the second and third digits are innervated by the median nerve.

Russell SM. Examination of Peripheral Nerve Injuries. New York: Thieme; 2006.

44. a

This patient has a common peroneal nerve injury, likely localized to the fibular head. Peroneal mononeuropathy at the fibular head has been associated with significant weight loss, prolonged bedrest or hospitalization, leg crossing, diabetes, and other compressive mechanisms in this area.

The common peroneal nerve is a division of the sciatic nerve, giving off the lateral cutaneous nerve of the calf before turning around the fibular head and passing through the fibular tunnel (Figure 9.9). This nerve then divides into superficial and deep peroneal nerves. The superficial peroneal nerve innervates the peroneus longus and brevis, as well as the skin in the lower two-thirds of the lateral aspect of the leg and dorsum of the foot. The deep peroneal innervates the tibialis anterior, extensor hallucis, extensor digitorum longus and brevis, and peroneus tertius. The sensory territory of the deep peroneal nerve is the web space between the first and second toes.

Foot drop can be seen with common or deep peroneal lesions, as well as with sciatic nerve lesions, L5 radiculopathies, and plexopathies. Localization is dependent on the distribution of motor abnormalities seen throughout the leg, especially of muscles not innervated by the deep peroneal nerve. In this case, the patient has abnormalities in both deep (tibialis anterior, extensor hallucis, and extensor digitorum brevis) and superficial peroneal nerve–innervated muscles (peroneus longus). Clinically, foot dorsiflexion weakness is attributed to the deep peroneal nerve–innervated muscles, whereas foot eversion weakness is attributed to superficial peroneal nerve–innervated muscles. Therefore, presence of weak dorsiflexion and eversion points toward a common peroneal nerve injury (as opposed to isolated superficial or deep peroneal nerve injuries) like in this patient. The fact that the short head of the biceps femoris is spared suggests that the lesion is distal to this level. The lack of tibial nerve involvement with abnormalities restricted to the peroneal nerve only makes sciatic neuropathy, tibial neuropathy, or L5 radiculopathy less likely. Sciatic nerve injury is discussed in question 32. L5 radiculopathy is discussed in question 86.

Tibial nerve injury is discussed in question 34.

Katirji B. Electromyography in Clinical Practice: A Case Study Approach, 1st ed. St. Louis: Mosby; 1998.

Russell SM. Examination of Peripheral Nerve Injuries. New York: Thieme; 2006.

45. b

The history and examination depicted in question 45 are consistent with mild ulnar neuropathy at the elbow. The ulnar nerve is most susceptible to entrapment at the post-condylar groove.

A truck driver who leans his arm against the window sill for prolonged periods of time while driving would be at risk for this type of compression. The symptoms and examination are not consistent with pathology in the median nerve. Similarly, the C6 and C7 myotomes would not be affected by this type of nerve injury, and there are not other historical points suggestive of a radiculopathy. This type of compression is best managed conservatively with avoidance of pressure on the elbow and avoidance of repetitive flexion and extension of the forearm. Surgery is indicated only in select severe cases.

Bradley WG, Daroff RB, Fenichel GM, et al. Neurology in Clinical Practice, 5th ed. Philadelphia, PA: Elsevier; 2008.

Russell SM. Examination of Peripheral Nerve Injuries. New York: Thieme; 2006.

46. e

Diabetic neuropathy has significant clinical implications. Patients with polyneuropathy are at risk for developing foot ulcers and ankle arthropathy (discussed also in Chapter 16).

Foot ulcers are a severe complication caused by a combination of factors, including loss of sensation from neuropathy leading to unnoticed trauma, poor vascular perfusion, and higher risk of infection.

Ankle arthropathy, known as "Charcot joint," is a joint deformity associated with loss of sensation and sensory ataxia resulting from neuropathy.

Mononeuropathies can involve peripheral or cranial nerves. A typical cranial nerve affected by diabetes is the third nerve, which can occur acutely, usually sparing the pupillary function (discussed in Chapter 1).

Bradley WG, Daroff RB, Fenichel GM, et al. Neurology in Clinical Practice, 5th ed. Philadelphia, PA: Elsevier; 2008.

Ropper AH, Samuels MA. Adams and Victor's Principles of Neurology, 9th ed. New York: McGraw-Hill; 2009.

47. a

This patient has meralgia paresthetica, which is caused by a mononeuropathy of the lateral femoral cutaneous nerve of the thigh. This nerve originates from L2 and L3, and is purely sensory. Patients with meralgia paresthetica complain of numbness, pain, and paresthesias on the anterolateral aspect of the thigh. Pain may be worse with standing and walking, and better with flexion at the hip or sitting. This condition results from compression of or trauma to this nerve. Predisposing factors include obesity, pregnancy, ascites, devices that compress the nerve at the waist (tight belts), diabetes, and rapid and significant weight loss.

Ropper AH, Samuels MA. Adams and Victor's Principles of Neurology, 9th ed. New York: McGraw-Hill; 2009.

Russell SM. Examination of Peripheral Nerve Injuries. New York: Thieme; 2006.

48. b

On the basis of the clinical and electrophysiologic findings, this patient has a femoral nerve injury that occurred in the intrapelvic region. Femoral nerve injury in the intrapelvic region can be caused by pelvic surgery, pelvic masses, or retroperitoneal hematomas. The history suggests a retroperitoneal hematoma, which can compress the femoral nerve in the intrapelvic region. This patient has pain with hip flexion and knee extension weakness, as well as absent patellar reflex. There are also sensory findings in the femoral nerve and saphenous nerve distribution. The presence of fibrillations in the iliacus and psoas muscles suggests an intrapelvic injury rather than an inguinal injury, given that these muscles are innervated by the femoral nerve in the intrapelvic region and prior to its course through the inguinal region. The anatomy of the femoral nerve is discussed in question 29 and shown in Figure 9.7.

Involvement of the psoas distinguishes intrapelvic injury from injury at the inguinal ligament (discussed also in question 29). The fact that thigh adductors and other muscle groups are spared suggests that this is not a plexopathy or radiculopathy as only the femoral nerve–innervated muscles are involved. The abnormal SNAPs point away from the diagnosis of a radiculopathy.

Katirji B. Electromyography in Clinical Practice: A Case Study Approach, 1st ed. St. Louis: Mosby; 1998.

Russell SM. Examination of Peripheral Nerve Injuries. New York: Thieme; 2006.

49. a

This patient has a small fiber diabetic neuropathy, which is characterized by painful paresthesias, burning sensations, and allodynia that typically affect both feet, but may affect other regions. There is preservation of vibratory sense and proprioception, as well as deep tendon reflexes. Strength is usually preserved as well. Small fiber neuropathy is commonly associated with autonomic neuropathy, and therefore these patients may have features of autonomic dysfunction.

Diabetic mononeuropathy can occur, affecting either the peripheral or cranial nerves, and usually involves one nerve. If several nerves are involved, the presentation is usually asymmetric, unlike in this case. Large fiber diabetic neuropathy is discussed in question 85. Diabetic polyradiculoneuropathy and diabetic amyotrophy are discussed in question 42.

Bradley WG, Daroff RB, Fenichel GM, et al. Neurology in Clinical Practice, 5th ed. Philadelphia, PA: Elsevier; 2008.

Ropper AH, Samuels MA. Adams and Victor's Principles of Neurology, 9th ed. New York: McGraw-Hill; 2009.

50. c

This patient's history and examination are consistent with posterior interosseus nerve palsy, which can occur as a diabetic mononeuropathy, but can also occur in the setting of posterior interosseus nerve compression (such as due to lipomas or nerve sheath tumors) or can be seen in Parsonage-Turner syndrome (discussed in question 52). The posterior interosseus nerve is a pure motor nerve. With a posterior interosseus nerve palsy, there is not an obvious wrist drop because radial nerve branches to extensor carpi radialis longus and brevis originate proximal to the posterior interosseus nerve; there is however weakness of wrist extension in an ulnar direction (see Table 9.6 for muscles innervated by the posterior interosseus nerve).

Strength of more proximal radial nerve–innervated muscles excludes a radial neuropathy at the spiral groove or elbow, and intact superficial sensory radial nerve responses on NCS further support this. Intact triceps reflex and normal strength of forearm extension exclude a C7 radiculopathy. Supinator syndrome causes a painful posterior interosseus nerve palsy due to compression or irritation of this nerve as it passes through the supinator muscle. Absence of pain on forced supination makes this uncommon disorder less likely.

Russell SM. Examination of Peripheral Nerve Injuries. New York: Thieme; 2006.

51. b

This patient has an L2-L3-L4 radiculopathy. Radiculopathies involving the upper lumbar roots are more difficult to assess and less common than those involving the lower lumbosacral roots.

L2-L3 radiculopathy manifests with pain in the hip and groin radiating down the anterior and medial thigh. If there is an L4 radiculopathy, the pain may also radiate down to the medial leg. L2-L3-L4 radiculopathy may affect hip flexion and knee extension, as well as ankle dorsiflexion due to involvement of the L4 root, which partially innervates the tibialis anterior along with L5. The patellar reflex is reduced or absent in L2-L3-L4 root lesions.

The iliacus muscle is innervated by L2-L3 roots. The quadriceps femoris is innervated by L3-L4 roots, and the tibialis anterior is innervated by L4-L5 roots.

L2-L3-L4 radiculopathies should be distinguished from a lumbar plexopathy and femoral neuropathy. The differences can be difficult to detect clinically, but may be further clarified with EMG. In radiculopathies, the SNAPs are normal, whereas in plexopathies, they are abnormal. Paraspinal fibrillations are seen in radiculopathies, but not in plexopathies. In femoral neuropathy, the manifestations should be restricted to the distribution and muscles supplied by this nerve. In this case, it should also be considered in the differential diagnosis. However femoral nerve injury does not involve the tibialis anterior muscle, which is an L4, peroneal nerve–innervated muscle.

L5 radiculopathy is discussed in question 86. S1 radiculopathy is discussed in question 40. Femoral neuropathy is discussed in questions 29 and 48.

Katirji B. Electromyography in Clinical Practice: A Case Study Approach, 1st ed. St. Louis: Mosby; 1998.

Russell SM. Examination of Peripheral Nerve Injuries. New York: Thieme; 2006.

52. b

The patient has a history and examination consistent with acute brachial plexitis, also known as neuralgic amyotrophy or Parsonage-Turner syndrome. This can occur following surgery, vaccination, or systemic viral illness; in some cases, it can be idiopathic. Symptoms of acute brachial neuritis include acute onset of severe shoulder and arm pain, which then resolve, with subsequent occurrence of weakness. This disorder can potentially affect any portion of the brachial plexus and can be isolated to a single upper extremity nerve, but frequently affects multiple nerves originating from the brachial plexus in a multifocal fashion. Nerves frequently affected include the suprascapular nerve, long thoracic nerve, and median nerve. It can also occur in the lumbosacral plexus. This disorder is most often monophasic with good recovery, but recurrent episodes may occur. There is a familial form, hereditary neuralgic amyotrophy, which is autosomal dominant in inheritance. Recovery typically occurs after each attack, though with time residual deficits may be incurred. Some cases of hereditary neuralgic amyotrophy have been linked to *SEPT9* gene on chromosome 17.

The fact that this patient had normal strength postoperatively argues against a nerve injury related to nerve traction, median sternotomy, or other procedure-related etiologies. Delayed weakness postoperatively should also place brachial plexus compression from a hematoma on the differential diagnosis. Infectious polyradiculitis would be unusual in this postoperative setting, and more often occurs in immunocompromised patients, such as cytomegalovirus polyradiculitis in HIV patients. The cervical-brachial-pharyngeal variant of Guillain-Barre is associated with neck and pharyngeal weakness as well, and the occurrence of pain which then resolves and is followed by weakness is more typical of acute brachial plexitis.

Bradley WG, Daroff RB, Fenichel GM, et al. Neurology in Clinical Practice, 5th ed. Philadelphia, PA: Elsevier; 2008.

Ropper AH, Samuels MA. Adams and Victor's Principles of Neurology, 9th ed. New York: McGraw-Hill; 2009.

53. a, 54. c

The patient in question 53 has a complete median nerve palsy at the level of the antecubital fossa. Brachial artery injury often occurs concomitantly, given its proximity to the median nerve in this area. Intact strength of the ulnar nerve–innervated muscles (see Table 9.5) is evidence that this is not a medial cord lesion. Ischemic monomelia, as can occur during placement of arteriovenous shunts for dialysis, is painful and causes circumferential sensory loss in multiple nerve distributions, a clinical picture not evident in this case. The sensory fibers of the median nerve are derived mainly from C6 and C7 through the lateral cord. Weakness of C6- and C7-innervated muscles, such as the pronators, is evidence that this is not a medial cord lesion because the medial cord carries predominantly C8 and T1 fibers. With complete median nerve palsy, on attempt to make a fist, the first digit does not flex, the second digit partially flexes, and the fourth and fifth digits flex normally, assuming a hand position similar to that used in religious blessings, termed the Benedictine sign.

The patient in question 54 has anterior interosseus nerve syndrome. The anterior interosseus nerve is a pure motor branch of the median nerve and innervates flexor digitorum profundus to the second and third digits, flexor pollicis longus, and pronator quadratus (Table 9.1). Weakness of these muscles, in the absence of sensory loss, suggests isolated involvement of the anterior interosseus nerve, as can occur with trauma, fracture, or in neuralgic amyotrophy (Parsonage-Turner syndrome; see question 52). Patients complain of weakness in grasping objects with their thumb and index finger, and on attempt to make an "okay sign," the distal phalanges are unable to flex, and instead, the fingertips touch.

In both cases, weakness of C8 and T1 median nerve–innervated muscles is evidence that this is not isolated to the C7 nerve root (see question 23 and Table 9.1 for more information on the course of the median nerve and action of median nerve–innervated muscles).

Bradley WG, Daroff RB, Fenichel GM, et al. Neurology in Clinical Practice, 5th ed. Philadelphia, PA: Elsevier; 2008.

Russell SM. Examination of Peripheral Nerve Injuries. New York: Thieme; 2006.

55. c, 56. c

In patients with Guillain-Barre syndrome (GBS), CSF typically shows albuminocytologic dissociation, which is the presence of increased proteins with low cell counts. The other options in question 55 are not CSF findings to be expected in patients with GBS.

Neurophysiologic studies should be performed early and repeated in 3 weeks if clinically indicated. The main findings are consistent with demyelination, and typically show prolonged or abnormal distal latencies and slow conduction velocities, with abnormal late responses, which are the F-response and the H-reflex. Although distal latencies may not be affected initially, they are almost always affected at some time in the disease process. There may also be evidence of motor conduction block.

Neurophysiologic data can help to evaluate GBS and determine the presence of other variants. The three possible variant subtypes are the following:

— Acute inflammatory demyelinating polyneuropathy: findings of demyelination, with prolonged latencies and slow conduction velocities.
— Acute motor and sensory axonal neuropathy: no features of demyelination, but reduced sensory and motor amplitudes.
— Acute motor axonal neuropathy: no features of demyelination, but reduced motor amplitudes.

MRI of the lumbar spine may show enhancement of the cauda equina.

Hughes RAC, Cornblath DR. Guillain-Barre syndrome. Lancet. 2005; 366:1653–1666.

Ropper AH, Samuels MA. Adams and Victor's Principles of Neurology, 9th ed. New York: McGraw-Hill; 2009.

57. c

This patient's history and examination are consistent with radiation-induced brachial plexopathy. Her examination suggests a pan-plexopathy. Radiation-induced plexopathy can occur months to years following exposure to radiation. Unlike carcinomatous invasion, radiation-induced plexopathy is painless. Myokymia on EMG further supports the diagnosis and distinguishes it from carcinomatous invasion. A paraneoplastic neuropathy as well as chemotherapy-induced neuropathy would more likely affect other limbs as well. Cervical spine stenosis would likely affect both limbs (though this is often asymmetric) and would also likely be associated with neck pain as well.

Russell SM. Examination of Peripheral Nerve Injuries. New York: Thieme; 2006.

58. d

This patient has a Miller-Fisher syndrome, which is associated with the presence of the antibody GQ1b. Miller-Fisher syndrome, described by C. Miller Fisher, is a variant of Guillain-Barre syndrome (GBS), characterized by the triad of ataxia, ophthalmoplegia, and areflexia. Antibodies to GQ1b are present in 90% of patients with Miller-Fisher syndrome. Antibodies to GQ1b can also lead to isolated ocular nerve abnormalities.

Other variants of GBS have been associated with antibodies to gangliosides. Gangliosides are glycosphingolipids with sugar residues on the extracellular surface bearing sialic acid molecules. Antibodies to GM1, GM1b, and GD1a have been detected in acute motor axonal neuropathy and acute motor and sensory axonal neuropathy. Antibodies to GalNAc-GD1a can be seen in patients with acute motor axonal neuropathy. Antibodies to GD1b can be seen in acute sensory neuronopathy.

Hughes RAC, Cornblath DR. Guillain-Barre syndrome. Lancet. 2005; 366:1653–1666.

Lee SH, Lim GH, Kim JS, et al. Acute ophthalmoplegia (without ataxia) associated with anti-GQ1b antibody. Neurology. 2008; 71:426–429.

59. b

Pronator teres syndrome results from compression of the median nerve as it passes between the two heads of pronator teres. It is uncommon, but occurs in people who perform repetitive forceful pronation and may be associated with medial epicondylitis, or "golfer's elbow." Symptoms include gradual onset of a deep ache in the forearm that may worsen with pronation and weakness in median nerve–innervated muscles. Because branches from the median nerve that innervate the pronator teres arise proximal to this muscle (before the nerve passes under this muscle), pronator teres strength is intact in this syndrome. Apparently normal strength in pronator teres excludes a complete median nerve palsy at the elbow. Weakness of muscles not innervated by the anterior interosseus nerve (such as finger flexors and thumb abductors) indicates that this is not isolated anterior interosseus nerve syndrome. Weakness of flexor carpi radialis, which is predominantly C6 and C7 in innervation (see Table 9.1), indicates that this is not a medial cord lesion.

Bradley WG, Daroff RB, Fenichel GM, et al. Neurology in Clinical Practice, 5th ed. Philadelphia, PA: Elsevier; 2008.

Russell SM. Examination of Peripheral Nerve Injuries. New York: Thieme; 2006.

60. d

Patients with carpal tunnel syndrome often have a history of repetitive motions at the wrist, as occurs in certain occupations. Some systemic illnesses predispose to carpal tunnel syndrome, including diabetes, rheumatoid arthritis, chronic renal failure, amyloidosis, acromegaly, obesity, and hypothyroidism. Testing for these conditions in the appropriate clinical setting may be indicated, especially in the absence of evident occupational risk factors or when the presentation is bilateral. Local compression by masses, such as ganglion cysts or neurofibromas, can cause median nerve compression as well. For mild carpal tunnel syndrome, in which sensory symptoms are intermittent and there is no evidence of axon loss on EMG, management includes wrist splinting, particularly at night, and minimization of provocative maneuvers. Surgical therapy is not indicated for asymptomatic cases, though measures to minimize further median nerve compression at the wrist are indicated. In more severe cases, surgery is indicated when there is significant sensory loss, motor weakness, and/or evidence of significant axon loss. Surgery may be indicated for milder cases if symptoms are significant and refractory to splinting and/or if the patient cannot avoid the provocative actions (due to, for example, employment).

Preston DC, Shapiro BE. Electromyography and Neuromuscular Disorders, 2nd ed. Philadelphia, PA: Elsevier; 2005.

Russell SM. Examination of Peripheral Nerve Injuries. New York: Thieme; 2006.

61. b, 62. d

The patient in question 61 has a history and examination consistent with a radial neuropathy at the axilla. Loss of sensation over the posterior arm (due to involvement of the posterior cutaneous nerve of the arm, the most proximal branch of the radial nerve), as well as weakness of the triceps (which receives innervation from the radial nerve proximal to the spiral groove), indicates that the lesion is proximal to the spiral groove. Proximal radial nerve lesions are not common, but can occur with repetitive pressure to the axilla, as occurs with prolonged crutch use, or with prolonged pressure otherwise on the axilla, as occurs in "Saturday night palsy," when a person sleeps with his or her arm hung over the back of a chair. Although the triceps reflex (C7) is absent, intact forearm pronation suggests that pronator teres, which is predominantly innervated by the C7 nerve root, is normal, excluding a C7 radiculopathy. Intact arm abduction, mediated in large part by axillary nerve–innervated muscles, excludes a posterior cord lesion. With posterior cord lesions, muscles innervated by both the axillary and radial nerves are weak.

The patient in question 62 has a history and examination consistent with a radial neuropathy at the spiral groove. Intact strength of the triceps and intact sensation on the posterior aspect of the arm support that the lesion is distal to origin of the posterior cutaneous nerve to the arm and branches to triceps, excluding a proximal radial nerve lesion or a posterior cord lesion; intact triceps strength and normal triceps deep tendon reflex are evidence that this not a C7 radiculopathy. Reduced sensation over the lateral aspect of the arm suggests that the lesion is more proximal than the elbow, as the lateral cutaneous nerve to the arm arises from the radial nerve within the spiral groove. The spiral groove is the most common location for radial nerve injury, and a common mechanism is humeral fracture. Other choices are excluded on the basis of the discussion above.

Russell SM. Examination of Peripheral Nerve Injuries. New York: Thieme; 2006.

63. d

This man's history and examination are consistent with injury to the spinal accessory nerve, which is rare in isolation, but can be an iatrogenic complication of radical neck dissection, because in the neck, it is interwoven among several lymph nodes. The spinal accessory nerve carries fibers from the lower medulla as well as C1 to C4. It exits the skull base through the jugular foramen and innervates the sternocleidomastoid, which turns the head contralaterally, as well as the trapezius, which is involved in shoulder shrug along with assisting in elevation of the scapula and assisting the deltoid in arm abduction beyond 90 degrees.

Jugular foramen syndrome, or Vernet's syndrome, results from compressive lesions of the foramen magnum, such as metastases or schwannomas, and there would be evidence of involvement of the vagus and glossopharyngeal nerves in addition to the spinal accessory nerve.

The cervical plexus consists of the ventral rami of C1 to C4. The cervical plexus provides innervation to several neck muscles including the levator scapula (C3 and C4), which significantly contributes to shoulder shrug (along with trapezius), allowing relatively preserved shoulder shrug strength in the setting of trapezial weakness. The cervical plexus is also the origin of the nerves that supply sensory innervation to the posterior head and neck regions, including the lesser occipital nerves that provide sensation to the area posterior to the ear, the greater occipital nerves, which carry predominantly C2 fibers and provide sensory innervation to most of the posterior head, the greater auricular nerves, and the transverse cervical nerves. Absence of sensory loss in this patient excludes the other choices listed.

Russell SM. Examination of Peripheral Nerve Injuries. New York: Thieme; 2006.

64. e

Diabetes mellitus involvement of the peripheral nervous system can present in various forms, with a distal symmetric polyneuropathy being the most common presentation. This polyneuropathy is commonly a large fiber length-dependent neuropathy, but small fiber neuropathy is also seen (discussed in question 49). Other presentations include autonomic neuropathy (discussed in question 20), polyradiculopathy (diabetic amyotrophy; discussed in question 42), mononeuropathy affecting either peripheral or cranial nerves, and multiple mononeuropathies.

Bradley WG, Daroff RB, Fenichel GM, et al. Neurology in Clinical Practice, 5th ed. Philadelphia, PA: Elsevier; 2008.

65. d

This patient has multifocal acquired demyelinating sensory and motor neuropathy(MADSAM). This is a demyelinating neuropathy with evidence of conduction block, presenting with asymmetric motor and sensory symptoms. The progression is gradual and slow, usually involving the upper limbs initially and later the lower limbs. Deep tendon reflexes are diminished in the distribution of the affected nerves. On CSF examination, the protein is usually elevated. Unlike multifocal motor neuropathy (discussed in questions 35 and 36), anti-GM1 antibodies are not present, and electrophysiologic studies show abnormalities in motor and sensory nerves, with features of demyelination and conduction block. Patients with MADSAM may improve on steroids.

Chronic inflammatory demyelinating polyneuropathy (CIDP) is discussed in questions 11, 12, and 38. Acute inflammatory demyelinating polyneuropathy (AIDP) is discussed in questions 15, 16, 24, 55, and 56. Subacute inflammatory demyelinating polyneuropathy is a controversial diagnosis that is not generally accepted, but some authors have used this term to define patients with manifestations similar to AIDP and CIDP, with a time evolution between 4 and 8 weeks.

Saperstein DS. Chronic acquired demyelinating polyneuropathies. Semin Neurol. 2008; 28:168–184.

66. d

This patient's history and examination are consistent with a superficial sensory radial neuropathy. This type of neuropathy, also called Wartenberg's syndrome, can result from compression or irritation of this nerve due to tight handcuffs or watches, venipuncture, or surgery. Rarely, compression may occur due to pinching of the nerve between the brachioradialis and extensor carpi radialis longus tendons as occurs with repetitive pronation. Symptoms include dysesthesias and numbness over the dorsolateral aspect of the hand. There is no motor weakness, as the superficial sensory radial nerve is a pure sensory nerve. Treatment is conservative, and includes avoidance of pressure to the nerve and medications for neuropathic pain (such as amitriptyline, pregabalin, or gabapentin) if necessary.

Russell SM. Examination of Peripheral Nerve Injuries. New York: Thieme; 2006.

67. e

This patient's history and examination are consistent with a musculocutaneous neuropathy. Such neuropathies in isolation are rare, but can occur with anterior shoulder dislocations and other types of trauma. The musculocutaneous nerve is a continuation of the lateral cord and carries predominantly C5 and C6 fibers. The musculocutaneous nerve innervates the coracobrachialis muscle that assists the deltoid in anterior flexion of the arm at the shoulder and stabilizes the humerus during forearm flexion. The musculocutaneous nerve then innervates the brachialis muscle and the biceps brachii, which flex the forearm at the elbow. The brachioradialis, innervated by the radial nerve, also contributes to forearm flexion. The biceps brachii also supinates the forearm, and is the main forearm supinator when the forearm is flexed.

The musculocutaneous nerve provides sensory innervation to the lateral half of the forearm via the lateral antebrachial cutaneous nerve, but this nerve does not provide any sensation below the wrist. The latter point, along with intact strength of the brachioradialis in the case (as evidence by stronger forearm supination with the forearm extended), is evidence that this is not a C6 radiculopathy. Absence of palpable contraction of the biceps during attempted forearm flexion is evidence that this is not biceps tendon rupture. A lateral cord lesion would lead to weakness in other C5- to C7-innervated muscles, such as flexor carpi radialis and pronator teres (see Tables 9.1 and 9.6). It would also lead to sensory loss over the palm, palmar aspect of the thumb, and second and third digits. Therefore, absence of weakness in wrist flexion and forearm pronation distinguishes a lateral cord lesion from musculocutaneous palsy. A median neuropathy would lead to weakness in muscles innervated by the median nerve (see Table 9.1), not evident in this case.

Russell SM. Examination of Peripheral Nerve Injuries. New York: Thieme; 2006.

68. e

EMG/NCS are normal in patients with pure small fiber neuropathy.

Small fibers include myelinated A-δ and unmyelinated C-fibers, which are involved in autonomic, temperature, and pain transmission. Patients with small fiber neuropathy present with painful burning sensations and dysesthesias distally (most frequently in the feet). Some patients may have autonomic manifestations that compromise sweating, vasomotor control, gastrointestinal, and genitourinary functions. In pure small-fiber neuropathy, besides sensory findings, the neurologic examination is normal, including motor and reflex examination, distinguishing it from large-fiber neuropathy.

A cause is not found in the majority of cases. There are multiple causes of small-fiber neuropathy that account for a small percentage of the cases and should be investigated. Of the cases in which an etiology is found, diabetes and impaired glucose tolerance are the most common. Others include alcohol, amyloidosis, vasculitis, sarcoidosis, HIV, hyperlipidemia, Sjogren's syndrome, and connective tissue disorders.

EMG/NCS are normal because these tests evaluate the integrity of large nerve fibers. Tests that help in making the diagnosis include quantitative sudomotor axon reflex test (QSART), thermoregulatory sweat test (TST) and skin biopsy (discussed also in Chapter 10). QSART evaluates postganglionic sympathetic cholinergic sudomotor function, and is performed by stimulation of sweat glands by iontophoresis of acetylcholine. TST assesses the pattern of sweating and dysfunction of sweating by placing the patient in a warming chamber while covered by a reactive powder that changes color with sweat. Skin biopsy determines if intraepidermal nerve fiber density is significantly reduced.

The treatment should target the underlying cause when determined. Symptomatic treatment includes medications for neuropathic pain, including gabapentin, pregabalin, carbamazepine, and amitriptyline, among others.

Al-Shekhlee A, Chelimsky TC, Preston DC. Small-fiber neuropathy. Neurologist. 2002; 8:237–253.

Hoitsma E, Reulen JPH, de Baets M, et al. Small fiber neuropathy: A common and important clinical disorder. J Neurological Sci. 2004; 227:119–130.

69. a

This patient's history and examination are consistent with an axillary neuropathy. Axillary neuropathies occur with fractures at the surgical neck of the humerus and with anterior shoulder dislocations. The axillary nerve is a continuation of the posterior cord, and carries predominantly C5 and C6 fibers. The axillary nerve innervates the deltoid muscle, which is the main arm abductor, particularly between 30 and 90 degrees (supraspinatus significantly contributes to arm abduction in the first 30 degrees of abduction and the trapezius contributes to greater than 90 degrees). The deltoid has three heads: (1) the anterior head, which is involved arm flexion (in front of the body), assisted by serratus anterior, (2) the lateral head, which along with the anterior head is mainly involved in arm abduction to the side and slightly anteriorly, and (3) the posterior head, which is involved in posterior movement of the abducted arm. The axillary nerve also innervates teres minor, which externally rotates the arm along with infraspinatus. The axillary nerve provides sensory innervation to the upper lateral arm through the upper lateral brachial cutaneous nerve.

Intact arm abduction in the first 30 degrees suggests the supraspinatus is of normal strength. In addition, there is intact sensation over the posterolateral arm, territory innervated by the C5 nerve root through the lateral and posterior cutaneous nerves to the arm (radial nerve branches). These findings make a C5 radiculopathy unlikely.

Intact strength of radial nerve–innervated muscles excludes a posterior cord lesion and a radial neuropathy; intact strength of predominantly C7-innervated muscles (see Tables 9.1 and 9.6) excludes a middle trunk lesion.

Russell SM. Examination of Peripheral Nerve Injuries. New York: Thieme; 2006.

70. b

This patient's history is consistent with Fabry's disease, an X-linked disorder that results from a deficiency in the enzyme α-galactosidase A, a lysosomal enzyme. Females can be affected, but the phenotype is milder than in males, with renal failure being less common. It is a lysosomal storage disease that results from accumulation of globotriaosylceramide in various organs. Commonly involved organs include the kidneys, heart, and skin. Typical skin findings include angiokeratomas, dark punctuate lesions that are often found on the trunk, and intertriginous areas such as the axilla and scrotum. Both central and peripheral nervous system complications can occur. Peripheral nervous system complications include small fiber neuropathy and autonomic neuropathy. Strokes in Fabry's disease can be cardioembolic or due to large or small vessel occlusion. Endothelial deposition of globotriaosylceramide can lead to dolichoectasia increasing risk for thrombosis. Enzyme replacement therapy for this disorder is available.

Deficiency of arylsulfatase A leads to metachromatic leukodystrophy (discussed in Chapter 14).

Bradley WG, Daroff RB, Fenichel GM, et al. Neurology in Clinical Practice, 5th ed. Philadelphia, PA: Elsevier; 2008.

Testaj FD, Gorelick PB. Inherited metabolic disorders and stroke part 1: Fabry disease and mitochondrial myopathy, encephalopathy, lactic acidosis and strokelike episodes. Arch Neurol. 2010; 67:19–24.

71. c

The distribution of muscle weakness and sensory loss, combined with the EMG findings, suggests a proximal lesion at the C5 and C6 root level. The key clue to this localization is involvement of the rhomboids, which are innervated by the dorsal scapular nerve, which arises from the C5 nerve root. With chronic denervation of the rhomboids, intrascapular wasting can occur. It is important to note that C5 has a significant contribution to the phrenic nerve, which also receives contributions from C3 and C4. A proximal lesion to C5 can lead to weakness of the ipsilateral diaphragm.

Bradley WG, Daroff RB, Fenichel GM, et al. Neurology in Clinical Practice, 5th ed. Philadelphia, PA: Elsevier; 2008.

Preston DC, Shapiro BE. Electromyography and Neuromuscular Disorders, 2nd ed. Philadelphia, PA: Elsevier; 2005.

72. b

The history and examination are consistent with suprascapular nerve entrapment, as can occur in athletes, but also due to trauma (shoulder dislocation or scapular fracture). The clinical picture is one of poorly localizable shoulder pain, and weakness of the supraspinatus, which abducts the arm, particularly during the first 30 degrees of abduction, and infraspinatus, which externally rotates the shoulder when the elbow is flexed and fixed at the patient's side.

The distribution of weakness in this patient is not consistent with long thoracic nerve injury. The long thoracic nerve arises from the C5, C6, and C7 roots and innervates serratus anterior, which acts to abduct the scapula. Injury to it causes winging of the scapula, which is most evident when the arms are extended and pressure is applied anteriorly (as if doing a push-up on a wall). Scapular winging also occurs with rhomboid weakness. Normal strength of forearm flexion suggests the biceps, a largely C5-innervated muscle, is normal; an intact biceps deep tendon reflex is further evidence that this is not a C5 radiculopathy. For similar reasons, an upper trunk lesion is also excluded.

The history is also not consistent with thoracodorsal nerve injury because arm adduction is normal in this patient; the thoracodorsal nerve arises from the posterior cord and innervates the latissimus dorsi, which acts to adduct the arm. The other two branches of the posterior cord are also involved in arm abduction (as well as internal rotation): (1) the upper subscapular nerve, which innervates the subscapularis muscle, and (2) the lower subscapular nerve, which innervates teres major as well as a portion of the subscapularis muscle.

Russell SM. Examination of Peripheral Nerve Injuries. New York: Thieme; 2006.

73. d

This patient has a thoracoabdominal polyradiculopathy, which is seen in patients with long-standing diabetes, and presents with pain and dysesthesias, patchy sensory and motor changes in thoracic and abdominal nerve root territories, usually unilateral but may be bilateral. It is commonly confused with intra-abdominal processes and extensive gastrointestinal work-ups are often undertaken before the diagnosis is made. The pathology is not known but thought to be an ischemic radiculopathy. EMG of the abdominal wall and paraspinals may assist with the diagnosis, showing fibrillations in the involved muscles in one or more adjacent myotomes. Recovery is protracted, and may occur spontaneously or with the treatment of the diabetes.

The clinical presentation in this patient is not consistent with spinal cord ischemia or a femoral neuropathy. The other options are not likely in this case.

Boulton AJ, Angus E, Ayyar DR, et al. Diabetic thoracic polyradiculopathy presenting as abdominal swelling. Br Med J (Clin Res Ed). 1984; 289:798–799.

Ropper AH, Samuels MA. Adams and Victor's Principles of Neurology, 9th ed. New York: McGraw-Hill; 2009.

74. c

This patient's history and physical examination are consistent with neurogenic thoracic outlet syndrome. The signs and symptoms result from compression on the C8 and T1 nerve roots. The brachial plexus passes through the scalene triangle, which is formed by the anterior scalene, middle scalene, and first rib. An anomalous fibrous band between the scalene muscles, a cervical rib, or an elongated C7 transverse process can lead to neural compression or irritation, resulting in neurogenic thoracic outlet syndrome. There is weakness of intrinsic hand muscles and sensory loss in a C8 and T1 distribution; the pattern of weakness distinguishes this disorder from the other disorders listed, which would lead to weakness in muscle groups innervated by the single nerves listed. Arm abduction and external rotation can precipitate symptoms and reduce the radial pulse. Sensory loss in both C8 and T1 dermatomes distinguishes thoracic outlet syndrome from C8 radiculopathy. Involvement of the medial antebrachial cutaneous nerve makes thoracic outlet syndrome more likely than ulnar neuropathy at the elbow.

Russell SM. Examination of Peripheral Nerve Injuries. New York: Thieme; 2006.

75. a, 76. d 77. e

The history and examination of the patient in question 75 suggest the diagnosis of hereditary sensory and autonomic neuropathy (HSAN) type 1. In question 76, the diagnosis is HSAN3. The patient in question 77 suffers from HSAN4.

The HSANs are a relatively rare, genetically and phenotypically heterogeneous group of hereditary neuropathies. As a group, they share in common prominent sensory signs and symptoms, including pain, sensory loss, and autonomic features with little motor involvement. Because of the sensory loss, patients with HSANs are prone to painful calluses, stress fractures, neuropathic (Charcot) joints, skin ulcerations that heal poorly, and infections with deep tissue involvement, such as osteomyelitis, leading to disfiguring acral mutilations.

Question 75 depicts HSAN1. HSAN1 is the most common HSAN. It is autosomal dominant. Presentation is typically in young adulthood. Painful sensory symptoms such as lancinating pains

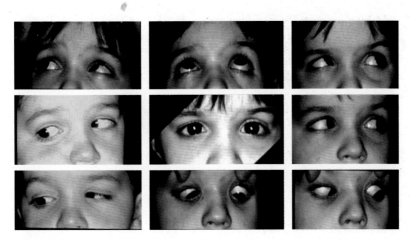

FIGURE 1.1 Directions of gaze. Courtesy of Dr. Gregory Kosmorsky

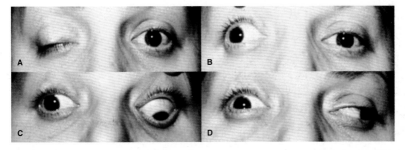

FIGURE 1.2 Directions of gaze. Courtesy of Dr. Gregory Kosmorsky. **A,** looking forward in primary gaze; **B,** looking forward in primary gaze with right eyelid lifted; **C,** looking down; **D,** looking left

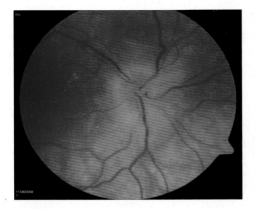

FIGURE 1.3 Courtesy of Anne Pinter

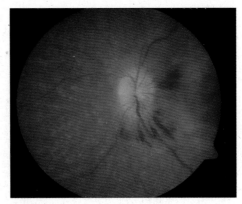

FIGURE 1.4 Courtesy of Anne Pinter

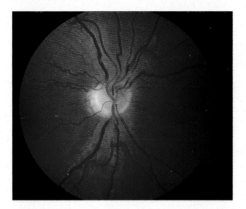

FIGURE 1.5 Courtesy of Anne Pinter

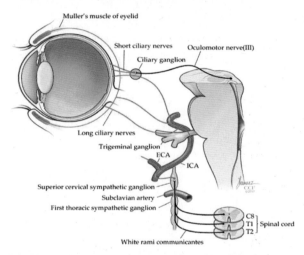

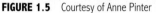

FIGURE 1.6 Sympathetic innervation to the eye. ECA; ICA. Illustration by Joseph Kanasz, BFA. Reprinted with permission of the Cleveland Clinic Center for Medical Art and Photography. © 2010. All rights reserved

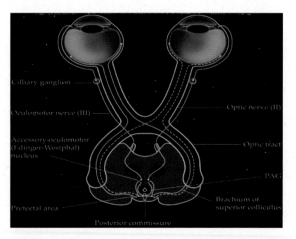

FIGURE 1.7 Pupillary light reflex. Periaqueductal gray (PAG). Illustration by Joseph Kanasz, BFA. Reprinted with permission of the Cleveland Clinic Center for Medical Art and Photography. © 2010. All rights reserved

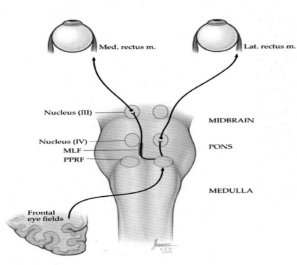

FIGURE 1.8 Pathways of horizontal gaze. MLF, medial longitudinal fasciculus; PPRF, paramedian pontine reticular formation. Illustration by Joseph Kanasz, BFA. Reprinted with permission of the Cleveland Clinic Center for Medical Art and Photography. © 2010. All rights reserved

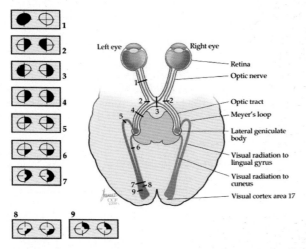

FIGURE 1.9 Visual pathways. Illustration by Joseph Kanasz, BFA. Reprinted with permission of the Cleveland Clinic Center for Medical Art and Photography. © 2010. All rights reserved

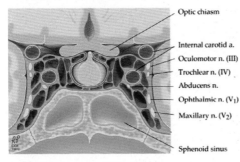

FIGURE 1.10 Cavernous sinus. Illustration by Ross Papalardo, BFA. Reprinted with permission of the Cleveland Clinic Center for Medical Art and Photography. © 2010. All rights reserved

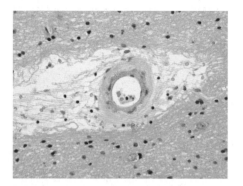

FIGURE 2.17   Brain specimen. Courtesy of Dr. Richard A. Prayson

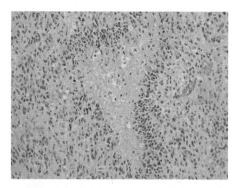

FIGURE 8.3   Brain specimen. Courtesy of Dr. Richard A. Prayson

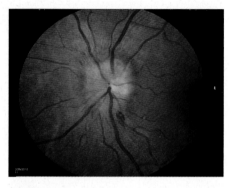

FIGURE 4.3   Fundoscopy of left eye. Courtesy of Anne Pinter

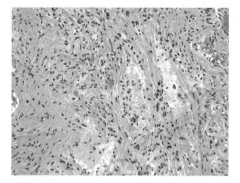

FIGURE 8.5   Brain specimen. Courtesy of Dr. Richard A. Prayson

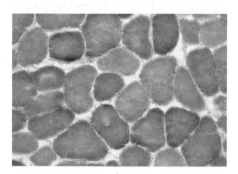

FIGURE 5.6   Muscle specimen. Courtesy of Dr. Richard A. Prayson

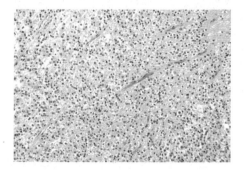

FIGURE 8.6   Brain specimen. Courtesy of Dr. Richard A. Prayson

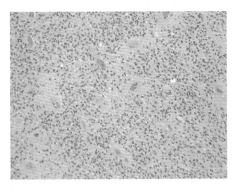

FIGURE 8.7   Brain specimen. Courtesy of Dr. Richard A. Prayson

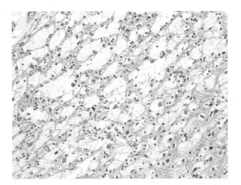

FIGURE 8.11   Brain specimen. Courtesy of Dr. Richard A. Prayson

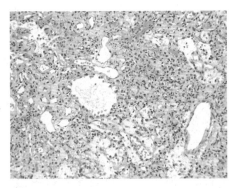

FIGURE 8.9   Brain specimen. Courtesy of Dr. Richard A. Prayson

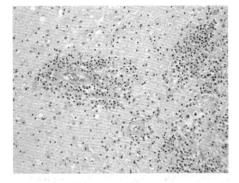

FIGURE 8.12   Brain specimen. Courtesy of Dr. Richard A. Prayson

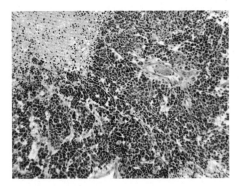

FIGURE 8.10   Brain specimen. Courtesy of Dr. Richard A. Prayson

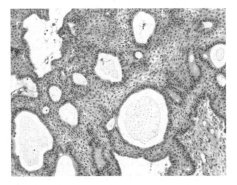

FIGURE 8.13   Suprasellar mass specimen. Courtesy of Dr. Richard A. Prayson

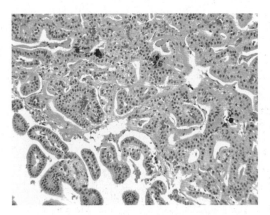

FIGURE 8.14   Intraventricular mass specimen. Courtesy of Dr. Richard A. Prayson

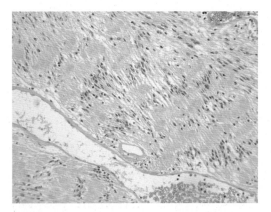

FIGURE 8.16   Pontocerebellar mass specimen. Courtesy of Dr. Richard A. Prayson

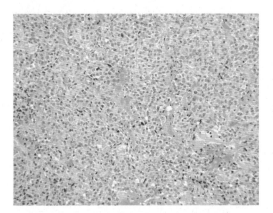

FIGURE 8.18   Pituitary mass specimen. Courtesy of Dr. Richard A. Prayson

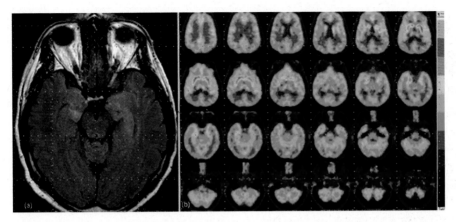

FIGURE 8.20 **(A)** Axial FLAIR MRI; **(B)** FDG-PET scan

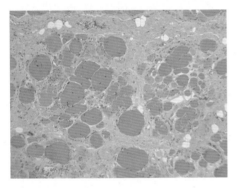

FIGURE 10.1 Muscle biopsy specimen. Courtesy of Dr. Richard A. Prayson

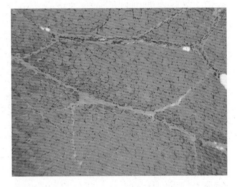

FIGURE 10.3 Muscle biopsy specimen. Courtesy of Dr. Richard A. Prayson

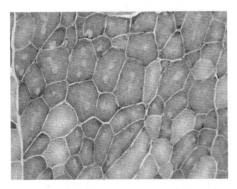

FIGURE 10.2 Muscle biopsy specimen. Courtesy of Dr. Richard A. Prayson

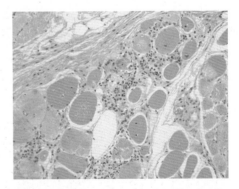

FIGURE 10.4 Muscle biopsy specimen. Courtesy of Dr. Richard A. Prayson

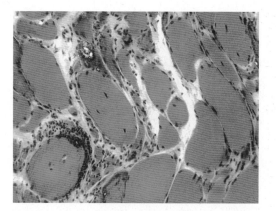

FIGURE 10.5   Muscle biopsy specimen. Courtesy of Dr. Richard A. Prayson

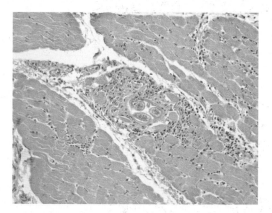

FIGURE 10.7   Muscle specimen. Courtesy of Dr. Richard A. Prayson

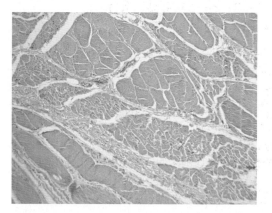

FIGURE 11.5   Muscle biopsy specimen. Courtesy of Dr. Richard A. Prayson

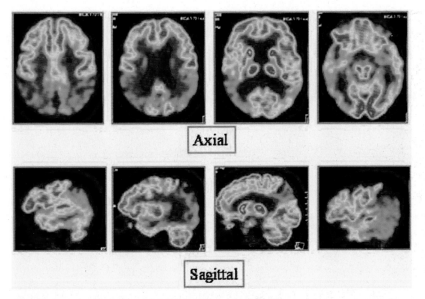

FIGURE 12.1   Axial and sagittal FDG-PET. Courtesy of Dr. Guiyun Wu

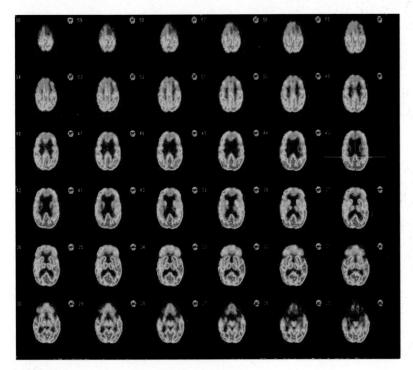

FIGURE 12.2   Axial FDG-PET. Courtesy of Dr. Guiyun Wu

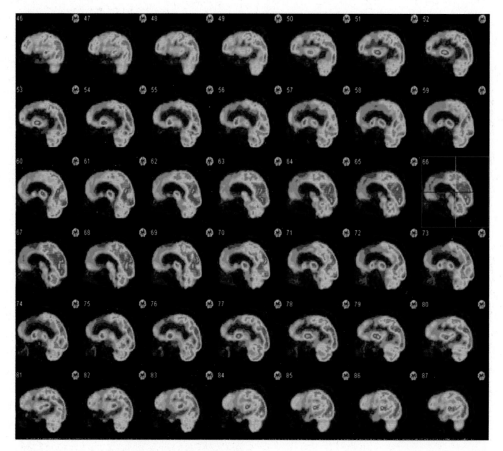

FIGURE 12.3 Sagittal FDG-PET. Courtesy of Dr. Guiyun Wu

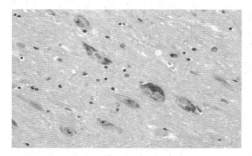

FIGURE 12.4 Brain specimen. Courtesy of Dr. Richard A. Prayson

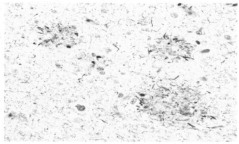

FIGURE 12.5 Brain specimen. Courtesy of Dr. Richard A. Prayson

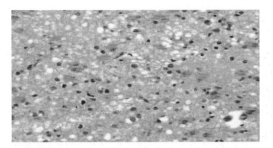

FIGURE 12.6 Brain specimen. Courtesy of Dr. Richard
A. Prayson

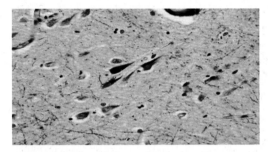

FIGURE 12.7 Brain specimen. Courtesy of Dr. Richard
A. Prayson

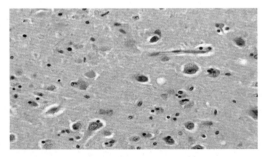

FIGURE 12.9 Brain specimen. Courtesy of Dr. Richard
A. Prayson

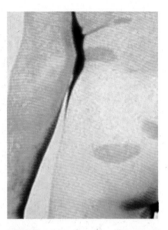

FIGURE 14.5 Courtesy of Dr. David
Rothner

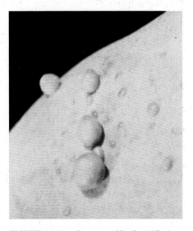

FIGURE 14.6 Courtesy of Dr. David Rothner

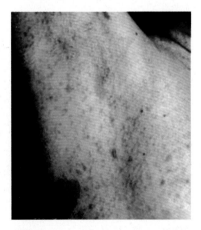

FIGURE 14.7 Courtesy of Dr. David Rothner

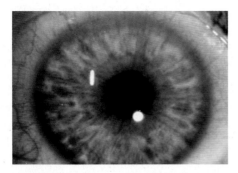

FIGURE 14.8 Courtesy of Dr. David Rothner

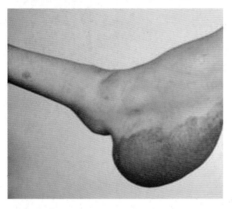

FIGURE 14.9 Courtesy of Dr. David Rothner

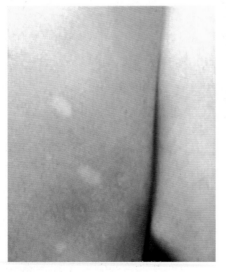

FIGURE 14.11 Courtesy of Dr. David Rothner

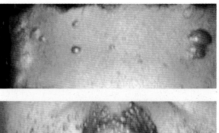
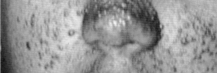

FIGURE 14.12 Courtesy of Dr. David Rothner

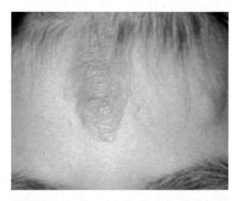

FIGURE 14.13 Courtesy of Dr. David Rothner

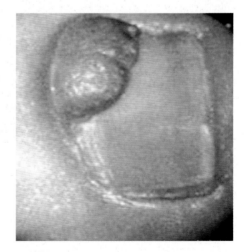

FIGURE 14.14 Courtesy of Dr. David Rothner

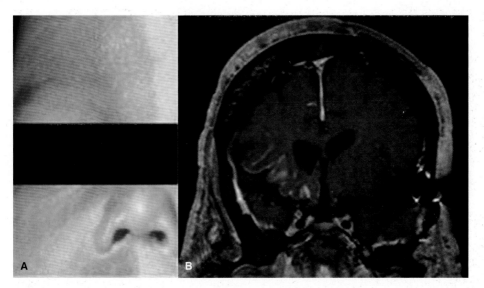

FIGURE 14.18 (**a**) Courtesy of Dr. David Rothner; (**b**) Coronal T1-weighted precontrast MRI

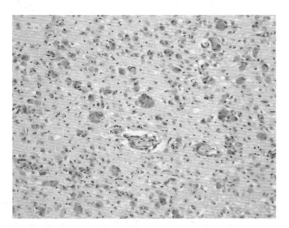

FIGURE 14.20 Brain specimen. Courtesy of Dr. Richard A. Prayson

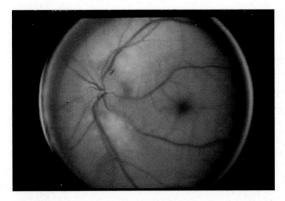

FIGURE 14.21   Courtesy of Dr. Gregory Kosmorsky

FIGURE 14.22   Brain specimen. Courtesy of Dr. Richard A. Prayson

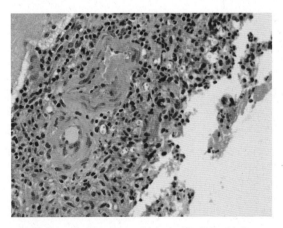

FIGURE 15.1   Brain specimen. Courtesy of Dr. Richard A. Prayson

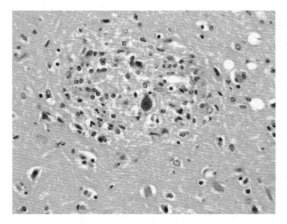

FIGURE 15.2 Brain specimen. Courtesy of Dr. Richard A. Prayson

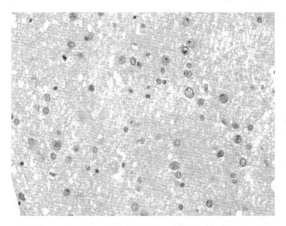

FIGURE 15.3 Brain specimen. Courtesy of Dr. Richard A. Prayson

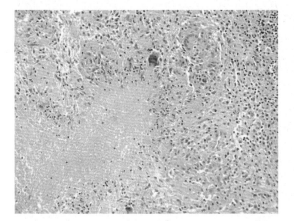

FIGURE 15.5 Leptomeningeal biopsy specimen. Courtesy of Dr. Richard A. Prayson

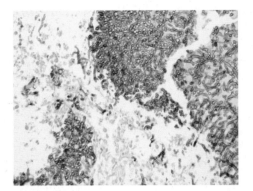

FIGURE 15.8 Pathologic specimen. Courtesy of Dr. Richard A. Prayson

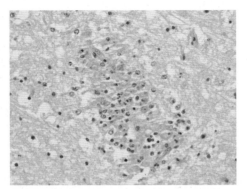

FIGURE 15.10 Brain specimen. Courtesy of Dr. Richard A. Prayson

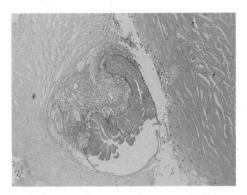

FIGURE 15.9 Brain specimen. Courtesy of Dr. Richard A. Prayson

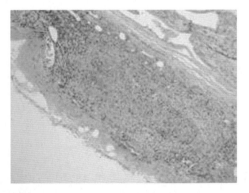

FIGURE 16.1 Nerve biopsy specimen. Courtesy of Dr. Richard Prayson

are prominent. There is relatively dissociated sensory loss, with pain and temperature affected more than dorsal column modalities. The main autonomic manifestation is hypohydrosis. Only in advanced cases do muscle weakness and atrophy occur. Hearing loss can rarely occur. HSAN1 results from a mutation in the gene encoding for serine palmitoyltransferase, which catalyzes the rate-limiting step of sphingolipid synthesis.

HSAN2 begins in infancy, and is characterized by generalized loss of sensation and insensitivity to pain, leading to significant risk of mutilation to the hands, feet, lips, and tongue. Autonomic symptoms are not prominent, and cognitive function is normal. Associated features include areflexia and retinitis pigmentosa. NCS show evidence of axon loss, with absence of SNAPs.

Question 76 depicts HSAN3, also known as familial dysautonomia or Riley-Day syndrome, an autosomal recessive HSAN with prominent autonomic features. Symptom onset is in infancy with dysphagia, vomiting, recurrent infections, and blood pressure lability. It is particularly prevalent among Ashkenazi Jews. With emotional stimulation, there is hyperhydrosis, skin flushing, and hypertension. Other autonomic features include absence of lacrimation. The tongue may be smooth due to absence of fungiform papillae. Later in life, evidence of a predominantly sensory neuropathy with insensitivity to pain occurs, as well as areflexia. Nerve biopsy shows a marked reduction in the density of unmyelinated axons and small myelinated axons, with a reduction in autonomic ganglia cell bodies. HSAN3 is due to a mutation in the *IKAP* gene, which results in abnormal mRNA splicing, leading to dysregulation of neural endocytosis.

Question 77 depicts HSAN4, or congenital insensitivity to pain. This is an autosomal recessive disorder marked by insensitivity to pain, leading to repeated injury and self-mutilation. Cognitive delay is also present, as are significant behavioral problems including hyperactivity. Autonomic features include anhidrosis, leading to heat intolerance and frequent fevers. There is little evidence of large fiber sensory or motor neuropathy on examination or EMG/NCS; diagnosis is made by demonstration of absent or a markedly reduced number of unmyelinated axons and small myelinated fibers on skin biopsy, absence of nerve endings in sweat glands, as well as absence of sweating by quantitative sudomotor axon-reflex test (discussed in Chapter 10). This disorder results from mutations in the tyrosine kinase receptor for nerve growth factor NTRK1, which plays a role in development of unmyelinated nociceptive and sudomotor fibers.

Prominence of sensory features with relatively few motor manifestations and the presence of autonomic signs and symptoms distinguish the HSANs from Charcot-Marie-Tooth (CMT).

CMT1A does not typically include features of early prominent dysphagia or autonomic dysfunction, but other features are present, as discussed in questions 21 and 22.

Bradley WG, Daroff RB, Fenichel GM, et al. Neurology in Clinical Practice, 5th ed. Philadelphia, PA: Elsevier; 2008.

Ropper AH, Samuels MA. Adams and Victor's Principles of Neurology, 9th ed. New York: McGraw-Hill; 2009.

78. C

The clinical presentation of Guillain-Barre syndrome is a symmetric ascending sensorimotor neuropathy, and not mononeuritis multiplex.

Multiple mononeuropathies or mononeuritis multiplex refers to the involvement of two or more nerves, usually with acute to subacute onset, in which subsequent nerves are involved at irregular intervals. Common causes of mononeuritis multiplex are vasculitic neuropathy, either isolated or caused by systemic conditions such as polyarteritis nodosa, Wegener granulomatosis, Sjogren's syndrome, or Churg-Strauss syndrome (discussed in Chapter 16). Cryoglobulinemia can also produce this presentation. Infectious processes such as Lyme disease and HIV can also produce mononeuritis multiplex.

Diabetes can present not only with a distal symmetric polyneuropathy, but can also be associated with mononeuritis multiplex. Other causes of mononeuritis multiplex include sarcoidosis, paraneoplastic processes, amyloidosis, leprosy, systemic lupus erythematosus, rheumatoid arthritis, and lymphoma.

Bradley WG, Daroff RB, Fenichel GM, et al. Neurology in Clinical Practice, 5th ed. Philadelphia, PA: Elsevier; 2008.

Ropper AH, Samuels MA. Adams and Victor's Principles of Neurology, 9th ed. New York: McGraw-Hill; 2009.

79. c

This patient has cryoglobulinemia, in which complement levels are reduced.

The clinical manifestation of cryoglobulinemia includes nonspecific constitutional symptoms, palpable purpura, arthralgias, lymphadenopathy, hepatosplenomegaly, and peripheral neuropathy, including mononeuritis multiplex. Cryoglobulins are immunoglobulins that precipitate when exposed to cold temperatures and redissolve on rewarming (discussed also in Chapter 16). This condition is frequently associated with hepatitis C, and sometimes has been found in patients with HIV. Other associated conditions are the monoclonal gammopathies, such as multiple myeloma, and connective tissue diseases. Treatment includes steroids and cyclophosphamide, and in some cases, plasmapheresis has shown beneficial results.

Ropper AH, Samuels MA. Adams and Victor's Principles of Neurology, 9th ed. New York: McGraw-Hill; 2009.

80. b

This patient's history is consistent with primary erythromelalgia, a rare autosomal dominant disorder characterized by episodes of severe burning and erythema of the distal extremities with heat exposure or exercise. Patients are asymptomatic between episodes. This disorder is due to mutations in the voltage-gated sodium channel *SCN9A* gene, which results in hyperactivity of the dorsal root ganglia.

Secondary erythromelalgia can be seen with polycythemia rubra vera and other myeloproliferative disorders; the family history and normal routine laboratory testing in this patient make primary erythromelalgia the more likely diagnosis. Similarly, there is no evidence of small fiber neuropathy due to glucose intolerance, and the episodic nature of the symptoms further excludes that diagnosis. The episodic nature of the symptoms with normal examination otherwise is evidence that this is not hereditary sensory and autonomic neuropathy type I. Fabry's disease can lead to painful acroparesthesias that are worsened with heat exposure and exercise, but evidence of small fiber neuropathy on examination and other findings on history and examination distinguish between these two disorders (discussed in question 70).

Bradley WG, Daroff RB, Fenichel GM, et al. Neurology in Clinical Practice, 5th ed. Philadelphia, PA: Elsevier; 2008.

81. e

This patient has a sensory neuronopathy or ganglionopathy, in which the dorsal root ganglia are involved, presenting with progressive sensory deficits that are usually non-length dependent, patchy, and asymmetric, and lead to global sensory loss. Sensory ataxia is a characteristic finding of sensory neuronopathy. Patients are also areflexic; however, strength tends to be normal. Some patients may also have autonomic dysfunction.

Sensory neuronopathy is frequently secondary to a primary pathology, and can be paraneoplastic, especially associated with small cell lung cancer, in which Anti-Hu antibodies are typically present. It may be associated with other neoplasms, such as neuroendocrine tumors, lymphomas, breast and ovarian cancers, and sarcomas. Another condition that typically can cause sensory neuronopathy is Sjogren's syndrome, which is a condition characterized by inflammation of the exocrine glands leading to keratoconjunctivitis sicca and xerostomia (discussed in Chapter 16). The diagnostic work-up includes Schirmer's test, SSA and SSB antibodies, and lip biopsy to detect inflammatory changes in small salivary glands. Other causes of sensory neuronopathy include HIV infection, HTLV-1, Epstein-Barr virus, varicella zoster virus, measles, monoclonal gammopathies, nicotinic acid deficiency, vitamin E deficiency, riboflavin deficiency, and drugs such as carboplatin, doxorubicin, suramin, thallium, and penicillin. Pyridoxine intoxication is one of the causes of sensory neuronopathy, and therefore should not be supplemented.

Ropper AH, Samuels MA. Adams and Victor's Principles of Neurology, 9th ed. New York: McGraw-Hill; 2009.

Sghirlanzoni A, Pareyson D, Lauria G. Sensory neuron diseases. Lancet Neurol. 2005; 4:349–362.

82. d

This patient's history and examination are consistent with a lower trunk lesion due to stretching, as occurs with excessive arm abduction such as when grabbing onto something during falling, motor vehicle accidents, or less commonly with birth injury. Lower trunk lesions lead to weakness in ulnar and median nerve–innervated muscles (see Table 9.1), leading to weakness of intrinsic hand muscles and sensory loss on the medial forearm and hand. Sensory loss occurs in a C8 and T1 distribution; the medial arm, innervated predominantly by T1 and T2, often has preserved sensation.

In the patient described in question 82, muscle weakness in the distribution of both of the median and ulnar nerves makes ulnar neuropathy and median neuropathy as isolated disorders unlikely; the distribution of weakness is not consistent with a radial neuropathy. A lateral cord lesion would lead to weakness of musculocutaneous-innervated muscles as well as C6- and C7-innervated median nerve muscles (see Table 9.1), which are not involved in this case.

Russell SM. Examination of Peripheral Nerve Injuries. New York: Thieme; 2006.

83. e

This patient's history is consistent with an acute hepatic porphyria. The acute hepatic porphyrias are autosomal dominant and involve multiple areas of the neuraxis. They result from enzymatic dysfunction in porphyrin metabolism with subsequent abnormalities in heme synthesis and metabolism. These disorders include acute intermittent porphyria (AIP), which results from various mutations that lead to reduced activity of the enzyme porphobilinogen deaminase, variegate porphyria, which results from reduced activity of the enzyme protoporphinogen IX oxidase, hereditary coproporphyria which results from reduced activity in the enzyme coprophorphinogen oxidase, and plumboporphyria, which results from reduced enzymatic activity of δ-aminolevulinic acid (ALA) dehydratase. Because the dysfunctional enzymes have some residual enzyme activity, symptoms often do not appear until adolescence or later, with some symptoms occurring in episodes with exposure to certain triggers. Common triggers include medications, menstruation, and alcohol exposure. With exposure to these triggers, activity of the hepatic enzyme ALA synthase increases, leading to overproduction of heme precursors that cannot be sufficiently metabolized by the involved downstream enzymes.

The different porphyrias differ in several biochemical aspects, but the neurologic manifestations of all four disorders are similar. Symptoms typically manifest in early adulthood, with females being more commonly and more severely affected as compared to males. Symptoms typically begin with abdominal pain and other gastrointestinal symptoms, followed by neurologic symptoms, including most prominently manifestations of autonomic instability (tachycardia, labile hypertension, orthostasis, and urinary retention). Neuropsychiatric symptoms including psychosis occur, and seizures may be present as well. In some patients, a subacute predominantly motor neuropathy occurs; the arms may be affected prior to the legs, and proximal muscles are involved more than distal muscles. Involvement of the radial nerve in isolation may occur. The neuropathy is both axonal and demyelinating. Cranial nerve involvement, and even respiratory muscle involvement leading to respiratory failure, may occur.

In AIP, photosensitivity is not present, whereas with variegate porphyria and hereditary coproporphyria, photosensitivity with skin blistering and hyperpigmentation occur.

During an attack, elevated levels of porphobilinogen and aminolevulinic acid are detectable in the urine and serum. Elevated protoporphyrinogen and coproporphyrinogen in the stool distinguish variegate porphyria and hereditary coproporphyria from AIP.

Management of the porphyrias involves prevention of attacks by avoidance of drugs that may precipitate the attack (including antiepileptics, particularly barbiturates) and other triggers. Treatment of attacks includes supportive care, a high-carbohydrate diet, and in some cases hematin, which suppresses δ-ALA synthase activity.

Although Wilson's disease is on the differential diagnosis of patients with neuropsychiatric symptoms, it does not typically lead to peripheral motor mononeuropathies or abdominal pain, except in the setting of hepatic impairment, and there is no evidence of liver disease in the case presented (see Chapter 6 for more on Wilson's disease). The history presented is not consistent with acute disseminated encephalomyelitis (discussed in Chapter 7), in which the MRI would be abnormal, or acute inflammatory demyelinating polyneuropathy (discussed in questions 15, 16, 24, 55, and 56). Although systemic lupus erythematosuis can lead to a similar clinical picture, normal MRI of the brain and CSF analysis make this less likely.

Bradley WG, Daroff RB, Fenichel GM, et al. Neurology in Clinical Practice, 5th ed. Philadelphia, PA: Elsevier; 2008.

Ropper AH, Samuels MA. Adams and Victor's Principles of Neurology, 9th ed. New York: McGraw-Hill; 2009.

84. b

This patient's history and examination are consistent with an upper trunk lesion. This type of injury is called Erb's palsy and commonly occurs when the shoulder is forcefully pulled down while the neck is flexed in the opposite direction, as can occur with birth injury. Other mechanisms of injury include falls and motorcycle accidents. The posture held by the patient depicted in question 84, "waiter's tip" position, is a classic example of Erb's palsy. Arm adduction and internal rotation result from unopposed action of the pectoralis major; the clavicular head of the pectoralis major is innervated by the lateral pectoral nerve that arises from the lateral cord and acts to adduct and internally rotate the arm. Forearm extension results from unopposed action of the triceps and forearm pronation from unopposed action of pronator teres; both of these muscles are predominantly C7 innervated, and normal strength in these muscles as well as a normal triceps deep tendon reflex excludes a C7 root lesion and a middle trunk lesion (because the middle trunk carries only C7 fibers).

Normal rhomboids on EMG suggest that the C5 and C6 nerve roots, which are the origin of the dorsal scapular nerves, are normal (discussed in questions 17 and 71). This patient's deficits, including weakness of wrist flexors, suggest the lesion is more extensive than just an axillary neuropathy.

Bradley WG, Daroff RB, Fenichel GM, et al. Neurology in Clinical Practice, 5th ed. Philadelphia, PA: Elsevier; 2008.

Preston DC, Shapiro BE. Electromyography and Neuromuscular Disorders, 2nd ed. Philadelphia, PA: Elsevier; 2005.

85. b

This patient has a large fiber diabetic neuropathy. This is usually a length-dependent neuropathy, in which the patient has numbness and paresthesias that are painless. The distribution is symmetric, affecting hands and feet in a glove and stocking distribution. On examination, there is loss vibratory sense and proprioception, as well as loss of deep tendon reflexes. Sensory ataxia may occur later in the course of the disease. Weakness may occur, but is not a prominent feature.

Diabetic mononeuropathy can affect either the peripheral or cranial nerves, and usually involves one nerve. If several nerves are involved, the presentation is usually asymmetric, unlike in this case. Small fiber diabetic neuropathy is discussed in question 49. Diabetic polyradiculoneuropathy and diabetic amyotrophy are discussed in question 42.

Bradley WG, Daroff RB, Fenichel GM, et al. Neurology in Clinical Practice, 5th ed. Philadelphia, PA: Elsevier; 2008.

Ropper AH, Samuels MA. Adams and Victor's Principles of Neurology, 9th ed. New York: McGraw-Hill; 2009.

86. a

L5 radiculopathy may manifest as pain from the buttock radiating down the lateral thigh, anterolateral leg, and dorsum of the foot, with sensory impairment in this dermatomal region extending to the big toe. The weakness is prominent on toe extension and ankle dorsiflexion, as well as inversion and eversion of the foot. The only reflex found to be abnormal is the hamstring reflex, which is not routinely checked. As foot drop is a frequent manifestation that may be seen with both an L5 root lesion and common peroneal neuropathy, one important means of distinguishing the two is seen on NCS. Superficial peroneal SNAPs are abnormal in common peroneal nerve lesions, but normal in L5 radiculopathies. Another key diagnostic feature is to detect abnormalities in L5-innervated muscles that are not innervated by the peroneal nerve, such as the tibialis posterior and flexor digitorum longus, both of which are innervated by the tibial nerve. The L5 nerve root provides innervation to the tensor fascia latae, gluteus medius, semitendinosus and semimembranosus, tibialis anterior, extensor hallucis, peroneus longus, extensor digitorum brevis, tibialis posterior, and flexor digitorum longus muscles (see Tables 9.2 and 9.4).

The distribution of the involvement in this patient does not correlate with an S1 radiculopathy, which is discussed in question 40. Common and deep peroneal neuropathies are discussed in question 44. A lesion affecting these nerves individually is not likely in this case, given the presence of involvement of other nonperoneal L5-innervated muscles.

In this case, the SNAPs are spared, which makes the possibility of a sciatic nerve injury unlikely as opposed to a radiculopathy. Sciatic nerve injury is discussed in question 32.

Katirji B. Electromyography in Clinical Practice: A Case Study Approach, 1st ed. St. Louis: Mosby; 1998.

Russell SM. Examination of Peripheral Nerve Injuries. New York: Thieme; 2006.

Buzz Phrases	Key Points
Orange tonsils and neuropathy	Tangier's disease
Albuminocytologic dissociation	Guillain-Barre syndrome
Acute motor and sensory axonal neuropathy	GM1, GM1b, GD1a
Finger abduction	Dorsal interossei (DAB: dorsal, abduct)
Finger adduction	Palmar interossei (PAD: palmar, adduct)
Benedictine sign	Median neuropathy. On attempt to make a fist, absent flexion of first digit, partial flexion of second digit, complete flexion of fourth and fifth digits
Claw hand	Ulnar neuropathy. On attempt to make a fist, the fourth and fifth digits hyperextend at the metacarpophalangeal joint and partially flex at the interphalangeal joint
Wartenberg's sign	Ulnar neuropathy. Fifth digit abduction at rest
Froment's sign	Ulnar neuropathy. During attempted forceful adduction of the thumb, as with attempt to hold a piece of paper between the thumb and index finger, thumb flexion occurs
Intrinsic hand weakness in frequent bicycle rider	Ulnar neuropathy due to compression in Guyon's canal
Wrist drop with strong forearm extension, reduced sensation over lateral arm	Radial neuropathy at the spinal groove
OK sign	Anterior interosseus neuropathy. On attempt to make an "okay sign," the distal phalanges are unable to flex, and instead, the fingertips touch. Weakness of flexor digitorum profundus to the second and third digits, flexor pollicis longus, and pronator quadratus, no sensory loss
Miller-Fisher syndrome	GQ1b
Acute sensory neuronopathy	GD1b
Multifocal motor neuropathy with conduction block	GM1
Sensory ataxia, asymmetric sensory loss, areflexia, normal strength, reduced SNAPs with normal CMAPs	Sensory neuronopathy
Paraneoplastic neuropathy and/or neuronopathy associated with small cell lung cancer	Anti-Hu
Inflammatory demyelinating polyneuropathy for more than 8 weeks	Chronic inflammatory demyelinating polyneuropathy
Inflammatory demyelinating polyneuropathy for less than 4 weeks	Acute inflammatory demyelinating polyneuropathy
Wrist drop with weak forearm extensors in an alcoholic	Saturday night palsy; proximal radial nerve injury, prior to spiral groove
Bilateral carpal tunnel, family history of carpal tunnel, mild sensory polyneuropathy (diagnosis, protein)	Familial amyloid polyneuropathy type 2, transthyretin

(*continued*)

Buzz Phrases	Key Points
Corneal dystrophy, multiple cranial neuropathies, peripheral sensorimotor neuropathy	Familial amyloid polyneuropathy type 4
Asymmetric demyelinating neuropathy affecting several motor nerves	Multifocal motor neuropathy
Asymmetric demyelinating neuropathy affecting several motor and sensory nerves	Multifocal acquired demyelinating sensory and motor neuropathy
Hammertoes, high-arched feet, pes cavus	Charcot-Marie-Tooth (CMT)
Most common type of CMT, mode of inheritance, type (axonal vs. demyelinating)	CMT1, autosomal dominant demyelinating (note: second most common type is X-linked CMT)
Duplication in peripheral myelin protein 22 (*PMP22*) gene on chromosome 17	CMT1A (note: CMT1 is also known as HSMN1)
Deletion in peripheral myelin protein 22 (*PMP22*) gene	Hereditary neuropathy with liability to pressure palsies
Gene mutated in X-linked CMT	Connexin 32 gene
Demyelinating neuropathy with monoclonal gammopathy	Anti-MAG
Sensory loss, acral mutilation, autonomic symptoms	Hereditary sensory and autonomic neuropathy
Episodes of painful burning in the hands and feet with heat exposure and exercise	Primary erythromelalgia (or Fabry's disease)
Acute motor axonal neuropathy	GM1, GM1b, GD1a, GalNac-GD1a
Painful sensory polyneuropathy, autonomic dysfunction, cardiac and renal involvement, family history of the same	Familial amyloid polyneuropathy type 1, transthyretin
Porphyria in which photosensitivity does not occur	Acute intermittent porphyria
Angiokeratoma	Purplish lesion seen on trunk, scrotum in Fabry's disease
Enzyme deficiency in Fabry's disease	α-galactosidase A
Mode of inheritance of Fabry's disease	X-linked
Retinitis pigmentosa, neuropathy	Refsum's disease
	Myoneurogastrointestinal encephalopathy
	Neurogenic muscle weakness, ataxia, and retinitis pigmentosa syndrome
	Abetalipoproteinemia
Retinitis pigmentosa, neuropathy, ataxia, low very low density lipoprotein, acanthocytes on peripheral smear	Abetalipoproteinemia, Bassen-Kornzweig syndrome, autosomal recessive

Chapter 10

Neuromuscular II

(Adult and Pediatric Muscle, Autonomic Nervous System, and Neuromuscular Junction Disorders)

Questions

Questions 1–3

1. A 25-year-old man presents frequently to the Emergency Department with episodes of weakness and inability to move his arms and legs. Extraocular movements and bulbar and respiratory muscles are spared. The patient says that he gets these episodes with emotional stressors, after exercise, or after eating heavy desserts. On further questioning, he says that his father has similar episodes. Which of the following is the most likely diagnosis?
   a. Hyperkalemic periodic paralysis
   b. Hypokalemic periodic paralysis
   c. Andersen-Tawil syndrome
   d. Paramyotonia congenita
   e. Myotonia congenita

2. A 42-year-old patient with chronic asthma has been treated with oral prednisone for over a year, given difficulties in controlling her illness. She comes with proximal weakness, and is noticed to have a cushingoid appearance. Which of the following is incorrect regarding the most likely cause of this patient's weakness?
   a. There is atrophy of type II fibers
   b. Steroid dose reduction is important in the treatment of this condition
   c. Creatine kinase levels are usually normal
   d. Patients with Cushing disease may have proximal weakness
   e. EMG shows specific findings that suggest this condition

3. A floppy baby is brought for evaluation, and on the basis of the biopsy, he is diagnosed with a centronuclear myopathy. Which of the following characteristics are incorrect regarding this condition?
   a. Respiratory failure occurs in severe forms
   b. The muscle fibers occurs show central nucleation
   c. Pharyngeal and laryngeal muscles may be affected

d. Extraocular movements are rarely affected

e. Could be autosomal dominant, autosomal recessive, or X-linked

Questions 4–6

4. A 32-year-old woman presents to the clinic complaining of double vision of 1-month duration. She also reports her speech slurs when she talks for prolonged periods of time, and her eyelids start to droop toward the end of the day. On examination, she has bilateral ptosis that worsens with sustained upward gaze, she is unable to hold air in her mouth against resistance, and her neck flexors are weak. Which of the following is incorrect regarding this patient's disease?

   a. It is more common in males, and females tend to present at an earlier age as compared with males

   b. The majority of patients have symptoms restricted to their extraocular muscles for the duration of their illness

   c. Patients with human leukocyte antigen DR2 and DR3 are at a higher risk of developing this disorder

   d. Family members of patients with this disease are at an increased risk of having this disorder

   e. Patients with this disorder are at an increased risk of developing other autoimmune disorders

5. Regarding the pathophysiology of myasthenia gravis, which of the following is correct?

   a. In its most common form, it is autoimmune due to antibodies against presynaptic voltage-gated calcium channels

   b. It is due to inhibition of exocytosis of presynaptic vesicles containing acetylcholine

   c. In its most common form, it is autoimmune due to antibodies against the acetylcholine receptor

   d. It results from increased degradation of acetylcholine at the neuromuscular junction

   e. In its most common form, it is due to mutations in the acetylcholine receptor gene

6. Which of the following is incorrect regarding the diagnosis of autoimmune myasthenia gravis?

   a. Improvement in muscle weakness after administration of edrophonium suggests the diagnosis of myasthenia gravis

   b. Anti-striational muscle antibodies are the most useful serologic test for the diagnosis

   c. Acetylcholine receptor binding antibodies have the highest sensitivity among all serologic tests for myasthenia gravis

   d. In a minority of patients with negative acetylcholine receptor binding antibodies, blocking or modulating antibodies may be positive

   e. Increased jitter seen on single-fiber EMG and more than 10% decrement seen on repetitive nerve stimulation are electrophysiologic findings in disorders of the neuromuscular junction

7. A 41-year-old man presents for evaluation of weakness. On examination, there is evidence of proximal weakness and very mild facial weakness. He also has early findings suggestive of cataracts. A genetic test was ordered, and he was found to have CCTG expansion in an intron of the zinc finger protein 9 gene. Which of the following is the most likely diagnosis?

   a. Becker muscular dystrophy

   b. Dystrophic myotonia type 1 (DM1) myotonic dystrophy

   c. Emery-Dreifuss muscular dystrophy

   d. Fascioscapulohumeral muscular dystrophy

   e. DM2 myotonic dystrophy

8. A baby is diagnosed with a congenital muscular dystrophy. He is floppy and weak, with contractures at the hip, knee, and ankles. As he grows, he has significant problems with cognitive and

speech development, and by 18 months, he starts having seizures. The muscle biopsy shows dystrophic changes and reduced α-dystroglycan. A mutation of the fukutin gene is detected. An MRI shows white matter changes in the frontal head regions. Which of the following is the most likely diagnosis?

   a. Fukuyama-type congenital muscular dystrophy
   b. Laminin-α-2 deficiency
   c. Bethlem myopathy
   d. Muscle-eye-brain disease
   e. Ullrich's congenital muscular dystrophy

9. A 20-year-old man presents for evaluation of weakness of his face and upper extremities, gradually progressing over the past few years. The patient has a nearly expressionless face, with difficulty closing his eyes tightly and pursing his lips. He has asymmetric proximal weakness of his upper extremities to the point where he has difficulty lifting his arms above his head. He also has peroneal weakness. On examination, there is muscle atrophy, more prominent proximally in the upper extremities, with evidence of winged scapula. Interestingly, his upper arms seem "thinner" than his forearms, but his deltoids are relatively spared. Creatine kinase is 510 IU/L (normal 220 IU/L). Which of the following is the most likely diagnosis?

   a. Becker muscular dystrophy
   b. Duchenne muscular dystrophy
   c. Emery-Dreifuss muscular dystrophy
   d. Fascioscapulohumeral muscular dystrophy
   e. Myotonic dystrophy

Questions 10–11

10. A 52-year-old man originally from Montreal presents to the clinic with gradually progressive dysphagia, dysphonia, and bilateral ptosis. There is no fatigability. Besides ptosis and the evident dysphonia, the rest of the neurologic examination is unremarkable. A Tensilon test is negative, as well as myasthenia gravis antibody studies. His brain MRI does not show abnormalities. Which of the following is the most likely diagnosis?

   a. Becker muscular dystrophy
   b. Inclusion body myositis
   c. Emery-Dreifuss muscular dystrophy
   d. Fascioscapulohumeral muscular dystrophy
   e. Oculopharyngeal muscular dystrophy

11. Which of the following is correct regarding this condition?

   a. The abnormality is caused by a GGG repeat expansion in the poly-A–binding protein gene
   b. It is inherited in an X-linked recessive fashion
   c. Histologically, there is variation in fiber size, rimmed vacuoles, and intranuclear tubular filaments
   d. Myotonia is an evident phenomenon in this condition
   e. Creatine kinase levels are elevated 10 to 100 times that of normal

12. A 25-year-old man was referred from the infertility clinic because of weakness. The patient has frontal balding, atrophy of the temporalis and masseter muscles, and weakness of the sternocleidomastoids and bilateral ptosis. He has also upper extremity weakness especially in forearm extensors, as well as atrophy in the anterior tibial muscles, with weakness of dorsiflexion of the

feet. After percussion of his thenar eminence, there is prolonged contraction and slow relaxation. Which of the following is the most likely diagnosis?

a. Becker muscular dystrophy
b. Dystrophic myotonia type 1 (DM1) myotonic dystrophy
c. Emery-Dreifuss muscular dystrophy
d. Fascioscapulohumeral muscular dystrophy
e. DM2 myotonic dystrophy

13. A 44-year-old otherwise healthy man is brought to the emergency department with an episode of loss of consciousness. He had dressed up to go to his niece's wedding and felt particularly uncomfortable in his suit and tie. He usually wore farming clothes, did not like to be formal, and felt his tie was very tight. He was leaving his house to head to the wedding when his wife called him from the kitchen. He turned his head around to see what she wanted, and suddenly, without warning, lost consciousness for a few seconds. His wife called emergency medical services, and when they arrived, his pulse was 40 bpm and his systolic blood pressure was 88 mm Hg. On arrival to the emergency department 20 minutes later, vital signs and physical examination were normal. What is the most likely diagnosis in this patient?

a. Vasovagal syncope
b. Asphyxiation from his tight tie
c. Carotid sinus hypersensitivity
d. Orthostatic hypotension with syncope
e. Severe aortic stenosis leading to syncope

14. A 10-year-old boy is brought for evaluation of muscle cramps. After exercise, the patient experiences muscle cramps, weakness, and contractures. After he rests for a few minutes, he can resume the activity. During the contractures, a needle EMG was obtained from an affected muscle, and it was electrically silent. A muscle biopsy with immunohistochemistry showed absence of myophosphorylase. Which of the following is the most likely diagnosis?

a. Tarui disease
b. McArdle's disease
c. Cori's disease
d. Andersen's disease
e. Pompe's disease

Questions 15–16

15. A 66-year-old man presents to the emergency department complaining of a 2-week history of marked slurring of speech, difficulty swallowing, and trouble holding his head up. He had been diagnosed with myasthenia gravis 2 years earlier, but symptoms had only included diplopia up until he had a flu-like illness 2 weeks earlier. On examination, he has bilateral ptosis and severe dysarthria. He cannot hold his head up off the bed when supine. He is tachypneic and is using accessory muscles to breathe. His negative inspiratory force is −15 cm H_2O. What is the most appropriate next step in the management of this patient?

a. Provide him with a prescription for pyridostigmine and arrange for outpatient follow-up for him
b. Administer intravenous methylprednisolone to him immediately while he is in the ED
c. Admit him to the hospital and observe him with frequent checks of respiratory function with forced vital capacity and negative inspiratory force measurements

    d. Admit him to the ICU, intubate him, and initiate therapy with intravenous immunoglobulin or plasma exchange

    e. Admit him and perform emergency thymectomy

16. Regarding the management of patients with myasthenia gravis, which of the following is incorrect?

    a. Thymectomy is indicated only in patients with thymoma

    b. There are several medications that should be avoided as they can exacerbate the disease, including aminoglycosides and β-blockers

    c. Pyridostigmine provides symptomatic relief but does not modify the course of the illness

    d. Corticosteroids can cause a transient worsening of symptoms in some patients

    e. Long-term immunosuppressive therapy, including azathioprine and mycophenolate mofetil, is used as steroid-sparing agents

17. An 8-year-old boy presents for evaluation of episodes of stiffness and difficulty relaxing his muscles. He has difficulty opening his eyes after closure and difficulty releasing after grasping with his hands. These symptoms are worse after exercising and performing the same task multiple times and also worsen with exposure to cold. His father also has similar symptoms. Which of the following is the most likely diagnosis?

    a. Paramyotonia congenita

    b. Becker's disease

    c. Thomsen's disease

    d. Hyperkalemic periodic paralysis

    e. Hypokalemic periodic paralysis

18. A 32-year-old woman requires blood testing as part of a pre-employment health evaluation. She goes to the laboratory and has her blood drawn without any problems. However, she starts to feel light-headed and begins sweating profusely, her vision dims and she loses consciousness and lies listless on the floor. There is no convulsive activity or loss of bowel or bladder control. Approximately 15 seconds later she regains consciousness. She feels slightly light-headed, but is not confused and is able to recall all the events preceding her loss of consciousness. A few minutes later she is feeling fine. What is the most likely diagnosis in this patient?

    a. Vasovagal syncope

    b. Glossopharyngeal neuralgia

    c. A seizure

    d. Carotid sinus hypersensitivity

    e. Third ventricular mass

Questions 19–20

19. An 8-year-old boy is brought by his parents to the clinic. His motor development has been significantly delayed, and he has difficulty walking. His weakness is predominantly in the proximal muscles, with severe weakness of hip flexors, quadriceps, gluteal, and pretibial muscles. He also has pectoral and shoulder weakness and winging of the scapulas. His calves are enlarged, with a "rubbery" texture. His intelligence quotient (IQ) is low. His serum creatine kinase is 11,560 IU/L (normal 220 IU/L). A muscle biopsy is obtained, which is shown in Figure 10.1. Which of the following is the most likely diagnosis?

    a. Becker muscular dystrophy

    b. Duchenne muscular dystrophy

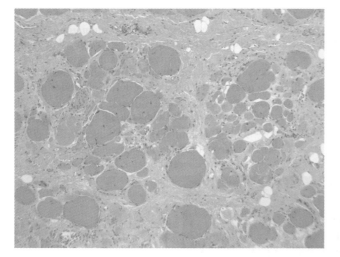

FIGURE 10.1   Muscle biopsy specimen (Courtesy of Dr. Richard A. Prayson). Shown also in color plates

c. Emery-Dreifuss muscular dystrophy
d. Fascioscapulohumeral muscular dystrophy
e. Limb-girdle muscular dystrophy

20. Which of the following is incorrect regarding this condition?
    a. It is autosomal recessive
    b. Cardiac involvement occurs in these patients
    c. Death commonly occurs from respiratory failure
    d. The dystrophin protein is completely absent from muscles
    e. Histopathologically, there is segmental degeneration and regeneration

21. A 21-year-old man from Japan is brought for evaluation of gait disturbance. He has bilateral foot drop and weakness, affecting the anterior leg compartment. There is mild weakness in the upper extremities, predominantly in the extensor muscles. Muscle biopsy shows rimmed vacuoles, and electron microscopy shows tubular filaments, resembling those seen in inclusion body myositis. His parents do not have a muscle disease. Which of the following is the most likely diagnosis?
    a. Miyoshi myopathy
    b. Nonaka myopathy
    c. Welander myopathy
    d. Markesbery-Griggs myopathy
    e. Scapuloperoneal muscular dystrophy

22. A 46-year-old woman presents with diplopia occurring predominantly in the afternoon or after prolonged reading or watching television. She is diagnosed with myasthenia gravis on the basis of serologic testing, and she is prescribed pyridostigmine 60 mg, to be taken three times a day as needed for diplopia. She presents to her physician 3 days later complaining of diarrhea and crampy abdominal pain that seem to occur in the afternoon, after she has taken a dose of pyridostigmine. Which of the following is correct regarding pyridostigmine?

d. Acetylcholine acts at nicotinic receptors in the heart to reduce heart rate

e. Acetylcholine acts at M_3-receptors in the salivary glands to increase secretions

29. Which of the following is not characteristic of congenital muscular dystrophies?
a. Decreased movements in utero
b. Hypotonia and weakness at birth
c. Autosomal dominant inheritance
d. Dystrophic changes on muscle biopsy
e. Frequent involvement of the brain

Questions 30–31

30. A 29-year-old man presents to the clinic for evaluation of weakness. He recalls that since he was a child, he was not able to keep up with his peers when running, biking, or in other sports, and recalls frequent falls that were attributed to clumsiness. He has proximal weakness, with difficulty standing from the sitting position, requiring the use of his arms to do so. He says he cannot lift objects above his head either. On examination, there is pseudohypertrophy of the calves. His creatine kinase is 10,490 IU/L (normal 220 IU/L). Needle EMG shows fibrillations, positive waves, and myopathic motor unit potentials. A biopsy is obtained, showing fibers of variable size, segmental degeneration and regeneration, and areas of fibrosis. The patient recalls that a maternal uncle had difficulty walking and was wheelchair-bound by age 40. Which of the following is the most likely diagnosis?
a. Becker muscular dystrophy
b. Duchenne muscular dystrophy
c. Emery-Dreifuss muscular dystrophy
d. Fascioscapulohumeral muscular dystrophy
e. Myotonic dystrophy

31. Which of the following is incorrect regarding this condition?
a. Cardiac involvement may occur
b. Intelligence quotient (IQ) is typically normal
c. The dystrophin protein is completely absent from muscles
d. It is X-linked recessive
e. The alteration of dystrophin makes the sarcolemma susceptible to rupture

Questions 32–33

32. A 40-year-old woman presents with weakness. She has difficulties standing from the sitting position and walking up the stairs. She also complains of difficulty lifting her arms above her head when she washes her hair. On examination, she has a purplish discoloration around her eyelids, and her face looks erythematous. She also has a purple scaly rash on the extensor surface of her hands, and her palmar region is thickened. Serum creatine kinase levels are elevated. A muscle biopsy is obtained, which is shown in Figure 10.3. Which of the following is the most likely diagnosis?
a. Dermatomyositis
b. Polymyositis
c. Inclusion body myositis
d. Mitochondrial myopathy
e. A muscular dystrophy

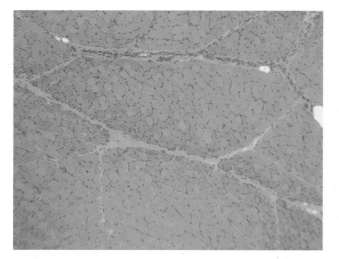

FIGURE 10.3   Muscle biopsy specimen (Courtesy of Dr. Richard A. Prayson). Shown also in color plates

33. Regarding this condition, which of the following is incorrect?
　　a. Methotrexate should be used, especially if there is interstitial lung disease
　　b. Age-appropriate malignancy work-up is indicated
　　c. Perifascicular atrophy is a characteristic histopathologic finding
　　d. It has been associated with interstitial lung disease
　　e. Steroids are the initial treatment of choice

34. A 62-year-old man presents with complaints of "whoozy" dizziness over the prior year. When he would wake up in the morning, while still lying in bed, he would feel fine. His wife had checked his blood pressure once in the early morning and had found it to be 180/90 mm Hg. As soon as he would get out of bed, the "whoozy" feeling would occur and would typically last throughout the day. His blood pressure during the day was as low as 80/60 mm Hg when standing. He felt particularly symptomatic after eating and when the weather was warm. He had lost consciousness twice in prior months; all episodes were triggered by changes in posture. He was otherwise relatively healthy, except for a 1-year history of impotence. He also reported frequent nocturia, urinary hesitancy, and urinary urgency. Besides demonstration of orthostasis on vital sign testing, his examination is entirely normal, with no evidence of ataxia or rigidity and normal sensory examination. What is the most likely diagnosis in this patient?
　　a. Multiple system atrophy
　　b. Autoimmune autonomic ganglionopathy
　　c. Familial amyloid neuropathy
　　d. Diabetic autonomic neuropathy
　　e. Pure autonomic failure

35. A 35-year-old man presents with progressive weakness in the proximal muscles of the upper and lower extremities. No skin rash is appreciated. Creatine kinase levels are elevated and a muscle biopsy is obtained, which is shown in Figure 10.4. Which of the following is incorrect?
　　a. Steroids are the initial treatment of choice
　　b. An association with malignancy is not well established

396   Chapter 10

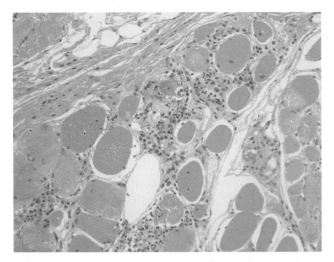

FIGURE 10.4   Muscle biopsy specimen (Courtesy of Dr. Richard A. Prayson). Shown also in color plates

    c. There is an association with interstitial lung disease
    d. The presence of rimmed vacuoles is very characteristic
    e. It is an inflammatory myopathy

36. A 65-year-old man with diabetes, hypertension, and hyperlipidemia suffered a stroke about 1 month ago. At that time, he was started on aspirin, clopidogrel, and a statin. He now presents with generalized weakness, myalgias, shortness of breath, and oliguria. He seems to be fluid overloaded, and his blood urea nitrogen and creatinine are very elevated. His creatine kinase (CK) is 15,460 IU/L (normal up to 220 IU/L). Which of the following is incorrect?
    a. Statins can produce rhabdomyolysis
    b. *SLCO1B* gene mutation is associated with predisposition to statin-induced myopathy
    c. Statins can produce myalgias without increased serum CK
    d. Statins can produce asymptomatic increases in serum CK
    e. Concomitant intake of statins and fibrates does not increase the risk of muscle toxicity

37. A 25-year-old woman with depression, migraines, and chronic fatigue syndrome presents to the clinic complaining of palpitations and light-headedness every time she stands from a seated position. These symptoms never occur while seated or supine. On vital sign testing, her pulse increases from 90-bpm while seated to 130 bpm while standing. Her examination is otherwise entirely normal. Tilt table testing confirms an increase of pulse from 80 bpm when supine to 150 bpm with head-up tilt (at approximately 70 degrees); blood pressure remains stable during the tilt. With the increase in heart rate she feels palpitations, light-headedness, and generalized weakness, without flushing or skin changes. Laboratory evaluation, echocardiography, and other testing are otherwise normal. What is the most likely diagnosis in this patient?
    a. Orthostatic hypotension
    b. Vasovagal response
    c. Systemic mastocytosis
    d. Postural orthostatic tachycardia syndrome
    e. Subclavian steal syndrome

38. A 45-year-old man originally from China has a history of palpitations and anxiety and presents with recent onset of episodes of weakness affecting arms and legs to the point that he feels paralyzed. There is sparing of respiratory and bulbar muscles. Which of the following should be done next?

a. EMG needle examination
b. Send genetic testing for *SCN4A* mutation
c. Refer to psychiatry
d. Obtain thyroid-stimulating hormone
e. Begin carbonic anhydrase inhibitors

Questions 39–40

39. A 59-year-old man presents with asymmetric atrophy and weakness of the wrist and finger flexor muscles, as well as the quadriceps femoris. There is also weakness of anterior tibial muscles. The deltoids are spared. Serum creatine kinase levels are slightly elevated. The muscle biopsy is shown in Figure 10.5. Which of the following is the most likely diagnosis?

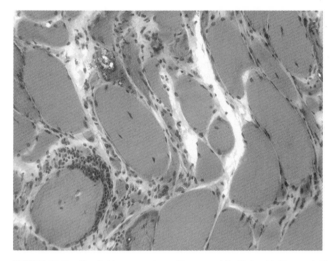

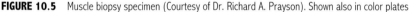

FIGURE 10.5   Muscle biopsy specimen (Courtesy of Dr. Richard A. Prayson). Shown also in color plates

a. Dermatomyositis
b. Polymyositis
c. Inclusion body myositis
d. Mitochondrial myopathy
e. A muscular dystrophy

40. Regarding the condition depicted in question 39, which of the following is correct?

a. Rimmed vacuoles are characteristic of this condition
b. There is perifascicular atrophy, but no inflammatory cells within the fascicles
c. Gottron's papules are characteristic
d. "Mechanic hands" are usually seen in these patients
e. This condition responds well to prednisone

41. Which of the following is incorrect regarding the limb-girdle muscular dystrophies (LGMD)?
    a. There is no cardiac involvement in any type of LGMD
    b. Muscle biopsy shows dystrophic changes
    c. Needle EMG shows myopathic changes
    d. Some types are associated with contractures
    e. The LGMD1 group is autosomal dominant

42. A 10-year-old boy is brought for evaluation of proximal weakness, affecting predominantly the pelvic girdle. A limb-girdle muscular dystrophy (LGMD) is suspected. Which of the following proteins is associated with its respective type of LGMD?
    a. Myotilin and LGMD2A
    b. Caveolin-3 and LGMD2B
    c. Dysferlin and LGMD1A
    d. Fukutin-related protein and LGMD2I
    e. Sarcoglycan and LGMD1C

Questions 43–44

43. A 52-year-old woman who has smoked since adolescence presented to the clinic complaining of weakness in her arms that she had noticed while blow-drying her hair and weakness in her legs when climbing stairs. Associated symptoms included constipation and a sensation of incomplete emptying of the bladder. On examination, she had Medical Research Council grade 4/5 weakness in proximal arm muscles and in hip flexors. Deep tendon reflexes were 1+ throughout. After brief sustained contraction of her biceps muscle, the biceps deep tendon reflexes increased to 2+. Medial nerve CMAPs are shown in Figure 10.6. EMG did not show evidence of denervation or myopathy. Serum creatine kinase was normal. What is the most likely diagnosis in this patient?

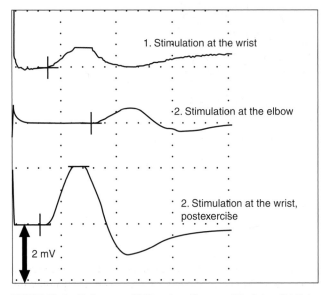

1. Stimulation at the wrist

2. Stimulation at the elbow

2. Stimulation at the wrist, postexercise

2 mV

FIGURE 10.6   Median nerve CMAP tracings (Courtesy of Dr. Robert Shields)

    a. Autoimmune myasthenia gravis
    b. Paraneoplastic Lambert-Eaton myasthenic syndrome
    c. Polymyositis
    d. Inclusion body myositis
    e. Acute demyelinating polyneuropathy

44. Regarding the condition described in question 43, which of the following is incorrect?
    a. It is due to antibodies against presynaptic P/Q-type voltage-gated calcium channels
    b. It can be either paraneoplastic or autoimmune
    c. It is more common in males
    d. Autonomic nervous system involvement occurs
    e. Symptoms respond well to acetylcholine esterase inhibitors

45. A 42-year-old man who was previously healthy presents with 1 week of puffy eyelids, diplopia, dysphagia, myalgias, and proximal greater than distal muscle weakness. Creatine kinase levels are only mildly elevated, but the serum eosinophil count is markedly increased. A muscle biopsy is obtained, which is shown in Figure 10.7. Which of the following is the most likely diagnosis?

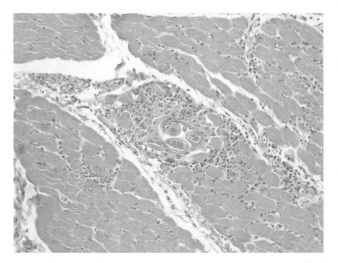

FIGURE 10.7 Muscle specimen (Courtesy of Dr. Richard A. Prayson). Shown in color plates

    a. Dermatomyositis
    b. Polymyositis
    c. Inclusion body myositis
    d. Trichinosis
    e. Muscular dystrophy

46. A baby is brought for evaluation of hypotonia, and on muscle biopsy, there are sarcoplasmic rods consistent with nemaline myopathy. Which of the following is incorrect regarding this condition?

a. There is great variability in age of onset, with presentations in the neonatal period as well as in adults
b. This condition can be inherited in an autosomal dominant or recessive fashion
c. Respiratory muscles are rarely affected in adult forms
d. α-actin, α-tropomyosin, and β-tropomyosin are genes implicated
e. Nebulin, troponin, and cofilin are genes implicated

47. Regarding testing of the autonomic nervous system, which of the following statements is incorrect?
a. Tilt table testing is a measure of autonomic function and assesses changes in blood pressure and heart rate that occur with changes in posture
b. Normally, with assumption of the upright posture, there is transient bradycardia and hypotension followed by blood pressure and heart rate normalization
c. In the evaluation of syncope, with upright tilt table testing, an abrupt reduction in blood pressure with bradycardia signifies a neurocardiogenic mechanism
d. The thermoregulatory sweat test is a qualitative test of sudomotor function, which can identify patterns of sweating abnormalities that may correspond to different forms of dysautonomia
e. The quantitative sudomotor axon reflex test is a measure of sudomotor function and specifically assesses the sympathetic postganglionic axon

Questions 48–49

48. A 1-month-old baby is evaluated for difficulty feeding and cyanosis. He is hypotonic and weak, and is noticed to have macroglossia, cardiomegaly, and hepatomegaly. A diagnosis of Pompe's disease is made. Which of the following is incorrect?
a. It is caused by acid maltase deficiency
b. There is glycogen accumulation in the affected tissues
c. This is type V glycogenosis
d. It is autosomal recessive
e. It is caused by deficiency of lysosomal α-1,4-glucosidase

49. A 29-year-old man has had a slowly progressive decline in exercise tolerance over the past year. The patient is currently in the ICU intubated for respiratory failure that started 2 days ago after acquiring an upper respiratory infection. An adult form of acid maltase deficiency is suspected. Which of the following is correct if this is the case?
a. Given the age of onset and the lack of cardiac and liver involvement, this patient does not have acid maltase deficiency
b. Muscle biopsy with vacuolated sarcoplasm with glycogen accumulation that stains strongly with acid phosphatase helps making the diagnosis of acid maltase deficiency
c. This patient has type III glycogenosis
d. Acid maltase deficiency is autosomal dominant
e. Mental retardation is common with presentations in this age group

50. Consultation is requested for a 6-month-old baby who in the neonatal period had required prolonged mechanical ventilation, tracheostomy, and percutaneous gastrostomy insertion. On examination, he has bilateral ptosis, and restricted eye movements are noted. Pupils are equal and briskly react to light. His mother is healthy, with no evidence of a neuromuscular disorder. On administration of edrophonium, his ptosis improves, his sucking reflex becomes stronger, and his eye movements achieve full range. What is the most likely diagnosis in this patient?

a. Transient neonatal myasthenia

b. Botulism

c. Congenital myasthenia due to congenital acetylcholine receptor deficiency

d. Congenital myasthenia due to choline acetyltransferase deficiency

e. A mitochondrial disorder

Questions 51–52

51. A 14-year-old boy has progressive weakness predominantly of the shoulders and upper arms, with milder involvement of the lower extremities. He has prominent contractures at the elbows and ankles, but no pseudohypertrophy of the calves. An electrocardiogram was obtained because he was found to be bradycardic, and a complete atrioventricular block was detected. Which of the following is the most likely diagnosis?

a. Becker muscular dystrophy

b. Duchenne muscular dystrophy

c. Emery-Dreifuss muscular dystrophy

d. Fascioscapulohumeral muscular dystrophy

e. Limb-girdle muscular dystrophy

52. Which of the following is/are the defective protein(s) in this condition?

a. Emerin

b. Laminin A/C

c. Dystrophin

d. a and b

e. a and c

53. A baby is diagnosed with a congenital muscular dystrophy. Clinically, he is weak and has multiple contractures with distal hyperlaxity. There are protrusions of the calcanei in the feet. Which is the most likely diagnosis?

a. Fukuyama-type congenital muscular dystrophy

b. Laminin-α-2 deficiency

c. Walker-Marburg syndrome

d. Muscle-eye-brain disease

e. Ullrich's congenital muscular dystrophy

54. Which of the following is correct regarding the anatomy of the sympathetic and parasympathetic systems?

a. Parasympathetic postganglionic neurons predominantly release norepinephrine

b. Cell bodies of neurons that provide innervation to the detrusor muscle of the bladder are located in L2 to L4

c. The intermediolateral cell column is present from T1 to L5 and is the source for preganglionic sympathetic fibers

d. Gray rami communicantes carry preganglionic fibers, and white rami communicantes carry postganglionic fibers

e. Parasympathetic ganglia are located close to the end organ, whereas sympathetic ganglia are distant from their end organ; sympathetic postganglionic fibers are longer as compared to parasympathetic postganglionic fibers

Questions 55–56

55. A 62-year-old woman with diabetes who has smoked since her teenage years is being evaluated during her annual examination. She has been doing relatively well except for a chronic cough, which she attributes to smoking. She fell a few days ago, but did not hit her head. During examination, her physician notices that her left eyelid is droopy. On further examination, in dim light, her left pupil is noted to be smaller than the right. The patient's left face appears to be clearly less moist as compared to the right and slightly paler. Extraocular movements are normal. What is the most likely diagnosis in this patient?

    a. An ICA dissection that she probably sustained when she fell

    b. An oculomotor palsy due to a lacunar infarct

    c. Ptosis due to levator dehiscence

    d. A partial third nerve palsy due to diabetic cranial neuropathy

    e. Horner's syndrome due to an apical lung mass (Pancoast tumor)

56. A 42-year-old man is involved in a motor vehicle accident. He experiences right-sided neck pain for 2 days following the accident and presents to his physician for further evaluation. On examination, he has drooping of his right eyelid. The right pupil is smaller than the left, and his right eye appears sunken. A carotid ultrasound is performed, and shows a right ICA dissection with an intact right ECA. Which of the following statements is correct?

    a. In this patient, there will be anhidrosis on the right side of the face

    b. His eyelid is droopy because of involvement of the levator palpebrae

    c. The eye abnormalities have resulted from extension of the dissection into the cavernous portion of the carotid artery, leading to involvement of cranial nerve III

    d. This patient's anisocoria will become more apparent in dim light

    e. This patient is likely to have reduced abduction of the right eye on attempted gaze to the right

57. Which of the following is not a distal muscular dystrophy?

    a. Dystrophic myotonia type 2 (DM2) myotonic dystrophy

    b. Miyoshi myopathy

    c. Welander myopathy

    d. Desmin myopathy

    e. Nonaka myopathy

Questions 58–60

58. Which of the following statements is incorrect regarding innervation of the genitourinary system?

    a. The intermediolateral cell column in the spinal cord at the level of L1 and L2 provides sympathetic innervation to the bladder

    b. Nerve roots S2 to S4 relay afferent sensory information from the genitourinary system, bladder, and anorectal area to the spinal cord

    c. Somatic efferents to the skeletal muscles of the pelvic floor arise from the anterior horn cells at S2 to S4 and are carried by the pudendal nerves

    d. Onuf's nucleus at S2 to S4 contains the cell bodies of neurons that control the urethral and anal sphincters

    e. Penile erection is mediated by the sympathetic nervous system and ejaculation by the parasympathetic nervous system

59. Which of the following pairs of urinary symptoms and associated bladder abnormalities are incorrect in the patients described?

    a. A 62-year-old man with cauda equina syndrome who involuntarily urinates when pressure is applied to his bladder—flaccid areflexic bladder leading to overflow incontinence

    b. A 72-year-old man with normal pressure hydrocephalus who has no control over urination—dysfunction of the medial frontal micturition centers in the paracentral lobule, leading to loss of voluntary suppression of the detrusor reflex

    c. A 17-year-old male who sustained a thoracic cord contusion 2 days ago and is unable to urinate—atonic bladder with reflex contraction of the urethral sphincter, leading to urinary retention

    d. A 32-year-old woman with multiple sclerosis who has multiple spinal cord lesions and sometimes has incontinence because she senses the need to urinate but has such urgency that she cannot always make it to the bathroom in time—detrusor hyperreflexia

    e. A 54-year-old man with multiple sclerosis who has severe painful pelvic cramps associated with a sensation that he needs to urinate, but after urination, feels he has not voided completely—detrusor-sphincter dyssynergia resulting from contraction of the detrusor muscle with excessive relaxation of the internal and external urethral sphincter

60. Regarding bladder function, which of the following statements is incorrect?

    a. There is normally voluntary inhibition of the detrusor reflex by the medial frontal micturition center located in the paracentral lobule

    b. External urethral sphincter tone is normally under voluntary control

    c. The internal urethral sphincter is under parasympathetic control

    d. The micturition center, located in the pons, regulates the detrusor reflex

    e. In detrusor-sphincter dyssynergia, the detrusor muscle contracts against an unrelaxed urethral sphincter

61. A 3-week-old child is brought to a pediatrician because of distended abdomen. His mother reports that he has had a few bowel movements, but that he was certainly not having the normal bowel movements that her other children at his age. On examination, he has a distended abdomen with hypoactive bowel sounds. X-ray of the abdomen shows dilated loops of bowel with excessive fecal material. A diagnosis of Hirschsprung's disease is suspected after additional testing. Which of the following is incorrect regarding the enteric nervous system?

    a. It consists of the myenteric plexus, located between the outer and inner smooth muscle layers of the gastrointestinal tract, and the submucous plexus, located between the circular muscle layer and the mucosa

    b. The myenteric plexus is predominantly involved in gut motility

    c. The submucous plexus is predominantly involved in secretory functions of the gastrointestinal tract

    d. Hirschsprung's disease is due to congenital absence of the submucous plexus

    e. Hirschsprung's disease is often focal, though rare cases involve the entire colon

62. Which of the following is incorrect regarding myofibrillar myopathy?

    a. Desmin is a protein implicated

    b. $\alpha\beta$-Crystallin is one of the proteins implicated

    c. There is no cardiac involvement

    d. Peripheral neuropathy can be seen in these patients

    e. There is focal dissolution of myofibrils and subsarcolemmal accumulation of dense granular and filamentous material

63. A 6-year-old boy is brought for evaluation of stiffness. His legs are stiff, and he has difficulty relaxing muscles after contracting them. For example, he cannot release objects easily once grasped with his hands, and when he closes his eyes, it takes a few seconds before he is able to open them completely. If he performs the same motor task multiple times, it becomes easier. When his thenar eminence is percussed, there is prolonged contraction and delayed relaxation. His father and grandfather have similar clinical features that started around the same age. Which of the following is the most likely diagnosis?

   a. Paramyotonia congenita
   b. Myotonia congenita, Becker' disease
   c. Myotonia congenita, Thomsen's disease
   d. Hyperkalemic periodic paralysis
   e. Hypokalemic periodic paralysis

64. A 39-year-old man with a history of alcoholism is admitted with pancreatitis and significant hyperglycemia. His hospital course is complicated by acute respiratory distress syndrome and sepsis. He requires prolonged intubation, and because he "fights" the ventilator, he required sedation and paralysis. Tracheostomy is required. After 3 weeks of being in the ICU, the neurology team is called because the patient does not move any of his limbs and his limbs are flaccid. NCS show that SNAPs are normal, with low CMAPs. Needle EMG study shows myopathic findings. Which of the following is incorrect?

   a. There is myosin loss
   b. This patient has critical illness polyneuropathy
   c. Systemic inflammatory response syndrome is associated with this condition
   d. Steroids and neuromuscular blocking agents are risk factors for this illness
   e. This is a potential cause for difficulty weaning patients from mechanical ventilation

65. A 10-year-old boy is brought for evaluation because of contractures. He has flexion contractures of the elbows and ankles, as well as hyperextensible interphalangeal joints. His father apparently also had contractures since adolescence. A diagnostic test demonstrates mutations associated with the gene that encodes collagen type VI. Which is the most likely diagnosis?

   a. Fukuyama-type congenital muscular dystrophy
   b. Laminin-α-2 deficiency
   c. Bethlem myopathy
   d. Muscle-eye-brain disease
   e. Walker-Marburg syndrome

Answer key

1. b	12. b	23. d	34. e	45. d	56. d
2. e	13. c	24. b	35. d	46. c	57. a
3. d	14. b	25. b	36. e	47. b	58. e
4. b	15. d	26. a	37. d	48. c	59. e
5. c	16. a	27. e	38. d	49. b	60. c
6. b	17. a	28. d	39. c	50. c	61. d
7. e	18. a	29. c	40. a	51. c	62. c
8. a	19. b	30. a	41. a	52. d	63. c
9. d	20. a	31. c	42. d	53. e	64. b
10. e	21. b	32. a	43. b	54. e	65. c
11. c	22. c	33. a	44. e	55. e	

Answers

1. **b**

This patient has hypokalemic periodic paralysis, which is inherited in an autosomal dominant fashion; however, sporadic cases have been reported. There are two types: type 1 caused by a mutation in the calcium channel gene *CACNA1S* on chromosome 1q31, and type 2 caused by a mutation in the sodium channel gene *SCN4A*. These patients present with episodes of weakness without myotonia that could be focal or generalized and ranges from mild to severe, associated with hyporeflexia during the attacks, each of which can last for hours, with some persistent mild weakness for a few days. During attacks, the creatine kinase level may be elevated and the serum potassium is usually reduced. These episodes are triggered by exercise, meals rich in carbohydrates, ethanol, cold exposure, and emotional stressors. Provocative testing can be done with glucose administration. The main treatment focus is to avoid triggers; carbonic anhydrase inhibitors such as acetazolamide and potassium-sparing diuretics are useful in treating this condition.

Hyperkalemic periodic paralysis, on the other hand, presents with episodes of weakness triggered by resting after exercise and fasting. This condition is autosomal dominant and is caused by a mutation in the sodium channel gene *SCN4A*. Provocative testing is done with administration of potassium. The treatment is focused on avoiding triggers. During attacks, glucose can be provided, and as prophylactic therapy, thiazide diuretics can be used.

Andersen-Tawil syndrome is also a channelopathy characterized by periodic paralysis, ventricular arrhythmias, and dysmorphic features. It is associated with a mutation in the potassium channel gene *KCNJ2*.

Paramyotonia congenita is discussed in question 17. Myotonia congenita is discussed in question 63.

Saperstein DS. Muscle channelopathies. Semin Neurol. 2008; 28:260–269.

2. **e**

This patient has steroid-induced myopathy, in which the needle EMG is nonspecific and creatine kinase levels are usually normal.

Steroid-induced myopathy can be caused by chronic use of exogenous corticosteroids used for the treatment of underlying inflammatory conditions or by endogenous hypercortisolism, such as in Cushing's disease. The weakness is typically mild or moderate and proximal. Histopathologically, there is atrophy of type II fibers. Management of this condition involves treatment of the underlying cause in case of endogenous hypercortisolism or reduction of exogenous steroids, as well as physical therapy.

Dalakas MC. Toxic and drug-induced myopathies. J Neurol Neurosurg Psychiatry. 2009; 80:832–838.

3. **d**

Centronuclear myopathy (also known as myotubular myopathy) is a congenital myopathy, manifesting characteristically with ptosis and ocular palsies, as well as weakness of facial, pharyngeal, laryngeal, and neck muscles. It typically presents with hypotonia and weakness at birth, or in early childhood. Proximal and distal weakness and hyporeflexia can be seen. Severe forms may be fatal due to respiratory failure in the first few months of life. Creatine kinase levels are mildly elevated. Needle EMG shows a myopathic pattern with positive waves and fibrillations. Pathologically, there are small muscle fibers and central nucleation, as well as predominance of type I fibers, which are small and hypotrophic.

This condition is inherited in an X-linked or autosomal dominant or recessive fashion. The X-linked form is severe and presents in the neonatal period, the autosomal dominant form is an adult-onset milder form, and the autosomal recessive form is intermediate in severity.

Cardamone M, Darras BT, Ryan MM. Inherited myopathies and muscular dystrophies. Semin Neurol. 2008; 28:250–259.

Ropper AH, Samuels MA. Adams and Victor's Principles of Neurology, 9th ed. New York: McGraw-Hill; 2009.

4. b

This patient has myasthenia gravis. As discussed below, the majority of patients with myasthenia gravis have generalized manifestations (not restricted to a single muscle group) within 2 years of symptom onset.

Myasthenia gravis is a neuromuscular junction transmission disorder. It is most commonly autoimmune in etiology, though there are rare cases of congenital myasthenia that are genetic (see question 50). It is more common in males and older adults. Women have an earlier age of onset, often presenting in the second or third decades of life, whereas men typically present in the sixth decade. Myasthenia gravis may present with a myriad of symptoms; the hallmarks are fluctuations and fatigability, with weakness worsening with increased muscle use. A proportion of patients present with predominantly extraocular muscle involvement, with diplopia and ptosis. The majority of such patients generalize to involve bulbar, limb, neck, and/or respiratory muscles within 2 years, though in a minority, involvement remains restricted to the eyes, so-called ocular myasthenia. Other patients present with predominantly bulbar symptoms due to involvement of muscles of mastication, speech, swallowing, and facial expression, leading to weakness and/or fatigability of chewing, dysphagia, and/or dysarthria. Limb and neck weakness also occur. Myasthenic crisis, or respiratory failure due to involvement of respiratory muscles, can be the presenting symptom, but more commonly occurs in those with exacerbation of symptoms in the setting of stressors such as infection or surgery. Myasthenia gravis is more common in family members of patients with this disorder. It has been associated with human leukocyte antigen types B8, DR1, DR2, and DR3. Patients with myasthenia gravis are at an increased risk of other autoimmune disorders including thyroid disorders, and these should be tested for as clinically indicated.

Bradley WG, Daroff RB, Fenichel GM, et al. Neurology in Clinical Practice, 5th ed. Philadelphia, PA: Elsevier; 2008.

5. c

The pathophysiology of autoimmune myasthenia gravis relates to the presence of circulating anti-acetylcholine receptor antibodies, which bind to the acetylcholine receptor causing immune-mediated destruction of the junctional folds that contain dense concentrations of this receptor, and a higher rate of internalization and destruction of acetylcholine receptor. In some cases, the antibodies might block binding of acetylcholine to its receptor at the neuromuscular junction. Antibodies against presynaptic voltage-gated calcium channels occur in Lambert-Eaton myasthenic syndrome (discussed in questions 43 and 44). Botulinum toxin inhibits exocytosis of presynaptic vesicles containing acetylcholine (discussed in Chapter 17). Rarely, myasthenia results from mutations in the acetylcholine receptor gene (discussed in question 50).

Bradley WG, Daroff RB, Fenichel GM, et al. Neurology in Clinical Practice, 5th ed. Philadelphia, PA: Elsevier; 2008.

6. b

Anti-striational muscle antibodies can be positive in myasthenia patients with thymoma, but they are much less sensitive and specific than acetylcholine receptor antibodies for the diagnosis of myasthenia gravis.

Edrophonium is an intravenous acetylcholine esterase inhibitor that increases the presence of acetylcholine at the neuromuscular junction. In patients with myasthenia, administration of edrophonium leads to transient improvement of weakness within minutes of administration; the edrophonium (Tensilon) test has therefore been used in the diagnosis of myasthenia gravis.

Laboratory testing for serum autoantibodies also aids in the diagnosis; positive tests confirm the diagnosis of autoimmune myasthenia gravis in the appropriate clinical setting, but their absence does not exclude it. Acetylcholine receptor binding antibodies can be detected by measuring binding to purified acetylcholine receptors radiolabeled with α-bungarotoxin. The sensitivity of this test is highest for generalized myasthenia, detecting antibodies in 70% to 95% of patients and lower for patients with ocular myasthenia. Patients who are initially seronegative for binding, blocking, or modulating antibodies may seroconvert later in the course of their disease. In a minority of patients with autoimmune myasthenia in whom the binding antibody is not detectable, modulating or blocking antibodies may be present. False-positive testing for these antibodies is rare, but can occur in patients with other autoimmune disorders. The patient's clinical picture, rather than antibody levels, is used to monitor response to therapy.

In approximately half of all patients who are seronegative for antibodies against the acetylcholine receptor, anti-muscle-specific tyrosine kinase antibodies are present (discussed in question 27).

EMG findings in myasthenia gravis include electrodecremental response and jitter. The presence of a 10% or greater decrement in amplitude of a CMAP between the first and fourth to fifth stimuli with repetitive nerve stimulation suggests a neuromuscular junction (NMJ) disorder (see Chapter 9). If there is not an abnormality present on repetitive nerve stimulation but there is a high clinical suspicion for myasthenia gravis and it cannot be confirmed with serologic testing, a single-fiber EMG can be performed. Single-fiber EMG is the most sensitive test of NMJ transmission. Jitter is the variability in the measure of interpotential difference between two muscle fiber action potentials during consecutive discharges of the same motor unit. Increased jitter (or increased interpotential time) is present in patients with NMJ abnormalities, but is not specific for myasthenia gravis. Blocking on single-fiber EMG is failure of a single muscle fiber action potential to appear during the motor unit discharge, and occurs when there is significantly increased jitter.

Bradley WG, Daroff RB, Fenichel GM, et al. Neurology in Clinical Practice, 5th ed. Philadelphia, PA: Elsevier; 2008.

7. e

This patient has Dystrophic myotonia type 2 (DM2) myotonic dystrophy. This condition is also known as PROMM or proximal myotonic myopathy. It is autosomal dominant and is characterized by proximal muscle weakness and myotonia. Cataracts and cardiac involvement are less frequent. Histopathologically, there are nonspecific findings of myopathy. The cause is a CCTG repeat expansion in an intron of the zinc finger protein 9 gene on chromosome 3q, and it is associated with intranuclear accumulation of the expanded RNA transcripts.

Becker muscular dystrophy is discussed in questions 30 and 31. DM1 myotonic dystrophy is discussed in question 12. Emery-Dreifuss muscular dystrophy is discussed in questions 51 and 52. Fascioscapulohumeral muscular dystrophy is discussed in question 9.

Cardamone M, Darras BT, Ryan MM. Inherited myopathies and muscular dystrophies. Semin Neurol. 2008; 28:250–259.

Ropper AH, Samuels MA. Adams and Victor's Principles of Neurology, 9th ed. New York: McGraw-Hill; 2009.

8. a

This patient has Fukuyama-type congenital muscular dystrophy. This condition is autosomal recessive, caused by a mutation of the fukutin gene on chromosome 9q. It is characterized by weakness and ocular and CNS abnormalities. Patients are hypotonic and floppy, with joint contractures at the hip, knee, and ankles. The weakness may be generalized, and these patients typically do not learn to walk. Creatine kinase levels are elevated, and muscle biopsy shows dystrophic changes and reduced α-dystroglycan. There is mental retardation and seizures are frequent. Brain MRI shows abnormalities in gyration and characteristic white matter changes in the frontal regions.

Laminin-α-2 deficiency is another muscular dystrophy, also known as merosin deficiency. These patients are hypotonic at birth, and have severe weakness of the trunk and limbs. Extraocular and facial muscles are spared. Contractures appear in the feet and hips. Some patients may have seizures; however, intelligence is generally preserved. MRI shows white matter changes and sometimes cortical abnormalities.

Ullrich myopathy and muscle-eye-brain disease are discussed in question 53. Bethlem myopathy is discussed in question 65.

Bradley WG, Daroff RB, Fenichel GM, et al. Neurology in Clinical Practice, 5th ed. Philadelphia, PA: Elsevier; 2008.

Cardamone M, Darras BT, Ryan MM. Inherited myopathies and muscular dystrophies. Semin Neurol. 2008; 28:250–259.

Ropper AH, Samuels MA. Adams and Victor's Principles of Neurology, 9th ed. New York: McGraw-Hill; 2009.

9. d

This patient has fascioscapulohumeral muscular dystrophy (FSHD). This condition is inherited in an autosomal dominant fashion and is caused by deletions in a 3.3 kb repeating sequences, termed D4Z4, located on chromosome 4q35.

FSHD is slowly progressive, and predominantly affects the face and shoulders, though later in the course of the disease, the lower extremities are affected as well. Age of onset is on average 16 in males and 20 in females, but can be variable, ranging between the first and sixth decades of life. These patients have weakness that can be asymmetric, and present with difficulty lifting their arms above their head, with prominent involvement of the upper arms (scapular muscles, biceps, triceps, trapezius, serratus anterior, and pectoralis), with relative sparing of the deltoids. The upper arm seems to be more atrophic than the forearms, making the bones of the shoulder appear prominent. Facial weakness is evident, with weakness of the orbicularis oculi, zygomaticus, and orbicularis oris. There is also weakness of the lower abdominal muscles, producing the "Beevor sign," in which the umbilicus moves upward with neck flexion. Pelvic muscles are compromised later, and involvement of peroneal muscles will manifest as foot drop. The masseters, temporalis muscle, extraocular muscles, and pharyngeal and respiratory muscles are usually spared. Cardiac involvement is rare and intelligence is typically normal. Creatine kinase levels are normal to slightly elevated.

The other options are unlikely in this case. Duchenne muscular dystrophy is discussed in questions 19 and 20. Becker muscular dystrophy is discussed in questions 30 and 31. Emery-Dreifuss muscular dystrophy is discussed in questions 51 and 52. Myotonic dystrophy is discussed in questions 7 and 12.

Bradley WG, Daroff RB, Fenichel GM, et al. Neurology in Clinical Practice, 5th ed. Philadelphia, PA: Elsevier; 2008.

Cardamone M, Darras BT, Ryan MM. Inherited myopathies and muscular dystrophies. Semin Neurol. 2008; 28:250–259.

Ropper AH, Samuels MA. Adams and Victor's Principles of Neurology, 9th ed. New York: McGraw-Hill; 2009.

10. e, 11. c

This patient has oculopharyngeal muscular dystrophy. This is an autosomal dominant late-onset muscular dystrophy with manifestations restricted to the ocular and pharyngeal regions. It is more frequent in patients with French-Canadian inheritance, and is caused by a GCG repeat expansion in the poly-A–binding protein 2 gene on chromosome 14q11. Patients present with dysphagia, dysphonia, and slowly progressive ptosis, and sometimes late involvement of extraocular muscles. There is no myotonia. Creatine kinase and aldolase levels are normal, and EMG is abnormal in affected muscles. Muscle biopsy demonstrates variation in fiber size, rimmed vacuoles, and intranuclear tubular filaments.

Cardamone M, Darras BT, Ryan MM. Inherited myopathies and muscular dystrophies. Semin Neurol. 2008; 28:250–259.

Ropper AH, Samuels MA. Adams and Victor's Principles of Neurology, 9th ed. New York: McGraw-Hill; 2009.

12. b

This patient has dystrophic myotonia type 1 (DM1) myotonic dystrophy, which is an autosomal dominant condition with high penetrance, caused by a CTG expansion in the myotonic dystrophy protein kinase gene on chromosome 19q. These patients present in early adult life with ptosis and facial weakness, and characteristic features such as frontal balding, atrophy of the masseters and temporalis, and weakness and atrophy of small muscles of the hands and extensors of the forearms and peroneal muscles. Pharyngeal and laryngeal weakness may be present, but this finding is rare. Patients have myotonia, which is a phenomenon of prolonged contraction and slow relaxation. Patients may also have diaphragmatic weakness, leading to respiratory failure, and cardiac abnormalities, especially conduction defects.

Various other tissues are also involved, and patients may exhibit esophageal dilatation, megacolon, lenticular opacities and cataracts, mental retardation, testicular atrophy with infertility, and androgen deficiency. Creatine kinase levels may be slightly elevated. EMG demonstrates myotonic discharges and short, rapidly recruiting motor unit potentials with fibrillations. Histopathologically, muscle biopsy demonstrates marked central nucleation, type 1 fiber atrophy, peripherally placed sarcoplasmic masses, ring fibers, and pyknotic nuclear clumps.

The other options are less likely to be the diagnosis in this patient. Becker muscular dystrophy is discussed in questions 30 and 31. Emery-Dreifuss muscular dystrophy is discussed in questions 51 and 52. Fascioscapulohumeral muscular dystrophy is discussed in question 9. DM2 myotonic dystrophy is discussed in question 7.

Cardamone M, Darras BT, Ryan MM. Inherited myopathies and muscular dystrophies. Semin Neurol. 2008; 28:250–259.

Ropper AH, Samuels MA. Adams and Victor's Principles of Neurology, 9th ed. New York: McGraw-Hill; 2009.

13. c

This patient most likely has carotid sinus hypersensitivity, as suggested by the triggering of symptoms with head movement in the setting of a tight collar. Carotid sinus hypersensitivity is defined by the occurrence of syncope associated with either a period of asystole of at least 3 seconds or a fall of at least 50 mm Hg in systolic blood pressure, or both, in response to pressure on the carotid sinus. In another form of carotid sinus hypersensitivity, hypotension without bradycardia may occur. Triggers can include a tight collar, turning of the head, or even swallowing, though no identifiable triggers may be present. Symptoms and changes in heart rate and/or blood pressure can be reproduced with carotid sinus massage. Treatment is avoidance of triggers, but when recurrent, pacemaker insertion may be necessary.

The carotid sinus, located at the bifurcation of the common carotid artery, is innervated by a branch of the glossopharyngeal nerve. The carotid sinus contains specialized mechanoreceptors that are capable of detecting changes in blood pressure (baroreceptors) and heart rate. With simulation, either mechanically (with applied pressure) or with elevations in blood pressure, mechanoreceptors send signals to the nucleus tractus solitarius in the medulla leading to a reduction in sympathetic tone (leading to a further reduction in blood pressure) and an increase in parasympathetic tone (leading to a reduction in heart rate). Carotid sinus hypersensitivity results from an exaggerated response to baroreceptor stimulation.

Vasovagal syncope is discussed in question 18; the absence of diaphoresis and nausea, and the presence of bradycardia, hypotension, and triggering by neck turning distinguish the two. Orthostatic hypotension, as most commonly occurs from dehydration leading to volume depletion and subsequent reduction in blood pressure with changes in posture, is usually preceded by warning symptoms such as light-headedness, which were not present in this case. Severe aortic stenosis can lead to syncope, but bradycardia would not be present, and other associated symptoms would include chest pain and shortness of breath.

Bradley WG, Daroff RB, Fenichel GM, et al. Neurology in Clinical Practice, 5th ed. Philadelphia, PA: Elsevier; 2008.

Morhman DE, Heller LJ. Cardiovascular Physiology, 6th ed. New York: McGraw-Hill; 2006.

14. b

This patient has McArdle's disease, or glycogenosis type V. This condition is an autosomal recessive disorder caused by myophosphorylase deficiency. This enzyme normally participates in the conversion of glycogen into glucose-6-phosphate; therefore, its deficiency will lead to glycogen accumulation and lack of glucose release from glycogen. The typical presentation is exercise-induced weakness, muscle cramps, and contractures, with electrical silence when needle EMG is performed in contracted muscles. Unlike normal muscles, when the muscle is exercised there is no production of lactic acid.

On exertion, a sensation of fatigue may ensue; however, if the patient slows down but does not stop, this sensation may disappear and the patient may be able to continue with the exercise. This is called a "second-wind phenomenon," which is typically seen in McArdle's disease, and may be related to a change in the blood supply, change in the muscle metabolism, and rise in fatty acid use.

Tarui disease (glycogenosis type VII) is caused by phosphofructokinase deficiency. This enzyme participates in the conversion of glucose-6-phosphate into glucose-1-phosphate, and therefore, it is similar to McArdle's disease from the clinical standpoint. Immunohistochemical analysis distinguishes these two disorders.

Cori's disease (glycogenosis type III) is caused by a deficiency in the debranching enzyme, leading to glycogen accumulation. These patients can present with a childhood form with liver disease and weakness or with an adult form characterized by myopathic weakness.

Andersen's disease (glycogenosis type IV) is caused by a deficiency in the branching enzyme, and is characterized by hepatomegaly from polysaccharide accumulation, cirrhosis, and liver failure. Pompe's disease (glucogenosis type II) is caused by acid maltase deficiency and is discussed in question 48.

Ropper AH, Samuels MA. Adams and Victor's Principles of Neurology, 9th ed. New York: McGraw-Hill; 2009.

15. d, 16. a

The patient depicted in question 15 is presenting in myasthenic crisis. In patients with signs of respiratory muscle involvement, negative inspiratory force and forced vital capacity should be monitored closely. Intubation and mechanical ventilation should be initiated when the negative inspiratory force is less then -20 cm of H_2O, forced vital capacity less than 15 mL/kg, or if there is a significant downward trend of spirometry measures with clinical evidence of respiratory muscle fatiguing.

The patient should be admitted to the ICU and intubated and mechanically ventilated. In patients with significant oculobulbar symptoms, neck flexor weakness (suggesting potential involvement of respiratory muscles), or respiratory muscle weakness, initial treatment is with either intravenous immunoglobulins or plasmapheresis.

Medications that exacerbate myasthenia gravis include aminoglycosides, β-blockers, and neuromuscular-blocking agents, among others. These should be avoided or used at the lowest possible dose in myasthenia gravis; symptom exacerbation with initiation of any medication should prompt investigation as to whether or not the medication is the culprit. Penicillamine can cause a seropositive myasthenic syndrome.

The majority of patients with myasthenia gravis, except some with purely ocular myasthenia, require immunosuppressive therapy. Patients are often treated with corticosteroids for several weeks to months until secondary immunosuppressive therapy has taken effect. Approximately one-third of patients will have worsening of their myasthenic symptoms at the onset of steroid therapy that lasts up to 10 days. Therefore, caution is required with the initiation of steroid therapy. When symptoms are severe, and there is concern for significant pharyngeal or respiratory muscle involvement, initiation of plasma exchange or intravenous immunoglobulins prior to starting corticosteroids may be necessary. Secondary immunosuppressive agents that may be used include azathioprine, mycophenolate mofetil, cyclophosphamide, and cyclosporine. Pyridostigmine provides symptomatic relief but does not modify the course of the illness. The acetylcholine esterase inhibitors are discussed in question 22.

In the majority of patients with autoimmune myasthenia gravis, thymic abnormalities are present, most commonly lymphoid follicular hyperplasia. In a minority of patients, benign thymoma is present, and rarely, malignant thymoma. Resection of the thymus (regardless of whether or not thymoma is present) can potentially induce remission of myasthenia gravis. In autoimmune myasthenia gravis, there are ongoing clinical trials to determine the utility of thymectomy. However, there is evidence that patients who undergo thymectomy are more likely to attain remission of their myasthenia gravis. Thymectomy is therefore recommended for patients with myasthenia gravis with symptom onset prior to the age of 60, especially in younger women who seem to show the most benefit. Response to resection may not be apparent for several months to years. Because myasthenic symptoms can worsen in the perioperative period, stabilization of symptoms with preoperative intravenous immunoglobulins or plasma exchange prior to operation may be indicated.

Bradley WG, Daroff RB, Fenichel GM, et al. Neurology in Clinical Practice, 5th ed. Philadelphia, PA: Elsevier; 2008.

Gronseth GS, Barohn RJ. Practice parameters: Thymectomy for autoimmune myasthenia gravis (an evidence-based review). Report of the Quality Standards Subcommittee of the American Academy of Neurology. Neurology. 2000; 55:7–15.

Ropper AH, Samuels MA. Adams and Victor's Principles of Neurology, 9th ed. New York: McGraw-Hill; 2009.

17. a

This patient has paramyotonia congenita, which is an autosomal dominant channelopathy caused by a mutation in the sodium channel gene *SCN4A*. The manifestations are very similar to those of myotonia congenita; however, there is no "warm-up" phenomenon and the symptoms are worsened with exercise and exposure to cold, features that help differentiate this condition from myotonia congenita. Percussion myotonia is rare, but can be seen after exposure to cold. EMG after cold exposure can also demonstrate fibrillation potentials followed by electrical inexcitability.

Becker's and Thomsen's disease are discussed in question 63. Hyperkalemia and hypokalemic periodic paralysis are discussed in questions 1 and 38.

Saperstein DS. Muscle channelopathies. Semin Neurol. 2008; 28:260–269.

18. a

This patient's history is consistent with vasovagal syncope, a form of neurally mediated syncope or neurocardiogenic syncope. Syncope is a sudden transient loss of consciousness with a loss of postural tone. There are several causes of syncope; one of the most common causes is vasovagal syncope. It can have many potential triggers, with phlebotomy being a common one. This type of syncope results from a combination of inhibition of normal vascular sympathetic tone and increased vagal tone. Clinical features that suggest vasovagal syncope include female sex, and preceding or concomitant diaphoresis, palpitations, and nausea.

The other options are all potential causes of syncope. Glossopharyngeal neuralgia is characterized by severe pain in the hypopharynx and pharynx, tongue, and ear, with hypotension and bradycardia that when severe may be associated with syncope. It is often posttraumatic, but can occur with neck tumors as well. There are no features in the case to suggest glossopharyngeal neuralgia. A lack of postictal confusion and absence of convulsions helps distinguish syncope from seizures in this case. Carotid sinus hypersensitivity is discussed in question 13; syncope in the latter disorder is triggered by maneuvers that increase pressure on the carotid sinus, such as a tight collar. A third ventricular tumor, such as a colloid cyst, can lead to syncope with postural changes if the change in posture leads to obstruction of the third ventricle, leading to increased intracranial pressure. The history in this case is more suggestive of vasovagal syncope.

Bradley WG, Daroff RB, Fenichel GM, et al. Neurology in Clinical Practice, 5th ed. Philadelphia, PA: Elsevier; 2008.

19. b, 20. a

This patient has Duchenne muscular dystrophy. This condition is a dystrophinopathy, inherited in an X-linked recessive fashion, and is the most common genetic muscle disease, affecting 1 in 3500 live male births. About a third of the cases are caused by spontaneous mutations in the dystrophin gene, so there may not be a positive family history. This condition presents early in life and manifests with weakness and delayed development of motor milestones. These children have frequent falls, and difficulty walking, running, and rising from supine and sitting positions. Weakness is significant in the proximal muscles, predominantly in the iliopsoas, quadriceps, and gluteals, as well as the shoulder girdle and upper limbs. It also tends to affect the pretibial muscles. These patients have pseudohypertrophy of the calves due to fibrosis. They also have scapular winging and contractures. Ocular, facial, and bulbar muscles are usually spared. Cardiac involvement includes arrhythmias, cardiomyopathy, and heart failure. Mild mental retardation with a subnormal intelligence quotient (IQ) may be seen. These children become wheelchair- or bed-bound, and may eventually die of respiratory failure and pulmonary infections. Creatine kinase values range from 10 to 100 times higher than normal. Needle EMG shows fibrillations, positive waves, and myopathic motor unit potentials.

The muscle biopsy findings in Figure 10.1 indicate a muscular dystrophy, showing endomysial fibrosis, loss of muscle fibers with residual fibers of different sizes, some of which are very large and eosinophilic, and others very small and atrophic. Degeneration and regeneration, as well as necrosis and macrophage invasion, may also be seen. In general, myofiber necrosis, degeneration, regeneration, increased fiber size variation, endomysial inflammation, and fibrosis are collectively called dystrophic changes, which are characteristic for Duchenne muscular dystrophy, but not specific, and can be seen in other dystrophies.

Dystrophin is the affected gene product and is absent in patients with Duchenne. Dystrophin is a cytoplasmic protein that binds and interacts with other intracytoplasmic proteins such as F-actin, and is linked to the trans-sarcolemmal dystroglycan protein complex, providing a structural link between the subsarcolemmal cytoskeleton and the extracellular matrix. If dystrophin is lost or altered, this sarcolemmal structure is affected, making it susceptible to rupture. The diagnosis of Duchenne muscular dystrophy is made by genetic testing of the dystrophin gene or by absent dystrophin immunostaining on muscle biopsy.

Becker muscular dystrophy is similar to Duchenne muscular dystrophy; however, it is much less severe, with a later onset (usually in adolescence or adulthood), which is not the case in this patient. Becker muscular dystrophy is discussed in questions 30 and 31. The other options are unlikely to be correct diagnosis in this case. Emery-Dreifuss muscular dystrophy is discussed in questions 51 and 52. Fascioscapulohumeral muscular dystrophy is discussed in question 9. Limb-girdle muscular dystrophy is discussed in questions 41 and 42.

Prayson RA, Goldblum JR. Neuropathology, 1st ed. Philadelphia, PA: Elsevier; 2005.

Ropper AH, Samuels MA. Adams and Victor's Principles of Neurology, 9th ed. New York: McGraw-Hill; 2009.

21. b

This patient has Nonaka myopathy, which is an autosomal recessive distal myopathy, with onset in early adulthood. It is characterized by foot drop associated with weakness of the anterior tibial muscles. Eventually, muscles of the upper extremities are affected, especially the extensors. Rarely, there is proximal weakness and no bulbar involvement. Histologically, the muscle biopsy shows rimmed vacuoles, and electron microscopy shows tubular filaments similar to those seen in inclusion body myositis, without inflammation. This condition is associated with a mutation in the *GNE* gene located on chromosome 9p.

Welander muscular dystrophy is a distal myopathy inherited in an autosomal dominant fashion, with an onset later in adult life usually between 40 and 60 years of age (not consistent with this case). Welander myopathy usually begins with weakness and atrophy in the distal muscles of the hands and later affects the legs. Muscle biopsy demonstrates myopathic changes and rimmed vacuoles.

Markesbery-Griggs is also an autosomal dominant distal myopathy with onset later in adult life, caused by mutations in the gene encoding titin on chromosome 2q. It is characterized by foot drop and the later development of wrist drop and weakness of extensor muscles of the forearms. The biopsy findings are similar to those seen in Welander myopathy.

Miyoshi myopathy and scapuloperoneal muscular dystrophy are not consistent with this case and are discussed in question 26.

Cardamone M, Darras BT, Ryan MM. Inherited myopathies and muscular dystrophies. Semin Neurol. 2008; 28:250–259.

Ropper AH, Samuels MA. Adams and Victor's Principles of Neurology, 9th ed. New York: McGraw-Hill; 2009.

22. c

Acetylcholine esterase inhibitors, including pyridostigmine and neostigmine, inhibit acetylcholine esterase, increasing levels of acetylcholine at the neuromuscular junction (NMJ). The most commonly used acetylcholine esterase inhibitor in myasthenia gravis is pyridostigmine. It improves symptoms, but does not alter the course of the disease. Side effects are due to activation of muscarinic receptors outside of the NMJ, and include diarrhea, nausea, abdominal cramps, and increased bronchial secretions. At therapeutic doses, pyridostigmine does not affect central cholinergic pathways, as it does not cross the blood-brain barrier.

With excessive dosing, cholinergic crisis can occur, with paradoxical worsening of weakness, even leading to respiratory failure. Patients with myasthenia presenting with significant worsening of symptoms with respiratory involvement should be assessed for the possibility of cholinergic crisis rather than myasthenic crisis. Cholinergic crisis results from overstimulation of muscarinic receptors not only at the NMJ but also systemically due to overdosing with pyridostigmine. Symptoms that distinguish cholinergic crisis from myasthenic crisis include the presence of nausea, vomiting, diaphoresis, sialorrhea, excessive bronchial secretions, miosis, bradycardia, and diarrhea (see also Chapter 3).

Bradley WG, Daroff RB, Fenichel GM, et al. Neurology in Clinical Practice, 5th ed. Philadelphia, PA: Elsevier; 2008.

Ropper AH, Samuels MA. Adams and Victor's Principles of Neurology, 9th ed. New York: McGraw-Hill; 2009.

23. d

The muscle biopsy shown in Figure 10.2 is consistent with a diagnosis of central core myopathy. This nicotinamide adenine dinucleotide-stained specimen demonstrates loss of oxidative activity within the center of muscle fibers, seen as paler areas where there is absence of mitochondria. These central cores run along the length of the muscle fiber, as opposed to multicore or minicore disease in which the cores are small, extending through only segments of the fiber length.

Central core myopathy is an autosomal dominant disease, caused by a mutation in the ryanodine receptor gene *RYR1* on chromosome 19q13.1. These patients are at risk for the development of malignant hyperthermia and this should be considered when general anesthesia is needed. The clinical presentation is that of weakness and hypotonia soon after birth, and subsequent delay in motor development. The weakness is proximal, and the pelvic girdle is usually more affected than the shoulder girdle. Facial, bulbar, and ocular muscles are usually spared. Creatine kinase levels are slightly elevated.

Cardamone M, Darras BT, Ryan MM. Inherited myopathies and muscular dystrophies. Semin Neurol. 2008; 28:250–259.

Prayson RA, Goldblum JR. Neuropathology, 1st ed. Philadelphia, PA: Elsevier; 2005.

Ropper AH, Samuels MA. Adams and Victor's Principles of Neurology, 9th ed. New York: McGraw-Hill; 2009.

24. b, 25. b

This patient's history and examination are consistent with an autonomic ganglionopathy. Symptoms develop over weeks, as opposed to pure autonomic failure, in which symptoms develop slowly over time. Symptoms of autonomic ganglionopathy are due to dysfunction in the parasympathetic and sympathetic nervous system, and include orthostatic hypotension, absent heart rate variability (see question 47 on tilt table testing), hypohidrosis or anhidrosis, dry mouth and eyes, pupillary abnormalities, sexual dysfunction, early satiety, constipation, and diarrhea due to abnormal gastric and intestinal motility. It results from impairment of transmission of impulses in the autonomic ganglia and affects both the parasympathetic and sympathetic nervous systems. In approximately half of patients, an antibody against the ganglionic nicotinic acetylcholine receptor can be identified in the serum. Autonomic ganglionopathy can be either autoimmune or paraneoplastic, with small cell lung carcinoma being a common associated malignancy; these cannot definitively be distinguished between clinically, and the antibody can be present in either form. In patients with the autoimmune form, other autoimmune disorders may be present, and symptoms may be preceded by antecedent viral illness.

Treatment of autoimmune autonomic ganglionopathy includes plasma exchange and intravenous immunoglobulins; typically, some improvement of symptoms occurs, but full recovery is unlikely.

Acetylcholine receptor binding antibodies are seen in autoimmune myasthenia gravis. Antistriational muscle antibodies can be detected in patients with autoimmune myasthenia gravis or thymoma. Antibodies against presynaptic P/Q-type voltage-gated calcium channel are seen in Lambert-Eaton syndrome. Anti-Jo 1 antibodies are seen in polymyositis.

In a patient without a known history of diabetes, autonomic neuropathy would unlikely be the sole manifestation of nervous system involvement from diabetes. Postural orthostatic tachycardia syndrome is described in question 37, amyloid autonomic neuropathy in Chapter 9, and pure autonomic failure in question 34.

Bradley WG, Daroff RB, Fenichel GM, et al. Neurology in Clinical Practice, 5th ed. Philadelphia, PA: Elsevier; 2008.

26. a

This patient has Miyoshi myopathy, which is an autosomal recessive condition presenting early in adult life and manifesting with weakness and atrophy in the distal leg muscles, predominantly in the posterior compartment. The weakness may eventually affect more proximal muscle groups. This condition is caused by a mutation in the gene encoding dysferlin on chromosome 2p. Dysferlin is also associated with limb girdle muscular dystrophy type 2B. Creatine kinase levels are markedly elevated in the range of 10 to 100 times that of normal. Biopsy shows dystrophic changes.

Scapuloperoneal muscular dystrophy is a disorder presenting with muscular weakness and wasting, affecting the muscles of the neck, shoulders, upper arms, and anterior leg compartment causing foot drop. It may be inherited in an autosomal dominant fashion, but can also be X-linked. It is not the case in this patient.

Nonaka, Markesbery-Griggs, and Welander myopathy are not consistent with this case, and are discussed in question 21.

Cardamone M, Darras BT, Ryan MM. Inherited myopathies and muscular dystrophies. Semin Neurol. 2008; 28:250–259.

Ropper AH, Samuels MA. Adams and Victor's Principles of Neurology, 9th ed. New York: McGraw-Hill; 2009.

27. e

This patient's history and examination are consistent with myasthenia gravis with anti-muscle specific tyrosine kinase (MuSK) antibodies. In approximately half of all patients who are seroneg-ative for antibodies against the acetylcholine receptor, anti-MuSK antibodies are present. In patients with anti-MuSK antibodies, the clinical picture may resemble the typical form of autoim-mune myasthenia gravis or ocular myasthenia, but more commonly, weakness involves pre-dominantly cranial and bulbar muscles, with prominent dysphagia, neck flexor weakness, and respiratory weakness, with relative sparing of ocular muscles (though eyelid and ocular mus-cle involvement may occur). This disorder is more common in young women, and typically does not respond to pyridostigmine. Treatment is with immune-modulating therapy, including intravenous immunoglobulins and plasmapheresis.

Anti-striational muscle antibodies would not be of utility in this case; they are discussed in question 6. Antibodies against the presynaptic calcium channel are seen in Lambert-Eaton syndrome (discussed in questions 43 and 44); features of this syndrome including hyporeflexia, transient improvement of symptoms with sustained contraction, and autonomic features are not present in this case. Anti-Jo 1 antibodies are seen in polymyositis; serum creatine kinase is often elevated, and EMG shows evidence of myopathy (discussed in question 35). Anti-GQ1b antibodies are seen in Miller-Fisher syndrome (discussed in Chapter 9).

Bradley WG, Daroff RB, Fenichel GM, et al. Neurology in Clinical Practice, 5th ed. Philadelphia, PA: Elsevier; 2008.

28. d

Acetylcholine acts at muscarinic M_2-receptors in the heart to reduce heart rate. The main neurotransmitters of the autonomic nervous system include norepinephrine and acetyl-choline, although several neuropeptide neurotransmitters colocalize with these neurotransmit-ters and exert actions that affect autonomic nervous system function as well. Epinephrine is released by the adrenal medulla, and exerts similar actions to norepinephrine at α-receptors. See Table 10.1 for some of the effects of acetylcholine and norepinephrine at various receptors.

Brunton LL. Goodman and Gilman's the Pharmacological Basis of Therapeutics, 11th ed. New York: McGraw-Hill; 2006.

Ropper AH, Samuels MA. Adams and Victor's Principles of Neurology, 9th ed. New York: McGraw-Hill; 2009.

TABLE 10.1	Actions of norepinephrine and acetylcholine at various receptors	
Neurotransmitter	**Receptor**	**Action**
Norepinephrine	α_1-receptors in smooth muscle in blood vessels and the genitourinary and gastrointestinal tract	Vasoconstriction, causing increases in blood pressure and increased tone in sphincter smooth muscles
Norepinephrine	Presynaptic α_2-receptors	Decreased presynaptic release of norepinephrine and other neurotransmitters
Norepinephrine	β_1-receptors in the sinus node of the heart and on blood vessels	Increased heart rate and vasoconstriction
Norepinephrine	β_2-receptors on bronchial smooth muscles and blood vessels	Bronchodilation and vasodilation. Activation of these receptors leads to dilation of skeletal muscle blood vessels in response to sympathetic activation
Acetylcholine	M_1-receptors on autonomic ganglia	Decreased presynaptic release of norepinephrine and acetylcholine
Acetylcholine	M_2-receptors in sinus node of the heart	Reduction in heart rate
Acetylcholine	M_3-receptors in salivary glands	Increase secretions and bronchodilation

29. c

The congenital muscular dystrophies are a group of disorders mostly inherited in an autosomal recessive fashion. In utero, there may be decreased movements. At birth, these children are hypotonic and weak, presenting with arthrogryposis, and may develop respiratory insufficiency and bulbar dysfunction. With time they may develop contractures and scoliosis. These patients also have mental retardation and developmental anomalies of the cerebral cortex. Creatine kinase is markedly elevated. EMG shows myopathic changes. Histopathologically, there are dystrophic changes with degeneration and regeneration of muscle fibers, and infiltration of connective tissue. The congenital muscular dystrophies are caused by genetic defects in sarcolemmal membrane proteins or membrane-supporting structures.

Cardamone M, Darras BT, Ryan MM. Inherited myopathies and muscular dystrophies. Semin Neurol. 2008; 28:250–259.

Ropper AH, Samuels MA. Adams and Victor's Principles of Neurology, 9th ed. New York: McGraw-Hill; 2009.

30. a, 31. c

This patient has Becker muscular dystrophy, which is a milder dystrophinopathy similar to Duchenne muscular dystrophy, but in which the dystrophin protein is not completely absent, but may be structurally abnormal or present in a smaller amount.

Becker muscular dystrophy is an X-linked recessive disorder, which presents with weakness and involvement of the same muscle groups as in Duchenne muscular dystrophy, as well as with pseudohypertrophy of the calves. However, patients with Becker muscular dystrophy present later in life, sometimes in childhood, but more frequently in adolescence or adulthood. Given the milder phenotype, these patients are able to ambulate beyond the second decade of life, cardiac involvement occurs but is less frequent, and intelligence quotient (IQ) is usually normal. Needle

EMG shows fibrillations, positive waves, and polyphasic motor unit potentials. The biopsy will detect similar findings as in Duchenne muscular dystrophy (see questions 19 and 20); however, dystrophin is not absent in Becker muscular dystrophy, but structurally abnormal or present in less amount.

The other options are not likely to be the diagnosis in this case. Duchenne muscular dystrophy is discussed in questions 19 and 20. Emery-Dreifuss muscular dystrophy is discussed in questions 51 and 52. Fascioscapulohumeral muscular dystrophy is discussed in question 9. The myotonic dystrophies are discussed in questions 7 and 12.

Prayson RA, Goldblum JR. Neuropathology, 1st ed. Philadelphia, PA: Elsevier; 2005.

Ropper AH, Samuels MA. Adams and Victor's Principles of Neurology, 9th ed. New York: McGraw-Hill; 2009.

32. a, 33. a

This patient has dermatomyositis. The use of methotrexate should be avoided if patients have interstitial lung disease because this medication can be toxic to the lung.

Dermatomyositis is an inflammatory condition of the muscle associated with skin findings. The muscle weakness is a typical myopathic weakness, predominantly proximal. Therefore, the patient will complain of being unable to stand from the sitting position, inability to walk up stairs, and difficulty lifting the arms above the head. Typical skin findings are the heliotrope rash (purplish discoloration of the eyelids), erythema of the face, neck, anterior chest, upper back, elbows and knees, Gottron's papules (purplish scaly papular rash on the extensor surface of the hands), and "mechanic's hands" (thickened skin on the dorsal and ventral surface of the hands. Serum creatine kinase levels may be normal or elevated. The muscle biopsy specimen shown in Figure 10.3 is characteristic for dermatomyositis, showing atrophic fibers in the borders of the fascicles, which is known as perifascicular atrophy.

Dermatomyositis is associated with malignancy and therefore these patients should have age-appropriate malignancy screening. Dermatomyositis is also associated with interstitial lung disease, especially if anti-Jo antibody is positive; this antibody is a marker of this association.

The initial treatment of choice is steroids; however, long-term steroid-sparing agents may be required, such as azathioprine or methotrexate. As mentioned above, methotrexate may be associated with pulmonary toxicity, and therefore if there is interstitial lung disease, this medication should be avoided.

On the basis of clinical and pathologic findings, this patient does not have polymyositis, inclusion body myositis, mitochondrial myopathy, or muscular dystrophy.

Greenberg SA. Inflammatory myopathies: Evaluation and management. Semin Neurol. 2008; 28:241–249.

Prayson RA, Goldblum JR. Neuropathology, 1st ed. Philadelphia, PA: Elsevier; 2005.

34. e

This patient's history is consistent with pure autonomic failure, also known as Bradbury-Eggleston syndrome, which has been attributed to loss of intermediolateral cell column neurons. It results from deposition of α-synuclein in the autonomic nervous system. Pathologically, Lewy bodies are seen (see Chapter 12). It presents in mid to late adulthood. In men, the earliest symptom is typically impotence. Orthostatic hypotension (defined as a reduction of systolic blood pressure by 20 mm Hg or diastolic blood pressure by 10 mm Hg), or a pulse rate increase of 20 bpm, is present, and is often worse in the morning, after meals, exertion, and with heat exposure. Supine hypertension may occur as well. Other features include hypohidrosis, nocturia, early satiety and nausea (due to gastrointestinal hypomotility), urinary hesitance and/or urgency with occasional incontinence, and neck and shoulder aching ("coat hanger" distribution) precipitated by standing.

In multiple system atrophy (discussed in Chapter 6), dysautonomia is typically more severe and disabling, and extrapyramidal or cerebellar findings are present on examination. Autoimmune autonomic ganglionopathy is discussed in questions 24 and 25. Familial amyloid polyneuropathy type I can lead to autonomic neuropathy (see Chapter 9), but the history and examination (specifically, absence of dissociated sensory loss on examination) make this less likely. This patient is not known to have diabetes, and a normal sensory examination further makes diabetic autonomic neuropathy unlikely.

Bradley WG, Daroff RB, Fenichel GM, et al. Neurology in Clinical Practice, 5th ed. Philadelphia, PA: Elsevier; 2008.

Ropper AH, Samuels MA. Adams and Victor's Principles of Neurology, 9th ed. New York: McGraw-Hill; 2009.

35. d

The muscle biopsy in Figure 10.4 demonstrates an inflammatory infiltrate composed of lymphocytes and macrophages surrounding muscle fibers. There are regenerating and necrotic fibers. These findings are characteristic of polymyositis, and neither rimmed vacuoles nor perifascicular atrophy are seen. Rimmed vacuoles are seen in inclusion body myositis. Perifascicular atrophy is seen in dermatomyositis.

Polymyositis is an inflammatory condition of the muscle in which there are no skin findings. The weakness is proximal, and this condition, similar to dermatomyositis, has been associated with interstitial lung disease, and anti-Jo antibody may be a marker of this association. On the other hand, polymyositis as opposed to dermatomyositis does not have a strong correlation with the presence of malignancy. The initial treatment of choice is steroids; however, in the long term, a steroid-sparing agent such as methotrexate or azathioprine may be required.

Greenberg SA. Inflammatory myopathies: Evaluation and management. Semin Neurol. 2008; 28:241–249.

Prayson RA, Goldblum JR. Neuropathology, 1st ed. Philadelphia, PA: Elsevier; 2005.

36. e

Concomitant use of statins and fibrates increases the risk of muscle toxicity.

Statins are lipid-lowering agents that inhibit the 3-hydroxy-3-methyl-glutaryl-coenzyme A reductase. Statins are known to have muscle toxic effects, and the possible mechanism of this adverse effect is by an action on the mitochondria and sarcoplasmic reticulum, especially in type II muscle fibers. A mutation in the gene *SLCO1B* has been associated with predisposition to develop statin-induced myopathy.

Various types of toxic muscle effects are seen clinically:

–Increased serum creatine kinase (CK) in asymptomatic patients, with mild elevations and rarely up to 10 times the upper limit of normal.
–Myalgia with or without increased serum CK levels. Usually, muscle strength is normal, and myalgias may improve after discontinuation of the medication.
–Muscle weakness with serum CK elevation.
–Rhabdomyolysis. In this condition, the CK levels are markedly elevated, sometimes above 15,000 IU/L (normal up to 220 IU/L). These CK elevations could lead to myoglobinuria and renal failure, such as in this case.

Concomitant use of fibrates can increase the risk of developing muscle toxicity. This risk can also be increased by the use of other drugs, such as azole antifungals, macrolides antibiotics, antiretrovirals, and amiodarone, among others. Therefore a careful assessment of the medications that the patient is taking is important when treating a patient with statins.

Dalakas MC. Toxic and drug-induced myopathies. J Neurol Neurosurg Psychiatry. 2009; 80:832–838.

37. d

This patient's history and tilt table test results are consistent with postural orthostatic tachycardia syndrome (POTS), the most common form of dysautonomia.

Tilt table examination is used to assess changes in heart rate and blood pressure that occur with changes in posture, increased vagal tone (as occurs with valsalva), and sometimes, in response to the administration of pharmacologic agents such as the β-agonist isoproterenol. In POTS, tilt table examination shows an increase in heart rate of at least 30 bpm from baseline, or up to more than 120 bpm within 10 minutes of head-up tilt, without significant changes in blood pressure, but with symptoms of orthostasis such as light-headedness, palpitations, generalized weakness, visual changes, headache, or tremor. The etiology of POTS is unclear; it is more common in females, and symptoms worsen around menses, suggesting a role for estrogen in the pathophysiology. Symptom onset may follow a variety of triggers, including viral infection, pregnancy, or surgery, and for this reason, autoimmune causes have also been postulated. POTS can rarely be a manifestation of a mutation in a norepinephrine transporter gene, which leads to elevated plasma levels of norepinephrine, with subsequent sympathetic overactivity. POTS may be comorbid with chronic fatigue syndrome; the significance of this relationship is not clear. In some patients with POTS, the symptoms are mild and do not require treatment. In others, treatment may include β-blockers, increased fluid and salt intake, fludrocortisone, and midodrine.

There is not a reduction in blood pressure in POTS, distinguishing it from orthostatic hypotension. With vasovagal response, there is no tachycardia but rather transient bradycardia due to parasympathetic overactivation. Systemic mastocytosis, a hematologic disorder in which mast cells are overactive, leading to excessive histamine release, can lead to POTS-like symptoms; skin changes such as flushing and an absence of clear postural component distinguish the two. Subclavian steal syndrome results in syncope in the setting of stenosis of the subclavian artery proximal to the origin of the left vertebral artery. With exercise of the left arm, blood flow steal from the vertebral arteries and basilar artery may occur, resulting in syncope and other symptoms of basilar insufficiency. There is no indication in the case that the syncope followed left arm exercise.

Bradley WG, Daroff RB, Fenichel GM, et al. Neurology in Clinical Practice, 5th ed. Philadelphia, PA: Elsevier; 2008.

Ropper AH, Samuels MA. Adams and Victor's Principles of Neurology, 9th ed. New York: McGraw-Hill; 2009.

38. d

This patient has manifestations suggesting a type of periodic paralysis. Adult-onset periodic paralysis suggests a possible secondary cause, of which thyrotoxic periodic paralysis is the best recognized. Therefore, thyroid-stimulating hormone (TSH) should be obtained, especially given the history of palpitations and possibly anxiety.

Thyrotoxic periodic paralysis is a condition associated with hyperthyroidism, thought to be present in genetically susceptible patients but without a known gene mutation detected to date. It is more common in Asians, with a male predominance. These patients have episodes of proximal weakness and other manifestations of thyrotoxicosis. During acute attacks, potassium should be provided. β-blockers may be of benefit as prophylaxis. Carbonic anhydrase inhibitors do not work.

In this case, the best next step is checking a TSH level. Needle EMG is not specific. Genetic testing is expensive and should only be done when a specific mutation is suspected, and in this case, a thyroid problem should be ruled out first. Referral to psychiatry is not indicated in this case, and as mentioned above, carbonic anhydrase inhibitors do not play a role in thyrotoxic periodic paralysis.

Saperstein DS. Muscle channelopathies. Semin Neurol. 2008; 28:260–269.

39. c, 40. a

This patient has inclusion body myositis, which is a myopathy that affects adults usually older than 50 years. It is characterized by asymmetric weakness and atrophy of the wrist and finger flexors, quadriceps, and anterior tibial muscles. Dysphagia can be present, and there are no skin manifestations. Creatine kinase may only be slightly elevated.

This biopsy specimen shown in Figure 10.5 demonstrates endomysial inflammation, groups of atrophic fibers, and intracytoplasmatic vacuoles with granular material known as rimmed vacuoles, which are characteristic of inclusion body myositis.

This condition does not respond to steroids, and effective therapies are currently not available.

Perifascicular atrophy, Gottron's papules, and "mechanic hands" are seen in dermatomyositis (discussed in questions 32 and 33), but not in inclusion body myositis.

Greenberg SA. Inflammatory myopathies: Evaluation and management. Semin Neurol. 2008; 28:241–249.

Prayson RA, Goldblum JR. Neuropathology, 1st ed. Philadelphia, PA: Elsevier; 2005.

41. a

Cardiac involvement is evident in various types of limb girdle muscular dystrophies (LGMD).

LMGD are a group of muscular dystrophies in which there is proximal weakness with involvement of the shoulder or pelvic girdle with sparing of the facial muscles. It can present in both sexes, and the inheritance is either autosomal dominant or recessive. The mode of inheritance determines the current classification, which has mainly been based on the genetic defects and gene products involved. Regarding classification by inheritance, LGMD1 is autosomal dominant and LGMD 2 is autosomal recessive. Needle EMG shows myopathic changes. Muscle biopsy shows dystrophic changes, with myofiber necrosis, degeneration, regeneration, increased fiber size variation, endomysial inflammation, and fibrosis.

Various types of LGMDs may be associated with cardiomyopathy, and some other types are associated with joint contractures.

Cardamone M, Darras BT, Ryan MM. Inherited myopathies and muscular dystrophies. Semin Neurol. 2008; 28:250–259.

Ropper AH, Samuels MA. Adams and Victor's Principles of Neurology, 9th ed. New York: McGraw-Hill; 2009.

42. d

As mentioned in the discussion to question 41, the limb girdle muscular dystrophies (LGMDs) are a large group of disorders in which patients present with proximal weakness. There is large variability in terms of presentation, and classification of the LGMDs has changed over time. Most recently, they have been classified on the basis of the gene product affected.

There are several types of LGMDs associated with various gene products (Tables 10.2 and 10.3).

TABLE 10.2 Autosomal dominant limb girdle muscular dystrophies (LGMDs)	
LGMD1 (Autosomal Dominant)	**Gene Product or Chromosome**
LGMD1A	Myotilin
LGMD1B	Lamin A/C
LGMD1C	Caveolin-3
LGMD1D	Chromosome 6p
LGMD1E	Chromosome 7q
Bethlem myopathy	Collagen VI

TABLE 10.3 Autosomal recessive limb girdle muscular dystrophies (LGMDs)	
LGMD2 (Autosomal Recessive)	**Gene Product or Chromosome**
LGMD2A	Calpain-3
LGMD2B	Dysferlin
LGMD2C-F	Sarcoglycans
LGMD2G	Telethonin
LGMD2H	E3-ubiquitin ligase
LGMD2I	Fukutin-related protein
LGMD2J	Titin
LGMD2K	Protein-I-mannosyltransferase 1
LGMD2L	Fukutin

Cardamone M, Darras BT, Ryan MM. Inherited myopathies and muscular dystrophies. Semin Neurol. 2008; 28:250–259.

Ropper AH, Samuels MA. Adams and Victor's Principles of Neurology, 9th ed. New York: McGraw-Hill; 2009.

43. b, 44. e

The history and examination of the patient depicted in question 43 are consistent with Lambert-Eaton myasthenic syndrome (LEMS). LEMS is a form of myasthenia. It is a neuromuscular junction (NMJ) disorder resulting from antibodies against presynaptic P/Q-type voltage-gated calcium channel, reducing the influx of calcium that normally leads to release of acetylcholine into the NMJ. It is more common in males. As compared to autoimmune myasthenia gravis, it is less likely to involve ocular or bulbar musculature; it predominantly affects proximal (shoulder and hip girdle) and trunk musculature. Proximal leg weakness is a common clinical presentation of LEMS, and the weakness perceived by the patient may be out of proportion to the examination. While in LEMS, worsening of muscle weakness with repetitive muscle use ultimately occurs, there is a transient improvement of muscle strength following repetitive muscle use prior to worsening weakness. This can sometimes be elicited on physical examination as well as electrophysiologically. Also, unlike myasthenia gravis, in LEMS, deep tendon reflexes are often diminished or absent. Autonomic features are prominent in LEMS, including constipation, urinary retention, and impotence.

LEMS may be either autoimmune or paraneoplastic; paraneoplastic LEMS is most commonly associated with small cell lung cancer. A diagnosis of autoimmune LEMS should be made only after excluding an occult malignancy with an extensive evaluation and after long-term surveillance for malignancy. The SOX antibody has been identified as being a useful marker to distinguish between squamous cell lung cancer–associated paraneoplastic LEMS (in which SOX antibody is present) and autoimmune LEMS.

Unlike myasthenia gravis, patients with LEMS respond little if at all to acetylcholine esterase inhibitors. Symptomatic treatment of LEMS may be achieved with 3,4-diaminopyridine (3,4-DAP), a drug which inhibits presynaptic potassium channels, prolonging depolarization and increasing acetylcholine vesicle exocytosis. Autoimmune LEMS is treated with immunosuppressive therapy, including corticosteroids as well as steroid-sparing agents, intravenous immunoglobulins, and plasmapheresis. Response to these treatments is variable and is typically not as successful as in myasthenia gravis. In paraneoplastic LEMS, treatment of the malignancy may improve the neuromuscular symptoms.

EMG shows low-amplitude CMAPs that increase in amplitude following exercise (as in Figure 10.6, in which there is a >50% increase in CMAP amplitude postexercise). This is a phenomenon known as facilitation. On high-frequency repetitive nerve stimulation, a prominent increment is seen, in contrast to the electrodecrement seen with low-frequency repetitive nerve stimulation in myasthenia gravis (discussed in question 6 and Chapter 9).

The history, examination, normal creatine kinase, and EMG/NCS findings make a myopathy or myositis unlikely. Similarly, a demyelinating polyneuropathy would have been detected on NCS, and facilitation of reflexes with both myopathies and demyelinating polyneuropathy does not occur.

Bradley WG, Daroff RB, Fenichel GM, et al. Neurology in Clinical Practice, 5th ed. Philadelphia, PA: Elsevier; 2008.

Sabater L, Titulaer M, Saiz A, et al. SOX1 antibodies are markers of paraneoplastic Lambert-Eaton myasthenic syndrome. Neurology. 2008; 70:924–928.

45. d

This patient has trichinosis. The patient was previously healthy, now with an acute to subacute onset of symptoms, mildly elevated creatine kinase (CK) and markedly elevated eosinophils, which make the other diagnoses less likely. Furthermore, the muscle biopsy demonstrates the presence of a parasite, confirming the diagnosis of trichinosis.

Trichinosis is caused by the intestinal nematode *Trichinella spiralis*, which is transmitted by the ingestion of uncooked pork containing the encysted larvae. Once ingested, the larvae are liberated from the cysts in the gastrointestinal tract, developing into adult worms in the duodenum or jejunum. The female worms deposit batches of larvae in the intestinal wall, which migrate via lymphatics into the bloodstream. These larvae invade all tissues, but survive only in muscles, where they become encysted and calcify.

Patients develop a mild gastroenteritis on ingestion of infected meat. About 1 week later and sometimes for up to 4 to 6 weeks, patients may experience low-grade fever, myalgias, fatigue, and edema of the conjunctiva and eyelids. Ocular muscle weakness occurs, resulting in strabismus and diplopia. Also, weakness of the tongue and masticatory as well as pharyngeal muscles occurs, which may cause dysarthria and dysphagia. Limb muscle weakness occurs, more prominent proximally. The diaphragm and cardiac muscles may also be involved. Myopathic symptoms eventually subside and patients generally improve completely. However, massive infections have been reported to cause CNS symptoms, including headaches, neck stiffness, and confusion.

Laboratory studies demonstrate eosinophilia and moderate elevations of CK. Enzyme-linked immunosorbent assay blood test for trichinella becomes positive after 1 to 2 weeks and may be helpful. Muscle biopsy, such as in this case, as shown in Figure 10.7, will demonstrate the parasite and sometimes an inflammatory infiltrate with eosinophils.

Treatment includes a combination of thiabendazole with steroids. Thiabendazole is an anti-helminthic that prevents larval reproduction and interferes with the metabolism of the larvae in the muscle. Albendazole is also effective.

Bradley WG, Daroff RB, Fenichel GM, et al. Neurology in Clinical Practice, 5th ed. Philadelphia, PA: Elsevier; 2008.

Ropper AH, Samuels MA. Adams and Victor's Principles of Neurology, 9th ed. New York: McGraw-Hill; 2009.

46. c

Nemaline myopathy has phenotypic variability, with presentations ranging from severe neonatal congenital forms to adult-onset forms in which patients have proximal weakness, cardiomyopathy, and prominent compromise of respiratory muscles. Neonatal forms present with dysmorphic features, contractures, arthrogryposis, generalized hypotonia, feeding difficulties, and respiratory problems. There are other intermediate forms with infantile onset, childhood- and adolescent-onset forms.

This condition is inherited in an autosomal dominant or recessive fashion, and the genes implicated include α-actin, α-tropomyosin, and β-tropomyosin, nebulin, troponin, and cofilin. Histopathologically, the fibers have rod-like structures that are seen beneath the sarcolemma, also known as nemaline bodies or nemaline rods. Type I fibers are smaller than normal and predominate.

Cardamone M, Darras BT, Ryan MM. Inherited myopathies and muscular dystrophies. Semin Neurol. 2008; 28:250–259.

Ropper AH, Samuels MA. Adams and Victor's Principles of Neurology, 9th ed. New York: McGraw-Hill; 2009.

47. b

Normally, with assumption of an upright posture, there is a transient reduction in blood pressure that is soon counteracted by an increase in heart rate mediated by inhibition of the parasympathetic nervous system and activation of the sympathetic nervous system. Splanchnic, renal, and skeletal muscle blood vessels vasoconstrict. The increase in heart rate is maximal at the 15th beat and a mild reflex bradycardia is noted at the 30th beat. In moderate or severe autonomic neuropathy, the compensatory increase in heart rate does not occur.

Upright tilt table evaluation is used to obtain objective measures of blood pressure and heart rate in various postures. In normal individuals, during the tilt table test, at 60 to 80 degrees of tilting for 10 minutes, there is a brief 5 to 15 mm Hg reduction in systolic blood pressure, a 5 to 10 mm Hg increase in diastolic blood pressure, and a 10 to 15 bpm increase in heart rate. If there is early, gradual, and sustained hypotension (>20 mm Hg reduction in systolic blood pressure) without compensatory tachycardia, this is an indication of insufficient sympathetic tone and impaired baroreceptor function. Hypotension with compensatory tachycardia suggests hypovolemia. If hypotension is delayed for several minutes but then occurs abruptly with bradycardia, this is more suggestive of a neurocardiogenic mechanism. Most neurogenic causes of syncope lead to gradual hypotension without a compensatory tachycardia that occurs within the first 5 to 10 minutes of tilting.

The thermoregulatory sweat test is a test of sudomotor function; it is a qualitative test of sweating in which an indicator powder is applied to the subject who is then exposed to elevated temperatures. Sweat interacts with the powder, indicating areas of normal sweating and identifying areas of absent or reduced sweating. Different patterns of anhidrosis can be identified that correspond to different autonomic disorders. In large and small fiber neuropathies, distal anhidrosis occurs. In patients with multiple system atrophy (see Chapter 6), pure autonomic failure (discussed in question 34), and autonomic neuropathies, global hypohidrosis or anhidrosis occurs.

The quantitative sudomotor axon reflex test is another test of sudomotor function. A sweat cell is applied to the skin and an electric current is then applied. Acetylcholine is iontophoresed into the skin, stimulating sweat glands. Sweat production is measured from adjacent sweat glands that are stimulated via an axon reflex. If there is a low or absent response following application of the electric current, this indicates a lesion of the postganglionic sympathetic axon.

Bolis CL, Licinio J, Govoni S. Handbook of the Autonomic Nervous System in Health and Disease, New York: Marcel Dekker; 2003.

Bradley WG, Daroff RB, Fenichel GM, et al. Neurology in Clinical Practice, 5th ed. Philadelphia, PA: Elsevier; 2008.

Ropper AH, Samuels MA. Adams and Victor's Principles of Neurology, 9th ed. New York: McGraw-Hill; 2009.

48. c, 49. b

These patients have glycogenosis type II or acid maltase deficiency.

Glycogenosis type II or acid maltase deficiency is an autosomal recessive condition caused by deficiency of acid maltase (also known as α-1,4-glucosidase) in lysosomes. This enzyme participates in the breakdown of glycogen to glucose; its deficiency leads to glycogen accumulation, causing the typical histopathologic findings on muscle biopsy, demonstrating vacuolated sarcoplasm with glycogen accumulation that stains strongly with acid phosphatase.

There are three forms of acid maltase deficiency:

1. Pompe's disease is the infantile form that presents in the first few months of life with difficulty feeding, cyanosis, dyspnea, macroglossia, hepatomegaly, cardiomegaly, and hypotonic weakness. This form progresses rapidly and patients die in the first few months.
2. Childhood form, which has an onset in the second year of life, manifests with proximal weakness, motor developmental delay, hypotonia, enlarged calves, and rarely with cardiomegaly, hepatomegaly, and mental retardation. These patients may die of pulmonary infections and respiratory failure.
3. Adult form, which presents in the second to fourth decades of life, manifests with slowly progressive proximal weakness and typically weakness of the diaphragm, leading to

neuromuscular respiratory problems. These patients do not typically have cardiomegaly, hepatomegaly, or mental retardation.

Glycogenosis type V is McArdle's disease. Glycogenosis type III is Cori's disease. Both are discussed in question 14.

Ropper AH, Samuels MA. Adams and Victor's Principles of Neurology, 9th ed. New York: McGraw-Hill; 2009.

50. c

This patient's history and examination are consistent with congenital myasthenia due to congenital acetylcholine receptor deficiency, a congenital myasthenic syndrome. The congenital myasthenic syndromes are a genetically heterogeneous group of neuromuscular junction disorders. They most commonly present at birth, but some forms do not present until childhood or early adulthood. They are more common in males. The typical presentation is one of ophthalmoparesis and ptosis in infancy, with facial diparesis. Limb weakness and hypotonia are often present, and respiratory involvement is rare but can occur. As in autoimmune myasthenia gravis, edrophonium injection transiently improves symptoms in congenital myasthenia, and there is symptomatic benefit from acetylcholine esterase inhibitors. Because the congenital myasthenic syndromes are not immune-mediated, there is no response to immunosuppressive therapy or thymectomy. Electrophysiologic findings are similar to other neuromuscular disorders, showing a decremental response on repetitive nerve stimulation studies and increased jitter on single-fiber EMG. The most common form of congenital myasthenia, congenital acetylcholine receptor deficiency, is due to an autosomal recessive or sporadic mutation in the acetylcholine receptor gene.

Choline acetyltransferase deficiency is another congenital myasthenia syndrome that differs from other congenital myasthenic syndromes in that extraocular muscle involvement is not prominent, and the clinical presentation is more typically generalized hypotonia, apneas, and feeding difficulties. Slow-channel congenital myasthenic syndrome is a rare congenital myasthenia syndrome that is autosomal dominant in inheritance and results from abnormally prolonged opening of the acetylcholine channel at the postsynaptic membrane.

In newborns of mothers with autoimmune myasthenia gravis, transient myasthenic symptoms can occur due to transfer of maternal antibodies to the fetus in utero. Signs of neonatal myasthenia include hypotonia and poor feeding, with symptoms improving typically within the first 2 weeks of life. This patient's symptoms were present at 6 months of age, and absence of evidence of a neuromuscular disorder in the patient's mother makes this less likely.

Other disorders that can lead to ophthalmoparesis, ptosis, and generalized weakness in infancy include mitochondrial disorders, botulism, and congenital myopathies, but the presence of fluctuating weakness and response to edrophonium distinguish congenital myasthenia from these.

Bradley WG, Daroff RB, Fenichel GM, et al. Neurology in Clinical Practice, 5th ed. Philadelphia, PA: Elsevier; 2008.

Ropper AH, Samuels MA. Adams and Victor's Principles of Neurology, 9th ed. New York: McGraw-Hill; 2009.

51. c, 52. d

This patient has Emery-Dreifuss muscular dystrophy. This condition is inherited in an X-linked fashion. The defect is in the gene encoding for the nuclear membrane protein emerin. There is an autosomal dominant form in which the gene affected, *LMNA*, encodes for the nuclear membrane protein laminin A/C.

Patients with Emery-Dreiffuss muscular dystrophy characteristically present with contractures, which can be seen at the elbows, ankles, and neck. Muscle weakness tends to affect the upper arms and shoulder girdle muscles first and later the pelvic girdle and distal leg muscles. There is no pseudohypertrophy of the calves, and intelligence quotient (IQ) is normal. Cardiac involvement is prominent, with serious conduction abnormalities, often requiring pacemaker placement.

Duchenne muscular dystrophy is discussed in questions 19 and 20. Becker muscular dystrophy is discussed in questions 30 and 31. Fascioscapulohumeral muscular dystrophy is discussed in question 9. Limb-girdle muscular dystrophy is discussed in questions 41 and 42.

Cardamone M, Darras BT, Ryan MM. Inherited myopathies and muscular dystrophies. Semin Neurol. 2008; 28:250–259.

Ropper AH, Samuels MA. Adams and Victor's Principles of Neurology, 9th ed. New York: McGraw-Hill; 2009.

53. e

This patient has Ullrich's congenital muscular dystrophy, which presents with neonatal weakness, contractures and distal hyperlaxity, as well as protrusion of the calcanei. It is associated with mutations of collagen type VI and is thought to be related to Bethlem myopathy.

Walker-Marburg syndrome is an autosomal recessive condition characterized by muscular dystrophy and brain and ocular abnormalities. Patients are hypotonic at birth with elevated creatine kinase levels. The ocular malformations include microphthalmia, colobomas, cataracts, glaucoma, corneal opacity, retinal dysplasia, and optic atrophy. There are multiple brain CNS malformations including hydrocephalus, aqueductal stenosis, cerebellar hypoplasia, and cortical abnormalities.

Muscle-eye-brain disease is an autosomal recessive condition in which there is also muscular dystrophy and brain and ocular abnormalities; however, the cortical changes are milder and the white matter changes are more focal. The eyes are also affected to a lesser degree than Walker-Marburg syndrome.

Fukuyama-type congenital muscular dystrophy and laminin-α-2 deficiency are discussed in question 8.

Bradley WG, Daroff RB, Fenichel GM, et al. Neurology in Clinical Practice, 5th ed. Philadelphia, PA: Elsevier; 2008.

Cardamone M, Darras BT, Ryan MM. Inherited myopathies and muscular dystrophies. Semin Neurol. 2008; 28:250–259.

Ropper AH, Samuels MA. Adams and Victor's Principles of Neurology, 9th ed. New York: McGraw-Hill; 2009.

54. e

The parasympathetic nervous system can be divided into cranial and sacral portions (Figure 10.8). The cranial portion includes fibers that originate in brain stem nuclei and are relayed to their target sites via four cranial nerves: (1) oculomotor, (2) facial, (3) glossopharyngeal, and (4) vagus. In the parasympathetic nervous system, the ganglia are located close to the target site, with long preganglionic fibers and short postganglionic fibers. Cells located in S2 to S4 of the spinal cord give rise to the sacral portion of the parasympathetic nervous system and innervate the genitourinary system and distal colon. The neurotransmitter for all sympathetic and parasympathetic preganglionic fibers is acetylcholine that acts at nicotinic receptors in

PARASYMPATHETIC DIVISION   SYMPATHETIC DIVISION

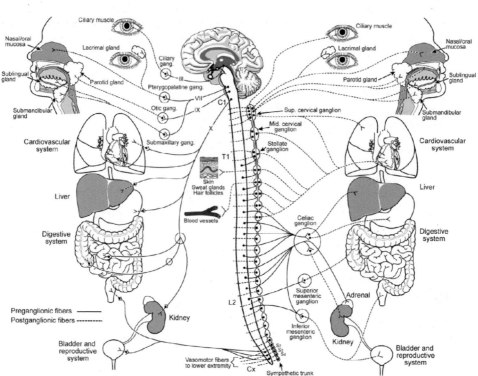

FIGURE 10.8   The autonomic nervous system (Illustration by David Schumick, BS, CMI. Reprinted with permission of the Cleveland Clinic Center for Medical Art & Photography. © 2010. All Rights Reserved)

the ganglia. Parasympathetic postganglionic neurons predominantly release acetylcholine. The parasympathetic nervous system leads to vasodilation, bradycardia, production of bronchial secretions, gastric acid production, lacrimation, salivation, pupillary constriction, and erection.

The intermediolateral cell column of the spinal cord, present from T1 to L2, contains the preganglionic neurons of the sympathetic nervous system. Small myelinated fibers known as white rami communicantes exit the intermediolateral cell column and synapse on sympathetic ganglia located in the paravertebral region. Postganglionic fibers known as gray rami communicantes are carried through spinal nerves T1 to T4 to supply thoracic regions and T5 to L2 to supply various subdiaphragmatic end organs including blood vessels, gastrointestinal organs, and genitourinary tract (Figure 10.8; sympathetic innervation to the head is carried by C8-T2, see questions 55 and 56 and Figure 10.9). The neurotransmitter released from postganglionic sympathetic fibers is norepinephrine, except in sweat glands, where acetylcholine is released and acts at muscarinic receptors. In the sympathetic nervous system, preganglionic fibers are short and postganglionic fibers are long (Figure 10.8).

Blumenfield H. Neuroanatomy through Clinical Cases. Sunderland, MA: Sinauer; 2002.

Ropper AH, Samuels MA. Adams and Victor's Principles of Neurology, 9th ed. New York: McGraw-Hill; 2009.

55. e, 56. d

Horner's syndrome results from a lesion in the sympathetic pathways (Figure 10.9; see also Figure 1.6). The sympathetic tracts originate in the hypothalamus and descend in the lateral brain stem to synapse with sympathetic neurons in the intermediolateral cell column in the spinal cord that is present from T1 to L2.

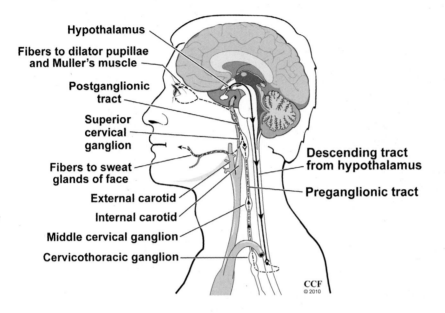

FIGURE 10.9   Cranial sympathetic innervation (Illustration by David Schumick, BS, CMI. Reprinted with permission of the Cleveland Clinic Center for Medical Art & Photography. © 2010. All Rights Reserved)

The face receives sympathetic innervation from intermediolateral cells at the C8 to T2 level. Preganglionic fibers synapse in the superior cervical ganglion. Postganglionic fibers travel along the common carotid artery. At the carotid bifurcation, fibers to the sphincter pupillae of the eye travel with the ICA, and are involved in pupillary dilation. Fibers to Muller's smooth muscles in the upper eyelid are also carried along this route. Sympathetic fibers destined for the eccrine glands of the face travel along the ECA.

Horner's syndrome, or oculosympathetic paresis, results from a lesion to the sympathetic pathways. Features include ptosis, due to loss of innervation of Muller's smooth muscle, miosis, due to loss of innervation of the pupillary dilator muscle, apparent enophthalmos, due to lack of input to the lid retractors (the eye appears sunken, though it is not), and loss of ciliospinal reflex (absence of pupillary constriction when painful stimulation is applied to the cervical region ipsilateral to the lesion). In preganglionic lesions, such as those occurring from medullary infarction, during thoracotomy, or with large lung masses that impinge on the preganglionic fibers as they course toward the superior cervical ganglion, facial anhidrosis occurs as well. Lesions in the area of the ICA spare the fibers destined for the eccrine glands of the face, and anhidrosis does not occur.

The patient in question 55 has a Horner's syndrome, and in the setting of chronic cough and the findings on examination, this suggests that this is due to an apical lung mass, or Pancoast tumor. The presence of anhidrosis makes an ICA dissection unlikely because fibers to facial sweat glands travel along the ECA (Figure 10.9). The patient in question 56 has an ICA dissection, and because the lesion is distal to branching of the sweat fibers to the face (which are, again, carried along the ECA), anhidrosis will not occur (see also Chapter 1 for further information on how lesions in different areas of the sympathetic pathways can be distinguished).

The ptosis and pupillary abnormalities seen in Horner's syndrome can be distinguished from a third nerve palsy by the presence of intact extraocular movements of cranial nerve III-innervated muscles (medial rectus, inferior oblique, superior rectus, and inferior rectus). In addition, with loss of sympathetic innervation to the pupil, the anisocoria will be more prominent in dim light, as the contralateral (normal) eye will normally dilate, whereas the eye that has lost sympathetic innervation will remain miotic. The miotic eye will still normally constrict to light and accommodation (because parasympathetics are not impaired). Levator dehiscence is a common cause of ptosis in older adults, but pupillary involvement and the other features of Horner's syndrome do not occur.

Blumenfeld H. Neuroanatomy through Clinical Cases. Sunderland, MA: Sinauer; 2002.

Bradley WG, Daroff RB, Fenichel GM, et al. Neurology in Clinical Practice, 5th ed. Philadelphia, PA: Elsevier; 2008.

57. a

Dystrophic myotonia type 2 myotonic dystrophy is a proximal myopathy and is also known as PROMM or proximal myotonic myopathy.

The distal myopathies are a group of disorders that are slowly progressive and with onset most commonly in adult life, though earlier presentations may occur. There are weakness and atrophy of the muscles of the hands, forearms, and lower legs. Some are autosomal dominant and others are autosomal recessive, each caused by mutations in different genes.

The distal myopathies are shown in Tables 10.4 and 10.5, including the mode of inheritance, age of presentation, as well as gene product affected (if known).

TABLE 10.4 Autosomal recessive distal myopathies

Myopathy	Onset	Gene
Miyoshi	Early adulthood	Dysferlin
Nonaka (myopathy with rimmed vacuoles)	Early adulthood	GND kinase—epimerase

TABLE 10.5 Autosomal dominant distal myopathies

Myopathy	Onset	Gene
Welander	Late adulthood	Unknown
Tibial muscular dystrophy	Late adulthood	Titin
Scapuloperoneal muscular dystrophy	Childhood-adulthood	Unknown
Desmin myopathy	Early adulthood	Desmin
Gower-Laing	Early adulthood	MYHC-1 (*MYH7*)
Markesbery-Griggs	Late adulthood	ZASP

Cardamone M, Darras BT, Ryan MM. Inherited myopathies and muscular dystrophies. Semin Neurol. 2008; 28:250–259.

Ropper AH, Samuels MA. Adams and Victor's Principles of Neurology, 9th ed. New York: McGraw-Hill; 2009.

58. e, 59. e, 60. c

Penile erection is mediated by the parasympathetic nervous system and ejaculation by the sympathetic nervous system. In detrusor-sphincter dyssynergia, the detrusor muscle contracts against an unrelaxed urethral sphincter. The internal urethral sphincter is under sympathetic control.

Micturition (urination) has both voluntary and involuntary components. Voluntary contraction of the external urethral sphincter is mediated by sympathetic innervation derived from the intermediolateral cell column in the spinal cord at the level of L1 and L2 (Figure 10.8). The detrusor muscle is under involuntary control by the parasympathetic nervous system. The pontine micturition center regulates the detrusor reflex. Nerve roots S2 to S4 relay afferent sensory information from the genitourinary system, bladder, and anorectal area to the spinal cord. Somatic efferents to the skeletal muscles of the pelvic floor arise from the anterior horn cells at S2 to S4 and are carried by the pudendal nerves.

Normally, individuals are able to maintain voluntary control over micturition through the medial frontal micturition centers located in the paracentral lobules (the medial continuation of the precentral gyrus). At the initiation of voluntary micturition, the detrusor reflex, which is mediated by spinal cord circuits, is initiated by voluntary external urethral sphincter relaxation and involuntary relaxation of the internal urethral sphincter with detrusor contraction. If the external urethral sphincter is voluntarily contracted during micturition, the detrusor muscle involuntarily relaxes and micturition stops.

Urinary incontinence can result from lesions along various areas of the neuraxis. With lesions of the cauda equina (discussed in Chapter 11), a flaccid bladder results from loss of detrusor tone, sensation of bladder fullness is lost, and voluntary control over urination is lost. Overflow incontinence may occur; these patients often require intermittent self-catheterization chronically. With lesions affecting the paracentral lobule, such as hydrocephalus or tumors, voluntary control over the external urethral sphincter is lost. Lesions above the conus medullaris lead initially to a flaccid bladder leading to urinary retention with or without overflow incontinence. Some time after a spinal cord lesion, the bladder may become hyperreflexic. Urge incontinence results from overactive detrusor contraction; this is a frequent occurrence in patients with multiple sclerosis, though flaccid bladder with requirements for intermittent catheterization can also occur.

Penile erection is mediated by parasympathetic fibers derived from S3 and S4 and carried by the pudendal nerve. Ejaculation is a sympathetically mediated reflex arc: the afferent pathway is via the dorsal nerve of the penis and pudendal nerve to S3 and S4, and the efferent pathway includes the perineal branch of the pudendal nerve.

Blumenfield H. Neuroanatomy through Clinical Cases. Sunderland, MA: Sinauer; 2002.

Bradley WG, Daroff RB, Fenichel GM, et al. Neurology in Clinical Practice, 5th ed. Philadelphia, PA: Elsevier; 2008.

61. d

Hirschsprung's disease is due to congenital absence of the myenteric plexus. The enteric nervous system consists of the myenteric (or Auerbach's) plexus that is located between the outer and inner smooth muscle layers of the gastrointestinal tract and the submucous (or Meissner's) plexus, which is located between the circular muscle layer and the mucosa. The myenteric plexus is predominantly involved in gut motility, whereas the submucous plexus is involved in secretory functions. Together, the myenteric and submucous plexus control the function of the gastrointestinal tract.

Hirschsprung's disease is due to maldevelopment of the myenteric plexus. Most commonly, focal congenital absence of the myenteric plexus in the internal anal sphincter or rectosigmoid junction occurs, though in rare cases, the myenteric plexus may be absent throughout the gastrointestinal system. Segments of the colon that lack myenteric plexus cannot relax, leading to fecal retention and distention of proximal colonic segments. Some cases of Hirschsprung's disease are due to mutations in the *RET* proto-oncogene.

Kandel ER, Schwartz JH, Jessel TM. Principles of Neural Science, 4th ed. New York: McGraw-Hill; 2000.

Ropper AH, Samuels MA. Adams and Victor's Principles of Neurology, 9th ed. New York: McGraw-Hill; 2009.

62. C

Cardiac involvement is present in about 25% of the patients with myofibrillar myopathy.

Myofibrillar myopathy is a congenital muscular dystrophy, which may be autosomal dominant or recessive, and affects males and females equally. It is characterized by slowly progressive weakness of the muscles of the limbs and trunk, affecting both proximal and distal muscles, but more the lower than the upper extremities. Cardiac involvement with conduction abnormalities is present in about 25% of the cases, and peripheral neuropathy can also be seen. Hyporeflexia is frequent.

Causative mutations involve the proteins myotilin, desmin, and $\alpha\beta$-crystallin. Pathologically, there is focal dissolution of myofibrils and subsarcolemmal accumulation of dense granular and filamentous material, variation of fiber sizes, rimmed vacuoles, and central nucleation.

Cardamone M, Darras BT, Ryan MM. Inherited myopathies and muscular dystrophies. Semin Neurol. 2008; 28:250–259.

Ropper AH, Samuels MA. Adams and Victor's Principles of Neurology, 9th ed. New York: McGraw-Hill; 2009.

63. C

This patient has myotonia congenita, more specifically Thomsen's disease.

There are two types of myotonia congenita: Thomsen's disease, which is autosomal dominant, and Becker's disease, which is autosomal recessive. This group of disorders is caused by a channelopathy secondary to a mutation in the chloride channel gene *CLCN1* on chromosome 7q. The main manifestation is myotonia, which is an impaired muscle relaxation as seen when the patients cannot relax their handgrip after grasping an object, and also manifested on percussion, leading to contraction and delayed relaxation. Myotonic potentials can be detected on EMG.

In myotonia congenita, as opposed to paramyotonia, there is a "warm-up" phenomenon, in which the myotonia improves after repetitive muscle activation.

Thomsen's disease, as mentioned above, is autosomal dominant and begins in the first decade of life manifesting with painless myotonia, but not weakness, and is milder than the recessive form. Becker's disease is the recessive form that presents later, usually in the second decade of life, is more severe than the dominant form, and may manifest with weakness after severe episodes of myotonia. Propofol and depolarizing neuromuscular blocking agents may aggravate the myotonia, and patients may have prolonged recovery. Mexiletine is the treatment of choice.

Paramyotonia congenita is discussed in question 17. Hyperkalemic and hypokalemic periodic paralysis are discussed in question 1.

Saperstein DS. Muscle channelopathies. Semin Neurol. 2008; 28:260–269.

64. b

This patient has critical illness myopathy (CIM) without polyneuropathy. CIM can occur independently or in combination with critical illness polyneuropathy (CIPN). The typical presentation is a flaccid weakness, which is diffuse and involves not only limb muscles but also the diaphragm, making these patients difficult to wean from mechanical ventilation. CIM occurs in severely ill patients, usually with systemic inflammatory response syndrome, and with risk factors including hyperglycemia, hypoalbuminemia, sepsis, exposure to steroids, neuromuscular-blocking agents, and certain antibiotics. Electrophysiologic studies show SNAP greater than 80% of the lower limit of normal and low-amplitude CMAPs, as well as myopathic findings on needle EMG. Pathologically, there is type II fiber atrophy and characteristic loss of thick myosin filaments.

CIPN presents in patients with similar risk factors as described above for CIM, and is characterized by the presence of axonal degeneration of motor and sensory fibers, as detected electrophysiologically by low SNAPs and CMAPs. Needle EMG may demonstrate neurogenic changes.

The management of these conditions begins with the treatment of the underlying cause and avoidance of risk factors. Adequate nutrition, physical therapy, and rehabilitation are necessary. Even though CIPN and CIM can occur independently, they are frequently seen together in critically ill patients. Because muscle regeneration is much faster than nerve regeneration, CIM improves earlier.

Bolton CF. Neuromuscular manifestations of critical illness. Muscle Nerve. 2005; 32:140–163.

65. c

This patient has Bethlem myopathy, which is an autosomal dominant condition associated with mutations affecting the gene encoding collagen type VI. These patients present with weakness and contractures of the elbow and ankles, as well as hyperextensible interphalangeal joints.

Walker-Marburg syndrome and muscle-eye-brain disease are discussed in question 53. Fukuyama-type congenital muscular dystrophy and laminin-α-2 deficiency are discussed in question 8.

Bradley WG, Daroff RB, Fenichel GM, et al. Neurology in Clinical Practice, 5th ed. Philadelphia, PA: Elsevier; 2008.

Cardamone M, Darras BT, Ryan MM. Inherited myopathies and muscular dystrophies. Semin Neurol. 2008; 28:250–259.

Ropper AH, Samuels MA. Adams and Victor's Principles of Neurology, 9th ed. New York: McGraw-Hill; 2009.

Buzz Phrases	Key Points
Acute onset of dysautonomia in a smoker with a lung mass	Paraneoplastic autonomic ganglionopathy, antibody against ganglionic nicotinic acetylcholine receptor
Horner's syndrome with intact facial sweating	Lesion distal to carotid bifurcation (as sweat fibers travel along external carotid)
Duchenne muscular dystrophy (protein, inheritance)	Absent dystrophin, X-linked recessive
Throat, tongue, ear pain associated with syncope	Glossopharyngeal neuralgia
Tilt table test showing increase in heart rate of at least 30 bpm from baseline, or up to more than 120 bpm within 10 minutes of head up tilt, without significant changes in blood pressure, but with symptoms of orthostasis	Postural orthostatic tachycardia syndrome, the most common form of dysautonomia
Emery-Dreifuss (gene, inheritance)	*LMNA*, autosomal dominant
Central core myopathy (gene, pathologic finding, clinical association)	*RYR1* / Central pale cores in NADH stains from absence of mitochondria / Associated with malignant hyperthermia
Tarui disease (enzyme)	Phosphofructokinase deficiency
Cause of Hirschsprung's disease	Maldevelopment of the myenteric plexus, sometimes due to *RET* proto-oncogene mutation
Becker's muscular dystrophy (protein, inheritance)	Abnormal or reduced dystrophin, X-linked recessive
Cori's disease (enzyme)	Debranching enzyme deficiency
Syncope with hypotension and bradycardia after putting on a tight neck tie	Carotid sinus hypersensitivity
Anti–muscle-specific tyrosine kinase antibodies	50% of seronegative myasthenics, predominantly involving swallowing, neck flexors
McArdle's disease (enzyme)	Myophosphorylase deficiency
Dermatomyositis (pathologic findings)	Perifascicular atrophy
Myotonic dystrophy DM1 (gene affected)	CTG repeat, *DMPK* gene
Presynaptic P/Q-type voltage-gated calcium channel antibodies	Lambert-Eaton myasthenic syndrome
Pompe's disease (enzyme)	Acid maltase deficiency
Emery-Dreifuss (protein, inheritance)	Emerin, X-linked
Oculopharyngeal dystrophy (gene affected)	GCG repeat, *PABP2* gene
Myotonic dystrophy DM2 (gene affected)	CCTG repeat, zinc finger protein gene
Inclusion body myositis (pathologic findings)	Rimmed vacuoles
Critical illness myopathy (pathologic finding)	Myosin loss
Andersen's disease (enzyme)	Branching enzyme deficiency

Chapter 11

Neuromuscular III
(Disorders of the Spinal Cord and Motor Neurons)

Questions

Questions 1–2

1. A 52-year-old man presents with a 6 month history of progressive weakness. He first noticed difficulty with fine motor coordination of the right hand, but this later progressed to involve the right arm and later all extremities. On examination, he has dysarthria and reduced gag reflex. There is generalized motor weakness and atrophy. Deep tendon reflexes are hyperactive in both upper and lower extremities. Sustained ankle clonus is present. Fasciculations are seen in the tongue, across the chest, and in all limbs proximally. Sensory examination is normal. There is no family history of neurologic disorders. What is the most likely diagnosis in this patient?
   a. Progressive muscular atrophy
   b. Amyotrophic lateral sclerosis
   c. Primary lateral sclerosis
   d. Adult-onset spinal muscular atrophy
   e. Kennedy's disease (X-linked spinobulbar muscular atrophy)

2. Which of the following statements is correct regarding the disorder depicted in question 1?
   a. Dysphagia and dysarthria are rare as presenting features and do not typically occur as the disease progresses
   b. Acute respiratory failure is a common initial presentation
   c. Urinary incontinence and impotence occur early
   d. Cognitive dysfunction is present in many patients with this disorder
   e. Pseudobulbar affect (pathologic laughter and crying) is not a feature of this disorder, and its presence should prompt evaluation for other causes

3. A 16-year-old boy presents with progressive bilateral lower extremity numbness and weakness, with difficulty walking for the past 2 months. He reports worsening over the past 5 days, and this morning when he woke up he was unable to move his legs and felt numb from his upper chest down. His examination shows mild weakness and areflexia in both upper extremities, and

significant weakness with spasticity and hyperreflexia in the lower extremities. He has a sensory level at T2. His MRI is shown in Figure 11.1. Which of the following is the most likely diagnosis?

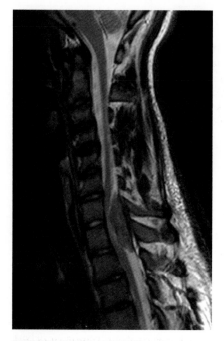

FIGURE 11.1   Sagittal STIR MRI

   a. Acute transverse myelitis
   b. Spinal cord infarct
   c. Cord compression from a metastatic tumor
   d. Epidural hematoma
   e. Meningioma with spinal cord compression

4. Which of the following statements is incorrect regarding the management of amyotrophic lateral sclerosis (ALS)?
   a. Periodic assessment of lung function is indicated in patients with ALS
   b. There is evidence to suggest that management of patients with ALS in multidisciplinary clinics is beneficial
   c. Riluzole is an inhibitor of glutamate release that modestly slows disease progression
   d. Frequent evaluation of swallowing function is important as patients with ALS are at increased risk of aspiration
   e. Parotid and submandibular botulinum toxin injections are ineffective in patients with ALS with refractory sialorrhea

5. A patient with a chronic progressive myelopathy presents for evaluation. You suspect vitamin B_{12} deficiency. Regarding this condition, which of the following is incorrect?
   a. Vitamin B_{12} levels may be within normal limits despite clinical manifestations of deficiency
   b. Elevated gastrin levels, anti-intrinsic factor antibodies, and anti-parietal cell antibodies may be associated with vitamin B_{12} deficiency

c. It can cause white matter vacuolization

d. Serum vitamin B_{12} level is the only laboratory test that needs to be followed when treating these patients

e. The most common cause of vitamin B_{12} deficiency is malabsorption

6. A 52-year-old woman from Ohio who has not traveled outside of the state her entire life presents with gait difficulties of 2 years' duration. There is no family history of a similar problem. On examination, she has significant lower extremity spasticity, with a scissoring gait. There is bilateral ankle clonus, Babinski signs are present bilaterally, and deep tendon reflexes are pathologically brisk throughout, especially at the knees and ankles. There are no fasciculations. Sensory examination is normal. MRI of the brain and spine are normal. What is the most likely diagnosis in this patient?

   a. Tropical spastic paraparesis
   b. Amyotrophic lateral sclerosis
   c. Hereditary spastic paraparesis
   d. Primary lateral sclerosis
   e. Cervical spondylosis

7. A 52-year-old man who is an intravenous drug user, HIV seropositive with a CD4 count of 120 and noncompliant with antiretrovirals, develops progressive neurologic symptoms over several months, including ataxia, spastic paraparesis, and sensory loss below his waist. After you examine him you suspect that he has a myelopathy. Which of the following is correct regarding HIV-related myelopathy?

   a. Copper deficiency is the most important factor for the development of this type of myelopathy
   b. Vitamin B_{12} deficiency is the most important cause of this type of myelopathy
   c. Pathologic analysis of the spinal cord shows lateral and posterior column demyelination with microvacuolar changes
   d. Pathologic analysis of the spinal cord shows axonal degeneration as the hallmark finding
   e. HTLV-1 is the most common etiology associated with this type of myelopathy

8. A 30-year-old man presents for evaluation of gradually progressive lower extremity spasticity, which has worsened slowly over the past 5 years. On examination he has spasticity of the lower extremities, with no evidence of lower motor neuron findings and no other neurologic abnormalities. He says that his father had a similar problem, and his younger brother is starting to have difficulty walking. Work-up has been negative, including an MRI of the brain and cervicothoracic spine that was unremarkable, normal vitamin B_{12} and copper levels, normal CSF studies for infectious and inflammatory conditions, negative HIV and HTLV-1 serologies, and nonreactive VDRL. Which of the following is the most likely diagnosis?

   a. Hirayama disease
   b. Hereditary spastic paraparesis
   c. Amyotrophic lateral sclerosis
   d. Progressive muscular atrophy
   e. Multiple sclerosis

9. A 78-year-old man who has a history of diabetes and hypertension presents in septic shock with a blood pressure of 60/40 mm Hg. He is admitted to the ICU, where antibiotics and pressors are started. Over the next few days he improves; however, it is noticed that he cannot move his legs, and has a sensory level approximately at T6. His MRI of the spine shows a midthoracic spinal cord T2 hyperintensity. The most common mechanism for this patient's condition is:

    a. Infarct in the territory of the artery of Adamkiewicz
    b. Watershed infarct
    c. Epidural abscess
    d. Aortic dissection
    e. Epidural hematoma

10. A 45-year-old woman presents with bilateral upper extremity weakness of 3 years' duration. She
    began experiencing weakness of finger flexors and extensors in the right hand 2 years earlier,
    with similar weakness later occurring in the left hand. Over the prior year, the weakness had
    progressed and she could no longer abduct her arms beyond 30 degrees or fully flex or extend
    her forearms. Physical examination revealed significant atrophy of proximal upper extremity
    muscles, occasional fasciculations in the deltoids and biceps bilaterally, diminished tone in the
    arms, and Medical Research Council 2/5 strength in most muscle groups of the upper extremities.
    Left hip flexors were 4/5; otherwise motor power in the lower extremities was 5/5. Legs had
    normal tone, no ankle clonus, and absent Babinski sign bilaterally. Deep tendon reflexes could not
    be elicited in the upper extremities and were 1+ in the lower extremities. EMG showed evidence
    of widespread motor neuron dysfunction. What is the most likely diagnosis in this patient?
    a. Progressive muscular atrophy
    b. Amyotrophic lateral sclerosis
    c. Postpolio syndrome
    d. Adult-onset spinal muscular atrophy
    e. Inclusion body myositis

11. Regarding the vascular supply of the spinal cord, which of the following is incorrect?
    a. There is one anterior spinal artery that supplies the anterior two-thirds of the spinal cord
    b. There is one posterior spinal artery that supplies the posterior one-third of the spinal cord
    c. Segmental arteries arising from the aorta and internal iliac arteries feed the circulation at the
       thoracic and lumbar levels
    d. There is an epidural venous plexus system that connects pelvic venous plexuses and the
       intracranial venous system
    e. The anterior spinal artery originates from the vertebral arteries

12. A 69-year-old man who has hypertension, hyperlipidemia, diabetes, coronary disease, and
    peripheral vascular disease undergoes an endovascular intervention for a thoracoabdominal
    aneurysm. After the procedure he has new neurologic findings attributed to an anterior spinal
    artery infarct of the spinal cord. On examination you expect to find:
    a. Paraplegia with bilateral loss of sensation to pain and temperature below the lesion, and
       preserved sensation to vibration and proprioception
    b. Paraplegia with bilateral loss of sensation to vibration and proprioception below the lesion,
       and preserved sensation to pain and temperature
    c. Loss of sensation to vibration and proprioception bilaterally, and preserved sensation to pain
       and temperature, with no weakness
    d. Loss of sensation to pain and temperature bilaterally, and preserved sensation to vibration
       and proprioception, with no weakness
    e. Weakness on one side with loss of sensation to vibration and proprioception ipsilaterally, and
       loss of sensation to pain and temperature on the contralateral side

13. A 70-year-old man complains of back pain, lower extremity weakness, and sensory deficit
    to all modalities below his mid-abdominal region for the past 3 days. Since onset, his

neurologic manifestations have progressed rapidly such that he is paraplegic on the day of evaluation. His MRI is shown in Figure 11.2. The most important risk factor for this patient's condition is:

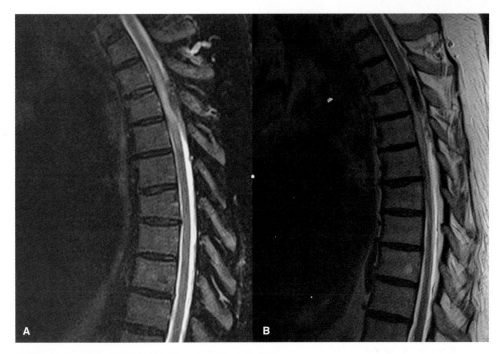

FIGURE 11.2   (**A**) Sagittal STIR MRI; (**B**) sagittal T2-weighted MRI

    a. An episode of hypotension
    b. Recent aortic manipulation
    c. Atherosclerosis
    d. The presence of a dural arteriovenous fistula
    e. Use of warfarin for atrial fibrillation

14. Which of the following statements is incorrect regarding the pathophysiology of amyotrophic lateral sclerosis (ALS)?
    a. Glutamate-induced excitotoxicity has been postulated as a cause
    b. Mutations in the superoxide dismutase gene account for approximately 20% of familial ALS
    c. No environmental exposures have been definitively identified to be associated with ALS
    d. A rare form of ALS with parkinsonism and dementia had been identified in a geographically restricted area in the Western Pacific island of Guam
    e. The majority of ALS cases are familial and most often X-linked

15. A 69-year-old man presents with 6 months of gradually progressive lower extremity weakness. His MRI is shown in Figure 11.3. Regarding this patient's condition, which of the following is correct?

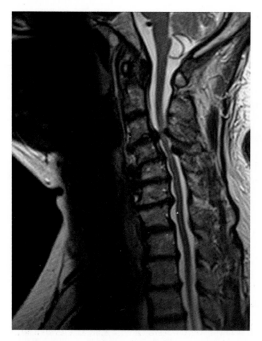

FIGURE 11.3 Sagittal T2-weighted MRI

    a. On examination there will be evidence of atrophy and fasciculations in the lower extremities

    b. On examination there will be evidence of spinal shock

    c. Steroids are indicated

    d. Radiation therapy should be started immediately

    e. On examination there will be spasticity in the lower extremities with hyperreflexia and upgoing toes

16. A 59-year-old man from Cape Town presents with progressive lower extremity weakness associated with numbness and paresthesias in both legs, as well as bladder and bowel incontinence. He has a history of diabetes, hypertension, chronic obstructive pulmonary disease with long-standing intermittent use of steroids, and prostate cancer with metastasis to the lower thoracic spine, treated with radiation 12 months prior. His MRI shows T2 hyperintensity in the thoracic spinal cord, with no evidence of compression or extradural mass. What is the most likely diagnosis?

    a. Lathyrism

    b. Transient radiation myelopathy *(3–6 month)*

    c. Epidural lipomatosis

    d. Delayed radiation myelopathy *> 6 months.*

    e. Konzo

17. A 45-year-old woman is evaluated for progressive spastic paraparesis. She also has anemia and leukopenia. Her vitamin B_{12} level is 300 pg/mL (220 to 700 pg/mL), folate level is 1.9 mg/mL (2 to 18 mg/mL), and copper is 90 μg/dL (85 to 155 μg/dL). Which of the following is correct in the treatment of this patient?

a. Start copper supplementation and observe for improvement before providing vitamin B_{12} or folate

b. Start folate supplementation

c. Check methylmalonic acid and homocysteine, and start vitamin B_{12} and folate supplementation

d. Start zinc supplementation

e. No therapies are needed because the test results are within normal limits

18. A 33-year-old man from Cleveland with unknown past medical history presents to the hospital in July with fever, mild lethargy, and bilateral lower extremity weakness, which has progressed over the past 5 days. On examination he is mildly confused with flaccid quadriparesis and areflexia. Which of the following is the most likely etiology?

a. An enterovirus

b. A flavivirus (West nile).

c. HTLV-1

d. HTLV-2

e. A herpesvirus

19. A previously healthy 36-year-old woman presents with rapidly progressive flaccid paraparesis. She recalls an episode of right-eye visual loss about 2 years ago, which resolved without treatment. Her spine MRI shows a large T2-hyperintense lesion extending from T5 to T11. MRI of the brain shows few scattered nonspecific white matter lesions. Her ESR is elevated and antinuclear antibody (ANA) is positive. CSF analysis shows 49 WBCs/mm³ (normal is up to 5 lymphocytes/mm³), half of which are polymorphonuclear leucocytes, a protein level of 92 mg/dL (normal is up to 45 mg/dL), normal immunoglobulin G (IgG) index, and no oligoclonal bands. Which of the following is incorrect regarding this condition?

a. In neuromyelitis optica, ANA positivity suggests a separate diagnosis of systemic lupus erythematosus

b. Neuromyelitis optica–IgG is an antibody against aquaporin-4

c. Asians and African populations are more frequently affected

d. Pathologic analysis of the spinal cord tissue will show inflammation, demyelination, and necrosis

e. Antibodies against aquaporin-4 are part of the diagnostic criteria

20. A 34-year-old man has progressive neurologic manifestations. He was a normal child and adolescent, and he was fine until he was about 23 years of age when he started noticing numbness and tingling in his feet and difficulty running. He has been diagnosed with a spastic paraparesis and has been getting gradually worse over the past few years to the point that now he needs a walker to walk. He also has very mild cognitive impairment, behavioral problems, mild hearing and visual impairment, as well as urinary incontinence. His past medical history is significant for at least five admissions to the ICU secondary to upper respiratory infections, leading to significant hypotension and hypoglycemia, for which he has required steroids. Regarding this condition, which of the following is correct?

a. He has amyotrophic lateral sclerosis

b. He has pure hereditary spastic paraparesis

c. The most likely diagnosis is neuromyelitis optica

d. He has adrenomyeloneuropathy

e. He has primary lateral sclerosis

21. A patient presents with a several months' history of gradually progressive sensory loss to pain and temperature over his shoulders and both arms bilaterally, with preserved sensation to light touch, vibration, and proprioception. On examination he has findings suggestive of multiple old injuries in both upper limbs. He also has weakness and atrophy in both upper extremities, with minimal findings in the lower extremities. Which of the following is correct regarding this condition?
    a. Syringomyelia can cause this syndrome
    b. MRI will likely show an infarct in the anterior spinal artery territory
    c. The syndrome is consistent with Brown-Séquard syndrome
    d. The findings suggest subacute combined degeneration of the spinal cord
    e. This patient has a watershed infarct of the spinal cord

22. Which of the following is correct regarding neoplastic disease of the spinal cord?
    a. Ependymomas are the most common intramedullary spinal cord tumor in children
    b. Astrocytomas are the most common intramedullary spinal cord tumor in adults
    c. Myxopapillary ependymomas originate from the filum terminale
    d. Meningioma is the most common extradural tumor of the spinal cord
    e. Intramedullary spinal cord metastases are more common than primary intramedullary neoplasms

23. A 12-year-old girl with no past medical history except a febrile illness about 1 week ago, presents with 3 days of headache, altered mental status, inability to move her legs, and urinary incontinence. On examination she is confused, has no meningeal signs, and has a flaccid paraplegia with areflexia and sensory loss below her waist. Her CSF shows 40 WBCs/mm^3 (normal up to 5 lymphocytes/mm^3) with lymphocytic predominance, a protein level of 70 mg/dL (normal up to 45 mg/dL) with normal glucose, and high immunoglobulin G index. MRI of the brain shows symmetric subcortical white matter lesions, and MRI of the spine shows an expanding intramedullary lesion between T5 and T10 with gadolinium enhancement. The most likely diagnosis is
    a. Multiple sclerosis
    b. Acute disseminated encephalomyelitis
    c. Neuromyelitis optica
    d. Idiopathic transverse myelitis
    e. Bacterial meningitis

24. A 50-year-old man presents with gradually progressive weakness in his upper extremities over the past 6 months. A cervical MRI is obtained, which is shown in Figure 11.4. On the basis of the location of the lesion, on examination you will find:
    a. Patellar and ankle areflexia
    b. Sensory level below the level of the nipples
    c. Sparing of superficial abdominal reflexes
    d. Horner's syndrome
    e. Flaccid weakness of his lower extremities

25. All of the following conditions are associated with atlantoaxial dislocation, except:
    a. Rheumatoid arthritis
    b. Klippel-Feil syndrome
    c. Systemic lupus erythematosus

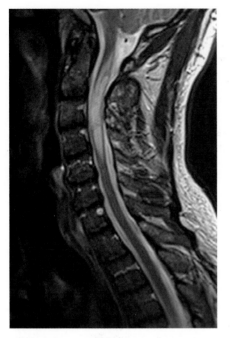

FIGURE 11.4 Sagittal T2-weighted MRI

d. Down's syndrome
e. Morquio syndrome

26. Regarding neoplastic spinal cord disease, which of the following is incorrect?
   a. Malignancies that may metastasize to the spine include those arising from the breast, lung, prostate, and kidney
   b. Radiation therapy can improve pain and neurologic symptoms in patients with lymphoproliferative neoplasia producing cord compression
   c. High-dose 24-hour treatment of continuous IV methylprednisolone is the treatment of choice
   d. Intradural extramedullary tumors causing cord compression include neurofibromas, schwannomas, and meningiomas
   e. Intramedullary tumors include ependymomas and astrocytomas

27. A 27-year-old man is involved in a motor vehicle accident and is ejected from the car. He suffers acute spinal cord injury with cord transection at the level of C5 to C6. The following findings would be present during the first week of injury, except:
   a. Flaccid weakness of his lower extremities
   b. Atonic bladder with overflow incontinence
   c. Decreased rectal tone
   d. Patellar and ankle areflexia
   e. Spontaneous reflex defecation

28. A 55-year-old man with slowly progressive gait ataxia, myelopathic findings, and mild cognitive impairment presents for follow-up. He has a diagnosis of superficial siderosis of the CNS. Regarding this condition, which of the following is incorrect?

a. There is hemosiderin deposition in the subpial layers of the brain and spinal cord
b. CSF analysis shows xanthochromia
c. Sensorineural hearing loss is a frequent manifestation
d. The source of hemorrhage is commonly not identifiable
e. MRI shows a T2-hyperintense rim around the brain, brain stem, and spinal cord

29. A 52-year-old patient with HIV on no antiretroviral treatment comes with a history of long-standing pain in his legs, spasticity in his lower extremities, and gait ataxia. Studies obtained show a positive serum rapid plasma reagin (RPR). Regarding spinal cord disease in syphilis, which of the following is incorrect?
    a. Syphilis does not present as a spinal cord infarction
    b. The treatment for neurosyphilis is penicillin G 24 million units/day intravenously for 14 days
    c. Syphilis can present as transverse myelitis
    d. Patients with tabes dorsalis have prominent sensory ataxia and proprioceptive loss
    e. Other presentations of syphilis affecting the spinal cord include pachymeningitis and gummas in the spinal cord

30. A 46-year-old woman with a history of pelvic cancer presents with severe radicular pain in the perineum radiating to both legs, right more than left. On examination she has asymmetric sensory loss in the lower extremities and perineal region, bilateral asymmetric lower extremity weakness, and areflexia. Which of the following is correct regarding this patient's condition?
    a. She has a cauda equina syndrome
    b. She has a lesion in the conus medullaris
    c. She has an intramedullary tumor
    d. She has transverse myelitis
    e. She has an epidural hematoma

31. A 56-year-old woman is referred to the clinic for evaluation of suspected amyotrophic lateral sclerosis (ALS). Her history and examination are for the most part consistent with ALS, but there has been recent rapid unexplained weight loss, serum calcium is mildly elevated, and she has chronic neck pain. Which of the following studies are indicated in evaluation of her disorder?
    a. EMG/NCS
    b. MRI of the brain and spine
    c. Anti-Hu antibody
    d. Serum parathyroid hormone
    e. All of the above

32. A 45-year-old morbidly obese woman undergoes gastric bypass surgery. She comes to the clinic 3 years later after having lost about 40 kg, with the complaint of difficulty walking. On examination she has manifestations consistent with a myelopathy, with a spastic gait and sensory ataxia. Laboratory tests show anemia with neutropenia and a normal vitamin B_{12} level, but a high methylmalonic acid. After treatment with vitamin B_{12} she does not improve. You suspect copper deficiency. Which of the following is incorrect regarding copper deficiency?
    a. Zinc deficiency is a risk factor
    b. Copper deficiency may coexist with vitamin B_{12} deficiency
    c. Optic nerve involvement may be caused by copper deficiency
    d. Findings of peripheral neuropathy may be present in patients with copper deficiency
    e. The spinal cord segment most commonly affected is in the cervical region

33. A 40-year-old man presents with complaints of inability to lift his arms above his head and difficulty climbing stairs. Examination shows Medical Research Council 4/5 weakness in shoulder and hip girdle muscles. He is also noted to have prominent fasciculations in his chin. A subtle high frequency postural tremor is present. His breast tissue is noted to be enlarged on examination. A family history of similar symptoms is present in his brother and two maternal cousins. His mother is apparently unaffected. Which of the following statements is correct regarding this disorder?
   a. It is autosomal recessive
   b. Precocious puberty commonly occurs
   c. Facial fasciculations are rare, but when present, suggest the diagnosis
   d. It typically presents in early childhood
   e. It results from a trinucleotide repeat expansion in the androgen receptor gene

34. Regarding the spinal cord, which of the following is incorrect?
   a. It has 31 pairs of spinal nerves: 8 cervical, 12 thoracic, 5 lumbar, 5 sacral, and 1 coccygeal
   b. It lies within the spinal canal ventral to the posterior longitudinal ligament
   c. In adults, it ends at the level of L1 to L2
   d. There are two enlargements, one at the cervical level and another at the lumbosacral level
   e. The denticulate ligament extends from pia mater to dura mater on both sides of the spinal cord

35. At birth, a male baby is noted to be hypotonic, admitted to the ICU and intubated for respiratory failure, and he eventually undergoes tracheostomy. He is noted to have little movement of the extremities and persistent head lag. Muscle biopsy is obtained and the findings are shown in Figure 11.5. What is the most likely diagnosis in this patient?

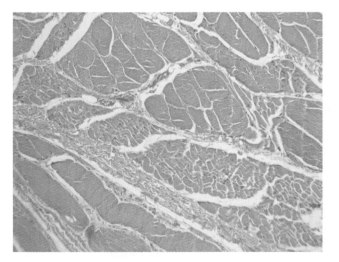

FIGURE 11.5 Muscle biopsy specimen (Courtesy of Dr. Richard A. Prayson). Shown also in color plates

   a. Spinal muscular atrophy (SMA) type 1
   b. SMA type 4
   c. Charcot-Marie-Tooth type 1a

d. Congenital myasthenia
e. Neonatal botulism

36. A 60-year-old anesthetist with obesity, hypertension, and diabetes undergoes gastric bypass surgery, and an inhaled anesthetic is used during the procedure. Around 5 days after the surgery he notices that he cannot move his legs, and he has a strange sensation below his waist. An MRI of the thoracic spine shows T2 cord signal hyperintensity with no evidence of an extradural collection. Which of the following is the most likely diagnosis?
    a. Copper deficiency
    b. Folate deficiency
    c. Spinal epidural hematoma
    d. Spinal epidural abscess
    e. Nitrous oxide toxicity

37. An 18-year-old man, originally from Hawaii, presents with a history of 2 years of progressive bilateral upper extremity weakness, right worse than left. He has no pain, and denies dysphagia or dysarthria. On examination he has weakness, atrophy, and fasciculations, more prominent in the hand muscles, right worse than left. His lower extremities are not affected. His sensory examination is normal. He also has a past medical history of seasonal allergies. On follow-up 3 years later, his hand weakness is stable to minimally improved, and no weakness has developed in other areas. What is the most likely diagnosis in this patient?
    a. Amyotrophic lateral sclerosis
    b. Primary lateral sclerosis
    c. Hirayama disease
    d. Spinal muscular atrophy
    e. Cervical osteoarthritis

38. A 77-year-old man with a history of hypertension, diabetes, hyperlipidemia, and coronary disease is admitted for open repair of a thoracoabdominal aortic aneurysm. When he wakes up from surgery, he is in pain, cannot move his legs, and does not have sensation to pinprick over his legs; however, he is able to feel vibration and proprioception in his toes. Which of the following is correct regarding this case?
    a. The patient has nitrous oxide toxicity–related myelopathy
    b. A spinal epidural hematoma is the most likely cause
    c. Vitamin B_{12} deficiency is the most likely cause
    d. Copper deficiency is the most likely cause
    e. This patient has a spinal cord infarct

39. A 22-year-old man, intravenous drug user, reports a history of 1 month of low-grade fevers and back pain, and over the past 3 days, he has developed progressive lower extremity weakness and urinary incontinence. His temperature is 39°C, and on examination he has paraplegia and a sensory level at T8. Rectal tone is decreased. Which of the following is correct regarding this patient's most likely condition?
    a. A lumbar puncture is indicated, and cultures are positive in the majority of the cases
    b. MRI of the spine is not very sensitive for the diagnosis of this condition
    c. Neurosurgical consultation may not be required if fever resolves with initial antibiotic therapy
    d. *Staphylococcus aureus* is the most common pathogen
    e. The treatment includes broad-spectrum antibiotic therapy for 2 weeks

Answer key

1. b	**8.** b	**15.** e	**22.** c	**29.** a	**36.** e
2. d	**9.** b	**16.** d	**23.** b	**30.** a	**37.** c
3. e	**10.** a	**17.** c	**24.** d	**31.** e	**38.** e
4. e	**11.** b	**18.** b	**25.** c	**32.** a	**39.** d
5. d	**12.** a	**19.** a	**26.** c	**33.** e	
6. d	**13.** e	**20.** d	**27.** e	**34.** b	
7. c	**14.** e	**21.** a	**28.** e	**35.** a	

Answers

1. b, 2. d

This patient's history and examination, including evidence of upper and lower motor neuron dysfunction, are suggestive of amyotrophic lateral sclerosis (ALS). ALS is a neurodegenerative disorder that affects motor neurons in the anterior horn of the spinal cord, but also the motor cortex and brain stem. Sporadic ALS affects men more than women. It can present at any age, but with a peak incidence in the sixth to seventh decades of life.

The hallmark of ALS is evidence of both upper motor neuron (UMN) disease (such as hyperreflexia, clonus, and presence of a Babinski sign) and lower motor neuron (LMN) disease (atrophy, fasciculations in the limbs, trunk, tongue, and occasionally face) in the absence of sensory symptoms or sensory abnormalities on examination.

Clinical presentation is variable, but most often muscle weakness begins focally, usually in the extremities (two-thirds of cases) and spreads to involve contiguous regions, though there is significant variability in the pattern of motor weakness. The split-hand phenomenon is a feature of ALS, characterized by weakness and atrophy of the lateral hand (thenar and first dorsal interosseous muscles) with relative sparing of the medial hand (hypothenar) muscles. About one-third of patients present with bulbar symptoms, such as dysarthria or dysphagia (bulbar-onset ALS). Other symptoms of bulbar involvement include sialorrhea. Pseudobulbar palsy (pathologic laughter and crying without a corresponding change in mood) and excessive yawning also occur in ALS and do not necessarily suggest an alternative diagnosis. Muscle cramps commonly occur. Only a minority of patients with ALS (approximately 1%) present with acute respiratory failure, though the majority progress to respiratory failure.

Cognitive impairment of some degree is present in up to 50% of patients with ALS; it is mostly subclinical, but can be detected on neuropsychologic testing. In a small proportion of cases, the cognitive dysfunction is more evident, manifesting as a dementia that is typically of the frontotemporal type, namely frontotemporal dementia (FTD). This tends to occur most frequently in patients who present with bulbar-onset ALS. On the other hand, a subset of patients presenting with FTD have clinical and electrodiagnostic features of motor neuron disease. The pathology of patients with so-called ALS-FTD includes atrophy in the frontal and temporal lobes and ubiquitin-positive, *TDP-43*-positive, *tau*-negative inclusions. Autosomal dominant forms have been linked to *TDP-43* gene mutations on chromosome 9.

Curiously (for unclear reasons), the region of motor neurons in the sacral spinal cord that are responsible for sphincter control, Onufrowicz nucleus (also known as Onuf's nucleus) is generally spared in ALS, and sphincter dysfunction is typically not a prominent problem. Sensory involvement and dysautonomia are also uncommon in ALS, but can occur.

ALS is relentlessly progressive and ultimately fatal within 2 to 5 years of symptom onset, although in approximately 20%, survival is longer than 5 to 10 years after symptom onset.

Primary lateral sclerosis (discussed in question 6), progressive muscular atrophy (discussed in question 10), Kennedy's disease (X-linked spinobulbar muscular atrophy, discussed in question 33), and spinal muscular atrophy (discussed in question 35) are all motor neuron disorders. In these disorders, either UMNs or LMNs alone are affected, not in combination, in contradistinction to ALS. In early ALS, however, combined UMN and LMN dysfunction may be subtle or absent until later stages when its presence is necessary for diagnosis (by definition; see question 31). In Kennedy's disease, there is often a family history of motor neuron disease in males and gynecomastia is present on examination.

Bradley WG, Daroff RB, Fenichel GM, et al. Neurology in Clinical Practice, 5th ed. Philadelphia, PA: Elsevier; 2008.

3. e

Figure 11.1 shows an intradural extramedullary tumor compressing the spinal cord. The tumor is located at the C7 to T1 vertebral level and is dural based. Meningiomas are one of the most common intradural extramedullary tumors. They are nonglial neoplasms that are usually benign and can cause neurologic problems due to compression. Because they grow slowly, neurologic manifestations progress very gradually and may compensate for the degree of compression. Patients may have very large tumors causing significant compression without prominent manifestations on clinical examination.

This patient does not have an acute transverse myelitis nor a spinal cord infarct because the presentation in both of these conditions is usually acute to subacute, with MRI findings showing a parenchymal cord lesion and not an extramedullary mass. Spinal cord infarct may be sudden in onset and usually affects the anterior cord (anterior spinal artery), causing primarily bilateral weakness and pain and temperature loss rather than vibration and position loss (dorsal columns are relatively spared). Acute transverse myelitis progresses over hours or a few days rather than months. A metastatic tumor usually has a more subacute presentation with prominent back pain. Because metastatic tumors develop more rapidly, the patient would have more symptoms and neurologic deficits than this patient has for the degree of compression seen on this MRI. An epidural hematoma also presents rapidly with an acute compressive myelopathy syndrome manifesting as spinal shock, usually with no evidence of spasticity or hyperreflexia on presentation.

Bradley WG, Daroff RB, Fenichel GM, et al. Neurology in Clinical Practice, 5th ed. Philadelphia, PA: Elsevier; 2008.

Jacob A, Weinshenker BG. An approach to the diagnosis of acute transverse myelitis. Semin Neurol. 2008; 28:105–120.

Ropper AH, Samuels MA. Adams and Victor's Principles of Neurology, 9th ed. New York: McGraw-Hill; 2009.

4. e

Parotid and submandibular botulinum toxin injections are effective in some patients with amyotrophic lateral sclerosis (ALS) with refractory sialorrhea, and should be offered when appropriate.

Guidelines have been issued by the American Academy of Neurology for the management of patients with ALS. The majority of patients experience hypoventilation, and orthopnea becomes significant in advanced stages. Nocturnal oximetry, supine forced vital capacity, and supine maximal inspiratory pressure should be periodically assessed in patients with ALS. Noninvasive ventilation should be offered as indicated, and it likely improves quality of life. Management of patients with ALS in multidisciplinary clinics, including experts in neurology, speech therapy, physical and occupational therapy, respiratory therapy, social work, and case management, is likely of benefit.

Pharmacologic treatment of ALS may include riluzole, an inhibitor of glutamate release, which slows disease progression, prolonging survival by approximately 3 months. Patients may experience side effects of dizziness, fatigue, and gastrointestinal upset, which are usually mild and transient; if intolerable, dosage can be reduced or taken with food prior to deciding to discontinue it. Importantly, blood count and liver enzymes should be checked routinely 1 month after beginning riluzole, monthly for 3 months, then every 3 months for the rest of the first year, and yearly afterward. Other medications being investigated as disease-modifying therapies include ceftriaxone, creatine monohydrate, and tamoxifen, but definitive data showing benefit are not available as of 2010. Management is therefore largely symptomatic.

Frequent evaluation of swallowing function is important as patients with ALS are at increased risk of aspiration. Placement of a percutaneous gastrostomy tube stabilizes body weight and maintains hydration in patients with ALS; although survival is probably not prolonged significantly, quality of life is improved. Treatment of pseudobulbar affect is off-label with tricyclic antidepressants or selective serotonin reuptake inhibitors, although an effective dextromethorphan-quinidine combination was FDA approved in October 2010.

Miller RG, Jackson CE, Kasarskis EJ, et al. Quality Standards Subcommittee of the American Academy of Neurology. Practice parameter update: The care of the patient with amyotrophic lateral sclerosis: drug, nutritional, and respiratory therapies (an evidence-based review): Report of the Quality Standards Subcommittee of the American Academy of Neurology. Neurology. 2009; 73:1218–1226.

Milller RG, Jackson CE, Kasarskis EJ, et al. Quality Standards Subcommittee of the American Academy of Neurology. Practice parameter update: The care of the patient with amyotrophic lateral sclerosis: Multidisciplinary care, symptom management, and cognitive/behavioral impairment (an evidence-based review): Report of the Quality Standards Subcommittee of the American Academy of Neurology. Neurology. 2009; 73:1227–1233.

5. d

Serum methylmalonic acid (MMA) and homocysteine levels should be obtained when following patients with vitamin B_{12} deficiency receiving treatment.

Vitamin B_{12} or cobalamin deficiency is a major cause of neurologic disease. Manifestations include subacute combined degeneration of the spinal cord, peripheral neuropathy, optic neuropathy, and even cognitive impairment.

Vitamin B_{12} as methylcobalamin is a cofactor for the enzyme methionine synthase in the conversion of homocysteine into methionine, which is then adenylated to S-adenosylmethionine. S-adenosylmethionine is required for methylation reactions, and decreased levels may lead to reduced myelin basic protein methylation and white matter vacuolization. Methionine also facilitates the formation of formyltetrahydrofolate, which is involved in purine and pyrimidine synthesis, and therefore low methionine levels secondary to vitamin B_{12} deficiency impair DNA synthesis. In another pathway, vitamin B_{12} as adenosylcobalamin is a cofactor in the conversion of methylmalonyl CoA to succinyl-CoA. Vitamin B_{12} deficiency will lead to the accumulation of methylmalonate and propionate, providing abnormal substrates for fatty acid synthesis, and therefore interfering with myelin synthesis.

In some cases of vitamin B_{12} deficiency, vitamin B_{12} levels may be within normal limits; however, MMA and homocysteine will be elevated, helping in the diagnosis.

Malabsorption is the most common cause of vitamin B_{12} deficiency, and achlorhydria in the setting of pernicious anemia is an important cause. Pernicious anemia is an autoimmune condition in which anti-intrinsic factor and anti-parietal antibodies may be present. Given that these patients have achlorhydria, gastrin levels may be elevated as well. Parenteral vitamin B_{12} supplementation is the treatment of choice in cases of malabsorption, and usually the hematologic abnormalities improve rapidly; however, the neurologic manifestations may not resolve completely. Vitamin B_{12} levels rise with treatment, regardless of the clinical effect; therefore, MMA and homocysteine levels should be followed.

Ropper AH, Samuels MA. Adams and Victor's Principles of Neurology, 9th ed. New York: McGraw-Hill; 2009.

6. d

Primary lateral sclerosis (PLS) is characterized by presence of upper motor neuron signs at least 3 years from symptom onset, without evidence of lower motor neuron dysfunction. PLS is considered along the spectrum of amyotrophic lateral sclerosis (ALS), although it is controversial as to whether or not it is a separate entity. It typically presents in the sixth decade of life with a progressive spastic tetraparesis and later cranial nerve involvement. Rarely, bulbar onset occurs. Spasticity, rather than muscle weakness or atrophy, is the most prominent feature. It typically progresses slowly over years. Autonomic involvement does not typically occur. Autopsy on patients with PLS has shown significant cell loss in layer 5 of the motor and premotor cortex, predominantly the large pyramidal Betz cells with corticospinal tract degeneration. The majority of patients with ALS who present with predominantly upper motor neuron signs and symptoms eventually develop lower motor neuron involvement within 3 to 4 years.

The differential diagnosis of PLS is broad and a thorough work-up to exclude any possibilities is indicated. It includes cervical myelopathy, although sensory abnormalities and other features of myelopathy such as bowel and bladder symptoms should be present, and a normal MRI of the spine excludes this. Similarly, multiple sclerosis is high on the differential diagnosis of PLS; the presence of sensory symptoms, changes on MRI of the brain and spine, and CSF findings (when CSF is available for analysis) distinguish between the two. Tropical spastic paraparesis due to HTLV-1 typically occurs in endemic regions (equatorial and south Africa, the Caribbean, parts of Asia, and Central and South America) and rarely in the United States. Patients with hereditary spastic paraparesis often, though not always, have a family history of similar symptoms and signs and have white matter abnormalities on MRI of the brain and spine. Another differential diagnosis is stiff person syndrome, which is associated with anti-glutamic acid decarboxylase antibodies, which should be assessed for in a patient with this presentation. Other disorders that can present with spastic quadriparesis that should be considered include hexosaminidase A deficiency, adrenomyeloneuropathy, a paraneoplastic process, and autoimmune processes (such as Sjögren's syndrome).

Treatment is symptomatic, and usually includes baclofen (a $GABA_B$ agonist) or tizanidine (an α_2 agonist) to reduce spasticity.

Bradley WG, Daroff RB, Fenichel GM, et al. Neurology in Clinical Practice, 5th ed. Philadelphia, PA: Elsevier; 2008.

7. c

This patient has HIV, is immunocompromised as evidenced by the low CD4 count, and has a progressive myelopathy. This population of patients should undergo an evaluation for various infectious agents as the potential cause of myelopathy, including syphilis, viruses such as herpes zoster and HTLV-1, mycobacteria, and fungal agents. However, the most common cause of spinal cord involvement in patients with HIV is primary HIV-related myelopathy. This is a vacuolar myelopathy, in which there is lateral and posterior column demyelination with microvacuolar changes and axonal preservation. Given that other potential conditions can cause myelopathic symptoms in patients with HIV, HIV-related vacuolar myelopathy should be a diagnosis of exclusion.

HIV-related vacuolar myelopathy presents in patients with AIDS, and affected patients have gradually progressive gait difficulty, spasticity, leg weakness, and impaired proprioception. There is no back pain and the upper extremities are typically spared. MRI may reveal spinal cord atrophy, but is most often normal. There is no effective treatment, and the initial goal is prevention with anti-retroviral therapy.

HTLV-1 is a cause of spinal cord disease in patients with HIV; however, it is not the cause of HIV-related vacuolar myelopathy. HTLV-1 causes tropical spastic paraparesis or HTLV-1-associated myelopathy. This is a chronic progressive myelopathy endemic in equatorial and south Africa, as well as in parts of Asia, Central and South America, and the Caribbean. This virus can be transmitted via contaminated blood, sexual activity, breast-feeding, and rarely in utero. Only 1% to 2% of infected individuals will develop neurologic disease. These patients will manifest with a slowly progressive spastic paraparesis, lower extremity paresthesias, painful sensory neuropathy, and bladder dysfunction. MRI reveals increased signal on T2-weighted images with atrophy of the thoracic cord, but these findings are not specific for this condition. The diagnosis is made with positive serology in blood and CSF to HTLV-1, as well as PCR. No antiviral agent is available for the treatment of HTLV-1.

Boisse L, Gill J, Power C. HIV infection of the central nervous system: Clinical features and neuropathogenesis. Neurol Clin. 2008; 26:799–819.

Bradley WG, Daroff RB, Fenichel GM, et al. Neurology in Clinical Practice, 5th ed. Philadelphia, PA: Elsevier; 2008.

Ropper AH, Samuels MA. Adams and Victor's Principles of Neurology, 9th ed. New York: McGraw-Hill; 2009.

8. b

On the basis of the family history and clinical findings of this patient, he most likely has hereditary spastic paraparesis (HSP), which is a group of disorders characterized by progressively worsening spasticity of the lower extremities, with variable weakness and difficulty walking. It is inherited most commonly in an autosomal dominant fashion, but it can occur in an autosomal recessive fashion, although X-linked and sporadic cases have also been reported. This condition can present at any age from childhood to late adulthood; however, more frequently the onset is between the second and fourth decades of life. Clinically, it has been divided into pure and complicated forms. The pure form presents only with lower extremity spasticity, whereas sensory and other neurologic functions are intact. The complicated form has other neurologic features, including optic neuropathy, deafness, amyotrophy, peripheral neuropathy, ataxia, dementia, mental retardation, and extrapyramidal dysfunction. Several genetic mutations have been identified involving various HSP loci and genes. The most common mutation is on chromosome 2p22 involved with the *SPAST* gene encoding for the protein spastin, which is inherited in an autosomal dominant fashion. Other proteins involved include atlastin, paraplegin, spartin, and maspardin, among others. Treatment is symptomatic, with pharmacologic treatment of spasticity and supportive care for disability.

This patient does not have Hirayama disease, amyotrophic lateral sclerosis (ALS), progressive muscular atrophy (PMA), or multiple sclerosis. Hirayama disease involves the upper extremities with predominant lower motor neuron findings (discussed in question 37). ALS manifests with a combination of upper and lower motor neuron findings. PMA (discussed in question 10) manifests with lower motor neuron findings, which are not seen in this patient. There are no features to support the diagnosis of multiple sclerosis on this patient.

Bradley WG, Daroff RB, Fenichel GM, et al. Neurology in Clinical Practice, 5th ed. Philadelphia, PA: Elsevier; 2008.

Ropper AH, Samuels MA. Adams and Victor's Principles of Neurology, 9th ed. New York: McGraw-Hill; 2009.

9. b

This patient has a watershed infarct of the spinal cord, which may occur after prolonged hypotension. The area of the spinal cord most susceptible to watershed infarcts is at the upper midthoracic levels (between T4 and T8), given that blood supply is scarce between the blood supply coming from the vertebral circulation and the aortic circulation, though watershed infarcts at lower levels have been described. Patients with vascular risk factors for atherosclerotic disease are at higher risk for developing this type of spinal cord infarct.

The artery of Adamkiewicz is a large radicular artery that arises between T8 and L3 and supplies the lower thoracic and upper lumbar regions. This patient most likely has an infarct in the watershed region rather than in the area supplied by the artery of Adamkiewicz. The patient does not have a history to suggest an aortic dissection.

In both epidural abscess and epidural hematomas, the MRI will show an epidural collection that was not present in this patient.

Blumenfeld H. Neuronatomy through Clinical Cases, 1st ed. Sunderland, MA: Sinauer Associates; 2002.

Ropper AH, Samuels MA. Adams and Victor's Principles of Neurology, 9th ed. New York: McGraw-Hill; 2009.

10. a

Progressive muscular atrophy (PMA) is considered along the spectrum of amyotrophic lateral sclerosis (ALS), although this is controversial; it is a motor neuron disease that affects only the lower motor neurons, distinguishing it from ALS, which affects both upper and lower motor neurons. PMA often presents with focal asymmetric distal weakness that later involves more proximal regions and other extremities, with lower motor neuron features on examination, such as atrophy, hyporeflexia, and fasciculations. PMA begins at an earlier age as compared to ALS, and survival is often longer than ALS, with a median survival of 5 years, though more rapidly progressive and more chronic forms of the disease occur. Bulbar and respiratory involvement occur later in the disease as compared to ALS. Laboratory evaluation may reveal moderately elevated creatine kinase, but never more than 10 times normal, and EMG shows evidence of motor neuron disease.

Patients with ALS can present with predominantly lower motor neuron features early in their disease, with upper motor neuron findings not occurring until later. Therefore, a diagnosis of PMA is usually reserved for patients who have electrodiagnostic evidence of motor neuron disease and isolated lower motor neuron findings at least 3 years from symptom onset. The poliovirus infects anterior horn cells, leading to a lower motor neuron pattern of weakness similar to PMA. In those who survive, a postpolio syndrome may emerge years after recovery, marked by progressive fatigue, and weakness in muscles previously affected minimally or seemingly not at all. The history provided in this case is not consistent with postpolio syndrome. Unlike PMA, which progresses, on average, over 3 to 5 years, adult-onset spinal muscular atrophy is even more indolent and often affects predominantly proximal muscles. Inclusion body myositis is on the differential diagnosis of PMA and has a very indolent onset; relatively selective weakness of deep finger flexors and knee extensors in the setting of normal or only slightly elevated (less than two times normal) serum creatine kinase should prompt work-up for this disorder, including EMG and muscle biopsy.

Bradley WG, Daroff RB, Fenichel GM, et al. Neurology in Clinical Practice, 5th ed. Philadelphia, PA: Elsevier; 2008.

11. b

There are two paired posterior spinal arteries.

The blood supply to the spinal cord is provided by an arterial network that runs longitudinally along the cord, and its core is conformed by one anterior and two posterior spinal arteries. The anterior spinal artery supplies the anterior two-thirds of the spinal cord and originates from the vertebral arteries just before they join to form the basilar artery. The two paired posterior spinal arteries supply the posterior third of the spinal cord and originate from the vertebral arteries as well. These three arteries receive contributions from multiple segmental and radicular arteries, which arise from intercostal and iliac arteries that originate from the aorta. The largest radicular artery is the artery of Adamkiewicz, which supplies the lower thoracic and upper lumbar regions of the spinal cord.

The cervical and upper thoracic regions receive multiple collaterals from the vertebral arteries and other cervical vessels. Similarly, the conus medullaris and cauda equina are also richly vascularized from the contribution of multiple radicular arteries. There is a watershed region in between these two well-perfused regions located between T4 and T8. Between the anterior and posterior spinal circulations there is a circumferential network as well.

There are anterior and posterior venous systems that drain into radicular veins and eventually into the epidural venous plexus system. This epidural venous plexus is a valveless system and extends from the pelvic region to the intracranial venous system. This could explain metastatic lesions in the CNS originating from the pelvic region.

Blumenfeld H. Neuronatomy through Clinical Cases, 1st ed. Sunderland, MA: Sinauer Associates; 2002.

Ropper AH, Samuels MA. Adams and Victor's Principles of Neurology, 9th ed. New York: McGraw-Hill; 2009.

12. a

The spinal cord has ascending and descending pathways distributed in the white matter funiculi. The corticospinal tract originates from the primary motor cortex. Approximately 85% of the fibers decussate at the level of the pyramids and descend in the lateral funiculi as the lateral corticospinal tract. Fifteen percent of the fibers descend uncrossed as the anterior corticospinal tract.

The dorsal columns of the spinal cord are formed by the fasciculi of gracilis and cuneatus, both carrying information related to vibration and proprioception. These fasciculi ascend ipsilaterally to the nucleus gracilis and cuneatus in the dorsal medulla. Fibers from these nuclei form the medial lemniscus, which decussates in the brain stem and ascends to the thalamus.

Sensation of pain, temperature, and crude touch is carried by the lateral spinothalamic tract. Peripheral sensory fibers enter the cord through the dorsal rami and cross over two to three segments above the level of entry to the contralateral side, where they enter the lateral spinothalamic tract. They ascend to synapse in the thalamus.

The anterior spinal artery provides blood supply to the anterior two-thirds of the spinal cord, perfusing the areas containing the corticospinal and spinothalamic tracts, but sparing the dorsal columns supplied by the posterior spinal arteries. Therefore, an anterior spinal artery infarct would manifest with paraplegia below the level of the infarct, as well as loss of sensation to pain and temperature, but spare the sensation to vibration and proprioception.

Option C can be produced by an infarct in the posterior spinal arteries territory, which is uncommon. Option E is consistent with Brown-Séquard (hemisection) syndrome, with ipsilateral loss of motor function and sensation to vibration and proprioception below the level of the lesion, and contralateral loss of sensation to pain and temperature. This happens because the lesion affects the spinothalamic tract after its decussation, and the corticospinal tracts and dorsal columns before the decussation. Options B and D are not likely in the setting of this patient.

Blumenfeld H. Neuronatomy through Clinical Cases, 1st ed. Sunderland, MA: Sinauer Associates; 2002.

Ropper AH, Samuels MA. Adams and Victor's Principles of Neurology, 9th ed. New York: McGraw-Hill; 2009.

13. e

Figure 11.2 shows an epidural collection consistent with an epidural hematoma. The most common initial symptom is back pain, followed by development of a myelopathic syndrome as the hematoma compresses the cord. It is more common in males and more frequent in the thoracolumbar region. Major risk factors for spinal epidural hematoma include anticoagulation either from medications or from coagulopathies and thrombocytopenia. Other factors that may increase the risk of this condition are trauma, neoplasms, pregnancy, and vascular malformations.

Dural arteriovenous fistula is the most common vascular malformation of the spinal cord, and presents with an insidious and slowly progressive myelopathic syndrome, sometimes with acute exacerbations. These manifestations are caused by increased venous congestion and mass effect in the spinal cord, leading to venous infarcts. Acute hemorrhages may occur; however, dural arteriovenous fistulas rarely produce epidural hematomas. MRI of the spine may show cord signal abnormalities and flow voids, but the definitive diagnostic procedure is conventional angiography.

Atherosclerosis, aortic dissection, and aortic manipulation (especially above the renal arteries) are associated with ischemic infarcts of the spinal cord. Prolonged hypotension may be associated with watershed infarcts of the spinal cord. Hypotension, atherosclerosis, and aortic manipulation are not typically associated with spinal epidural hematomas.

Kreppel D, Antoniadis G, Seeling W. Spinal hematoma: A literature survey with meta-analysis of 613 patients. Neurosurg Rev. 2003; 26:1–49.

Ropper AH, Samuels MA. Adams and Victor's Principles of Neurology, 9th ed. New York: McGraw-Hill; 2009.

14. e

The majority of amyotrophic lateral sclerosis (ALS) cases are sporadic. Familial ALS is usually autosomal dominant in inheritance, although autosomal recessive forms occur and X-linked inheritance is rare.

The cause of ALS is unknown; there are various hypotheses and several environmental exposures postulated and investigated as causative but without definite evidence of associations. The majority of ALS cases are sporadic; approximately 10% are familial. Several gene mutations or deletions have now been identified, resulting in differing patterns of inheritance (most frequently autosomal dominant, but also autosomal recessive and rarely X-linked), age of onset, and phenotypic variability. Mutations in the copper/zinc superoxide dismutase (*SOD1*) gene on chromosome 21 account for approximately 20% of cases of familial ALS and less than 5% of sporadic ALS cases. The abnormal SOD1 protein usually maintains its dismutase function, but appears to damage motor neurons through other mechanisms, including a toxic gain of function of the mutant protein. More than 160 mutations have been identified, most often inherited in an autosomal dominant fashion. A rare form of ALS associated with parkinsonism and frontotemporal dementia was identified in a geographically restricted area in the Western Pacific island of Guam. Several theories abound regarding this rare syndrome, including exposure to cyanobacterial toxins and the presence of specific genetic mutations in the indigenous population.

Bradley WG, Daroff RB, Fenichel GM, et al. Neurology in Clinical Practice, 5th ed. Philadelphia, PA: Elsevier; 2008.

15. e

The patient's history and MRI shown in Figure 11.3 are consistent with a cervical spondylotic myelopathy with spinal cord compression, which has occurred slowly over months. This condition is the most common cause of spinal cord compression in the elderly. Spondylosis is a degeneration of the spinal column, in which there is formation of osteophytes that eventually lead to compression of the spinal cord and nerve roots. Along with this, there are also disc herniations and ligamentum flavum hypertrophy, leading to narrowing of the spinal canal. Because the degenerative process progresses slowly, the neurologic manifestations develop insidiously, unlike acute cord compressions in which the patient has manifestations of spinal shock, which include weakness below the level of the lesion with flaccidity and hyporeflexia, sensory loss, and sphincteric dysfunction.

Patients with cervical spondylotic myelopathy gradually develop neck stiffness and pain, weakness at and below the compression level, and unsteady gait. The examination shows findings of upper motor neuron signs below the level of compression, with spastic paraparesis, hyperreflexia, and upgoing toes. In the upper extremities there may be evidence of lower motor neuron signs, such as areflexia and atrophy, mainly at the same level of the compression. Patients have sensory deficits and may experience L'hermitte's phenomenon, an electric sensation radiating down the back that occurs following neck flexion. The diagnostic test of choice is MRI of the spine. Goals of treatment include prevention of further neurologic deficits and therapies to help improve existing ones. Surgical decompression is the treatment of choice. Nonoperative options may provide pain relief; however, once myelopathic findings are evident surgical intervention may be required.

Radiation therapy plays no role in the treatment of cervical spondylotic myelopathy, and is reserved for the treatment of radiosensitive neoplasms. Steroid therapy is not indicated and is mainly used in patients with traumatic spinal injury and in neoplastic cord compression.

Ropper AH, Samuels MA. Adams and Victor's Principles of Neurology, 9th ed. New York: McGraw-Hill; 2009.

16. d

This patient has had radiation to the spine with development of radiation-induced myelopathy. There are two types of radiation-induced myelopathy, a transient and a delayed form. The transient form happens early, approximately 3 to 6 months after the radiation treatment, and presents with dysesthesias in the extremities that eventually resolve without sequelae. The delayed form occurs 6 months or greater following radiation therapy, as in this case. The presentation is insidious with paresthesias and dysesthesias of the feet, L'hermitte's phenomenon, and progressive weakness of the legs. Eventually, bowel and bladder can be affected. The MRI shows increased T2 signal in the affected regions, sometimes with heterogeneous gadolinium enhancement. Steroids have been tried; however, the key is prevention by minimizing the dose of radiation used.

Lathyrism is a neurotoxic disorder presenting as a myelopathy with subacute spastic paraparesis. It is endemic in certain parts of Ethiopia, India, and Bangladesh, and occurs from consumption of *Lathyrus sativus*, a legume (grass pea or chick pea) that contains the toxin β-N-oxalylamino-L-alanine. It is more prevalent in poor populations.

Konzo is a type of myelopathy that presents with a spastic paraparesis of abrupt onset, sometimes associated with involvement of the visual pathways. It is most commonly seen in certain parts of Africa and results from consumption of poorly processed *Cassava*, which contains cyanide. It is more prevalent in droughts and in poor populations.

Epidural lipomatosis is a condition in which there is hypertrophy of extramedullary adipose tissue in the epidural space, and is usually associated with chronic use of steroids. Patients present with back pain and myelopathic findings. The treatment involves stopping steroids, and sometimes even surgical decompression. MRI of the spine demonstrates the fatty tissue within the spinal canal producing spinal stenosis, which was not described in this patient.

Bradley WG, Daroff RB, Fenichel GM, et al. Neurology in Clinical Practice, 5th ed. Philadelphia, PA: Elsevier; 2008.

Ropper AH, Samuels MA. Adams and Victor's Principles of Neurology, 9th ed. New York: McGraw-Hill; 2009.

17. c

This patient likely has a myelopathy and hematologic disturbances from a metabolic cause. Deficiency of vitamin B_{12} and/or copper can lead to this clinical picture and it is difficult to differentiate the etiology; therefore, blood levels of these vitamins and trace elements should be checked. Methylcobalamine acts as a cofactor for methionine synthase in the reaction where homocysteine is converted into methionine. This enzyme also requires folate as a cosubstrate. This metabolic pathway is important for DNA synthesis, and when there is lack of the cofactors or substrates, there is dysfunction leading to the clinical manifestations including myelopathy and hematologic disturbances.

Folate deficiency can lead to neurologic disturbances like those seen in vitamin B_{12} deficiency; however, they are less frequent and less severe. When patients have vitamin B_{12} and folate deficiency, and only folate is supplemented, hematologic abnormalities improve, but not the neurologic manifestations. Therefore, both should be supplemented at the same time. In this case, folate levels are low but vitamin B_{12} levels are within the normal range. However serum vitamin B_{12} levels can be normal in some patients with vitamin B_{12} deficiency, and serum methylmalonic acid (MMA) and total homocysteine levels should be checked because they are more sensitive in detection of these deficiencies.

Patients with copper deficiency can also have these clinical manifestations; however, this deficiency is encountered less frequently than that of vitamin B_{12} and folate. In this case, the copper level is borderline low and should be rechecked in the future; this level would in all likelihood not explain all the manifestations in this patient.

Zinc induces the synthesis of metallothionein in enterocytes. Copper has high affinity for metallothionein and will bind to it, entering the enterocytes that eventually are sloughed off the mucosa, leading to loss of copper. Therefore, zinc ingestion may be associated with copper deficiency and may decrease copper levels.

In this patient, MMA and homocysteine should be checked, and vitamin B_{12} along with folate should be started.

Bradley WG, Daroff RB, Fenichel GM, et al. Neurology in Clinical Practice, 5th ed. Philadelphia, PA: Elsevier; 2008.

Ropper AH, Samuels MA. Adams and Victor's Principles of Neurology, 9th ed. New York: McGraw-Hill; 2009.

18. b

This patient has West Nile virus (WNV) infection. WNV is a flavivirus transmitted by mosquitoes. It causes an illness characterized by meningitis, encephalitis, and myeloradiculitis. Cases in the United States present during summer months, and the initial symptom is fever, progressing to altered mental status, gastrointestinal symptoms, back pain, and flaccid weakness with areflexia, more often proximal and asymmetric and sometimes affecting all limbs. The progression to nadir occurs in 3 to 8 days.

The diagnosis is made with serology, CSF antibodies, and/or PCR. CSF shows neutrophilic pleocytosis, with high protein and normal glucose. MRI shows cauda equina, spinal cord, and/or leptomeningeal enhancement. Pathologic studies have shown perivascular inflammation with anterior horn cell loss in the spinal cord.

Many enteroviruses and herpesviruses are associated with a transverse myelitis, usually as a post-infectious phenomenon; there are no features of transverse myelitis in this case. Poliovirus is an enterovirus that can lead to areflexic flaccid paralysis from damage to anterior horn cells; however, poliovirus does not cause the encephalopathic changes seen in WNV, and furthermore, it has been eradicated from the United States.

This patient does not have a history to suggest HIV, which causes a gradually progressive myelopathy characterized by spastic paraparesis with impaired vibration and proprioception sensation, and sensory gait ataxia. The pathologic finding in HIV myelopathy is microvacuolar changes. Myelopathy from HIV is usually a late disease manifestation, and does not seem to be the case in this patient.

HTLV-1 is a virus transmitted via sexual, parenteral, or maternal routes, which causes a chronic progressive myelopathy known as tropical spastic paraparesis. The myelopathy is usually localized in the thoracic region, and pathologically, there is neuronal cell loss, microvacuolization, and long tract degeneration. The diagnosis is made by detecting antibodies to HTLV-1 in the serum and CSF, as well as PCR. This virus is also associated with adult T-cell lymphoma and leukemia. HTLV-2 is also associated with a progressive myelopathy and can be seen in native Americans, intravenous drug users, and patients with HIV, but this is much less common than HTLV-1.

Jeha LE, Sila CA, Lederman RJ, et al. West Nile virus infection: A new acute paralytic illness. Neurology. 2003; 61:55–59.

Ropper AH, Samuels MA. Adams and Victor's Principles of Neurology, 9th ed. New York: McGraw-Hill; 2009.

19. a

This patient has neuromyelitis optica (NMO) or Devic's disease, which is an inflammatory demyelinating disease of the CNS affecting the optic nerves and spinal cord. It is nine times more common in women than in men, and unlike multiple sclerosis, it tends to affect more Asian and African populations. Patients present with a combination of optic neuritis and myelitis. The myelitis usually presents acutely as a longitudinally extensive transverse myelitis extending over three or more segments. This commonly causes bilateral signs and symptoms, which can be severe.

MRI of the spinal cord demonstrates T2 hyperintensity and gadolinium enhancement. MRI of the brain may show white matter changes; however, these changes are nonspecific and not necessarily diagnostic for multiple sclerosis. There are sometimes unusual brain changes in areas where aquaporin channels are common, such as in the brain stem and hypothalamus. Occasionally posterior reversible encephalopathy syndrome changes will be present.

CSF is frequently abnormal, showing increased WBCs and increased protein with normal glucose. Oligoclonal bands are rarely present in the CSF, in contrast to multiple sclerosis. Pathologic analysis of the spinal cord tissue will show inflammation and demyelination, with polymorphonuclear infiltrates and eosinophils, associated with necrosis.

The NMO-IgG antibody helps make the diagnosis and is part of the diagnostic criteria. It has a sensitivity of 64% and a specificity of 99%. This antibody is directed against aquaporin-4, which is a protein found in astrocyte foot processes around cerebral microvessels located at the blood-brain barrier.

A majority of patients will have nonspecific seropositivity to other autoantibodies, including the antinuclear antibody. The presence of these antibodies does not establish the presence of other autoimmune disease nor does it establish causality. It is possible that these seropositivities are a result of a general predisposition to autoimmunity.

Matiello M, Jacob A, Wingerchuk DM, et al. Neuromyelitis optica. Curr Opin Neurol. 2007; 20:255–260.

Wingerchuk DM, Lennon VA, Pittock SJ, et al. Revised diagnostic criteria for neuromyelitis optica. Neurology. 2006; 66:1485–1489.

20. d

This patient has adrenomyeloneuropathy, which is one of the phenotypes of adrenoleukodystrophy. This is a peroxisomal disorder transmitted in an X-linked fashion and associated with a mutation in the *ABCD1* gene on chromosome Xq28, which encodes a peroxisomal adenosine triphosphate-binding cassette transporter protein. Because of this mutation there is an impaired ability to oxidize very long chain fatty acids (VLCFAs), especially hexacosanoic acid, leading to the accumulation of VLCFAs in tissues and plasma.

In adrenoleukodystrophy there are four main phenotypes; an early onset cerebral white matter disease (adrenoleukodystrophy), adrenomyeloneuropathy, isolated Addison's disease, or asymptomatic. In adrenomyeloneuropathy, male patients begin having manifestations around age 20, with slowly progressive paraparesis, sensory neuropathy, problems with sphincter control, mild hypogonadism, and mild cognitive impairment. Some patients may develop hearing and visual impairment as well. Most patients also develop adrenal insufficiency. Increased levels of VLCFAs in plasma and cultured fibroblasts help in the diagnosis. Patients require steroids for the adrenal insufficiency; however, this medication does not have an effect on the CNS involvement. Very early bone marrow transplantation may be a therapeutic option.

Neither amyotrophic lateral sclerosis, primary lateral sclerosis, hereditary spastic paraparesis, nor neuromyelitis optica lead to adrenal insufficiency or the cognitive, behavioral, or sensory features that the patient in the case has.

Fenichel GM. Clinical Pediatric Neurology: A Signs and Symptoms Approach, 6th ed. Philadelphia, PA: Saunders Elsevier; 2009.

21. a

This patient has a dissociated sensory loss with loss of sensation to pain and temperature and preserved sensation to light touch, vibration, and proprioception in his upper extremities. This clinical syndrome is seen with central spinal cord lesions in which there is compromise of crossing fibers in the midline anterior to the central canal, which carry sensory input related to pain and temperature. Usually the distribution of this sensory loss is described as "cape-like" or "shawl-like". Because it does not affect the posterior columns, the sensory modalities carried by this pathway are not affected. This dissociated sensory loss is seen in syringomyelia, in which there is a cavitation in the central parts of the spinal cord, usually in the cervical region, sometimes extending upward to the brain stem or downward to the thoracic region. It has been described that patients with syringomyelia, given their lack of sensory input in their upper extremities, may experience repeated trauma and recurrent injuries. Syringomyelia may be associated with other developmental anomalies of the vertebral column or skull, as well as with Chiari malformations.

This patient does not have a spinal cord infarct, because the history is that of a gradually progressive illness, and there is no significant motor disturbance, such as that seen from infarcts affecting the anterior horns and corticospinal tracts.

Brown-Séquard syndrome, or hemisection of the spinal cord, is a characteristic syndrome in which there is loss of pain and temperature sensation contralateral to the side of the lesion due to interruption of the crossed spinothalamic tract. There is also ipsilateral loss of proprioception and vibration sensation below the level of the lesion from interruption of the ipsilateral posterior columns, as well as ipsilateral weakness below the lesion from corticospinal tract involvement.

Blumenfeld H. Neuronatomy through Clinical Cases, 1st ed. Sunderland, MA: Sinauer Associates; 2002.

Ropper AH, Samuels MA. Adams and Victor's Principles of Neurology, 9th ed. New York: McGraw-Hill; 2009.

22. c

Neoplasms of the spinal cord can be divided into primary or metastatic. Also they can be divided anatomically into extradural, intradural extramedullary, and intradural intramedullary.

Primary neoplasms accounting for intramedullary spinal cord metastases include small cell lung cancer, breast cancer, renal cell cancer, lymphoma, and melanoma. However, metastatic intramedullary disease is not very common, and primary intramedullary tumors are more frequent.

Meningioma is a common intradural extramedullary tumor, which has predilection for the thoracic spine, and with its growth can produce spinal cord compression. Nerve sheath tumors such as schwannomas and neurofibromas are also intradural and extramedullary.

The most frequent intradural intramedullary tumors found include ependymoma and astrocytoma. Astrocytomas are most common in children and are usually slow-growing low-grade tumors. Ependymomas are the most common intramedullary tumors in adults, usually arising from the central canal and expanding outward. Myxopapillary ependymoma is a type of ependymoma that arises from the ependymal cells in the filum terminale, and is the most common tumor in this location.

Fenichel GM. Clinical Pediatric Neurology: A Signs and Symptoms Approach, 6th ed. Philadelphia, PA: Saunders Elsevier; 2009.

Ropper AH, Samuels MA. Adams and Victor's Principles of Neurology, 9th ed. New York: McGraw-Hill; 2009.

23. b

This patient has an acute neurologic disorder temporally associated with a recent febrile illness, with findings suggestive of an inflammatory myelopathy and encephalopathy. At the time of presentation, the illness was apparently monophasic, with symmetric involvement of cerebral white matter and simultaneous spinal cord involvement. CSF findings support an inflammatory cause. In this case the most likely explanation for her clinical picture is acute disseminated encephalomyelitis (ADEM).

ADEM is an inflammatory demyelinating disorder of childhood in which there is a monophasic immunologic reaction to a viral illness. Patients have an encephalopathy, with confluent white matter changes on MRI and inflammatory markers in the CSF. Occasionally, the spinal cord is also affected with features of a transverse myelitis, in which the lesion affects more than three segments of the spinal cord. The treatment is intravenous steroids in high doses.

Encephalopathy is not a feature of neuromyelitis optica; the patient may have some white matter lesions, but in contrast to ADEM, they are not symmetric or confluent.

Multiple sclerosis is an inflammatory demyelinating disorder that presents with a relapsing and remitting or a progressive course. When it affects the spinal cord, the lesions are usually in short segments, not like in this case. Acute encephalopathy is not common in multiple sclerosis.

The diagnosis of idiopathic transverse myelitis is made when the patient has a transverse myelitis with no other explanation, and usually without other features. This patient has encephalopathy and white matter brain lesions, making transverse myelitis unlikely.

The clinical, imaging, and CSF findings do not correlate with bacterial meningitis.

Fenichel GM. Clinical Pediatric Neurology: A Signs and Symptoms Approach, 6th ed. Philadelphia, PA: Saunders Elsevier; 2009.

Ropper AH, Samuels MA. Adams and Victor's Principles of Neurology, 9th ed. New York: McGraw-Hill; 2009.

24. d

Horner's syndrome is seen in patients with spinal cord lesions above T1, where the spinal sympathetic tract synapses before exiting the spinal cord (discussed in Chapters 1 and 10). This patient has a lesion above T1, and will likely have a Horner's syndrome.

As shown in Figure 11.4, this patient has an intramedullary lesion producing signal abnormality in the cervical cord from C1 to C6. Because the lesion has developed gradually, the patient will likely have myelopathic findings with upper motor neuron manifestations below the lesion. Therefore, the patient will likely have increased tone with spasticity and hyperreflexia below the level of the lesion. Some cases will demonstrate lower motor neuron findings at the same level of the lesion due to involvement of anterior horn cells, in this case probably in the upper extremities. A sensory level is helpful for clinical localization of the level of the lesion. The level of the nipple line correlates with T4. Other levels that are useful landmarks are the base of the neck (C4), umbilicus (T10), groin (L1), and anal region (S5). In this case the lesion is in the cervical region; therefore, the patient's sensory level is likely above the nipple line. The presence of superficial abdominal reflexes is a normal finding, and their absence indicates a corticospinal tract lesion above the T6 segment.

Blumenfeld H. Neuroanatomy through Clinical Cases, 1st ed. Sunderland, MA: Sinauer Associates; 2002.

25. c

The ligaments between the atlas and the axis, as well as the odontoid process, are important in maintaining the stability of this articulation. When this articulation fails, or the odontoid is absent or damaged, atlantoaxial dislocation can occur, leading to neck pain and other manifestations of spinal cord compression including quadriplegia and death.

Rheumatoid arthritis is known to produce a destructive inflammatory process of the ligaments that attach the odontoid process to the atlas and the skull, therefore causing atlantoaxial dislocation.

Other causes of this condition include Klippel-Feil syndrome, Down's syndrome, and Morquio syndrome. Klippel-Feil syndrome is a condition in which there is decreased number and abnormal fusion of cervical vertebrae. Morquio syndrome is a skeletal disease in which the odontoid process may be aplastic or absent, leading to secondary spinal cord disease.

Systemic lupus erythematosus has been associated with syndromes consistent with myelitis or myelopathy, but not atlantoaxial dislocation.

Fenichel GM. Clinical Pediatric Neurology: A Signs and Symptoms Approach, 6th ed. Philadelphia, PA: Saunders Elsevier; 2009.

Ropper AH, Samuels MA. Adams and Victor's Principles of Neurology, 9th ed. New York: McGraw-Hill; 2009.

26. C

Neoplastic disease of the spinal cord can be intrinsic to the cord or metastatic disease. Tumors affecting the spinal column and spinal cord can be anatomically divided into extradural or intradural, the latter further classified into intramedullary or extramedullary. All of these tumors can also be divided into metastatic or nonmetastatic disease. The most common nonmetastatic extramedullary tumors include neurofibromas, schwannomas, and meningiomas. The most frequent nonmetastatic intramedullary tumors are spinal cord astrocytomas and ependymomas.

Metastatic disease to the spinal cord most commonly originates from breast, lung, prostate, and kidney cancer, although it is not limited to these. Other invading neoplastic lesions include lymphoma and multiple myeloma.

Spinal cord neoplastic disease usually presents with pain and focal neurologic manifestations resulting from spinal cord compression or dysfunction. Patients have findings consistent with myelopathy, along with other manifestations of the underlying cancer.

The diagnostic test of choice to determine the presence of neoplastic disease is MRI of the spinal cord with gadolinium.

There are multiple treatment options that are selected depending on the underlying neoplasm, degree of neurologic disease, timing of presentation, functional status, and prognosis. Steroids are frequently used, especially in the acute phase of cord compression, with dexamethasone being the most commonly used. Methylprednisolone with a 30 mg/kg bolus and an infusion of 5.4 mg/kg/hour for 23 hours is a formulation used more commonly in spinal cord traumatic injury, but not for neoplastic disease.

Radiation therapy is used for radiosensitive neoplasias, such as lymphoproliferative disease and germ cell tumors, and for various types of metastases, particularly in the setting of cord compression. It may be used as a palliative measure to improve symptoms of pain and other symptoms of cord compression.

Surgical resection should be entertained when feasible, even in cases of metastatic disease, where it has shown superiority when combined with radiotherapy as compared to radiotherapy alone. However surgical treatments may not be possible in some neoplasms, such as in intramedullary lesions.

Bradley WG, Daroff RB, Fenichel GM, et al. Neurology in Clinical Practice, 5th ed. Philadelphia, PA: Elsevier; 2008.

Ecker RD, Endo T, Wetjen NM, et al. Diagnosis and treatment of vertebral column metastases. Mayo Clinic Proc. 2005; 80:1177–1186.

Ropper AH, Samuels MA. Adams and Victor's Principles of Neurology, 9th ed. New York: McGraw-Hill; 2009.

27. e

Spinal cord trauma is a significant cause of myelopathy and common cause of severe disability after trauma, especially in young adults. Trauma produces spinal cord injury by multiple mechanisms, including direct transection of the cord, displacement of spinal column structures, disruption of axons, interruption of blood flow to the cord, hemorrhage, inflammation, and/or edema.

After spinal cord injury there are two phases: an initial phase of spinal shock followed by a second phase of increased reflex activity with spasticity. The acute spinal shock phase occurs soon after the injury and lasts for a few weeks (between 1 and 6, but with no exact limits). It is manifested by suppression of spinal segmental activity below the level of the lesion. With complete spinal cord injury, the patient has a flaccid weakness with areflexia below the lesion, atonic bladder with overflow incontinence, distention of the bowel with absence of peristalsis and constipation, depressed rectal tone, and abolished genital reflexes. There is autonomic dysfunction below the lesion explaining the labile blood pressure seen in these cases.

A few weeks after spinal cord injury, the patient will start presenting features of increased reflexic activity below the lesion. There is no clear chronologic boundary between this stage and the previous one of spinal shock. In this second stage, there are upper motor neuron findings with increased tone, leading to spasticity and hyperreflexia. Plantar responses are upgoing; triple flexion response commonly occurs. Patients will have detrusor spasms and hyperactivity with urinary loss secondary to spontaneous bladder contraction as well as spontaneous reflex defecation. These bladder and bowel reflexes are probably explained by the lack of inhibition of the sacral neurons by rostral centers, leading to spontaneous contraction secondary to a local reflex arc. Neither spontaneous reflex defecation nor detrusor contraction are present in the spinal shock phase.

Ropper AH, Samuels MA. Adams and Victor's Principles of Neurology, 9th ed. New York: McGraw-Hill; 2009.

28. e

Superficial siderosis of the CNS is the result of hemosiderin deposition in the subpial layers of the brain and spinal cord, which is secondary to recurrent bleeding into the subarachnoid space. The bleeding source is undetermined in most cases. Some risk factors have been reported, such as previous subarachnoid hemorrhage, head trauma, and previous intradural surgery; however, the significance of these historical aspects is not clear.

The most common manifestations include gait ataxia, dysarthria, and sensorineural hearing loss. Other clinical manifestations include anosmia, cognitive decline, and myelopathic findings. Xanthochromia and/or the presence of red blood cells is a common CSF finding. MRI shows T2 hypointensity around the brain, brain stem, and spinal cord, and sometimes intraspinal fluid collections are detected.

If a possible etiology for the recurrent bleeding is found, endovascular or surgical repair may be entertained; however, it is unclear if this approach has a significant impact on progression of the disease.

Kumar N, Cohen-Gadol AA, Wright RA, et al. Superficial siderosis. Neurology. 2006; 66:1144–1152.

29. a

Syphilis is caused by the spirochete *Treponema pallidum* and is associated with a wide variety of neurologic manifestations. Myelopathy is frequently encountered and can be produced by various mechanisms, including spinal cord infarction. Tabes dorsalis is the classic myelopathic syndrome described in neurosyphilis.

Tabes dorsalis is characterized by dysfunction of the posterior columns with prominent sensory ataxia and proprioceptive loss, along with other manifestations such as sphincter dysfunction, L'hermitte's sign, lancinating pain, and areflexia.

The natural history of tabes dorsalis has been described in three different phases:

- The preataxic phase in which the patient has lancinating pain of his legs, along with sphincter and sexual dysfunction
- The ataxic phase with prominent proprioceptive loss, sensory ataxia leading to the development of Charcot joints
- The postataxic or paralytic phase characterized by spastic paraparesis, autonomic dysfunction, worsening of the pain and sphincter dysfunction, and cachexia

Pathologic findings demonstrate inflammation, demyelination, and gliosis of the posterior columns and dorsal roots of the spinal cord.

Syphilis can also produce spinal cord disease by other mechanisms, such as spinal cord infarction from vasculitis, meningomyelitis manifested as an inflammatory transverse myelitis, hypertrophic pachymeningitis, and gummas, which can be intramedullary or extramedullary.

The treatment of neurosyphilis is penicillin G intravenously, with a dose of 24 million units daily in divided doses for 14 days.

Ropper AH, Samuels MA. Adams and Victor's Principles of Neurology, 9th ed. New York: McGraw-Hill; 2009.

30. a

The conus medullaris is at the lower end of the spinal cord, beyond which the lumbar and sacral spinal nerve roots descend within the spinal canal as a bundle of fibers, called the cauda equina (meaning horse's tail), to reach their corresponding exit foramina. Lesions in the lumbar or lumbosacral region can compress either the conus medullaris and/or the cauda equina, producing a distinctive clinical syndrome.

A lesion affecting primarily the conus medullaris presents with perineal sensory deficit in a saddle distribution, which is usually bilateral and symmetric. Pain is often symmetric, but is not typically radicular. There is usually lower extremity symmetric weakness and sometimes decreased or absent ankle reflexes, but this may be mild. Bowel and bladder dysfunction occur early in the course of the disease, as well as sexual dysfunction.

A lesion that affects the cauda equina presents with distinctive radicular pain and sensory loss with an asymmetric distribution. Motor deficits are also asymmetric with evidence of hyporeflexia. Bowel and bladder function may be affected, but usually this occurs later in the course and less frequently than with conus lesions. Spasticity and other upper motor neuron signs will not be present as this is a lower motor neuron disorder.

This patient has features of cauda equina syndrome. This condition is produced by compression or irritation of the fibers, with causes including disc herniations, tumors, hematomas, or trauma, as well as infectious and inflammatory disorders (e.g., tuberculosis, cytomegalovirus, and sarcoidosis). There are no clinical features to suggest an intramedullary tumor, transverse myelitis, or an epidural hematoma.

Brazis PW, Masdeu JC, Biller J. Localization in Clinical Neurology, 5th ed. Philadelphia, PA: Lippincott Williams & Wilkins; 2007.

Ropper AH, Samuels MA. Adams and Victor's Principles of Neurology, 9th ed. New York: McGraw-Hill; 2009.

31. e

The diagnosis of amyotrophic lateral sclerosis (ALS) is made on the basis of the history, examination, and electrophysiologic testing. The El-Escorial diagnostic criteria for definite ALS as defined by the World Federation of Neurology include clinical and/or electrophysiologic evidence of both upper and lower motor neuron involvement in at least three of the four following regions: bulbar, cervical, thoracic, and lumbosacral.

Electrodiagnostic features of ALS include evidence of ongoing denervation indicated by the presence of spontaneous activity (fibrillation potentials) and chronic denervation (reduced recruitment and polyphasic motor units). Other variable features include fasciculation potentials and motor unit instability (variability of motor unit amplitude and presence of repetitive discharges). Reduced motor unit recruitment with a rapid firing rate on EMG reflects compensation of existing motor units for those that are no longer functional, and only a single motor unit may be seen to be activated during voluntary contraction in a severely denervated muscle. Sensory NCS are normal. EMG/NCS is indicated in the evaluation of a patient with suspected ALS, and should include evaluation of cervical, thoracic, and lumbosacral regions routinely, and of bulbar region when clinically affected.

The differential diagnosis of ALS is broad, and investigations into alternative, especially treatable, causes are indicated when there are features suggesting the possibility of another diagnosis. In the evaluation of an ALS patient, laboratory and imaging studies are done as indicated to exclude mimickers of ALS. There are a variety of other disorders that lead to clinical signs and symptoms of both upper and lower motor neuron involvement that are on the differential diagnosis of ALS, including Machado-Joseph disease (spinocerebellar ataxia type 3), adrenoleukodystrophy, multifocal motor neuropathy, hyperparathyroidism, cervical spondylosis, GM2 gangliosidoses, polyglucosan body disease, paraneoplastic motor neuron disease, HIV-associated motor neuron disease, West Nile virus infection, and others. Laboratory tests may include evaluation of parathyroid hormone, paraneoplastic autoantibodies (such as anti-Hu), GM1 autoantibodies, and others depending on the suspicion. MRI of the brain and spinal cord are indicated to exclude other potential causes masquerading clinically as ALS, such as cervical spondylosis. MRI in ALS may show increased signal in the corticospinal tract on T2-, proton density-, and FLAIR-weighted images, possibly due to Wallerian degeneration.

Bradley WG, Daroff RB, Fenichel GM, et al. Neurology in Clinical Practice, 5th ed. Philadelphia, PA: Elsevier; 2008.

32. a

Copper is a trace element that functions as a prosthetic group in metalloenzymes that have a role in maintaining the structure and function of the CNS. Copper deficiency causes a myelopathy similar to that seen in vitamin B_{12} deficiency. It also produces multiple other neurologic manifestations, including peripheral neuropathy, CNS demyelination, myopathy, and optic neuropathy. Hematologic manifestations are also seen in copper deficiency, with anemia, neutropenia, and left shift in granulocytic and erythroid maturation. MRI of the spine may show T2-signal hyperintensity in the paramedian cord, most frequently in the cervical region.

Copper deficiency results from malabsorption, one of the most common causes being previous gastric surgery, especially bariatric surgery for weight loss. It is frequent to find vitamin B_{12} deficiency along with copper deficiency, and in most cases in clinical practice, vitamin B_{12} is supplemented, whereas copper is usually overlooked. Lack of improvement with vitamin B_{12} supplementation should prompt evaluation for copper deficiency.

Excessive zinc ingestion may also contribute to copper deficiency, because zinc induces the synthesis of metallothionein in enterocytes, which has a high affinity to copper, leading to internalization of copper into the enterocytes and its eventual loss when they are sloughed off from the mucosa.

Kumar N. Copper deficiency myelopathy (Human Swayback). Mayo Clin Proc. 2006; 81(10): 1371–1384.

Ropper AH, Samuels MA. Adams and Victor's Principles of Neurology, 9th ed. New York: McGraw-Hill; 2009.

33. e

This patient's history and examination are consistent with Kennedy's disease (X-linked spinobulbar muscular atrophy). Kennedy's disease typically presents in males beginning the fourth decade of life. The clinical presentation includes motor weakness often starting in proximal muscles associated with features of lower motor neuron dysfunction, such as atrophy and hyporeflexia. Tremor, muscle cramps, and fasciculations, particularly involving the face and perioral region, are other features. Later in the course of the disease, evidence of bulbar dysfunction becomes apparent. Examination may reveal gynecomastia, but its absence does not preclude this diagnosis. Endocrine abnormalities, including hypogonadism with sterility and diabetes, occur in some patients. This disorder rarely manifests in females, likely due to random X-inactivation, but has been reported, presenting with bulbar dysfunction. Kennedy's disease results from expansion of a CAG repeat in the androgen receptor protein gene on the X chromosome. Genetic testing for this disorder is commercially available. Treatment is supportive.

Bradley WG, Daroff RB, Fenichel GM, et al. Neurology in Clinical Practice, 5th ed. Philadelphia, PA: Elsevier; 2008.

34. b

The spinal cord lies dorsal to the posterior longitudinal ligament.

The vertebral column is composed of vertebral bodies, pedicles, and laminae. Two pedicles arise from the posterior aspect of each vertebral body. Two laminae fuse posteriorly leaving the spinal canal in the middle within which the spinal cord lies. Multiple ligaments attach and give support to the vertebral column. The anterior longitudinal ligament runs along the anterior surface of the vertebral bodies, whereas the posterior longitudinal ligament runs along the posterior surface and ventral to the spinal cord. The ligamentum flavum runs in the posterior aspect of the spinal canal, and the denticulate ligament extends on both sides of the spinal cord between the pia mater and the dura mater. Between each vertebral body there is an intervertebral disc, which is composed of a central nucleus pulposus and a surrounding annulus fibrosus.

The spinal cord has 31 segments and a corresponding number of pairs of spinal nerve roots, with 8 cervical, 12 thoracic, 5 lumbar, 5 sacral, and 1 coccygeal. The cervical nerve roots exit the spinal column above the vertebral body of the same number, except for C8, which exit between the C7 and T1 intervertebral foramen. The subsequent nerve roots below this level exit the spinal column below the corresponding vertebral body.

In adults, the spinal cord extends from the foramen magnum to the level of L1 to L2. It has two major enlargements, one in the cervical region and another one in the lumbosacral region. These enlargements correlate with the areas related to innervation of the arms and legs.

Blumenfeld H. Neuronatomy through Clinical Cases, 1st ed. Sunderland, MA: Sinauer Associates; 2002.

Ropper AH, Samuels MA. Adams and Victor's Principles of Neurology, 9th ed. New York: McGraw-Hill; 2009.

35. a

This patient's history and muscle biopsy are consistent with spinal muscular atrophy (SMA) type 1. The SMAs are a group of four disorders of anterior horn cell degeneration. SMA type 1, infantile SMA, or Werdnig-Hoffman disease presents with decreased fetal movements, neonatal hypotonia, and weak cry. Patients with SMA type 1 exhibit head lag and frog-leg posture when supine, and are never able to sit up or achieve anti-gravity strength in the arms or legs. Diffuse areflexia is often present. Bulbar involvement leads to dysphagia, and respiratory involvement occurs. Death usually occurs by 2 years of age.

In SMA type 2, intermediate SMA, symptoms begin in the first 1 to 2 years of life, with motor delay and tremor in some cases. This form is less severe than SMA type 1, with most children being able to sit unsupported, but significant contractures develop, and most are not able to ambulate.

SMA type 3, juvenile SMA or Kugelberg-Welander disease, typically presents in childhood (between ages 5 and 15 years) with difficulty walking. The clinical picture is one of proximal muscle weakness, a fine action tremor, and fasciculations. Patients often remain ambulatory into adulthood.

SMA type 4, adult-onset SMA or pseudomyopathic SMA, is the least common and least severe. Symptoms typically begin in the third to fourth decades of life and include proximal muscle weakness, with the quadriceps being prominently involved, and fasciculations. Ambulation into late adulthood is common. Cranial nerve and respiratory involvement is rare.

Commercially available molecular analysis of the survival motor neuron (SMN) gene is available. Serum creatine kinase may be significantly elevated (more than 10 times normal), particularly in the younger-onset forms. Sensory NCS are normal; EMG shows evidence of acute and chronic denervation and reinnervation, with large polyphasic motor units. Complex repetitive discharges occur in SMA type 3. Muscle biopsy shows atrophy of the entire fascicles or groups of fascicles, with normal or hypertrophied neighboring fascicles, as depicted in Figure 11.5.

The majority of cases of SMA are due to mutations in the SMN1 gene on chromosome 5. Inheritance is autosomal recessive in most cases, though a minority of cases involving other genes with autosomal dominant or X-linked inheritance have been identified. The gene product, SMN1 protein, is involved in RNA processing. In later-onset forms, some residual functional protein is present, leading to the milder phenotype.

As mentioned, SMA type 4 presents in adulthood. Charcot-Marie-Tooth type 1 typically presents in childhood (rather than the neonatal period), and will not be associated with the muscle biopsy findings shown in Figure 11.5. Congenital myasthenia and botulism are on the differential diagnosis of neonatal hypotonia but would not lead to the muscle biopsy findings shown in Figure 11.5.

Aminoff MJ. Neurology and General Medicine, 4th ed. Philadelphia, PA: Elsevier; 2008.

Bradley WG, Daroff RB, Fenichel GM, et al. Neurology in Clinical Practice, 5th ed. Philadelphia, PA: Elsevier; 2008.

36. e

This patient has nitrous oxide toxicity, causing a neurologic manifestation that has been termed "anesthesia paresthetica." Nitrous oxide is an inhalational anesthetic agent that produces irreversible oxidation of cobalamin and makes the methylcobalamin inactive. The manifestations occur in patients with underlying cobalamin deficiency even after a single exposure to nitrous oxide, usually with a rapid onset of symptoms. However, chronic exposure can lead to similar manifestations, and this has been described among anesthetists, dentists, or medical personnel working with nitrous oxide, either from occupational exposure or from abuse. Patients with chronic exposure can have an acute exacerbation during an acute exposure to larger amounts of nitrous oxide.

The neurologic manifestations include myelopathy, neuropathy, or even cognitive changes and encephalopathy. MRI changes with T2 hyperintensity can be detected. Prophylactic vitamin B_{12} can help prevent this condition.

This patient does not have copper deficiency, which usually produces a more protracted course, usually related to malabsorption. In cases of malabsorption after gastric bypass, the manifestations usually occur gradually over months or years. Folate deficiency causes neurologic manifestations in very rare instances, and usually gradually over long periods of time in patients who have other nutrient deficiencies.

In cases of spinal epidural abscess or hematomas causing myelopathy, the MRI images usually are distinct, showing spinal cord compression, which is not the case in this patient.

Kinsella LJ, Green R. "Anesthesia paresthetica": Nitrous oxide-induced cobalamin deficiency. Neurology. 1995; 45:1608–1610.

Kumar N. Copper deficiency myelopathy (Human Swayback). Mayo Clin Proc. 2006; 81:1371–1384.

Ropper AH, Samuels MA. Adams and Victor's Principles of Neurology, 9th ed. New York: McGraw-Hill; 2009.

37. c

This patient has Hirayama disease, also known as monomelic amyotrophy. This condition presents in young patients of Asian origin, and it is characterized by progressive asymmetric wasting of one or both hands and forearms. Examination shows atrophy and fasciculations with no sensory deficits. These patients have a high incidence of atopic disorders. The pathophysiology is not understood, but some have suggested a chronic progressive compression of the cervical cord, associated with dynamic changes of the cervical dural sac and spinal cord induced by neck flexion. MRI of the cervical spine in flexion demonstrates cervical cord thinning with signal changes. A cervical collar may be used to prevent neck flexion, and surgical intervention may have an impact in some patients.

Amyotrophic lateral sclerosis (ALS) is a progressive degenerative motor neuron disease in which there are upper and lower motor neuron signs in multiple segments of the neuraxis. This patient has only lower motor neuron findings in his upper extremities, which is usually not consistent with ALS.

Primary lateral sclerosis is a disorder in which the predominant feature is the presence of upper motor neuron signs, without lower motor neuron signs, which is not consistent with the case depicted.

Spinal muscular atrophy is a group of genetic disorders that affect the anterior horn cells of the spinal cord and motor nuclei of the brain stem. Usually there are findings affecting upper and lower limbs, as well as bulbar muscles.

This patient is not in the age group and does not have other clinical features to suggest the diagnosis of cervical osteoarthritis.

Fenichel GM. Clinical Pediatric Neurology: A Signs and Symptoms Approach, 6th ed. Philadelphia, PA: Saunders Elsevier; 2009.

Hirayama K. Juvenile muscular atrophy of distal upper extremity (Hirayama disease). Inter Med. 2000; 39:283–290.

Ropper AH, Samuels MA. Adams and Victor's Principles of Neurology, 9th ed. New York: McGraw-Hill; 2009.

38. e

This patient has a spinal cord infarction in the territory of the anterior spinal artery. The spinal cord's blood supply consists of one anterior spinal artery and two posterior spinal arteries. The former supplies the anterior two-thirds of the spinal cord, whereas the two posterior spinal arteries supply the posterior one-third. Therefore patients with an anterior spinal artery syndrome present with weakness below the lesion, with sensory deficit to pain and temperature due to involvement of the lateral spinothalamic tracts, but because the dorsal columns are not involved, there is preservation of vibratory sense and proprioception.

Spinal cord infarction may occur after aortic aneurysm surgical repair. Endovascular approaches have a lower rate of overall complications as compared to open surgical approaches, including lower rates of spinal cord ischemia.

In this case there is no history or clinical findings to support a spinal epidural hematoma as the cause. Patients with copper and vitamin B_{12} deficiency usually present rather gradually and not rapidly as in this case. Furthermore, vitamin B_{12} deficiency is associated with posterior column degeneration affecting proprioception and vibratory sensation, which was not present in this case. Patients with vitamin B_{12} deficiency are at risk for nitrous oxide toxicity.

Ropper AH, Samuels MA. Adams and Victor's Principles of Neurology, 9th ed. New York: McGraw-Hill; 2009.

39. d

This patient most likely has a spinal epidural abscess. This condition occurs when an infectious process extends into the epidural space, either from local extension or from a remote source via hematogenous spread. Risk factors include diabetes mellitus, intravenous drug use, previous infection, history of spine injury or spine surgery, renal disease, and multiple medical comorbidities. The most common presenting symptoms are fever, low back pain, and progressive neurologic symptoms attributed to cord or root compression. Myelopathic findings develop over time, and patients may have upper motor neuron findings below the level of the lesion. Sometimes the patient worsens rapidly and examination may show findings of spinal shock. The symptoms may ascend over time as the epidural abscess propagates cranially.

MRI of the spine is the standard test for diagnosis and has high sensitivity. An LP is not usually performed, and may be contraindicated due to risk of spread of infection to the intrathecal compartment. Furthermore, CSF cultures are positive only in 25% of cases.

The most common organism is *S. aureus*, followed by streptococci, gram-negative bacilli, and anaerobic organisms. Empiric broad-spectrum antibiotics should be started early, with narrowing of the spectrum once a specific organism is identified. The usual duration of antibiotic therapy is between 4 and 6 weeks; however, antibiotics alone may not be effective. Once this condition is suspected, urgent neurosurgical consultation should be obtained. If the patient has findings of cord compression, surgical evacuation should be performed. Epidural spinal abscess is a true neurosurgical and neurologic emergency.

Ropper AH, Samuels MA. Adams and Victor's Principles of Neurology, 9th ed. New York: McGraw-Hill; 2009.

Buzz Phrases	Key Points
Motor neuron disease with both upper and lower motor neuron involvement	Amyotrophic lateral sclerosis
Survival motor neuron 1 gene	Spinal muscular atrophy
Motor neuron diseases with only lower motor neuron involvement	Progressive muscular atrophy, spinal muscular atrophy, benign focal amyotrophy
Subacute combined degeneration of the spinal cord	Vitamin B_{12} deficiency
Post-gastric bypass neurologic syndrome	Copper deficiency
Anterior two-thirds of the spinal cord	Anterior spinal artery
Posterior third of the spinal cord	Posterior spinal arteries
Aquaporin-4	Neuromyelitis optica (Devic's disease)
Nitrous oxide toxicity	Anesthesia paresthetica, associated with vitamin B_{12} depletion
HIV-related myelopathy	Vacuolar myelopathy
Large radicular artery supplying lower thoracic and upper lumbar region	Adamkiewicz
Ipsilateral loss of motor function and sensation to vibration and proprioception below the level of the lesion, with contralateral loss of sensation to pain and temperature	Brown-Séquard syndrome
Tabes dorsalis	Syphilis
Adrenomyeloneuropathy: gene, chromosome	*ABCD1* gene on chromosome Xq28
Epidural lipomatosis	Chronic steroid use

Chapter 12

Cognitive and Behavioral Neurology

Questions

Questions 1–2

1. A 77-year-old man presents to the office with a complaint of difficulty remembering things such as names and directions. His wife has noticed this more than he has. He denies any other cognitive complaints and his memory impairment has not interfered with his daily activities. On examination, you note that he recalls zero out of three objects on the Mini-Mental Status Examination at 5 minutes, and his Mini-Mental Status Examination score is 27. Which of the following is the most likely diagnosis?
    a. Alzheimer's disease
    b. Mild cognitive impairment
    c. FTD
    d. Normal aging
    e. DLB

2. Your suspected diagnosis for the patient depicted in question 1 is defined by impairment in:
    a. One or more cognitive domains
    b. Two or more cognitive domains
    c. Three or more cognitive domains
    d. Four or more cognitive domains
    e. Five or more cognitive domains

Questions 3–6

3. A 60-year-old man is brought to your office by his daughter and wife because of prominent memory loss, several recent automobile accidents near his home, and lack of insight regarding these recent events. There is a family history of early dementia in his uncle. You decide to proceed with an evaluation. According to the American Academy of Neurology guidelines, which of the following is not recommended in the routine evaluation of patients presenting with dementia?

a. Vitamin B$_{12}$
b. Complete blood count
c. VDRL
d. Depression screening
e. Electrolytes

4. You suspect that the patient depicted in question 3 has Alzheimer's disease. With that in mind, which chromosome is linked to presenilin-2?
   a. 14
   b. 1
   c. 21
   d. 19
   e. 2

5. Which of the following is not a structure involved in the formation of new memories within the circuit of Papez?
   a. Hippocampus
   b. Mamillary bodies
   c. Fornix
   d. Mediodorsal nucleus of the thalamus
   e. Entorhinal cortex

6. Which of the following symptoms is typically the earliest symptom of Alzheimer's disease?
   a. Immediate memory impairment
   b. Recent memory impairment
   c. Remote memory impairment
   d. Procedural memory impairment
   e. Apraxia

Questions 7–9

7. A 74-year-old woman is brought to your office for memory problems and neuropsychiatric symptoms. An FDG-PET scan was completed, which is shown in Figure 12.1. What diagnosis do you suspect on the basis of this?
   a. Parkinson's disease
   b. Alzheimer's disease
   c. DLB
   d. FTD
   e. Huntington's disease

8. On the basis of your suspected diagnosis in question 7, which of the following would be the least commonly associated histopathologic finding in the brain of this patient?
   a. Neurofibrillary tangles and neuritic plaques
   b. Amyloid deposition in cortical and leptomeningeal blood vessel walls
   c. Lewy bodies
   d. Granulovacuolar neuronal degeneration
   e. Hirano bodies

9. In the neurodegenerative disease suspected in the patient depicted in question 7, there is loss of cholinergic neurons in which of the following structures?

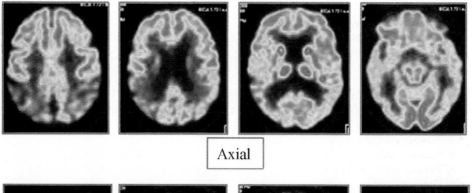

Axial

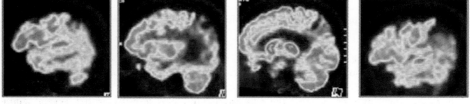

Sagittal

FIGURE 12.1 Axial and sagittal FDG-PET (Courtesy of Dr. Guiyun Wu). Shown also in color plates

a. Locus coeruleus
b. Raphe nuclei
c. Nucleus accumbens
d. Substantia nigra pars reticulata
e. Nucleus basalis of Meynert (substantia innominata)

Questions 10–11

10. A 78-year-old man is seen in the office, brought in by nursing home personnel for progressively worsening agitation and other neurologic features. On the basis of your findings and history provided, you diagnose DLB. The three primary clinical findings in DLB are:
    a. Parkinsonism, impaired memory, visual hallucinations
    b. Visual hallucinations, aphasia, parkinsonism
    c. Fluctuating cognitive function, parkinsonism, aggression
    d. Parkinsonism, fluctuating cognitive function, visual hallucinations
    e. Visual hallucinations, auditory hallucinations, fluctuating cognitive function

11. Which of the following medications would not be recommended to treat severe agitated psychotic symptoms in this patient?
    a. Quetiapine
    b. Risperidone
    c. Haloperidol
    d. Olanzapine
    e. Clozapine

12. Depression is least likely to be seen in:
    a. Alzheimer's disease
    b. Parkinson's disease
    c. Huntington's disease
    d. Multiple sclerosis
    e. Pick's disease

13. Impairment in which of the following structures would be least likely to be associated with personality changes?
    a. Orbitofrontal cortex
    b. Temporal lobe
    c. Dorsolateral frontal lobe
    d. Occipital lobe
    e. Caudate nucleus

Questions 14–15

14. A 59-year-old woman is brought to your office by her family for progressively offensive speech, inappropriate behavior, and impaired social functioning over the past year. She pays no attention to her personal hygiene and sometimes urinates in her pants without even noticing anything is wrong. Her family reports that these behaviors are highly unusual for her. Several family members have reportedly been diagnosed with FTD. Given a possible case of familial FTD, which chromosome may be involved?
    a. 14
    b. 17
    c. 19
    d. 21
    e. 1

15. Regarding FTD, which of the following is not commonly associated with one of the FTD variants?
    a. Anomia
    b. Motor neuron disease
    c. Progressive supranuclear palsy
    d. Corticobasal degeneration
    e. Visual hallucinations

16. The FDG-PET scan in Figures 12.2 and 12.3 are suggestive of which neurodegenerative disease?
    a. Parkinson's disease
    b. Alzheimer's disease
    c. DLB
    d. FTD
    e. Huntington's disease

17. A 65-year-old woman presents with abrupt onset akinetic mutism, lack of motivation, apathy, leg weakness, and incontinence. You suspect she may have had a stroke. Which of the following could explain her symptoms?
    a. Pontine infarct
    b. Dominant temporal lobe infarct
    c. Nondominant parietal lobe infarct

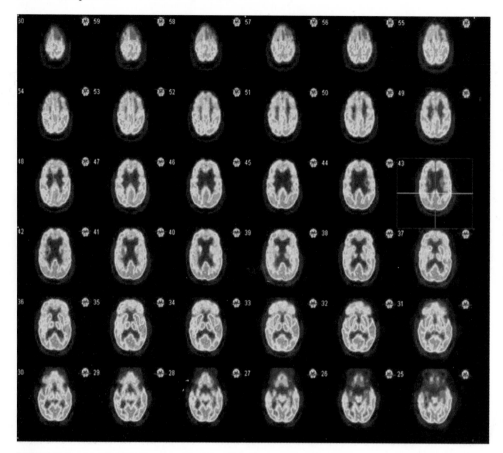

FIGURE 12.2 Axial FDG-PET (Courtesy of Dr. Guiyun Wu). Shown also in color plates

d. Nondominant temporal lobe infarct
e. Bilateral ACA infarcts

18. Lesions in which thalamic nucleus would most likely cause symptoms of abulia, anterograde amnesia, social disinhibition, and motivation loss?
    a. Anterior nucleus
    b. Ventral posteromedial nucleus
    c. Pulvinar nucleus
    d. Dorsomedial nucleus
    e. Ventral posterolateral nucleus

19. Akinetic mutism can be caused by lesions to which of the following structures?
    a. Bilateral globus pallidus interna
    b. Bilateral globus pallidus externa
    c. Bilateral putamen
    d. Bilateral caudate
    e. Bilateral amygdala

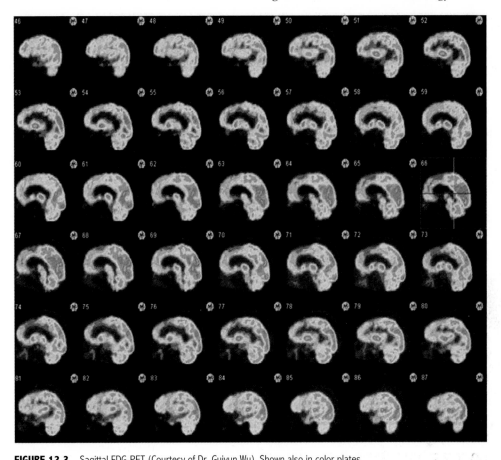

FIGURE 12.3   Sagittal FDG-PET (Courtesy of Dr. Guiyun Wu). Shown also in color plates

20. Huntington's disease is a neurodegenerative disease resulting from genetic changes to which chromosome?
   a. 14
   b. 4
   c. 17
   d. 21
   e. 19

21. Features of Kluver-Bucy syndrome may occur as part of which of the following neurodegenerative disorders?
   a. Alzheimer's disease
   b. Schizophrenia
   c. DLB
   d. Pick's disease
   e. Parkinson's disease

22. In traumatic brain injury, which of the following signs or symptoms is most likely to persist and interfere with rehabilitation?
a. Memory loss
b. Motor deficit
c. Altered personality
d. Sensory deficit
e. Language dysfunction

23. You are consulted on a 39-year-old woman for significant memory loss following an uncomplicated medical procedure. You suspect transient global amnesia. This disorder typically affects what aspect of memory?
a. Immediate memory
b. Procedural memory
c. Recent (short-term) memory
d. Remote memory
e. Personal identity

Questions 24–26

24. A 79-year-old man is brought to your office by his daughter. She says he has been getting increasingly confused, although his periods of confusion seem to fluctuate. Some days he seems much better than others. He often complains that there are squirrels and rodents in his bedroom. On examination, he appears bradykinetic, and you notice a fine resting tremor in both hands. What is your suspected diagnosis?
a. Progressive supranuclear palsy
b. Alzheimer's disease
c. Pick's disease
d. DLB
e. Parkinson's disease

25. What would you expect to find on an FDG-PET scan in the patient depicted in question 24?
a. Occipital hypometabolism > temporoparietal hypometabolism
b. Occipital hypometabolism < temporoparietal hypometabolism
c. Frontotemporal hypometabolism > temporoparietal hypometabolism
d. Frontotemporal hypometabolism > occipital hypometabolism
e. Global hypometabolism of cortex and deep brain structures

26. Two years later, the daughter of the patient depicted in question 24 calls you and says that her father died and had an autopsy. On the basis of the histopathology in Figure 12.4, what is your final diagnosis?
a. Alzheimer's disease
b. DLB
c. CJD
d. Progressive supranuclear palsy
e. Pick's disease

27. A 32-year-old alcoholic woman presents to the emergency department. She says she cannot remember how she got there or even what her name is. On examination, you find that she has intact new learning ability with loss of remote memory, including autobiographical memory. What is your diagnosis?

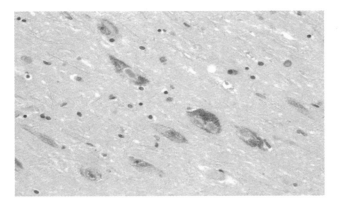

FIGURE 12.4   Brain specimen (Courtesy of Dr. Richard A. Prayson). Shown also in color plates

    a. Wernicke's encephalopathy
    b. Korsakoff's disease
    c. Transient global amnesia
    d. Psychogenic amnesia
    e. Retrograde amnesia

Questions 28–32

28. A 76-year-old man with a clinical diagnosis of Alzheimer's disease (AD) is brought to your office by his family. They are here today and have been reading up on different AD medications and have many questions. Which of the following is not an acetylcholinesterase inhibitor used to treat AD?
    a. Donepezil
    b. Memantine
    c. Rivastigmine
    d. Galantamine
    e. Tacrine

29. The mechanism of action of donepezil is:
    a. NMDA receptor antagonist
    b. Acetylcholinesterase agonist
    c. Butyrylcholinesterase inhibitor
    d. Allosteric nicotinic modulator
    e. Acetylcholinesterase inhibitor

30. The mechanism of action of rivastigmine is:
    a. Allosteric nicotinic modulator
    b. Acetylcholinesterase agonist
    c. Acetylcholinesterase and butyrylcholinesterase inhibitor
    d. NMDA receptor antagonist
    e. Acetylcholinesterase antagonist and allosteric nicotinic modulator

31. The mechanism of action of galantamine is:
    a. Acetylcholinesterase and butyrylcholinesterase inhibitor
    b. Pure acetylcholinesterase inhibitor

c. Acetylcholinesterase inhibitor and allosteric nicotinic modulator
d. NMDA receptor antagonist
e. NMDA receptor agonist

32. The mechanism of action of memantine is:
   a. NMDA receptor agonist
   b. Acetylcholinesterase and butyrylcholinesterase inhibitor
   c. Acetylcholinesterase inhibitor and allosteric nicotinic modulator
   d. NMDA receptor antagonist
   e. Acetylcholinesterase inhibitor

33. Immediate recall (digit span) is preserved in all of the following, except:
   a. Korsakoff's encephalopathy
   b. Mild cognitive impairment
   c. Transient global amnesia
   d. Major depression
   e. Early Alzheimer's disease

Questions 34–35

34. You are called to the bedside of a previously healthy 79-year-old man who underwent a total knee replacement yesterday. The nurse states his level of alertness has been fluctuating and he has been slurring his speech, has been very drowsy at times, and mentioned seeing a large colorful eye on the wall looking at him. What is the most likely explanation for these symptoms?
   a. Posterior circulation stroke
   b. Occipital lobe seizures
   c. Delirium
   d. Dementia
   e. Schizophrenia

35. Which of the following will likely give the most useful information in your evaluation of this patient?
   a. CT brain
   b. EEG
   c. Lumbar puncture
   d. Psychiatry consult
   e. Checking the patient's medications list and laboratory studies

36. Which of the following diseases is considered a synucleinopathy?
   a. Corticobasal ganglionic degeneration
   b. Multiple system atrophy
   c. Progressive supranuclear palsy
   d. FTD
   e. Pick's disease

37. What disease do you suspect on the basis of the histopathologic findings seen in Figure 12.5?
   a. Parkinson's disease
   b. Alzheimer's disease
   c. Pick's disease

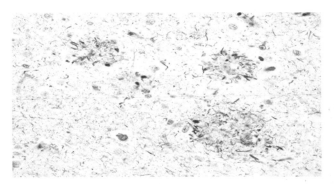

FIGURE 12.5   Brain specimen (Courtesy of Dr. Richard A. Prayson). Shown also in color plates

    d. CJD
    e. DLB

Questions 38–40

38. Which of the following diseases would you suspect on the basis of the histopathology in Figure 12.6?

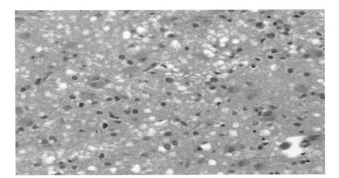

FIGURE 12.6   Brain specimen (Courtesy of Dr. Richard A. Prayson). Shown also in color plates

    a. Rabies
    b. DLB
    c. Sphingolipidosis
    d. CJD
    e. Alzheimer's disease

39. The disease that you suspect from the histopathologic slide shown in Figure 12.6, has been associated with which of the following chromosomes?
    a. 1
    b. 19
    c. 14
    d. 20
    e. 21

40. Which of the following is not typically an associated finding on MRI in patients with the histopathologic findings seen in Figure 12.6?
   a. Cortical ribbon sign
   b. Pulvinar sign
   c. Increased T2 signal in the neocortex and thalamus
   d. Increased T2 signal in the caudate and putamen
   e. Increased T2 signal in the globus pallidus

Questions 41–43

41. What is the pathologic finding in Figure 12.7?

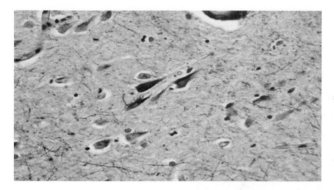

FIGURE 12.7   Brain specimen (Courtesy of Dr. Richard A. Prayson). Shown also in color plates

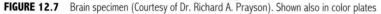

   a. Lewy bodies
   b. Negri bodies
   c. Pick bodies
   d. Bunina bodies
   e. Neurofibrillary tangles

42. Which of the following has not been suggested to be a risk factor for the disease associated with the pathologic finding in Figure 12.7?
   a. Low level of education
   b. Male gender
   c. Age
   d. Repeated head trauma
   e. Family history

43. Which of the following would be the most consistent finding on an FDG-PET scan in patients with the disease associated with the pathologic finding in Figure 12.7?
   a. Occipital hypometabolism greater than temporoparietal hypometabolism
   b. Posterior temporal and parietal hypometabolism
   c. Frontotemporal hypometabolism
   d. Temporoparietal hypermetabolism
   e. Global hypometabolism of cortex and deep brain structures

Questions 44–46

44. A 76-year-old woman with a history of successfully-treated breast cancer is brought in by her daughter for progressive memory loss and cognitive difficulties. Her daughter is very concerned by this and also mentions that the patient has difficulty with walking and seems to have a problem with lifting her feet off the floor. She wonders if you can also give a referral to a urologist because her mother has been requiring the use of adult diapers in the last 6 months. On the basis of the history, which of the following is the best next step for diagnosis?

   a. Formal neuropsychiatric/cognitive testing
   b. Trial of levodopa
   c. Lumbar puncture
   d. MRI brain
   e. MRI spine

45. A brain MRI was obtained in this patient. What diagnosis do you suspect based on the findings in Figure 12.8?

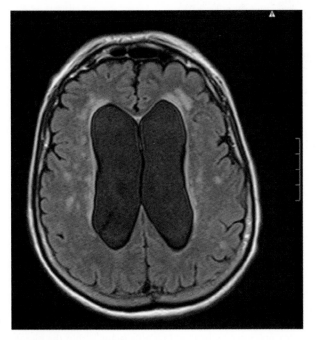

FIGURE 12.8 Axial FLAIR MRI

   a. Parkinson's disease
   b. Advancing Alzheimer's disease
   c. Normal-pressure hydrocephalus
   d. Metastatic disease to central nervous system
   e. Transverse myelitis

46. What would be your first choice in the approach and management of this patient?

   a. Levodopa
   b. Lumbar puncture

c. Schedule a CSF shunt procedure
d. Referral to oncology for further evaluation
e. A course of intravenous steroids

47. What is the pathologic finding in Figure 12.9?

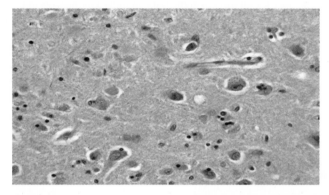

FIGURE 12.9 Brain specimen (Courtesy of Dr. Richard A. Prayson). Shown also in color plates

a. Negri bodies
b. Bunina bodies
c. Pick bodies
d. Granulovacuolar degeneration
e. Lewy bodies

48. A woman with Alzheimer's disease stopped being able to recognize her son after he shaved his moustache. She could recognize her husband only when she heard his voice. The term used to describe this type of agnosia is:
a. Topographagnosia
b. Prosopagnosia
c. Asomatognosia
d. Misoplegia
e. Somatoparaphrenia

49. A 69-year-old man was noted to have difficulty looking at objects that were brought into his visual field. He could also not reach for objects placed in front of him, though he could see them. When presented with a picture of a complex scene, he could identify items within the picture but could not describe the picture as a whole. This syndrome localizes to:
a. Bilateral temporooccipital region
b. Bilateral primary visual cortices
c. Bilateral parietooccipital region
d. Anterior thalamus
e. Bilateral anterior cingulate gyrus

50. A 52-year-old woman is brought to the emergency department by her family with disorientation. On further questioning, her family reported that she had been walking into walls and into furniture, and then she would make up absurd excuses as to why this occurred. On examination, she had complete visual loss on confrontation testing and loss of optokinetic nystagmus. She confabulated when asked to name objects or count fingers. She categorically denied there being anything wrong with her vision. This presentation is most consistent with:

a. Delusional disorder
b. A receptive aphasia
c. Anton's syndrome
d. Balint's syndrome
e. Psychogenic blindness

51. An 87-year-old gentleman who is legally blind due to severe macular degeneration reports seeing images of people and colorful animals. He realizes that he is blind and clearly understands that these are hallucinations. This man has:

a. Anton's syndrome
b. Balint's syndrome
c. Psychosis with visual hallucinations
d. Charles Bonnet syndrome
e. Delusional disorder

52. A 63-year-old college professor is brought to a neurologist after she is noted to have difficulty reading her slides during a lecture she was giving. On examination, she has speech hesitation, but speech output is otherwise normal. She is able to read individual letters, but not entire words. She can write a full sentence to dictation, but cannot read what she has written. Her comprehension, repetition, writing, and naming are normal. Visual acuity is normal. On visual field testing to confrontation, she has a right homonymous hemianopia. Cranial nerve, motor, and sensory examinations are normal. Her MRI is shown in Figure 12.10. This patient's symptoms are consistent with:

a. Wernicke's aphasia
b. Psychogenic dyslexia
c. Alexia without agraphia
d. A selective neglect syndrome
e. Cortical blindness

53. A woman cannot understand others when they speak to her. She can speak normally and her reading comprehension is intact. She has:

a. Wernicke's aphasia
b. Anomia
c. Conduction aphasia
d. Nonverbal auditory agnosia
e. Pure word deafness

54. A man is able to write normally, but his speech is fragmented and effortful. He can speak only in brief phrases, and exhibits multiple paraphasic errors. He is unable to repeat. Comprehension is intact. This is most consistent with:

a. Aphemia
b. A receptive aphasia
c. Conduction aphasia
d. Transcortical motor aphasia
e. Alexia without agraphia

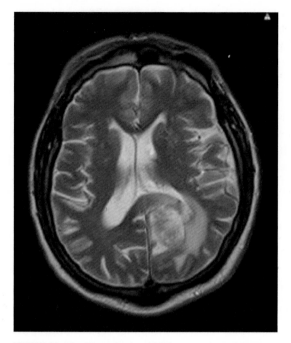

FIGURE 12.10 T2-weighted axial MRI

55. A 72-year-old woman with atrial fibrillation has suffered multiple strokes over the past several years. On examination, she is noted to have severe dysarthria and is able to utter only a few unintelligible sounds. She has severe dysphagia and bilateral near-total paralysis of both upper and lower parts of her face. She cannot voluntarily smile, but in response to a joke, will smile symmetrically. During yawning and sneezing, there is no evidence of facial or pharyngeal weakness. This syndrome localizes to:
   a. Bilateral anterior operculum
   b. Anterior cingulate
   c. Bilateral occipital lobes
   d. Medulla
   e. Pons

56. A 67-year-old woman is seen in the medical ICU, where she is being treated for sepsis with profound hypotension. On examination, she is speaking fluently but nonsensically, and comprehension is markedly impaired. However, she can repeat, and exhibits significant echolalia throughout the examination. This constellation of findings is consistent with:
   a. A Broca's (expressive) aphasia due to a dominant hemisphere posteroinferior frontal gyrus lesion
   b. A Wernicke's (receptive) aphasia due to a dominant hemisphere posterosuperior temporal gyrus lesion
   c. A conduction aphasia due to a lesion to the internal arcuate fasciculus
   d. A transcortical sensory aphasia due to a watershed infarct involving the MCA-PCA distribution
   e. Aphemia due to a lesion in the dominant hemisphere anteroinferior frontal gyrus

57. On examination, an 88-year-old man has impaired speech marked by inability to verbalize, except for a few single- or two-word phrases, and he cannot write. His language comprehension is intact, and he can repeat. This aphasic syndrome localizes to:
    a. The frontal operculum of the dominant hemisphere, involving Broca's area
    b. The posterior aspect of the superior temporal gyrus in the dominant hemisphere, involving Wernicke's area
    c. The right anterior cingulate gyrus
    d. The middle frontal gyrus of the nondominant hemisphere
    e. Dominant hemisphere ACA-MCA watershed territory, involving connections from the supplementary motor area to Broca's area

58. On examination, a patient is found to have normal speech, normal language comprehension, and normal naming abilities. However, he is unable to repeat. The aphasia this patient exhibits is:
    a. Broca's aphasia due to a dominant hemisphere posteroinferior frontal gyrus lesion
    b. Wernicke's aphasia due to a dominant hemisphere posterosuperior temporal gyrus lesion
    c. Conduction aphasia due to a lesion in the internal arcuate fasciculus
    d. Wernicke's aphasia due to a dominant hemisphere posterosuperior temporal gyrus lesion
    e. Thalamic aphasia due to right anterior thalamic infarction

59. A 39-year-old right-handed woman loses the ability to vary her speech according to her emotional state. Her speech becomes monotonous. This localizes to:
    a. Right posteroinferior frontal gyrus
    b. Left posteroinferior frontal gyrus
    c. Caudate
    d. Superior temporal gyrus
    e. Internal arcuate fasciculus

Questions 60–61

60. A 58-year-old man with a 20-year history of relapsing-remitting multiple sclerosis presents for follow-up in an outpatient clinic. His wife reports that he has been having episodes of involuntary laughter and crying during which he does not feel associated mirth or sadness. These episodes occur suddenly and are causing significant social embarrassment. He has also developed progressive dysarthria and dysphagia. It can be expected that this man has lesions in the:
    a. Right occipital lobe
    b. Bilateral frontal operculum
    c. Bilateral corticobulbar pathways
    d. Cerebellum
    e. Bilateral anterior thalamic nuclei

61. Which of the following medications have been shown in randomized controlled trials to be effective in treating the disorder depicted in question 60?
    a. Levodopa
    b. Risperidone
    c. Dextromethorphan-quinidine
    d. Prochlorperazine
    e. Morphine

62. A 68-year-old man with an infarction in the territory of the superior division of the left MCA is undergoing inpatient rehabilitation. Following his infarction, he had significant right arm weakness, could speak only a few words and exhibited marked paraphasic errors, and could not write, but his comprehension was intact. His speech has been steadily improving, as is the strength in his right hand. However, he is noticed to have significant difficulty performing simple, previously known motor tasks on command with his left hand, though his hand is not weak per se and he understands the command. This is explained by:

   a. A new infarction in the left middle cerebral artery territory
   b. A disconnection syndrome resulting from impaired transmission from his left receptive speech area to his right-hand motor area
   c. Neglect of his left hand due to his MCA infarction
   d. Sympathy weakness, in which his left hand is weak because his right hand is weak
   e. A receptive aphasia due to a dominant posterosuperior temporal gyrus infarct

63. A 72-year-old woman is brought to a neurology clinic by her family members for memory impairment and a decline in functional abilities. On examination, when she is asked to pantomime brushing her teeth, she uses her finger as the toothbrush, instead of pretending to hold a toothbrush. When asked to show how she would open a letter with a letter opener, she uses her finger as the blade instead of pretending to hold a letter opener. This is consistent with:

   a. Ideomotor apraxia
   b. Conduction apraxia
   c. Ideational apraxia
   d. Disassociation apraxia
   e. Conceptual apraxia

64. Dressing apraxia localizes to the

   a. Left frontal lobe
   b. Left parietal lobe
   c. Right parietal lobe
   d. Anterior cingulate
   e. Splenium of the corpus callosum

Questions 65–67

65. A 54-year-old woman was brought to a psychiatry clinic by her family with a 2-month history of odd behavior. She was previously a reserved, pious woman, but in recent days, she had been found at a bar singing karaoke in leather pants and had a tattoo placed on her arm. She was also irritable, and had been sleeping less than 4 hours a night. On examination, she seemed distinctly restless and her speech was pressured. She made lewd remarks and joked inappropriately. She would imitate the gestures of the examiner, and pretended to be holding a stethoscope and auscultating the examiner with it. This presentation is most consistent with dysfunction in the:

   a. Dorsolateral prefrontal cortex
   b. Dorsomedial prefrontal cortex
   c. Anterior cingulate
   d. Caudate
   e. Orbitofrontal cortex

66. Following an infarct, an 81-year-old previously gregarious and active gentleman became socially withdrawn. He no longer conversed with loved ones or laughed at jokes. He would spend his day sitting in his armchair and staring at the wall. This presentation is most consistent with dysfunction in the:

a. Dorsolateral prefrontal cortex
b. Dorsomedial prefrontal cortex
c. Anterior cingulate
d. Caudate
e. Orbitofrontal cortex

67. A 72-year-old chief executive officer of a multinational corporation was brought to a neuropsychiatry clinic by his wife. She reported that he had been a highly functioning person for years, was adept at multitasking, and single-handedly built his corporation from a small business over a decade. In the past year, he had become disorganized, and several of his affiliates were concerned because he kept missing scheduled meetings. He had made some poor investments in the prior year and his company was nearing bankruptcy. He did not seem particularly concerned about these mishaps, and had lost interest in social activities. He had previously been a cheese connoisseur, but he seemed to have lost all interest in food and had lost a significant amount of weight. This presentation is most consistent with dysfunction in the:

a. Dorsolateral prefrontal cortex
b. Dorsomedial prefrontal cortex
c. Anterior cingulate
d. Caudate
e. Orbitofrontal cortex

68. Regarding the utilization of neuropsychologic tests in the evaluation of various cortical functions, which of the following is incorrect:

a. The Trail-Making Tests are used to assess attention
b. The Wisconsin Card Sorting Test can be used as a measure of prefrontal cortical function
c. The Random Cancellation Test can be used to assess attention
d. The Clock-Drawing Test is a test of visuospatial function
e. The Grooved Pegboard Test is a test of verbal registration

69. A 28-year-old man is brought to a psychiatrist's office by his fiancée. She reports that he is convinced that the man who "claims to be his father" is in fact a double, identical-looking imposter. This is known as:

a. Fregoli's syndrome
b. Intermetamorphosis
c. Pseudocyesis
d. Capgras' syndrome
e. Cotard's delusion

70. A 62-year-old man is brought to the emergency department by his wife because he was acting "funny." He had been paying bills that morning and could not seem to calculate simple sums. He was also having trouble writing. On examination, he had right-left confusion and finger agnosia. This man's syndrome localizes to the:

a. Nondominant superior parietal lobule
b. Dominant inferior parietal lobule
c. Nondominant frontal operculum
d. Dominant dorsolateral prefrontal cortex
e. Nondominant superior temporal gyrus

71. A 52-year-old woman presents with acute left hemiparesis, with predominant involvement of the left face and arm. On examination, she has extinction to double simultaneous visual and tactile stimulation, impaired two-point discrimination, and agraphesthesia. Her lesion is most likely in the:

    a. Right MCA distribution
    b. Right internal capsule area with thalamic involvement
    c. Left pons
    d. Right pons
    e. Right ACA-MCA watershed territory

72. A 13-year-old male undergoes resection of a large hemispheric tumor. He is undergoing inpatient rehabilitation, and his therapy is being hindered by his lack of awareness of the left side of his body. He barely acknowledges the presence of weakness on the left side of his body; in fact, he largely does not recognize the left side of his body as being his own. This is consistent with:

    a. A lesion in the dominant hemisphere parietal region involving the primary somatosensory cortex
    b. A lesion in the nondominant hemisphere primary visual cortex
    c. A lesion in the nondominant frontal lobe
    d. A lesion in the nondominant hemisphere parietal region involving the primary somatosensory cortex
    e. A lesion in the dominant hemisphere angular gyrus

73. A 52-year-old woman is brought to the emergency department after sudden onset of left hemiparesis. On examination, she has forced gaze deviation to the right that can be overcome by oculocephalic maneuver. Her lesion most likely involves:

    a. The left frontal eye fields in the middle frontal gyrus
    b. The right frontal eye fields in the middle frontal gyrus
    c. The right parapontine reticular formation
    d. The left parapontine reticular formation
    e. The right parapontine reticular formation

74. A 73-year-old man suffers from an acute infarction leading to right arm and leg hemianesthesia. Three months later, he presents to an outpatient clinic with severe right-sided hyperesthesia and allodynia. Which of the following would not be a likely explanation for this man's symptoms?

    a. A left thalamic lesion
    b. A lesion in the left parietal operculum
    c. A lesion in the primary somatosensory cortex
    d. A lesion in the medial lemniscus
    e. A lesion in the cervical dorsal columns

75. Regarding the different types of memory, which of the following is incorrect?

    a. Memory of high school graduation is an example of declarative, or explicit, memory
    b. Ability to drive a car or ride a bicycle after years of having not done so is an example of nondeclarative, or implicit, memory
    c. Lesions to the bilateral medial temporal lobes lead largely to loss of declarative (explicit) memory, with relative preservation of nondeclarative (implicit) memory
    d. Lesions to the bilateral parietal lobes lead to loss of nondeclarative (implicit) memory
    e. Nondeclarative memory does not localize to one specific area of the cerebral hemispheres

76. An 18-year-old man is admitted to a neurologic ICU with herpes simplex encephalitis. A brain MRI shows hyperintensities on T2 sequences involving extensive areas of the bilateral temporal lobes. He is treated with acyclovir and is discharged to a rehabilitation center for several weeks. As his encephalopathy begins to improve, he is noted to constantly ask for food, place any objects that come into sight into his mouth, and make sexual advances, lewd comments, and obscene gestures to all female staff in the rehabilitation center. He is otherwise calm and easily appeased. At times he is noted to focus for prolonged periods of times on minute visual stimuli, such as a piece of lint on his pajamas. This syndrome is due to:
    a. A hypothalamic lesion
    b. Bilateral mamillary body necrosis
    c. Bilateral medial frontal lesions
    d. Bilateral amygdala lesions
    e. Bilateral thalamic lesions

77. A 59-year-old man was brought to a neurology clinic by his family with complaints of abnormal posturing of his right arm. A few months prior to presentation, he had been involved in a motor vehicle accident because he reported his "right hand was driving the steering wheel on its own" and he could not control it. On physical examination, he was found to have rigidity in the right arm with dystonic posturing. Sensory examination showed intact sensation to light touch, but impaired graphesthesia in the right hand. This presentation is most consistent with:
    a. Progressive supranuclear palsy
    b. Huntington's disease
    c. DLB
    d. Pick's variant of frontotemporal dementia
    e. Corticobasal ganglionic degeneration

78. Which of the following lesions would not lead to a significant alteration in level of consciousness?
    a. Bilateral hemispheric lesions
    b. Bilateral midbrain infarct
    c. Bilateral thalamic infarct
    d. Bilateral dorsal pontine infarct
    e. Bilateral occipital infarct

79. An 82-year-old man with moderate Alzheimer's dementia is brought to the emergency department in respiratory distress due to aspiration pneumonia. He is intubated and mechanically ventilated, and has a prolonged ICU stay due to multiorgan failure in the setting of sepsis, and is now considered to be in a terminal state. After 6 days in the ICU, his physicians approach the family about goals of care. The patient's best friend, who is his legal durable power of attorney for health care (and has the paperwork to prove it), states that the patient would not want to be on long-term mechanical ventilation and would not want to have a feeding tube. A living will to that effect is available that the patient had made several years earlier, when he had mild memory problems, but was otherwise cognitively normal. The patient's son, who lives in another country and had flown in when his father was hospitalized, states that he wants "everything done" for the patient. Which of the following statements is most appropriate in the management of this patient?
    a. The patient's wishes as communicated by his power of attorney will be upheld though communication with the son in order to reconcile him with his father's wishes if possible

b. Because the patient's son is his next of kin, the wishes of the son will be followed
c. Consultation with a lawyer is necessary because there is discrepancy between the patient's power of attorney and the family members
d. Because the patient had dementia, his living will is not valid even if he was of sound mind when the living will was made
e. Decisions regarding this patient's management will be taken strictly by the medical team because there is disagreement among the patient's friend and son

Answer key

1. b	15. e	29. e	43. b	57. e	71. a
2. a	16. d	30. c	44. d	58. c	72. d
3. c	17. e	31. c	45. c	59. a	73. b
4. b	18. d	32. d	46. b	60. c	74. c
5. d	19. a	33. d	47. d	61. c	75. d
6. b	20. b	34. c	48. b	62. b	76. d
7. b	21. d	35. e	49. c	63. a	77. e
8. c	22. c	36. b	50. c	64. c	78. e
9. e	23. c	37. b	51. d	65. e	79. a
10. d	24. d	38. d	52. c	66. b	
11. c	25. a	39. d	53. e	67. a	
12. e	26. b	40. e	54. a	68. e	
13. d	27. d	41. e	55. a	69. d	
14. b	28. b	42. b	56. d	70. b	

Answers

1. b, 2. a

Mild Cognitive Impairment (MCI) is defined by cognitive impairment that does not interfere with activities of daily living, is not severe enough to classify the patient as demented, and patients retain general cognitive function. MCI is characterized by memory complaints (especially when noticed by friends and family), objective memory impairment for age and education, intact activities of daily living, and preserved general cognition. Impairments may be in one or more cognitive domains, such as attention, memory, language, executive, or visuospatial function. In general, MCI is classified as amnestic MCI (primarily memory), nonamnestic MCI (cognitive domain other than memory, such as language), or multiple-domain MCI (more than one cognitive domains affected). A gradual decline in cognition can be characteristic of normal aging, but it can often be differentiated from MCI by the degree of cognitive impairment. Amnestic MCI is often an early stage of Alzheimer's disease, with a conversion rate to dementia of about 10% to 15% per year.

Petersen RC, Smith GE, Waring SC, et al. Mild cognitive impairment: Clinical characterization and outcome. Arch Neurol. 1999; 56:303–308.

Petersen RC, Stevens JC, Ganguli M, et al. Practice parameter: Early detection of dementia: Mild cognitive impairment (an evidence-based review). Report of the Quality Standards Subcommittee of the American Academy of Neurology. Neurology. 2001; 56:1133–1142.

Tierney MC, Szalai JP, Snow WG, et al. Prediction of probable Alzheimer's disease in memory-impaired patients: A prospective longitudinal study. Neurology. 1996; 46:661–665.

3. c, **4.** b, **5.** d, **6.** b

According to the American Academy of Neurology guidelines, routine dementia screening should include assessment for vitamin B_{12}, complete blood count, electrolytes, glucose, blood urea nitrogen, creatinine, liver function tests, thyroid function tests, and depression screening. Further testing including HIV, VDRL, lumbar puncture, and heavy metals are not recommended unless there is a specific clinical indication.

Alzheimer's disease (AD) is the most common cause of dementia. Most inherited forms of AD are autosomal dominant and typically present before age 65, although these cases account for less than 5% of all cases of AD. Presenilin-2 is in chromosome 1 and leads to early-onset familial AD. Presenilin-1 is in chromosome 14 and accounts for 80% of early-onset aggressive familial cases of AD. Apolipoprotein E4 is in chromosome 19 and triples the risk of AD, as well as leads to an early age of onset, but does not lead to AD per se (only modifies the risk of AD). Amyloid precursor protein (APP) is in chromosome 21. Chromosome 2 is not related to AD.

Injury to any of the structures within the circuit of Papez will interrupt formation of new memories. The mediodorsal nucleus of the thalamus is not part of the circuit of Papez. The circuit of Papez is: entorhinal cortex → hippocampus → fornix → mamillary bodies → anterior nucleus of thalamus → cingulate gyrus → entorhinal cortex → hippocampus. Clinical neurologists often divide memory into stages. Immediate memory is the amount of information someone can keep in conscious awareness without active memorization. Immediate memory can be tested by forward digit span. Normal human beings can retain seven digits in active memory span. Working memory is tested by manipulation of information retained in immediate memory (such as adding two of the digits repeated in a number series). Recent memory involves the ability to register and recall specific items after a delay of minutes or hours. It requires the hippocampus and parahippocampal areas of the medial temporal lobe for storage and retrieval, which is why this type of memory is usually impaired first in early AD and is evident by impaired word recall. Remote memory is tested by asking about historical life events and long-known information.

Memory impairment is the essential and earliest clinical feature of AD. Declarative memory (facts and events) is significantly affected in AD. Of declarative memory, episodic memory (specific events and contexts) is the most impaired in early AD. Within episodic memory, memory for recent events is more prominently impaired in early AD compared with immediate or remote memory. Memory for facts such as vocabulary and concepts (semantic memory) is spared until later. Likewise, procedural memory and motor learning are also spared until later. Loss of visuospatial skills is also often an early feature of AD, which manifests as navigational difficulty in unfamiliar and later familiar areas and misplacement of items. Verbal dysfluency and anomia are also commonly early features and may be the presenting symptom. Other features often associated with later stages of AD include progressive language dysfunction, impaired executive function, lack of insight, neuropsychiatric symptoms, and apraxia. Inability to recognize objects and faces, or visual agnosia and prosopagnosia, respectively (see discussion to question 48), are a late feature.

Ahmed S, Mitchell J, Arnold R, et al. Memory complaints in mild cognitive impairment, worried well, and semantic dementia patients. Alzheimer Dis Assoc Disord. 2008; 22:227–235.

Guerin F, Belleville S, Ska B. Characterization of visuoconstructional disabilities in patients with probable dementia of Alzheimer's type. J Clin Exp Neuropsychol. 2002; 24:1–17.

Knopman DS, DeKosky ST, Cummings JL, et al. Practice parameter: Diagnosis of dementia (an evidence-based review): Report of the quality standards subcommittee of the American Academy of Neurology. Neurology. 2001; 56:1143–1153.

Peters F, Collette F, Degueldre C, et al. The neural correlates of verbal short-term memory in Alzheimer's disease: An fMRI study. Brain. 2009; 132:1833–1846.

Ropper AH, Samuels MA. Adams and Victor's Principles of Neurology, 9th ed. New York: McGraw-Hill; 2009.

7. b, 8. c, 9. e

The FDG-PET scan in Figure 12.1 shows bilateral parietotemporal hypometabolism, consistent with Alzheimer's disease (AD). FDG-PET scanning may reveal decreased glucose metabolism in parietotemporal regions in AD, in the frontal and anterior temporal regions in FTD, in the head of the caudate in Huntington's disease, and in the occipital regions in DLB. FDG-PET scanning in Parkinson's disease usually does not show a decrease in metabolism.

All of the listed items in question 8 are commonly associated histopathologic findings seen in AD except for Lewy bodies, which would be the least commonly associated finding. Neuritic plaques and neurofibrillary tangles are the most specific, although granulovacuolar degeneration, amyloid deposition, and Hirano bodies are also commonly seen. Cortical Lewy bodies are classically found primarily in DLB, although there are occasionally overlapping histopathologic features between different types of dementia.

In AD, along with loss of cholinergic neurons in the nucleus basalis of Meynert, there is loss of choline acetyltransferase activity throughout the cortex, which correlates with the severity of memory loss. The locus coeruleus contains noradrenergic neurons, the median and dorsal raphe nuclei contain serotonergic neurons, the nucleus accumbens and ventral tegmental area contain dopaminergic neurons, and the substantia nigra pars reticulata contain GABAergic neurons (as opposed to the pars compacta, which contain dopaminergic neurons).

Bradley WG, Daroff RB, Fenichel GM, et al. Neurology in Clinical Practice, 5th ed. Philadelphia, PA: Elsevier; 2008.

Hoffman JM, Welsh-Bohmer KA, Hanson M, et al. FDG PET imaging in patients with pathologically verified dementia. J Nucl Med. 2000; 41:1920–1928.

Prayson RA, Goldblum JR. Neuropathology, 1st ed. Philadelphia, PA: Elsevier; 2005.

10. d, 11. c

Parkinsonism, fluctuating cognitive impairment, and visual hallucinations make up the classic triad of DLB. Auditory hallucinations are not a typical finding in DLB. DLB is considered the second most common type of degenerative dementia after Alzheimer's disease. In addition to dementia, other clinical features may include dysautonomia, sleep disorders, and neuroleptic sensitivity. Treatment is generally symptomatic and targeted toward specific disease manifestations. Acetylcholinesterase inhibitors may be of benefit. Typical neuroleptics are generally avoided due to significant sensitivity reactions, such as neuroleptic malignant syndrome, worsening parkinsonism, confusion, or autonomic dysfunction. If absolutely necessary, especially for agitated psychotic symptoms, atypical neuroleptics should be tried cautiously in low doses. Of the choices in question 11, haloperidol is the only typical neuroleptic listed, and should not be used.

Ballard CG, O'Brien JT, Swann AG, et al. The natural history of psychosis and depression in dementia with Lewy bodies and Alzheimer's disease: Persistence and new cases over 1 year of follow-up. J Clin Psychiatry. 2001; 62:46–49.

Ropper AH, Samuels MA. Adams and Victor's Principles of Neurology, 9th ed. New York: McGraw-Hill; 2009.

Stavitsky K, Brickman AM, Scarmeas N, et al. The progression of cognition, psychiatric symptoms, and functional abilities in dementia with Lewy bodies and Alzheimer disease. Arch Neurol. 2006; 63:1450–1456.

12. e

Pick's disease is a disorder grouped under the FTDs (see discussion to questions 14–15). Of the listed choices, depression is least likely to be seen in Pick's disease, although it can occur. Pick's disease is manifested predominantly by frontal lobe symptoms such as personality changes, behavioral problems, apathy, abulia, and poor judgment. Aphasia can be present with temporal lobe involvement as well as features of Kluver-Bucy syndrome (see discussion to questions 21 and 76). Cognitive decline does occur, but memory impairment is not the most prominent feature, distinguishing the FTDs from Alzheimer's disease.

Josephs KA. Frontotemporal lobar degeneration. Neurol Clin. 2007; 25:683–696.

Mendez MF, Shapira JS. Loss of insight and functional neuroimaging in frontotemporal dementia. J Neuropsychiatry Clin Neurosci. 2005; 17:413–416.

13. d

Lesions in the occipital lobe would not be associated with personality changes. Lesions in the dorsolateral frontal lobe cause symptoms such as personality changes, perseveration, apathy, and depression. Lesions in the orbitofrontal cortex may cause obsessive compulsive disorder traits, disinhibition, hypersexuality, anxiety, depression, impulsiveness, and antisocial behavior. Temporal lobe lesions can cause psychosis and memory disturbances. Caudate nucleus lesions can occasionally affect behavior. The occipital lobe underlies visual processing (see discussion to question 49), and is least likely to be associated with personality change (see discussion to questions 65 to 67 for a more extensive review of the frontal lobe syndromes).

Bradley WG, Daroff RB, Fenichel GM, et al. Neurology in Clinical Practice, 5th ed. Philadelphia, PA: Elsevier; 2008.

Ropper AH, Samuels MA. Adams and Victor's Principles of Neurology, 9th ed. New York: McGraw-Hill; 2009.

14. b, 15. e

Visual hallucinations are not a common finding in FTD. In familial FTD, the most common genetic association is to chromosome 17q21, although chromosomes 3 and 9 have also been implicated in autosomal dominant inheritance. Most sporadic cases of FTD have not been linked to specific chromosomal sites. Linkage to the remaining chromosomes listed has been identified in some patients with familial Alzheimer's disease.

In FTD, mean age of symptom onset is between 55 and 60 years. There are three major distinct clinical phenotypes of FTD. The behavioral variant FTD is the most common phenotype and symptoms include personality changes, abulia, apathy, social withdrawal, disinhibition, impulsivity, lack of insight, poor personal hygiene, stereotyped or ritual behaviors, change in eating patterns, suddenly new artistic abilities or hobbies, emotional blunting, loss of empathy, mental rigidity, distractibility, impersistence, perseverative behavior, and impaired organizational and executive skills. The patient depicted in question 14 appears to have this phenotype.

The second phenotype is progressive nonfluent aphasia and is characterized in early stages by anomia, word-finding difficulty, impaired object naming, and effortful speech with preserved comprehension. Spontaneous speech becomes increasingly dysfluent and speech errors become frequent. Behavior and social interaction remain unaffected until late in the disease at which point the patient becomes globally aphasic.

The third phenotype is semantic dementia, also called progressive fluent aphasia or the temporal variant of FTD. It is characterized by a progressive speech disturbance with normal fluency, but impaired comprehension, anomia, and semantic paraphasias. It may clinically resemble a transcortical sensory aphasia. There is typically a predominance of left temporal dysfunction, and/or in face and object recognition, reflecting right temporal dysfunction.

In addition, some patients with FTD may develop variant syndromes of motor impairment including motor neuron disease, progressive supranuclear palsy and corticobasal degeneration.

Josephs KA. Frontotemporal lobar degeneration. Neurol Clin. 2007; 25:683–696.

Kertesz A. Clinical features and diagnosis of frontotemporal dementia. Front Neurol Neurosci. 2009; 24:140–148.

Knibb JA, Xuereb JH, Patterson K, et al. Clinical and pathological characterization of progressive aphasia. Ann Neurol. 2006; 59:156–165.

Liu W, Miller BL, Kramer JH, et al. Behavioral disorders in the frontal and temporal variants of frontotemporal dementia. Neurology. 2004; 62:742–748.

McKhann GM, Albert MS, Grossman M, et al. Clinical and pathological diagnosis of frontotemporal dementia: Report of the Work Group on Frontotemporal Dementia and Pick's Disease. Arch Neurol. 2001; 58:1803–1809.

16. d

These FDG-PET scan images are consistent with FTD. FDG-PET reveals decreased glucose metabolism in the frontal and anterior temporal regions in FTD, parietotemporal regions in Alzheimer's disease, the head of the caudate in Huntington's disease, and the occipital regions in DLB. FDG-PET scanning in Parkinson's disease usually does not show a decrease in cortical metabolism.

Hoffman JM, Welsh-Bohmer KA, Hanson M, et al. FDG PET Imaging in Patients with Pathologically Verified Dementia. J Nucl Med. 2000; 41:1920–1928.

17. e

These symptoms would be most consistent with bilateral ACA infarcts. The key is identifying symptoms of frontal lobe dysfunction (such as those listed in the question) along with ACA territory dysfunction in terms of motor weakness. Recall the vascular distribution and the homunculus in which the legs are supplied by the ACA, where they are represented along the medial frontal cortex. Pontine infarcts can result in leg weakness and incontinence, but not frontal lobe symptoms. Lesions in the dominant temporal lobe could cause amnesia for verbal information and sensory, or Wernicke's, aphasia. Lesions in the nondominant temporal lobe can cause amnesia for nonverbal and visuospatial information, as well as amusia.

Bradley WG, Daroff RB, Fenichel GM, et al. Neurology in Clinical Practice, 5th ed. Philadelphia, PA: Elsevier; 2008.

Ropper AH, Samuels MA. Adams and Victor's Principles of Neurology, 9th ed. New York: McGraw-Hill; 2009.

18. d

The dorsomedial nucleus has projections to dorsolateral prefrontal, orbitofrontal, anterior cingulate gyrus, and temporal lobe/amygdala. Dysfunction of this nucleus can result in the symptoms listed. The anterior nucleus is mostly involved in limbic relay and memory formation (part of the circuit of Papez). The pulvinar is involved in processing visual information and sensory integration. The ventral posterolateral nucleus is involved in sensory relay from the body, whereas the ventral posteromedial nucleus is involved in sensory relay from the face, both of which project to the somatosensory cortex.

Carrera E, Bogousslavsky J. The thalamus and behavior effects of anatomically distinct strokes. Neurology. 2006; 66:1817–1823.

19. a

Bilateral globus pallidus interna lesions can cause akinetic mutism. In akinetic mutism, the patient generally has preserved awareness with open eyes, but remains immobile and mute and does not respond to commands. The globus pallidus interna is part of the anterior cingulate-frontal-subcortical circuit. Bilateral ACA infarcts and other lesions to the medial frontal lobes are other causes of akinetic mutism.

Bradley WG, Daroff RB, Fenichel GM, et al. Neurology in Clinical Practice, 5th ed. Philadelphia, PA: Elsevier; 2008.

Ropper AH, Samuels MA. Adams and Victor's Principles of Neurology, 9th ed. New York: McGraw-Hill; 2009.

20. b

Huntington's disease is an autosomal dominant trinucleotide repeat disorder resulting from expansion of CAG repeats on chromosome 4p in a region that codes for the Huntingtin protein. The disease is associated with choreoathetosis and dementia. Chromosome 17 has been linked to FTD. Chromosomes 14, 19, and 21 are linked to some familial forms of Alzheimer's disease.

Bradley WG, Daroff RB, Fenichel GM, et al. Neurology in Clinical Practice, 5th ed. Philadelphia, PA: Elsevier; 2008.

Ropper AH, Samuels MA. Adams and Victor's Principles of Neurology, 9th ed. New York: McGraw-Hill; 2009.

21. d

Pick's disease has been associated with Kluver-Bucy syndrome (KBS), and is discussed in question 12. KBS is caused by lesions to bilateral anterior temporal lobes/amygdala and is characterized by hyperorality (tendency to explore objects with mouth), hypermetamorphosis (preoccupied with minute environmental stimuli), blunted emotional affect, hypersexuality, and visual agnosia (see discussion to question 76 for further review of KBS).

Bradley WG, Daroff RB, Fenichel GM, et al. Neurology in Clinical Practice, 5th ed. Philadelphia, PA: Elsevier; 2008.

Ropper AH, Samuels MA. Adams and Victor's Principles of Neurology, 9th ed. New York: McGraw-Hill; 2009.

22. c

Disorders of higher cortical function often confer more disability than focal neurologic deficits after traumatic brain injury (TBI) and interfere with rehabilitation. Of these, alterations in personality interfere with rehabilitation the most. The other listed options frequently result from TBI, and may affect rehabilitation, but to a lesser degree. In addition, TBI can cause overlapping cognitive, physical, emotional, and behavioral symptoms. TBI is the result of a traumatic external force to the skull, injuring the brain. Causes include motor vehicle accidents, falls, sports injuries, and violence. It is a major cause of death and disability worldwide, especially in children and young adults because they are more likely to be involved in these scenarios. The trauma to the brain can be caused either by direct impact or acceleration, or both, which may lead to alterations in cerebral blood flow and intracranial pressure. Outcome can range from death or permanent disability to complete recovery.

Brooks N, Mckinlay W, Symington C, et al. Return to work within the first seven years of severe head injury. Brain Inj. 1987; 1:5–19.

Lezak MD, O'brien K. Longitudinal study of emotional, social, and physical changes after traumatic brain injury. J Learn Disabil. 1988; 21(8):456–463.

23. c

In transient global amnesia (TGA), recent memory is impaired. The pathophysiology of TGA is not well understood, but in at least some cases, it is thought to result from functional alterations in the bilateral medial temporal lobes. It has been associated with migraine, hypertension, medical procedures, and stressful events, among others. It typically lasts 12 to 24 hours and usually resolves without deficit. Clinically, the patients may ask the same questions over and over each time the examiners come into the room. They often forget meeting the examiner if the examiner leaves the room briefly and then returns. Immediate memory is usually spared and can be tested by digit span. Remote and procedural memory and personal identity are also retained. The primary clinical impairment in TGA is in recent (short-term) memory.

Rae-Grant AD. Neurology for the House Officer. Philadelphia, PA: Lippincott Williams and Wilkins; 2008.

Sander K, Sander D. New insights into transient global amnesia: Recent imaging and clinical findings. Lancet Neurol. 2005; 4:437–444.

24. d, 25. a, 26. b

This patient exhibits symptoms of DLB. Parkinsonism, fluctuating cognitive impairment, and visual hallucinations make up the classic triad of DLB. This disorder is discussed further in questions 10 and 11.

FDG-PET imaging of DLB reveals bilateral occipital hypometabolism greater than temporoparietal hypometabolism. Progressive supranuclear palsy (PSP) is associated with global metabolic reduction in various regions including the anterior cingulate, basal ganglia (especially caudate and putamen), thalamus, and upper brain stem. FTD shows frontotemporal hypometabolism. Alzheimer's disease shows temporoparietal hypometabolism. FDG-PET scan is not typically useful in CJD; specific MRI findings are characteristic, making MRI a useful imaging modality in the diagnosis of CJD.

The histopathologic specimen obtained from the brain of this patient shows Lewy bodies, which are seen in DLB. Lewy bodies are cytoplasmic inclusions with anti-ubiquitin and anti-α-synuclein immunohistochemistry. Pick's disease is defined pathologically by the presence of silver-staining, spherical aggregations of tau protein in neurons (Pick bodies). PSP is characterized by globose neurofibrillary tangles in neurons of subcortical nuclei and tufted astrocytes. The histopathology of Alzheimer's disease is discussed in questions 37, 41, and 47, and CJD in question 38.

Gold G. Dementia with Lewy bodies: Clinical diagnosis and therapeutic approach. Front Neurol Neurosci. 2009; 24:107–113.

Hoffman JM, Welsh-Bohmer KA, Hanson M, et al. FDG PET imaging in patients with pathologically verified dementia. J Nucl Med. 2000; 41:1920–1928.

Prayson RA, Goldblum JR. Neuropathology, 1st ed. Philadelphia, PA: Elsevier; 2005.

27. d

Psychogenic amnesia has the characteristic finding of loss of autobiographical memory, sometimes with preserved ability for new learning. Wernicke's encephalopathy, which results from deficiency in thiamine (vitamin B_1), as occurs in malnourishment, such as in alcoholism, is defined by the triad of confusion, ataxia, and ophthalmoplegia. Korsakoff's disease, the chronic phase of thiamine deficiency, presents with anterograde and retrograde amnesia, and is classically associated with confabulation as a result of the poor memory. Transient global amnesia is transient and impairs recent memory while sparing immediate memory and remote memory.

Bradley WG, Daroff RB, Fenichel GM, et al. Neurology in Clinical Practice, 5th ed. Philadelphia, PA: Elsevier; 2008.

Ropper AH, Samuels MA. Adams and Victor's Principles of Neurology, 9th ed. New York: McGraw-Hill; 2009.

28. b, 29. e, 30. c, 31. c, 32. d

Memantine is the only listed drug that is not an acetylcholinesterase inhibitor. Memantine is a low-to-moderate affinity noncompetitive NMDA receptor antagonist and is approved for moderate-to-severe dementia in Alzheimer's disease (AD). The other listed drugs in question 28 are acetylcholinesterase inhibitors. Tacrine is no longer available in United States due to hepatotoxicity.

Patients with AD have reduced cerebral production of choline acetyltransferase, which leads to a decrease in acetylcholine synthesis and impaired cortical cholinergic function. Donepezil, rivastigmine, galantamine, and memantine are all medications used in the treatment of dementia, most commonly AD. Donepezil is a pure acetylcholinesterase inhibitor. Rivastigmine is a combined acetylcholinesterase and butyrylcholinesterase inhibitor, both of which result in limiting the breakdown of acetylcholine. Galantamine is a combined acetylcholinesterase inhibitor and allosteric nicotinic modulator. Memantine is an NMDA receptor antagonist that inhibits glutamate stimulation and thus theoretically limits overactivation and toxicity to remaining cholinergic neurons. Memantine also has some antagonistic action at the $5\text{-}HT_3$ serotonin receptor.

Qaseem A, Snow V, Cross JT Jr, et al. Current pharmacologic treatment of dementia: A clinical practice guideline from the American College of Physicians and the American Academy of Family Physicians. Ann Intern Med. 2008; 148:370–378.

Raina P, Santaguida P, Ismaila A, et al. Effectiveness of cholinesterase inhibitors and memantine for treating dementia: Evidence review for a clinical practice guideline. Ann Intern Med. 2008; 149(5):358–359.

33. d

Major depression results in poor attention, and subsequently, immediate recall is often impaired, whereas short-term memory is typically preserved. Early Alzheimer's disease and Korsakoff's disease preserve immediate recall and show impaired learning and recall of new information. Transient global amnesia is also associated with retrograde and anterograde amnesia with preserved immediate recall.

Bradley WG, Daroff RB, Fenichel GM, et al. Neurology in Clinical Practice, 5th ed. Philadelphia, PA: Elsevier; 2008.

Schatzberg AF, Posener JA, DeBattista C, et. al. Neuropsychological deficits in psychotic versus nonpsychotic major depression and no mental illness. Am J Psychiatry. 2000; 157(7):1095–1100.

34. c, 35. e

This elderly man fits the typical clinical scenario of delirium, and checking his medications and recent laboratory testing would be the first step in evaluation. Delirium is classically differentiated from dementia by its waxing and waning course as opposed to the steady cognitive impairment seen in dementia. His age, combined with the stress of major surgery, and probable exposure to postoperative pain medications are all contributors to this common occurrence. Infections such as urinary tract infection and pneumonia, as well as hypoxia (such as from pulmonary embolus), are also potential causes of delirium. Assessing his medications to look for contributors (especially narcotics, antihistamines, and anticholinergics) and routine metabolic studies should be checked. An arterial blood gas should be checked if hypoxia is suspected. Visual hallucinations are most often related to metabolic derangements and medications. Although stroke should be ruled out, it is unlikely on the basis of this constellation of symptoms (especially positive visual hallucinations). Seizures are also unlikely, although occipital lobe seizures can cause colorful geometric shapes to be seen. EEG would most likely show diffuse slowing, which would be typical of delirium. In this case, his symptoms are unlikely to be related to schizophrenia, as there is no prior history. In addition, hallucinations in schizophrenia are typically auditory, rather than visual. Therefore, there is no need for a psychiatry consult at this time. A lumbar puncture is not indicated at this time, although can be considered in the future if symptoms progress or do not improve, despite an unrevealing work-up.

Bradley WG, Daroff RB, Fenichel GM, et al. Neurology in Clinical Practice, 5th ed. Philadelphia, PA: Elsevier; 2008.

Ropper AH, Samuels MA. Adams and Victor's Principles of Neurology, 9th ed. New York: McGraw-Hill; 2009.

36. b

Multiple system atrophy (MSA) is considered a synucleinopathy, whereas the other listed choices represent tauopathies. The synucleins are a family of proteins that includes α-synuclein, β-synuclein, and γ-synuclein. Abnormal accumulation of these proteins results in the synucleinopathies and include Parkinson's disease, DLB, MSA, and neuroaxonal dystrophies. The tauopathies are associated with the microtubule-associated protein, tau. Tau promotes microtubule polymerization and stabilization. Accumulation of this protein results in the tauopathies.

Dickson DW. Neuropathology of non-Alzheimer degenerative disorders. Int J Clin Exp Pathol. 2010; 3(1):1–23.

Prayson RA, Goldblum JR. Neuropathology, 1st ed. Philadelphia, PA: Elsevier; 2005.

37. b

The photomicrograph in Figure 12.5 shows histopathology consistent with Alzheimer's disease (AD). It shows amyloid (neuritic) plaques, which are extracellular collections of amyloid protein deposited on dendrites and axons. They are composed of β-amyloid proteins. Amyloid plaques are a characteristic finding in AD. The other histopathologic findings in AD include intraneuronal neurofibrillary tangles (paired helical filaments made up of abnormally hyperphosphorylated tau protein), granulovacuolar degeneration (neuronal intracytoplasmic granule-containing vacuoles), amyloid angiopathy (amyloid deposition in the walls of small- and medium-sized arteries), and Hirano bodies (cytoplasmic inclusions composed mainly of actin and actin-associated proteins).

Bradley WG, Daroff RB, Fenichel GM, et al. Neurology in Clinical Practice, 5th ed. Philadelphia, PA: Elsevier; 2008.

Prayson RA, Goldblum JR. Neuropathology, 1st ed. Philadelphia, PA: Elsevier; 2005.

38. d, 39. d, 40. e

The histopathology shown in Figure 12.6 is consistent with CJD. The five human prion diseases are kuru, CJD, variant CJD ("mad cow disease"), Gerstmann-Sträussler-Scheinker syndrome, and fatal familial insomnia. These diseases share the neuropathologic features of neuronal loss, glial cell proliferation, absent inflammatory response, and vacuolization of the neuropil, which produces the characteristic spongiform appearance.

Sporadic CJD occurs at a rate of approximately 1/1,000,000 population per year. CJD is a rapidly progressive dementia associated with variable extrapyramidal/pyramidal tract signs, myoclonus, and ataxia, and death typically ensues within 1 year. Sporadic cases account for 85% to 95%, whereas 5% to 15% are familial, with an autosomal dominant pattern of inheritance. The pathology occurs when the normal prion protein (PrP), which is primarily an α-helical structure, converts into an abnormal form containing a higher percentage of β-pleated sheets. The abnormal form is insoluble, polymerizes and accumulates intracellularly, and is resistant to proteolysis. The prion protein gene (*PRNP*) coding for PrP is located on chromosome 20p. The other chromosomes listed all relate to Alzheimer's disease. Polymorphism at codon 129 of the *PRNP* is believed to determine susceptibility for CJD, and homozygosity for either methionine or valine at codon 129 has a strong correlation with the various forms of CJD, including sporadic, iatrogenic, variant ("mad cow disease") and familial forms. Neuroimaging findings in CJD include cortical ribbon sign, pulvinar sign, and increased T2 signal in the neocortex, thalamus, caudate, and putamen (see Chapter 15). Increased T2 signal in the globus pallidus is not a typical finding in CJD.

Bradley WG, Daroff RB, Fenichel GM, et al. Neurology in Clinical Practice, 5th ed. Philadelphia, PA: Elsevier; 2008.

Lewis V, Hill AF, Klug GM, et al. Australian sporadic CJD analysis supports endogenous determinants of molecular-clinical profiles. Neurology. 2005; 65:113–118.

Parchi P, Giese A, Capellari S, et al. Classification of sporadic Creutzfeldt-Jakob disease based on molecular and phenotypic analysis of 300 subjects. Ann Neurol. 1999; 46:224–233.

Prayson RA, Goldblum JR. Neuropathology, 1st ed. Philadelphia, PA: Elsevier; 2005.

Ropper AH, Samuels MA. Adams and Victor's Principles of Neurology, 9th ed. New York: McGraw-Hill; 2009.

41. e, 42. b, 43. b

Figure 12.7 reveals neurofibrillary tangles (NFTs) associated with Alzheimer's disease (AD). NFTs are intraneuronal collections of paired helical filaments made up of hyperphosphorylated tau protein. Negri bodies are seen in rabies, pick bodies are seen in Pick's disease, and Bunina bodies are seen in amyotrophic lateral sclerosis.

Low level of education, repeated head trauma, and family history of dementia have been associated with increased risk of developing AD. The major risk factor for AD is aging. Gender has also been associated with risk, with female gender conferring a greater risk than male gender.

AD reveals hypometabolism of the posterior temporal and parietal regions on FDG-PET scan (discussed in question 7 and shown in Figure 12.1). To review, FDG-PET imaging of DLB reveals occipital hypometabolism greater than temporoparietal hypometabolism. Progressive supranuclear palsy is associated with global metabolic reduction, including anterior cingulate, basal ganglia (especially caudate and putamen), thalamus, and upper brain stem. FTD shows frontotemporal hypometabolism.

Bradley WG, Daroff RB, Fenichel GM, et al. Neurology in Clinical Practice, 5th ed. Philadelphia, PA: Elsevier; 2008.

Dickson DW. Neuropathology of non-Alzheimer degenerative disorders. Int J Clin Exp Pathol. 2010; 3(1):1–23.

Prayson RA, Goldblum JR. Neuropathology, 1st ed. Philadelphia, PA: Elsevier; 2005.

Ryans NS, Fox NC. Imaging biomarkers in Alzheimer's disease. Ann NY Acad Sci. 2009; 1180: 20–27.

44. d, 45. c, 46. b

This patient demonstrates the classic triad of normal pressure hydrocephalus (NPH): cognitive dysfunction, gait impairment (often termed "magnetic gait"), and urinary incontinence. A brain MRI would be the best diagnostic test to start with and should reveal ventriculomegaly, which is out of proportion to cortical atrophy. It should be done prior to lumbar puncture to rule out intracranial masses, atrophy (with resultant ex-vacuo ventriculomegaly), and other pathology. In NPH, there may also be transependymal edema seen on MRI. A large-volume lumbar puncture (30 to 50 cc) with subsequent improvement in symptoms predicts a better chance of improvement from a shunting procedure. Therefore, the first choice of treatment should be a lumbar puncture, possibly followed by shunt procedure (depending on positive response to lumbar puncture). Patients with dementia for more than 2 years are less likely to improve with shunting.

Shprecher D, Schwalb J, Kurlan R. Normal pressure hydrocephalus: Diagnosis and treatment. Curr Neurol Neurosci Rep. 2008; 8(5):371–376.

Sudarsky L, Simon S. Gait disorder in late-life hydrocephalus. Arch Neurol. 1987; 44:263–267.

47. d

This histologic slide reveals granulovacuolar degeneration, associated with Alzheimer's disease. Granulovacuolar degeneration results from the formation of abnormal neuronal intracytoplasmic granule-containing vacuoles. Lewy bodies are seen in DLB and are characterized by cytoplasmic inclusions with anti-ubiquitin and anti-α-synuclein immunohistochemistry. Pick bodies occur in Pick's disease, and are characterized by silver staining, showing spherical aggregations of tau protein in neurons. Bunina bodies are seen in amyotrophic lateral sclerosis, and Negri bodies are seen in rabies.

Bradley WG, Daroff RB, Fenichel GM, et al. Neurology in Clinical Practice, 5th ed. Philadelphia, PA: Elsevier; 2008.

Dickson DW. Neuropathology of non-Alzheimer degenerative disorders. Int J Clin Exp Pathol. 2010; 3(1):1–23.

Prayson RA, Goldblum JR. Neuropathology, 1st ed. Philadelphia, PA: Elsevier; 2005.

48. b

Agnosia is loss of ability to recognize stimuli while the specific sense to detect the stimuli is not impaired. Prosopagnosia is the inability to recognize faces. Ability to recognize people using other cues is often preserved. Face recognition is thought to be a function of the right hemisphere, but prosopagnosia most commonly occurs with bilateral lesions of the temporo-occipital regions (bilateral fusiform gyri), as occurs with bilateral PCA infarction. It can also be seen as part of more diffuse processes that preferentially affect the temporal lobes, such as Alzheimer's disease. Associated features may include achromatopsia (a disorder of color perception) and visual field deficits.

Topographagnosia, a defect in spatial orientation, is marked by inability to navigate in familiar places, read maps, draw floor maps of familiar places, and perform similar functions. It localizes to the nondominant posterior parahippocampal region, infracalcarine cortex, or nondominant parietal lobe.

Asomatognosia is marked by an indifferent inability to recognize one's own body part. It most often localizes to the contralateral (usually nondominant) superior parietal lobule, the supramarginal gyrus, and/or its connections. In somatoparaphrenia, a form of asomatognosia, the patient denies ownership of a limb(s) and claims the limb is missing, or has been stolen.

Misoplegia is severe hatred of a limb, a rare form of agnosia seen in hemiparetic or hemiplegic patients following stroke. The patient may attempt to cut off the limb or damage it otherwise.

Campbell W. Dejong's The Neurological Examination, 6th ed. Philadelphia, PA: Lippincott Williams and Wilkins; 2009.

Ropper AH, Samuels MA. Adams and Victor's Principles of Neurology, 9th ed. New York: McGraw-Hill; 2009.

49. C

The case describes Balint's syndrome (also known as Balint-Holmes syndrome), which localizes to the bilateral parieto-occipital region. This syndrome consists of a triad of optic ataxia (a deficit of reaching for objects under visual guidance), oculomotor apraxia (gaze apraxia, inability to voluntarily move the eyes to a new point of visual fixation despite normal extraocular muscle function), and simultanagnosia (inability to visually perceive more than one object at a time). This syndrome has been described with a variety of pathologies, including neurodegenerative disorders, progressive multifocal leukoencephalopathy, bilateral watershed infarcts, and malignancy.

In general, though there are exceptions, lesions of the dorsal visual pathways that pass through the parieto-occipital regions can be thought of as leading to an abnormality in detecting "where": where an object is in space, how to reach that object while looking at it. Lesions of the ventral, temporo-occipital pathways lead to an abnormality of detecting "what": what an object is.

Blumenfeld H. Neuroanatomy through Clinical Cases, 1st ed. Sunderland, MA: Sinauer Associates; 2002.

Ropper AH, Samuels MA. Adams and Victor's Principles of Neurology, 9th ed. New York: McGraw-Hill; 2009.

50. C

Anton's syndrome, also known as Anton-Babinski syndrome or visual anosognosia, manifests as cortical blindness with denial of visual loss and confabulation. This syndrome results from bilateral lesions of the medial occipital lobes (primary visual and visual association cortices). A delusional disorder is not suspected. In psychogenic blindness, confabulation does not typically occur and optokinetic nystagmus is typically preserved. A language disorder is not depicted here; receptive aphasia is discussed in question 53. Balint's syndrome is discussed in question 49.

Blumenfeld H. Neuroanatomy through Clinical Cases, 1st ed. Sunderland, MA: Sinauer Associates; 2002.

51. d

Charles Bonnet syndrome, a form of release hallucinations, is a condition marked by vivid hallucinations that occur in people with severe visual impairment due to a variety of reasons, most commonly ophthalmologic. Patients acknowledge that these images are hallucinations. This may be mistaken for a delusional disorder or psychosis, but the patient's insight into the fact that these are hallucinations helps rule this out. Anton's syndrome is discussed in question 50. Balint's syndrome is discussed in question 49.

Cammaroto S, D'Aleo G, Smorto C, et al. Charles Bonnet syndrome. Func Neurol. 2008; 23(3):123–127.

52. c

This patient exhibits the syndrome of alexia without agraphia. Alexia is a loss of reading comprehension despite normal visual acuity. Ability to read individual letters of a word is often retained. Writing and language comprehension are normal in alexia without agraphia. It is a disconnection syndrome, due to lesions in the dominant (usually left) PCA territory, commonly involving the medial and inferior occipitotemporal region and splenium of the corpus callosum. The patient has a contralateral (usually right) homonymous hemianopia. Although the ipsilateral visual field is intact, words that are seen cannot be effectively read, as the lesion in the splenium of the corpus callosum prevents them from being transmitted to Broca's area. This is not a disturbance of language per se, unlike Wernicke's aphasia (discussed in question 53), and is not a neglect syndrome. Given the history, examination, and MRI findings, a psychogenic disorder is highly unlikely. Cortical blindness, or Anton's syndrome, is associated with vision loss (see question 50).

Blumenfeld H. Neuroanatomy through Clinical Cases, 1st ed. Sunderland, MA: Sinauer Associates; 2002.

Ropper AH, Samuels MA. Adams and Victor's Principles of Neurology, 9th ed. New York: McGraw-Hill; 2009.

53. e

Pure word deafness, or verbal auditory agnosia, is marked by impaired auditory comprehension of language, though hearing per se (of tones and other nonverbal sounds) is intact; audiogram is normal in these patients. There is normal comprehension of written language, distinguishing it from Wernicke's (sensory) aphasia; Wernicke's aphasia is characterized by inability to comprehend, read, or repeat, with fluent, nonsensical speech. The lesion causing pure word deafness is most often in the bilateral middle portion of the superior temporal gyri, sparing Wernicke's area, but disrupting its connections with the primary auditory cortex (Heschl's gyrus) and temporal lobe association cortices. Cases have been reported with unilateral dominant temporal lobe lesions. This may be associated with amusia, or agnosia for music.

In nonverbal auditory agnosia, there is agnosia to sounds, such as the sounds animals make or environmental sounds. This most often occurs with bilateral anterior temporal lesions, though nondominant temporal lobe lesions can lead to this as well.

Anomia is inability to name objects with otherwise relative preservation of language expression and comprehension. Patients are able to recognize objects but cannot name them. Anomia usually occurs in association with other features of Broca's (expressive) aphasia (see question 54), though it may occur in isolation, particularly during recovery of a Broca's (expressive) aphasia. Anomia may occur with a variety of lesions, including dominant hemisphere posteroinferior frontal gyrus and temporal lesions. It has also been reported to occur in angular gyrus syndrome, due to lesions of the dominant angular gyrus, in association with Gertsmann's syndrome (discussed in question 70) and constructional difficulties.

Bradley WG, Daroff RB, Fenichel GM, et al. Neurology in Clinical Practice, 5th ed. Philadelphia, PA: Elsevier; 2008.

Ropper AH, Samuels MA. Adams and Victor's Principles of Neurology, 9th ed. New York: McGraw-Hill; 2009.

54. a

Aphemia, or pure word mutism, also referred to as verbal apraxia, is marked by an inability to speak fluently, impaired repetition, and intact auditory comprehension. A pure Broca's (expressive) aphasia is characterized by inability to speak, write, name, or repeat, but intact comprehension. In aphemia, there is retained ability to write and comprehend written language. The lesion is in the dominant frontal operculum, anterior and superior to Broca's area (posteroinferior frontal gyrus). Receptive aphasia is discussed in question 53; conduction aphasia is discussed in question 58; transcortical motor aphasia is discussed in question 57; and alexia without agraphia is discussed in question 52.

Blumenfeld H. Neuroanatomy through Clinical Cases, 1st ed. Sunderland, MA: Sinauer Associates; 2002.

55. a

Foix-Chavany-Marie syndrome, also known as anterior opercular syndrome, is characterized by severe dysarthria, bilateral voluntary paralysis of the lower cranial nerves with preserved involuntary and emotional innervation. This syndrome is associated with bilateral anterior opercular lesions, frequently in the setting of multiple infarcts.

Mao CC, Coull BM, Golper LAC, et al. Anterior operculum syndrome. Neurology. 1989; 39:1169–1172.

Ropper AH, Samuels MA. Adams and Victor's Principles of Neurology, 9th ed. New York: McGraw-Hill; 2009.

56. d

Transcortical sensory aphasia can be thought of as a Wernicke's (receptive) aphasia, but with intact repetition. Transcortical sensory aphasia may be seen in dominant hemisphere MCA-PCA territory watershed infarction, thalamic lesions (thalamic aphasia), and in neurodegenerative disorders such as Alzheimer's disease. Transcortical aphasias are also seen in the stages of recovery from other aphasia syndromes. Broca's (expressive) aphasia is discussed in question 54; Wernicke's (receptive) aphasia is discussed in question 53; conduction aphasia is discussed in question 58; and aphemia is discussed in question 54.

Blumenfeld H. Neuroanatomy through Clinical Cases, 1st ed. Sunderland, MA: Sinauer Associates; 2002.

57. e

This man exhibits a transcortical motor aphasia, which can be thought of as a Broca's (expressive) aphasia, but with intact repetition. This aphasic syndrome is seen with a variety of cortical and subcortical dominant hemisphere lesions in the frontal lobe, but is most commonly seen in two general settings. The first occurs in the setting of watershed infarcts in the dominant hemisphere ACA-MCA watershed territory, sparing connections between Wernicke's and Broca's area, but impairing speech output due to disruption of connections between Broca's area and the supplementary motor area. The supplementary motor area is located in the medial aspect of the superior frontal gyrus and can be thought of as the pacemaker for speech output. Second, transcortical motor aphasia is seen in the recovery phases of a Broca's (expressive) aphasia.

Goetz CG. Textbook of Clinical Neurology, 3rd ed. Philadelphia, PA: Saunders Elsevier; 2007.

Ropper AH, Samuels MA. Adams and Victor's Principles of Neurology, 9th ed. New York: McGraw-Hill; 2009.

58. c

The internal arcuate fasciculus connects Wernicke's area in the superior temporal gyrus to Broca's area in the inferior frontal gyrus. Lesions in this fasciculus lead to conduction aphasia, in which repetition is impaired but other aspects of language are intact. Broca's (expressive) aphasia is discussed in question 54 and Wernicke's (receptive) aphasia is discussed in question 53. Aphasia resulting from thalamic lesions is often a transcortical sensory aphasia (discussed in question 56).

Blumenfeld H. Neuroanatomy through Clinical Cases, 1st ed. Sunderland, MA: Sinauer Associates; 2002.

59. a

Amelodia or affective motor aprosodia localizes to the nondominant posteroinferior frontal gyrus, the nondominant hemisphere's analogue to Broca's area. Similarly, the inability to perceive and understand the emotional content of others' speech, sensory or receptive aprosodia, localizes to the nondominant posterosuperior temporal gyrus, the nondominant hemisphere's analogue to Wernicke's area.

Mesulam M. Principles of Behavioral and Cognitive Neurology, 2nd ed. New York: Oxford University Press; 2000.

Ropper AH, Samuels MA. Adams and Victor's Principles of Neurology, 9th ed. New York: McGraw-Hill; 2009.

60. c, 61. c

This man suffers from pseudobulbar affect, also known as involuntary emotional expression disorder. The pathophysiology of pseudobulbar affect is complex, but it most often occurs in patients with bilateral lesions that disconnect the corticobulbar tracts from the brain stem cranial nerve nuclei. It is commonly seen in patients with diffuse subcortical dysfunction, as occurs with amyotrophic lateral sclerosis, multiple sclerosis, and following traumatic brain injury, but has also been reported in patients with focal mass lesions or acute infarctions. A dextromethorphan-quinidine combination has been shown to reduce and sometimes even eliminate pseudobulbar affect in patients with a variety of neurologic disorders.

Blumenfeld H. Neuroanatomy through Clinical Cases, 1st ed. Sunderland, MA: Sinauer Associates; 2002.

Brooks BR, Thisted RA, Appel SH, et al. Treatment of pseudobulbar affect in ALs with dextromethorphan/quinidine: A randomized trial. Neurology. 2004; 63(8):1364–1370.

Panitch HS, Thisted RA, Smith RA, et al. Randomized, controlled trial of dextromethorphan/quinidine for pseudobulbar affect in multiple sclerosis. Ann Neurol. 2006; 59(5):780–787.

62. b

In this patient, an infarct in the superior division of the left middle cerebral artery resulted in a Broca's aphasia combined with right arm weakness. His left Wernicke's area is intact, but because of disconnection between Wernicke's area, left premotor cortex, and right premotor cortex, left-hand apraxia occurred. This is a rare disconnection syndrome.

Blumenfeld H. Neuroanatomy through Clinical Cases, 1st ed. Sunderland, MA: Sinauer Associates; 2002.

63. a

Apraxia is characterized by an impaired ability to execute a previously known movement. This woman exhibits ideomotor apraxia, which is suggested by use of a body part as an object during pantomime. Patients with ideomotor apraxia understand the movement that they are supposed to execute and achieve the general, overall movement, but exhibit abnormal postures and spatial errors. Ideomotor apraxia is seen with lesions in the dominant parietal cortex, in or around the area of the superior marginal and angular gyrus.

The dominant feature of conduction apraxia is impairment in imitation of movements. The localization of conduction apraxia is not well defined.

Ideational apraxia is characterized by impairment in the sequence of motions needed to carry out a specific movement. When asked to pantomime pouring a glass of water and drinking from it, patients with ideational apraxia will, for example, drink from the cup before pouring water into it. Ideational apraxia is seen in patients with bifrontal or biparietal dysfunction, as occurs in neurodegenerative disorders.

Disassociation apraxia is characterized by inability to execute a movement on command, but with normal ability to imitate. It has most commonly been reported to occur in the left hand in left hemispheric language-dominant patients who have left MCA territory lesions.

Conceptual apraxia is characterized by misconception of the function of objects in the environment. For example, a patient with conceptual apraxia may use a fork to eat soup or may pretend to use a screwdriver when asked to pantomime hammering a nail into a wall. Conceptual apraxia is seen with diffuse neurodegenerative processes, as well as with lesions in the nondominant hemisphere.

Bradley WG, Daroff RB, Fenichel GM, et al. Neurology in Clinical Practice, 5th ed. Philadelphia, PA: Elsevier; 2008.

Goetz CG. Textbook of Clinical Neurology, 3rd ed. Philadelphia, PA: Saunders Elsevier; 2007.

64. c

Dressing apraxia localizes to the right parietal lobe. It often occurs in the setting of a neglect syndrome.

Brazis PW, Masdeu JC, Biller J. Localization in Clinical Neurology, 5th ed. Philadelphia, PA: Lippincott Williams & Wilkins; 2007.

65. e, 66. b, 67. a

The prefrontal cortices (the areas of the frontal lobes anterior to the primary motor cortex) have extensive connections with various cortical and subcortical areas including the limbic system, basal ganglia, thalamus, and brain stem. The prefrontal cortex can be functionally divided into orbitofrontal, dorsolateral, and dorsomedial areas. Lesions of the frontal lobes, or disruptions in frontal-subcortical pathways, lead to a variety of syndromes that have extensive overlap, but can be broadly categorized on the basis of the most prominent features occurring with lesions to the different prefrontal regions.

The orbitofrontal cortex is located on the ventral aspect of the frontal lobes. It is involved in judgment, inhibition of socially inappropriate behaviors, as well as emotional and visceral functions. Lesions to this area, which commonly include trauma and olfactory groove or sphenoid wing meningiomas, lead to changes in personality, social disinhibition, facetiousness, inappropriate jocularity (*witzelsucht*), echopraxia, and utilization behavior (mimicking of use of objects in the environment), as depicted in question 65.

The dorsomedial prefrontal cortex is involved in motor initiation, goal-directed behavior, and motivation. Lesions to this area and bilateral lesions to the anterior cingulate, which commonly result from ACA infarcts and tumors, lead to apathy, indifference, loss of initiative, amotivation, and abulia, or a reduction (or in severe cases abolition) of movement and communication due, in part, to involvement of the supplementary motor area, as depicted in question 66. In extensive bilateral lesions to the dorsomedial prefrontal cortex, the most severe form of this nonparalytic akinesia, akinetic mutism, results. Because the paracentral lobule (the mesial projection of the somatosensory cortex) is involved in voluntary urinary continence, lesions to this area are often associated with urinary incontinence.

The dorsolateral prefrontal cortex is involved in the planning of motor activity and behavior, executive functioning, judgment, and problem solving. Lesions to this area lead to impaired judgment, impaired ability to plan, multitask, and problem solve, and anhedonia, or a lack of interest in previously pleasurable activities, as depicted in question 67.

Associated physical examination findings with frontal lobe pathology include frontal release signs, including grasp, suck, palmomental, snouting, and rooting reflexes.

Goetz CG. Textbook of Clinical Neurology, 3rd ed. Philadelphia, PA: Saunders Elsevier; 2007.

Ropper AH, Samuels MA. Adams and Victor's Principles of Neurology, 9th ed. New York: McGraw-Hill; 2009.

68. e

The Grooved Pegboard Test is a test of finger dexterity. The patient is timed as he/she places pegs into small grooved holes in a board. The grooves are oriented in different directions, requiring the patient to rotate the peg in their fingers, which increases the demands for distal dexterity. Right and left hands are performed separately, and the patient's time is compared to normative data.

The Trail-Making Test part A times the patient as he/she connects numbers on a page, and is a test of simple speed of processing, visual search, and attention. The Trail-Making Test part B requires the patient to connect consecutive numbers and letters; in addition to the demands of Trails A, it requires set shifting (shifting between numbers and letters) and working memory (maintaining the correct sequence).

The Wisconsin Card Sorting Test requires the patient to arrange cards on the basis of a specific concept. It is a test of frontal lobe function, and assesses visual conceptualization and set shifting.

The Random Cancellation Test, a measure of visual attention and processing speed, assesses the ability to visually scan and identify specific targets in a large array of similar items.

In the Clock-Drawing Test, a test of visuospatial function but also auditory comprehension, attention, and executive function, the patient is asked to draw a clock (including the numbers) with the hands set at a specific time.

Bradley WG, Daroff RB, Fenichel GM, et al. Neurology in Clinical Practice, 5th ed. Philadelphia, PA: Elsevier; 2008.

Goetz CG. Textbook of Clinical Neurology, 3rd ed. Philadelphia, PA: Saunders Elsevier; 2007.

69. d

The case describes Capgras' syndrome, which is characterized by the delusional belief that a person, often a member of the patient's immediate family, is an identical-looking imposter.

Other delusional misidentification disorders include Fregoli's syndrome (in which the patient believes that the same person exists in several disguises), intermetamorphosis (the belief that individuals have swapped identities with each other while maintaining the same external appearance), reduplicative paramnesia (which overlaps significantly with Capgras' syndrome, but there is a delusion that there are identical places/objects rather than just people), and Cotard's delusion (a person's belief that they are dead or dying). Pseudocyesis is not classified under the delusional misidentification disorders, but is a delusion that a person is pregnant when they are in fact not; the patient may manifest the signs and symptoms of pregnancy. It is more common in females, but has been reported in males.

Delusional misidentification disorders and other types of delusions can be seen in neurodegenerative disorders such as Alzheimer's dementia and Lewy body dementia, as well as in patients with structural brain lesions such as traumatic brain injury and cerebral infarction. Lesions are usually bifrontal or right hemispheric. Delusional misidentification disorders are also seen in primary psychiatric disorders such as schizophrenia, affective disorders, and delusional disorder.

Devinsky O. Delusional misidentifications and duplications. Right brain lesions, left brain delusions. Neurology. 2009; 72:80–87.

Forstl H, Almeida OP, Owen AM, et al. Psychiatric, neurological and medical aspects of misidentification syndromes: A review of 260 cases. Psychol Med. 1991; 21:905–910.

Sadock BJ, Sadock VA, Ruiz P, eds. Kaplan and Sadock's Comprehensive Textbook of Psychiatry, 9th ed. Philadelphia, PA: Lippincott Williams and Wilkins; 2009.

70. b

This man exhibits the features of Gerstmann's syndrome, which is characterized by the tetrad of finger agnosia (inability to identify fingers bilaterally), right-left confusion, dyscalculia (inability to carry out calculations), and dysgraphia (inability to write). It localizes to the dominant inferior parietal lobule, particularly the dominant angular gyrus. Common causes include infarction of the inferior division of the MCA, in which case there may be associated contralateral visual field deficits.

Ropper AH, Samuels MA. Adams and Victor's Principles of Neurology, 9th ed. New York: McGraw-Hill; 2009.

71. a

An infarct in the right MCA territory would be the best explanation for this patient's physical examination findings. Lesions to the primary somatosensory cortex lead to cortical sensory loss, manifesting as loss of two-point discrimination, agraphesthesia (inability to perceive letters or numbers drawn on the hand), astereognosis (inability to recognize shapes manipulated in the hand), and extinction to bilateral simultaneous stimulation. These findings localize the lesion to the cortex, as opposed to brain stem or subcortical areas.

Brazis PW, Masdeu JC, Biller J. Localization in Clinical Neurology, 5th ed. Philadelphia, PA: Lippincott Williams & Wilkins; 2007.

72. d

This boy exhibits anosognosia, or a lack of awareness of an acquired neurologic deficit, and hemispatial neglect syndrome, consistent with a lesion in the nondominant hemisphere involving the primary somatosensory cortex (area SI). A lesion in the thalamus can also lead to a neglect syndrome.

Blumenfeld H. Neuroanatomy through Clinical Cases, 1st ed. Sunderland, MA: Sinauer Associates; 2002.

73. b

The frontal eye fields are located in the middle frontal gyrus, and each frontal eye field is responsible for conjugate eye movement to the contralateral side. A lesion to the right frontal eye fields causes unopposed activity of the left frontal eye fields, leading to eye deviation to the right. A left hemiparesis with conjugate eye deviation to the right suggests a lesion in the right MCA territory. Focal motor seizures that involve the frontal eye fields lead to contralateral hemibody convulsions with conjugate gaze deviation to the side of the seizure manifestations (contralateral to the seizure focus). The parapontine reticular formation leads to ipsilateral conjugate gaze, and a lesion in the right pons would lead to a left hemiparesis and left gaze deviation due to unopposed action of the left parapontine reticular formation. A lesion in the left pons would lead to right hemiparesis with gaze deviation to the right. Gaze deviation with pontine lesions is not overcome by oculocephalic maneuver.

Brazis PW, Masdeu JC, Biller J. Localization in Clinical Neurology, 5th ed. Philadelphia, PA: Lippincott Williams & Wilkins; 2007.

74. c

Damage to the posterolateral thalamus gives rise to Dejerine-Roussy syndrome, or thalamic pain syndrome, which is characterized by initial contralateral hemianesthesia followed weeks later by pain, hyperesthesia, and allodynia. A similar delayed central pain syndrome can occur with a lesion to the medial lemniscus, dorsal columns, or with lesions to the parietal operculum (the latter is also termed pseudothalamic syndrome). The spinothalamic tract projects to the ventral posterolateral nucleus of the thalamus, which in turn projects to the secondary somatosensory cortex (area SII). A lesion to the primary somatosensory cortex (area SI) would lead to contralateral loss of sensation to touch, joint position sense, and vibration, but would spare pain and temperature sensation, and would not cause a delayed pain syndrome.

Ropper AH, Samuels MA. Adams and Victor's Principles of Neurology, 9th ed. New York: McGraw-Hill; 2009.

75. d

Declarative, or explicit memory, involves memory for facts or experiences. Declarative memory includes semantic knowledge, or knowledge for facts and objectives, and episodic knowledge, or knowledge of events. Nondeclarative, or implicit, memory involves memory of skills and other acquired behaviors. Lesions to the bilateral medial temporal lobes leads to loss of predominantly declarative (explicit) memory, leading to an anterograde amnesia, with a retrograde amnesia involving a specific period prior to injury, but usually with preservation of more remotely formed memories. On the other hand, there is not a specific lesion that would lead to loss of nondeclarative memory in general.

Blumenfeld H. Neuroanatomy through Clinical Cases, 1st ed. Sunderland, MA: Sinauer Associates; 2002.

76. d

This man exhibits features of Klüver-Bucy syndrome, which is seen with bilateral medial temporal lobe lesions, involving the amygdala. Clinical features may include hyperorality, visual agnosia, hypersexuality, blunted emotional affect (docility), hypokinesia, and hypermetamorphosis (over-attention to minute stimuli in the environment). It is seen following herpes simplex encephalitis, with neurodegenerative disorders such as FTD, following anoxic-ischemic injury to the temporal lobes, and after bilateral temporal lobectomy (a historical procedure) (see question 21 for further discussion of Klüver-Bucy syndrome).

Bradley WG, Daroff RB, Fenichel GM, et al. Neurology in Clinical Practice, 5th ed. Philadelphia, PA: Elsevier; 2008.

Brazis PW, Masdeu JC, Biller J. Localization in Clinical Neurology, 5th ed. Philadelphia, PA: Lippincott Williams & Wilkins; 2007.

77. e

The vignette most likely describes corticobasal ganglionic degeneration (CBGD), in which alien limb syndrome occurs. The phenomenon of alien limb is marked by movement of a limb, sometimes seemingly purposefully, but not under voluntary control. Alien limb syndrome also occurs with lesions to the contralateral ACA territory, involving the corpus callosum or sup-plementary motor area. Progressive supranuclear palsy, Huntington's disease, and CBGD are discussed further in Chapter 6. DLB is discussed in questions 10 and 11, and Pick's disease in question 12.

Ropper AH, Samuels MA. Adams and Victor's Principles of Neurology, 9th ed. New York: McGraw-Hill; 2009.

Rowland LP. Merritt's Neurology, 11th ed. Philadelphia, PA: Lippincott Williams and Wilkins; 2005.

78. e

Consciousness is maintained by the function of a variety of structures, including the reticular activating system in the brain stem, the thalamus (particularly the intralaminar nuclei), and the frontal lobes, particularly the medial aspects. In order to significantly affect consciousness, these areas must be involved. Lesions to the occipital cortices would not be expected to affect consciousness per se, but would rather cause various visual disturbances including visual field deficits and cortical blindness.

Brazis PW, Masdeu JC, Biller J. Localization in Clinical Neurology, 5th ed. Philadelphia, PA: Lippincott Williams & Wilkins; 2007.

79. a

This patient has a living will that clearly states his wishes, and has appointed a durable power of attorney for health care to make decisions on his behalf. The wishes of the patient, as com-municated by his power of attorney, should be upheld. The history suggests that the patient had full mental capacity at the time of drafting of the living will, and in such cases, it should be upheld even if he later loses capacity to make decisions for himself. Even though the son is next of kin, legal appointment of a durable power of attorney supersedes the word of the next of kin. Although continued communication with the son is important, in order for him to better accept his father's wishes and the management plans for him, his father's wishes will be enforced regardless of the son's ultimate acceptance. Involvement of the courts is not necessary because there is evidence that the patient has appointed his best friend as power of attorney and because a living will is available. Advanced directives, including living wills and durable power of attorney for health care, allow patients to exercise autonomy in their medical care even when they are unable to communicate at a specific time of medical decision making.

Jonsen A, Siegler M, Winslade W. Clinical Ethics: A Practical Approach to Ethical Decisions in Clinical Medicine, 6th ed. New York: McGraw-Hill; 2006.

Buzz Phrases	Key Points
Chromosome 1 gene associated with Alzheimer's Disease	Presenilin-2
Chromosome 14 gene associated with Alzheimer's Disease	Presenilin-1
Chromosome 19 gene associated with Alzheimer's Disease	Apolipoprotein E4
Chromosome 21 gene associated with Alzheimer's Disease	Amyloid precursor protein
Neuritic plaques, amyloid plaques, amyloid angiopathy, neurofibrillary tangles, granulovacuolar degeneration, Hirano bodies	Alzheimer's Disease
Lewy bodies	DLB
Fluctuating cognition, visual hallucinations, and parkinsonism	DLB
CAG repeat on chromosome 4, autosomal dominant	Huntington's disease
Waxing and waning mental status	Delirium
Synucleinopathies	Multiple system atrophy, Parkinson's disease, DLB, neuroaxonal dystrophy
Tauopathies	Alzheimer's Disease, corticobasal ganglionic degeneration, progressive supranuclear palsy, FTD
Globose neurofibrillary tangles and tufted astrocytes	Progressive Supranuclear Palsy
Spongiform encephalopathy	CJD
Cognitive dysfunction, gait impairment, and urinary incontinence	Normal pressure hydrocephalus
Gerstmann's syndrome	Finger agnosia, right-left confusion, dysgraphia, dyscalculia. Localization: dominant inferior parietal lobule, angular gyrus
Where? (where is an object in space?)	Parieto-occipital pathways
What? (what is an object?)	Parietotemporal pathways
Balint's syndrome	Optic ataxia, oculomotor apraxia, and simultagnosia. Localization: bilateral parieto-occipital cortices

(*continued*)

Buzz Phrases	Key Points
Anton's syndrome	Denial of cortical blindness. Bilateral medial occipital lesions.
Kluver-Bucy syndrome	Hyperorality, visual agnosia, hypersexuality, blunted emotional affect (docility), hypokinesia, and hypermetamorphosis. Localization: bilateral medial temporal lobe lesions, involving amygdala
Dressing apraxia	Nondominant parietal cortex
Hemisensory neglect	Nondominant parietal cortex
Conjugate gaze deviation in direction contralateral to hemiparesis	Lesion in frontal eye fields
Expressive aphasia, but with intact repetition	Transcortical motor aphasia; MCA-ACA watershed territory, disconnecting SMA from Broca's area
Receptive aphasia, but with intact repetition	Transcortical sensory aphasia; MCA-PCA watershed territory or thalamic infarct
Ideomotor apraxia	Patient understands the movement to be executed, but has difficulty with postural and spatial orientation. Dominant parietal cortex (superior marginal/angular gyrus)
Ideational apraxia	Patient struggles with temporal sequence of events needed to execute a movement. Bifrontal or biparietal cortex

Chapter 13

Psychiatry

Questions

Questions 1–2

1. A 33-year-old woman is brought to a psychiatrist's clinic by her husband. She was previously a quiet lady, but enjoyed social activities and loved her job. Over the past 4 weeks, she had stopped going to work and was spending most of her time at home, often in bed in her pajamas. She was constantly complaining of feeling tired. She was barely eating, and had lost 7 kg. Her husband would frequently find her lying in bed crying. She stated to him several times that she thought she would be better off dead. What is the most likely diagnosis in this patient?
    a. Major depressive disorder
    b. Major depressive episode
    c. Dysthymic disorder
    d. Bipolar disorder
    e. Depressive personality disorder

2. The woman in question 1 is treated with medications and her symptoms improve over a few months. She returns to work and resumes her social activities. Three years later, her symptoms recur: she stops going to work, cries frequently, sleeps most of the time, and stops eating. She attempts suicide unsuccessfully. What is the most likely diagnosis at this time?
    a. Major depressive disorder
    b. Major depressive episode
    c. Dysthymic disorder
    d. Bipolar disorder
    e. Depressive personality disorder

3. Which of the following statements regarding depression is incorrect?
    a. Psychosis cannot be a feature of depression; if psychotic symptoms are present, a diagnosis of depression cannot be made
    b. Depression may present with cognitive dysfunction, rather than the typical symptoms of depression, particularly in older adults

c. Excessive eating and sleeping are a feature of atypical depression

d. A seasonal pattern to depression can occur

e. Either insomnia or hypersomnolence may occur in depression

4. Regarding the epidemiology of depression, which of the following statements is incorrect?

a. Depression is more common in females as compared to males

b. Depression is the most common mood disorder

c. Depression is more common in Caucasians compared to other races

d. Depression is more common among those of low socioeconomic status

e. Depression is more common among urban-dwelling individuals as compared to those who live in rural areas

5. Which of the following statements regarding the genetics of mood disorders is incorrect?

a. Mood disorders are familial: depression and bipolar disorder are more common among family members of a patient with either depression or bipolar disorder

b. The mood disorders are genetically complex as compared to single-gene Mendelian disorders

c. Mood disorders are entirely explained by genetic factors, and environmental factors have little role to play in the occurrence of mood disorders

d. Alcoholism is more common in family members of patients with mood disorders

e. Specific polymorphisms of a serotonin transporter have been associated with an increased chance of developing a mood disorder

6. Regarding the neuroanatomic substrates of major depression, which of the following is incorrect?

a. The subcallosal cingulate gyrus has been implicated in depression, and is a potential target for treatment of depression with deep brain stimulation

b. Hippocampal abnormalities have been demonstrated in patients with depression, and these relate to abnormalities in the hypothalamic-pituitary-adrenal axis

c. The pathophysiology of depression in part relates to dysfunction of cortical-subcortical circuits connecting the frontal cortex and limbic regions

d. Patients with untreated depression show hypometabolism of the orbitofrontal cortex

e. Hypometabolism of the dorsal prefrontal cortex occurs in depression

Questions 7–8

7. A 39-year-old woman reports that over the prior month she has had several episodes that occur "out of the blue," in which she develops, over a 5-minute period, pounding sensation in her chest, chest tightness, choking sensation, and sweating all over, associated with a sense of fear, "as if something terrible was going to happen." She underwent an extensive cardiac work-up that did not show any abnormalities. She cannot identify any specific triggers for the episodes. She continues about her usual activities despite these attacks, but frequently worries about having more attacks and worries that one day the attacks will kill her. Which of the following is the most likely explanation for this patient's symptoms?

a. She is suffering from post-traumatic stress disorder

b. She is a hypochondriac

c. She has generalized anxiety disorder

d. She is suffering from panic attacks

e. She is malingering

8. A 41-year-old man suffers from similar episodic attacks as those described in question 7. He becomes so worried that one of these attacks will kill him that he has his wife undergo basic life support training, and he starts refusing to go anywhere without her. He also refuses to go to malls or other crowded places where he may not be able to get to help in sufficient time if one of these attacks occurs. What is the most likely diagnosis in this patient?
   a. Generalized anxiety disorder
   b. Post-traumatic stress disorder
   c. Panic disorder with agoraphobia
   d. Social phobia
   e. Separation anxiety

9. The mother of a 22-year-old man attempts unsuccessfully to reach him by telephone for 8 days. She finally goes over to his apartment building and finds him sitting on his couch. He appears disheveled, dazed, and has multiple bruises, abrasions, and dried blood on various body parts. She asks him repeatedly what had happened, but he does not know. In fact, the last thing he could recall was coming home from work 9 days prior. A police investigation is initiated, and from surveillance camera footage, it is surmised that a group of men had broken into his apartment and beaten him repeatedly and tortured him. This man's inability to recall these events is known as:
   a. Dissociative fugue
   b. Dissociative amnesia
   c. Depersonalization disorder
   d. Dissociative identity disorder
   e. Post-traumatic stress disorder

Questions 10–11

10. A 52-year-old man is brought for an urgent visit to a psychiatrist's clinic. He was in general a level-headed, calculating person, but had changed over the prior 2 weeks. He had not slept more than a few hours in prior days, secretly quit the job he had as a bank manager for 15 years, and stayed up all night designing websites for three separate Internet companies he had decided to launch. His wife found out that he had invested their entire life's savings in these companies during the prior week. His speech had become fast, and he was speaking almost constantly. He kept jumping from one topic to another and barely made any sense. This man's history is most consistent with which of the following?
   a. Acute depressive episode
   b. Acute psychotic episode
   c. Acute manic episode
   d. Acute hypomanic episode
   e. A mixed episode

11. The man depicted in question 10 had a history of depression, with one episode of severe depression associated with suicide attempt 7 years earlier, but had recovered well from that. What diagnosis can be made in this patient?
   a. Bipolar I disorder
   b. Bipolar II disorder
   c. Cyclothymic disorder
   d. Borderline personality disorder
   e. Major depression and schizophrenia combined

12. A 44-year-old man, previously divorced twice, presents with his third wife for marriage counseling. They had been married for 10 years, and as far back as she could remember, living with him had always been "a roller coaster." There were weeks to months that he would be happy and energetic, and would sometimes stay up all night working on many projects that eventually earned him promotions at work. There were other months during which he would be either irritable and unapproachable or sullen and disinterested in participating in social activities. What is the most likely diagnosis in this man?
    a. He is normal; his wife is just too critical
    b. Dysthymic disorder
    c. Bipolar I disorder
    d. Borderline personality disorder
    e. Cyclothymic disorder

Questions 13–14

13. An 8-year-old girl is typically well behaved and rarely acts out. She loves visiting her neighbors' houses, except for one neighbor's house where she categorically refuses to go to because they have a dog. Whenever she sees a dog, she begins screaming, becomes flushed, starts sweating, and will not calm down until the dog is removed. Which of the following best describes this patient's history?
    a. Panic disorder
    b. Generalized anxiety disorder
    c. Post-traumatic stress disorder
    d. Social phobia
    e. Specific phobia

14. A 33-year-old woman has been particularly productive at work, and her boss asks her to present the data on her department's performance at a meeting. This fills her with a sense of dread, as she has struggled with speaking in public all her life. During the days prior to the meeting, she is unable to sleep and stays up all night imagining all the possible things that could go wrong during her presentation. On the day of the presentation, she feels nauseous and can barely concentrate. As she begins the presentation, she starts to sweat, has palpitations, feels light-headed, experiences chest tightness, and has a syncopal event. What is the most likely diagnosis in this patient?
    a. Panic disorder
    b. Generalized anxiety disorder
    c. Agoraphobia
    d. Social phobia
    e. Specific phobia

15. Which of the following is incorrect regarding penetration of medications into the CNS?
    a. Serum concentrations of a medication are always a good indication of the CNS concentration
    b. The blood-brain barrier and blood-CSF barrier result from tight junctions between brain capillary endothelial and choroid plexus epithelial cells, respectively
    c. Uncharged particles and lipophilic substances have higher penetration into the CNS than ionized particles, drugs with low lipid solubility, and protein-bound drugs
    d. The blood-brain barrier is absent in certain parts of the brain
    e. Neurotransmitter metabolites are cleared through an acid transport system in the choroid plexus

16. A 33-year-old woman is brought to a psychiatrist's office by her family. They report that for the past 3 months she has changed significantly, with several new and concerning occurrences. She has been trying to convince family members that she is a prophet sent to earth to spread the word of God. In the office, she appears to be speaking up at the ceiling, and when questioned, reports she is conversing with God. She has stopped bathing so as not to wash off any of her holiness. On mental status examination, her affect is blunted, she jumps from one topic to another in response to simple questions, and she uses unusual words that make no sense. What is the most likely diagnosis?
    a. Obsessive-compulsive disorder
    b. Brief psychotic disorder
    c. Schizophreniform disorder
    d. Schizoid personality disorder
    e. Schizoaffective disorder

17. A 22-year-old man is brought to his family physician by his parents for worrisome behaviors. He wakes up at 6:03 AM every morning and spends more than 40 minutes making his bed so that "the lines on his cover align perfectly." He then spends more than 2 hours in the shower, and his skin has multiple abrasions on it where he has scrubbed repeatedly. When he leaves his room in the morning, he always has to tap on the doorknob just the right way, and does so more than 100 times before it "feels right." He has to skip specific steps on the staircase, and does not let anyone prepare his breakfast because he will eat only from unopened and perfectly sealed containers. Because of his morning routine, he has repeatedly been late to work and his boss has threatened to terminate his employment. He admits to a consuming fear of contamination and to an "indescribable urge" to arrange things in specific ways, but says he cannot help it. Which of the following disorders is most consistent with this history?
    a. Generalized anxiety disorder
    b. Post-traumatic stress disorder
    c. Obsessive-compulsive personality disorder
    d. Obsessive-compulsive disorder
    e. Bipolar disorder

18. A 16-year-old is brought to a psychiatrist by her father. He reports that his daughter had always been a "worrywart," but that things were getting out of control. She worried about "everything and everyone." She was so concerned that her father would die unexpectedly that during the day she would call him at least once an hour to make sure he was okay. She constantly worried that she would not have enough to pay for her college education, though funds had already been secured for that. She admitted to being tired all the time, to neck pain because she was "tensed up" all day, to poor sleep because she stayed up most of the night worrying, and to difficulty with concentrating on her schoolwork. What is the most likely diagnosis in this patient?
    a. Hypochondriasis
    b. Post-traumatic stress disorder
    c. Panic disorder
    d. Social phobia
    e. Generalized anxiety disorder

19. An 18-year-old girl is mugged by a tall blond man while walking on the streets of Cleveland. She is held at gunpoint, on her knees, while her purse, jacket, and watch are taken from her. She is hit on the head and left on the concrete bleeding until a police officer on patrol finds her and

provides her with assistance. In subsequent months, she refuses to sleep alone in a room, and she constantly looks toward the window, scared that her assailant has found her again. On the rare occasion that she falls asleep, she wakes up screaming due to a terrible nightmare during which she sees the entire event unfold in front of her. She rarely leaves her house, and when she does, every time she sees a tall blond man, she experiences palpitations, diaphoresis, and an intense sense of fear. This woman's history is most consistent with:

a. Acute stress reaction
b. Generalized anxiety disorder
c. Post-traumatic stress disorder
d. Night terrors
e. Panic disorder

Questions 20–22

20. A 29-year-old woman presents to the emergency department for the third time in 3 months. She reports severe abdominal pain of 2 years' duration that had intensified earlier that day. On review of systems, she endorses multiple other complaints that have been present for years, including headache, knee pains, and eye pains. She also reports painful, irregular menses, and tingling and numbness in her hands, feet, and face. Review of her medical records reveals multiple visits to various specialists, with extensive diagnostic testing including CT of the chest, abdomen, and pelvis, pelvic ultrasound, full cardiac evaluation, MRI of the brain and spine, and EMG/NCS in addition to extensive laboratory evaluation for rheumatologic disorders, vitamin deficiencies, and endocrinologic disorders. After social work and psychiatric consultation, no secondary gain can be identified, but a history of physical abuse in childhood is revealed. What is the most likely diagnosis in this patient?

a. Hypochondriasis
b. Somatization disorder
c. Generalized anxiety disorder
d. Body dysmorphic disorder
e. Factitious disorder

21. A 42-year-old right-handed man is brought to the emergency department by ambulance. He had sudden onset of left hemiparesis earlier that day. On examination, he cannot move his left arm or leg and has no sensation to any modality. His plantar responses are flexor, and his reflexes are symmetric, and remain as such for several days. He has two MRIs of the brain, which show no abnormalities on diffusion weighted images or on any other sequences. During psychiatric consultation, he reports his fiancée had recently broken up with him. He is sincerely concerned about his deficits, and wants them to resolve so that he can return to work. No secondary gains can be identified. What is the most likely diagnosis in this patient?

a. Factitious disorder
b. Somatization disorder
c. Generalized anxiety disorder
d. Body dysmorphic disorder
e. Conversion disorder

22. A 33-year-old woman presents to a plastic surgeon for consultation. She reports that her nose is too large and insists that the surgeon correct it. On examination, her nose is small but deformed, with multiple scars apparent. She reports that she has had three prior surgeries, but that "not enough was taken off." The patient's driver license picture, taken prior to any of the surgeries, shows that the patient's nose had been of normal size. The surgeon declines to offer her surgery; she storms out of his office and requests a second opinion from another plastic surgeon. What is the most likely diagnosis in this patient?

a. Hypochondriasis
b. Somatization disorder
c. Conversion disorder
d. Body dysmorphic disorder
e. Munchausen's syndrome

23. Regarding the pathogenesis of depression, which of the following is incorrect?

a. The monoamine hypothesis of depression postulates that depression results from a deficiency of or dysfunction in cortical and limbic catecholaminergic pathways
b. Support for the monoamine hypothesis comes from evidence that reserpine, which depletes catecholamines, leads to depression
c. Data showing that carriers of specific serotonin transporter promoter gene polymorphisms are more susceptible to depression and suicidal behavior in response to stress support the monoamine hypothesis of depression
d. Deficiencies in the monoamines have unequivocally been demonstrated in patients with depression, proving the monoamine hypothesis
e. Antidepressants act by increasing availability of catecholamines and otherwise enhance catecholaminergic transmission

Questions 24–25

24. A 27-year-old man is brought to a clinic by his mother with a 1-year history of slowly, but distinctly, progressive changes in behavior. He had always been shy and had difficulty making friends at school, but over the past year, he had become significantly withdrawn. He never smiled anymore; he was "emotionless" according to his mother. His mother would find him sitting alone in his room seemingly talking to someone. He was also becoming increasingly paranoid, and was convinced that the government was controlling his mind with high-frequency satellite waves. What is the most likely diagnosis in this patient?

a. Delusional disorder
b. Brief psychotic episode
c. Schizophrenia
d. Schizoaffective disorder
e. Schizoid personality disorder

25. Regarding the disorder depicted in question 24, which of the following is incorrect?

a. It is more common in males
b. It usually manifests after the age of 40
c. Both positive and negative symptoms are seen, with negative symptoms prevailing later in the disease course
d. It affects 1% of the world's population
e. It is more prevalent in lower socioeconomic populations

26. A 72-year-old woman suffers from a major depressive episode. She has a history of coronary artery disease, atrial fibrillation on anticoagulation therapy, sick sinus syndrome, glaucoma, and chronic obstructive pulmonary disease. Which of the following medications is most appropriate for the treatment of her depression?

a. Amitriptyline
b. Nortriptyline
c. Doxepin
d. Fluvoxamine
e. Escitalopram

Questions 27–28

27. A 13-year-old boy is seen by a psychiatrist while he is at a juvenile correctional facility. He had reportedly always been a troublemaker, but he had just gotten expelled from school and charged in court after for putting a dead rabbit on his teacher's desk and then on the same day setting a fire in the school library. He had a history of multiple detentions and suspensions for getting into fights and bullying his classmates and for skipping school. At home, he had enucleated his sister's pet gerbil's eyes, and once, when his mother grounded him for staying out all night (though he had a 10:00 PM curfew), he had threatened her with a kitchen knife. He had robbed their 91-year-old neighbor, threatening to strangle her if she did not give him money, and had been arrested at the mall repeatedly for shoplifting. Which of the following disorders does this child's history suggest?
a. Oppositional defiant disorder
b. Conduct disorder
c. Antisocial personality disorder
d. Acute manic episode
e. Borderline personality disorder

28. An 8-year-old boy is brought to a child psychiatrist by his parents. For the past 2 years, and increasingly over time, he had been showing significant hostility toward his parents and teachers. He was irritable, would lose his temper at the slightest things, would argue with his parents over everything, and would never abide by parents' or teachers' rules. He would blame his little brother for everything and frequently get his little brother in trouble. Which of the following disorders does this child's history suggest?
a. Oppositional defiant disorder
b. Conduct disorder
c. Antisocial personality disorder
d. Acute manic episode
e. Borderline personality disorder

29. A 45-year-old man presents to a psychiatry clinic with complaints of depression. He reports that he has always been depressed since as far back as he could remember. He reports that although some days are better than others, for most days over the prior several years, he was always tired, and had difficulty falling asleep almost every night. He reports that he had not felt like leaving the house much and had to force himself to get out of bed to go to work, where he had difficulty concentrating and barely got by on performance measures. At the end of the interview, he states he is not sure why he even came to the clinic because he did not think anything could be done to change the way he feels. This man's history is most consistent with:
a. Major depressive disorder
b. Chronic depression
c. Dysthymic disorder
d. Depressive personality disorder
e. Cyclothymic disorder

30. Which of the following is incorrect regarding the neurotransmitter serotonin?
    a. Serotonin is synthesized from tryptophan, with the rate-limiting step being catalyzed by tryptophan hydroxylase
    b. Serotonin is metabolized through action of monoamine oxidase (MAO) into 5-hydroxy-indoleacetic acid; the MAO-B isoform is the principle isoform involved in serotonin metabolism and is inhibited by selegiline
    c. In the CNS, the highest density of serotonergic neuron cell bodies is in the raphe nuclei of the brain stem
    d. There are multiple subtypes of the serotonin receptor, some that are ligand-gated ion channels and others that are metabotropic, linked to G-proteins
    e. Serotonin has multiple actions, including platelet aggregation, increased intestinal motility, vasoconstriction, and bronchoconstriction

31. A 69-year-old man who went to college with the first lady has claimed for the past 3 months that she is madly in love with him. He tells everyone he meets about how much she is in love with him, and he is convinced that she winks at him and smiles just for him when she is giving speeches on television. He works as a bank manager, and is very productive at his job. He is liked by all, and has many friends, who take his supposed love affair with the first lady as an amusing joke. There really is nothing particularly unusual about him, except for his belief regarding the first lady. What is the most likely diagnosis in this case?
    a. Brief psychotic disorder
    b. Schizophrenia
    c. Delusional disorder
    d. Schizoaffective disorder
    e. Atypical depression

32. Regarding the epidemiology and risk factors for suicide, which of the following is incorrect?
    a. Death due to suicide is three times more common in males as compared to females, but females attempt suicide three times more than males
    b. In Caucasians, suicide rates increase with increasing age
    c. Native Americans have the highest rates of suicide among all ethnicities in the United States
    d. More than half of all patients who commit suicide were suffering from a mood disorder prior to their death
    e. Among patients with personality disorders, those with schizoid personality disorder are the most likely to attempt suicide

33. The selective serotonin reuptake inhibitors (SSRIs) are commonly used antidepressants. Which of the following is correct regarding the SSRIs?
    a. The SSRIs act by inhibiting reuptake of serotonin and, through various pre- and postsynaptic effects, have antidepressant activity that may take several weeks to take effect
    b. Unlike the tricyclic antidepressants, the SSRIs have no drug-drug interactions
    c. The SSRIs are conveniently available in various formulations and can be administered through subcutaneous, sublingual, and intravenous routes
    d. The SSRIs have little use beyond depression
    e. The SSRIs have few systemic side effects because they only inhibit serotonin reuptake centrally

34. Regarding the pathophysiology of schizophrenia, which of the following is incorrect?
    a. The dopamine hypothesis of schizophrenia postulates that in this disorder, there is excessive limbic dopaminergic activity

b. Support for the dopamine hypothesis comes from evidence that postsynaptic blockade of D_2 (dopamine) receptors is useful in the treatment of schizophrenia

c. Overactivity of the nigrostriatal and tuberoinfundibular dopaminergic pathways forms the basis of the dopamine hypothesis

d. Patients with schizophrenia have increased dopamine receptor density, and imaging studies have shown increased striatal D_2 receptor occupancy by extracellular dopamine

e. The dopamine hypothesis does not fully account for the manifestations of schizophrenia and other psychotic disorders

35. A 19-year-old man is arrested after he is denied seating at a restaurant and proceeds to break all the plates and glasses in his sight and push over tables and chairs. He has a long history of detentions at school for angry outbursts. He has gotten into multiple fights, and had been previously arrested for physical aggression against a classmate. After each of these occurrences, he expresses regret, though he often attempts to justify his actions. When not aggravated, he is usually a pleasant person. What is the most likely diagnosis in this man?

a. Antisocial personality disorder
b. Bipolar disorder
c. Intermittent explosive disorder
d. Oppositional defiant disorder
e. Borderline personality disorder

36. A 16-year-old girl has always been considered short tempered and "moody," but does well in school. One day, she is arrested at the mall for attempted theft of a pair of shoes. When contacted, her distraught parents, wealthy and prominent members of society who have always given their daughter everything she wants, admit that she has a history of multiple prior thefts. The patient is taken to a therapist, to whom she admits to theft over the years on almost a daily basis because it gives her a "rush." She reports that she usually has no specific interest in the objects she has stolen. She knows her parents could buy these objects for her. Which of the following best describes this patient's disorder?

a. Borderline personality disorder
b. Antisocial personality disorder
c. Trichotillomania
d. Kleptomania
e. Pyromania

Questions 37–38

37. A 17-year-old girl is brought to the emergency department after being found unconscious on the floor of her dormitory. She is found to have a potassium level of 2.2 mmol/L (normal 2.5-5.0) and a sodium level of 120 mmol/L (normal 135-148). Her body mass index (BMI) is 16 (normal 18.5-24.9). Her roommate, who had been friends with her for several years, reported the patient had always been thin, but had a dramatic weight loss over the prior 2 years. The patient frequently ate; in fact, she would binge on junk food several times a day, and though she never admitted to it, her friends had noticed several signs, indicating the patient was self-inducing vomiting multiple times a day. She had not menstruated in over 1 year. What is the most likely diagnosis in this patient?

a. Bulimia nervosa
b. Anorexia nervosa, restricting type
c. Anorexia nervosa, binge eating/purging type

    d. Eating disorder not otherwise specified

    e. Impulse control disorder

38. An 18-year-old woman is referred to her college's health counselor after a pharmacist detects several unusual prescriptions for laxatives purchased by the patient. Her body mass index had been in the range of 23 to 24 since adolescence (normal 18.5-24.9). The patient admits to an intense fear of being fat for years, wishing to be thinner. She reported trying not to eat, but then gets so hungry that several times a week she would binge for hours, would subsequently feel guilty, and would take 30 to 40 pills of laxatives at once. What is the most likely diagnosis in this patient?

    a. Bulimia nervosa

    b. Anorexia nervosa, restricting type

    c. Anorexia nervosa, binge eating/purging type

    d. Eating disorder not otherwise specified

    e. Impulse control disorder

39. Tricyclic antidepressants are commonly used to treat depression. Which of the following statements is correct regarding the tricyclic antidepressants?

    a. The mechanism of action of all types of tricyclic antidepressants includes inhibition of reuptake of both norepinephrine and serotonin

    b. They have effects at muscarinic, histaminergic, and α_1-adrenergic receptors

    c. They directly inhibit reuptake of dopamine

    d. The action of tricyclic antidepressants is relatively specific, and there is little activity at non-catecholaminergic receptors

    e. They have little use beyond the treatment of depression and anxiety

40. A 16-year-old boy, a star athlete at his school, is noticed by his teachers to significantly struggle in activities that require reading. He is further assessed and found to be reading at less than the 10th percentile of normal for his age. He does relatively well in other subjects that do not heavily rely on reading, such as mathematics and geography, and his intelligence quotient is determined to be 90. What is the most like diagnosis in this boy?

    a. Reading disorder

    b. Mild mental retardation

    c. Mathematics disorder

    d. Disorder of written expression

    e. Acquired dyslexia

Questions 41–43

41. A 42-year-old man works as an accountant. As a child and adolescent, he made a few friends, but has lost touch with most of them because he always felt that they were friends with him only because they wanted money from him. He would frequently have arguments with the friends he maintained because he felt they were always making fun of him and criticizing him. As a student in college, he had multiple issues with his teachers, who he accused of grading him poorly because they hated him or were judging him. He had a few girlfriends, but only for brief periods, because he was convinced each of them was having an affair. At work, he had requested that human resources add a lockable door to his cubicle, because he was convinced that fellow office employees went through his drawers, stole his supplies, and logged into his computer and read his e-mails. Which of the following disorders best describes this man?

a. This man does not have a diagnosable disorder
b. Schizoid personality disorder
c. Schizotypal personality disorder
d. Schizophrenia, paranoid subtype
e. Paranoid personality disorder

42. A 38-year-old man had always been a "loner." He had few friends in childhood, and as a teenager and young adult, he had no interest in getting to know others. He stuck to a strict daily schedule, consisting mainly of meals, work, and sleep. He visited his parents once a week, for Sunday dinner. He rarely went to social events, and when he had to, he would spend most of his time staring at the floor and would appear annoyed if someone attempted to converse with him. He had no interest in romantic relationships or friendships. Which of the following disorders best describes this man?

a. This man does not have a diagnosable disorder
b. Schizoid personality disorder
c. Schizotypal personality disorder
d. Schizophrenia, paranoid subtype
e. Paranoid personality disorder

43. A 61-year-old woman has always been told she was weird. She is a fortune teller and is convinced that the spirits speak to her. She is very superstitious, and creates significant annoyance among family members because of all the rituals she makes them follow when they visit her house to avoid the wrath of the "evil eye." She has not had a haircut in over 10 years because she feels her hair gives her healing powers, and wears several necklaces and bracelets all the time, because she thinks they bring her good luck. She has few friends, and although she loves her siblings and spends time with them, she is always paranoid that they are planning to try to take away her spiritual powers. Which of the following disorders best describes this woman?

a. This woman does not have a diagnosable disorder; she is just eccentric
b. Schizoid personality disorder
c. Schizotypal personality disorder
d. Schizophrenia, paranoid subtype
e. Paranoid personality disorder

44. A 48-year-old woman, mother of six troublemaking children and an unloving husband, presents to the emergency department with severe abdominal pain. She is a poor historian and offers only vague information about time of onset and nature of the pain. General surgical consultation is immediately requested for her presentation of acute abdomen. She seems almost pleased when an exploratory laparotomy is suggested to her. During examination, she screams when her abdomen is initially palpated, but when she is distracted, deep palpation of her abdomen does not seem to bother her. Her husband and children gather around her bed, with concerned, guilty looks on their faces, tears streaming down their faces. When family members or physicians are in her room, she writhes in pain and cries, but when she is alone and thinks she is not being observed, she appears comfortable and makes a few phone calls and watches television. Extensive laboratory and radiologic testing is normal. What is the most likely diagnosis in this patient?

a. Factitious disorder
b. Malingering

c. Hypochondriasis

d. Ischemic bowel

e. Generalized anxiety disorder

45. Regarding the subtypes of schizophrenia, which of the following is correct?

   a. In the catatonic subtype, patients most commonly have psychomotor agitation with restlessness, excessive movement, and nonsensical speech

   b. The residual subtype is marked predominantly by disorganized speech and behavior and flat, inappropriate affect

   c. The disorganized subtype is diagnosed when visual and auditory hallucinations are the most prominent residual symptoms after an acute psychotic exacerbation

   d. The paranoid subtype is characterized by prominent auditory hallucinations and delusions with relative preservation of cognitive function and affect

   e. Undifferentiated schizophrenia is diagnosed when the diagnostic criteria for schizophrenia have never been met but there are some psychotic symptoms

Questions 46–48

46. A 33-year-old man is brought to a psychologist by his mother. His mother reported that her son is "crazy" and that she wanted the psychologist to "talk some sense into him." Apparently, the man had been offered a promotion at work into a more prestigious, higher paying job with several perks that he had declined because he was scared that as soon as his work load increased, his employers would start criticizing him, think he could not handle it, and fire him. His mother reported he had always been like that: always avoided any situation where he might get criticized, was overly sensitive, and was convinced that people hated him. As a teenager, he was shy and made only a few friends because he felt no one would want to hang out with him, though there were many people in his class he wished he could have been friends with. He would date girls only after his mother repeatedly ensured him that they would like him. She said she was tired of having opportunities pass him because he felt he was never good enough for them. Which of the following disorders best describes this man?

   a. Schizoid personality disorder

   b. Panic disorder with agoraphobia

   c. Dependent personality disorder

   d. Obsessive-compulsive personality disorder

   e. Avoidant personality disorder

47. A man meets a woman, and in a whirlwind romance, they are married within 4 weeks of meeting; he justifies this to his friends by stating that she is "very low maintenance," never arguing with him and letting him do things his own way. However 2 months later, he is cursing the day he ever met her. She apparently could not make any decision on her own, and had to consult with him on everything. Within weeks of being married, he found himself doing almost everything for her because she would say she did not know how or was scared of messing things up. He would become upset and yell at her and insult her, but she would just sit there and take it because she did not want him to leave her. According to the woman's family members, she had always been very clingy, and "couldn't take care of herself." Which of the following disorders best describes this woman?

   a. Schizoid personality disorder

   b. Panic disorder with agoraphobia

   c. Dependent personality disorder

d. Obsessive-compulsive personality disorder

e. Avoidant personality disorder

48. A 52-year-old man is asked to assume the role of a team leader at his office. The team members dread the experience; they have known the man for years. He is best known for having his entire office filled with filing cabinets because he files every single paper he has ever come across, regardless of whether or not it is important or needed for the future. As expected, during the first 2 days of his leadership, he makes all the team members reorganize their offices so that everything is in order and there is no clutter on any of the office desks. During meetings, he has everyone write down the minutes of the meeting and then at the end of the meeting, has every person read them out in order to make sure they are all accurate and as similar to each other as possible. By the end of the day, little has been done in terms of productive work because of the time spent on such activities. He makes everyone in the office stay over hours, is dismissive if anyone suggests that they should spend their time more efficiently, and when one of the team members tells him she needs to leave to pick her children up from day care, he scoffs at her for not having good work ethic and having deranged priorities. Which of the following disorders best describes this man?

a. Schizoid personality disorder

b. Obsessive-compulsive disorder

c. Dependent personality disorder

d. Obsessive-compulsive personality disorder

e. Avoidant personality disorder

49. A 32-year-old man wakes up one morning convinced that he had been abducted by aliens overnight. He reports that sperm was extracted from him and injected into the queen of the galaxies, and that she is now carrying his baby. He meets a 28-year-old woman, and when she hears his story, she is skeptical, but interested. Soon after they meet, they marry, and she soon becomes convinced of his story. The couple travels around the country trying to lobby for funding for a space mission to rescue the man's extraterrestrial son from outer space. Which of the following statements is correct?

a. They both have schizophrenia

b. They are both just eccentric, but do not meet criteria for any one type of psychiatric disorder

c. They both have histrionic personality disorder

d. They suffer from a somatoform disorder, which can be contagious

e. They have shared psychotic disorder (folie à deux)

50. Which of the following is not an adverse effect of tricyclic antidepressants?

a. Overactive bladder

b. Xerostomia

c. Sedation

d. Weight gain

e. Seizures

51. A 7-year-old boy, Matt, and his 9-year-old brother, Tom, are being seen by their pediatrician for their annual checkup. Their mother appears worn out and reports to the physician that her sons have always kept her busy, but that over the past year, Matt has been giving her extensive trouble with his school work. She thinks he is smart, but he just cannot seem to pay attention to anything, cannot seem to concentrate for more than 5 minutes on his homework, is easily distractible, and never does what he is told, is constantly misplacing things, and even forgets to brush his teeth and shower sometimes if she does not remind him. Tom is also giving her trouble with his school work, but his main problem is that he "just can't seem to sit still." At home, he fidgets at the dinner table and while doing homework, and at school there have been multiple complaints about him leaving his seat and even the classroom. He talks constantly, jumping from one topic to another, cannot wait in turn, and is constantly butting into conversations. What is the most likely diagnosis in Matt and Tom?

a. There is no diagnosis; their behavior is age appropriate
b. Conduct disorder
c. Oppositional defiant disorder
d. Attention-deficit/hyperactivity disorder
e. Generalized anxiety disorder

52. Which of the following are potential side effects of selective serotonin reuptake inhibitor therapy?
a. Nausea
b. Irritability
c. Suicidal thoughts, particularly in younger age groups
d. Erectile dysfunction
e. All of the above

Questions 53–55

53. Which of the following is incorrect regarding the first generation of antipsychotics, so-called typical antipsychotics or neuroleptics?
a. Chlorpromazine and thioridazine are examples of low-potency typical antipsychotics, and have higher levels of side effects related to antagonism at nondopamine receptors
b. The typical antipsychotics exert their antipsychotic effect predominantly by antagonism at D_2 receptors
c. Haloperidol and other high-potency typical antipsychotics, such as fluphenazine, have the highest risk of extrapyramidal side effects among the antipsychotic agents
d. Some of the typical antipsychotics are available in intravenous or intramuscular formulations
e. The typical antipsychotics are rarely used in the treatment of schizophrenia and other psychotic disorders because newer, more efficacious, and cost-effective medications are now available

54. An 18-year-old man is diagnosed with schizophrenia and started on an antipsychotic agent. Six weeks later, he has multiple complaints, including dry mouth, sleepiness, and dizziness when he stands from a seated position. Which of the following medications is he most likely being treated with?
a. Chlorpromazine
b. Haloperidol
c. Fluphenazine
d. Perphenazine
e. Prochlorperazine

55. A 32-year-old man has been treated with typical antipsychotic medications for more than 10 years. He has been well controlled on medications, with only residual negative symptoms. During a routine follow-up visit with his psychiatrist, he is noticed to have constant chewing movements, occasional tongue protrusion, and jaw thrusting. His medication is stopped, but these movements persist. Which of the following medications is most likely to lead to these manifestations?

a. Chlorpromazine
b. Haloperidol
c. Thioridazine
d. Benztropine
e. Prochlorperazine

56. The fiancé of a 32-year-old woman ends their relationship of 4 years' duration. In the following 2 months, she can barely sleep at night, and some nights she will stay up all night watching romantic movies and crying. She continues to go to work, but can barely concentrate, and is frequently found at her desk crying. She finally seeks psychologic counseling, and within 4 months of the breakup, she starts to feel better again and is able to date. What disorder was this woman exhibiting?

a. Bereavement
b. Major depressive episode
c. Adjustment disorder
d. There is no disorder; this was a normal reaction to a breakup
e. Acute stress reaction

57. Regarding the anxiolytics, which of the following statements is incorrect?

a. Benzodiazepines may be used for brief periods of time in the treatment of anxiety disorders
b. Chronic use of benzodiazepines leads to tolerance and dependence
c. Selective serotonin reuptake inhibitors are used for chronic therapy of anxiety disorders
d. Buspirone is an anxiolytic that acts as a dopamine D_1 receptor antagonist
e. Benzodiazepines are available in various oral, sublingual, intravenous, and intramuscular formulations

58. Which of the following is correct regarding imaging findings in schizophrenia?

a. Slit-like ventricles, due to reduced volume of the lateral ventricles, is often seen
b. There is evidence of gyral hypertrophy with sulcal narrowing
c. There is atrophy of areas of the frontal and temporal lobes
d. Positron emission tomography studies have shown significant hypermetabolism at rest in the cingulate cortex
e. There is bilateral symmetric caudate head atrophy

59. A 69-year-old man is brought to the emergency department by his family for altered mental status. For the prior few weeks, he had been increasingly sleepy, and that morning, he could barely be aroused. He has a chronic history of depression and was started on fluoxetine 2 months earlier. He also suffers from coronary artery disease, hypertension for which he is on a thiazide diuretic, and cirrhosis. In the emergency department, his serum sodium is found to be 118 (normal 132-148 mmol/L). Which of the following statements is incorrect in relation to this patient's presentation?

a. Hyponatremia occurs as an adverse effect from selective serotonin reuptake inhibitors (SSRIs)
b. Coadministration of an SSRI with a diuretic increases the risk of hyponatremia
c. The hyponatremia occurring with SSRIs is thought to be due to syndrome of inappropriate antidiuretic hormone
d. Treatment of hyponatremia due to SSRIs involves discontinuation of the SSRI as well as other usual measures for hyponatremia
e. Hyponatremia resulting from SSRIs typically occurs after 3 months of therapy

60. Regarding the genetics of schizophrenia, which of the following is correct?
   a. Family members of patients with schizophrenia are not at a higher risk of developing schizophrenia than the general population
   b. Schizophrenia is likely a result of the presence of predisposing genes combined with exposure to various environmental factors
   c. Schizophrenia is a monogenic, autosomal dominant disorder that localizes to chromosome 4
   d. Monozygotic twins and dizygotic twins have similar concordance rates for schizophrenia
   e. No specific genetic abnormalities have been associated with schizophrenia as yet

61. A 52-year-old woman has a long history of depression. She has had a partial response to fluoxetine combined with duloxetine, but continues to feel depressed, so her psychiatrist adds amitriptyline to her regimen. Two weeks later, she is brought to the ED where she is found to be obtunded, diaphoretic, and tachycardic. On examination, multifocal myoclonus and sustained ankle clonus are noted. What is the most likely diagnosis in this patient?
   a. Neuroleptic malignant syndrome
   b. Thyroid storm
   c. Serotonin withdrawal syndrome
   d. Serotonin syndrome
   e. Psychogenic coma, due to her depression

62. A 38-year-old man was brought to the emergency department by his family for a 3 day history of auditory hallucinations, paranoid delusions, and disorganized speech. Symptoms had started after he had witnessed the murder of his wife. He was admitted to an inpatient psychiatry unit and treated with medications. His psychotic symptoms resolved over 8 days. At the time of discharge, he was appropriately mourning the death of his wife. At 1-year follow-up, he continued to express sadness about the death of his wife, but showed no features of depression, psychosis, or any other psychiatric conditions. He did not have further recurrences of psychosis. The occurrence of psychotic symptoms in this man is most consistent with a diagnosis of:
   a. Schizophrenia
   b. Schizophreniform disorder
   c. Delusional disorder
   d. Schizoaffective disorder
   e. Brief psychotic disorder

63. Regarding the neurotransmitter GABA, which of the following is incorrect?
   a. GABA is the main excitatory neurotransmitter in the central and peripheral nervous system, along with glycine
   b. The $GABA_A$ receptor is an ionotropic receptor and the $GABA_B$ receptor is a metabotropic receptor
   c. The medication baclofen is a selective agonist at $GABA_B$ receptors
   d. Benzodiazepines act at the $GABA_A$ receptor
   e. GABA is an example of an amino acid that acts as a neurotransmitter

Questions 64–67

64. A coworker of yours is disliked by everyone who works in the office because, as is frequently said, he is "so full of himself" and "thinks he's God's gift to women." He thinks he is smarter than everyone and constantly takes credit for all successes within the company. He acts as though he is doing others a favor when he speaks to them and tells stories of how women throw themselves at his feet. When others make comments to him about his conceitedness, he claims that they are jealous of him and not even worth his time. Which of the following disorders best describes this man?

a. Antisocial personality disorder
b. Borderline personality disorder
c. Histrionic personality disorder
d. Narcissistic personality disorder
e. This man does not have a diagnosable disorder; he is just too conceited

65. The distraught parents of a 23-year-old man bail their son out of jail for the fourth time. He had always been "a troublemaker," but this had worsened over time, and in the prior 6 years, he had been arrested for assaulting a police officer, theft, reckless driving, and most recently for vandalism. He had dropped out of school at the age of 16 and had never maintained legitimate employment for more than a few weeks. He sustained his income by stealing, selling drugs, selling weapons, and conning older frail and ill women in their neighborhood out of thousands of dollars. He expressed no remorse or regret for any of his actions and seemed amused by his parents' tears and pleas. Which of the following disorders best describes this man?

a. Antisocial personality disorder
b. Borderline personality disorder
c. Histrionic personality disorder
d. Narcissistic personality disorder
e. Conduct disorder

66. The boyfriend of a 19-year-old woman broke up with her because "there's just too much drama" in their relationship. Two days later, she called him and told him she was calling to say goodbye because she was planning to take 100 pills of acetaminophen to "end the pain" because she loved him and could not imagine living without him. After she is treated in the hospital for suicidal ideation and released, she vandalizes her ex-boyfriend's house and assaults him, yelling at him repeatedly about how much she hates him. She has had two other suicide gestures previously, once when another boyfriend had broken up with her and another time when she had a fight with her best friend. She has multiple scars on her arms and chest from self-inflicted cuts with a knife, and when asked about them states, "I feel empty and dead, and it makes me feel alive." She is sexually promiscuous, and engages in sexual activity with strangers because they "help fill the emptiness." Which of the following disorders best describes this woman?

a. Antisocial personality disorder
b. Borderline personality disorder
c. Histrionic personality disorder
d. Narcissistic personality disorder
e. Impulse control disorder

67. A 26-year-old woman frequents several bars and clubs on a regular basis, and prides herself on being the "life of the party." At social events, she frequently partially undresses and then dances on tables and chairs in a dramatic and sometimes indecent manner. When a man that she has danced with starts speaking with another woman, she may confront the woman for "stealing her man" (though often she has not known the man for more than a few hours). When she does not receive the attention she would like, she becomes tearful and creates a scene about the smallest occurrence, until the majority of those present have contributed efforts in soothing her and calming her down. Which of the following disorders best describes this woman?

a. Antisocial personality disorder
b. Borderline personality disorder
c. Histrionic personality disorder
d. Narcissistic personality disorder
e. Impulse control disorder

68. Which of the following statements is incorrect regarding the mechanism of action of the antidepressants listed?

a. Duloxetine and venlafaxine strictly inhibit reuptake of norepinephrine
b. Mirtazapine, by acting as an antagonist at presynaptic α_2-receptors, enhances presynaptic release of norepinephrine and serotonin, and also acts as an antagonist at 5-HT$_2$ and 5-HT3 receptors
c. Bupropion may act by inhibiting reuptake of norepinephrine and dopamine, and increases presynaptic release of norepinephrine and dopamine
d. Trazodone works primarily through antagonism at the 5-HT$_2$ receptor
e. Phenelzine and isocarboxazid are monoamine oxidase inhibitors and are rarely used in clinical practice

69. A 27-year-old man is living with his parents after losing his job. His parents notice that he has started collecting different types of wires and antennas, claiming that he has assembled a device that is communicating with extraterrestrial beings, which have designated him as their leader on earth. His parents would find him carrying on discussions while he was alone in his room. At the time of onset of these delusions and hallucinations, he did not show any depressive symptoms, but 2 months later, he began to show significant symptoms of depression, in addition to the psychotic symptoms. Three months later, he attempts suicide. He is admitted to an inpatient psychiatric unit and is treated pharmacologically; his depression resolves, but his delusions persist, though attenuated, and he continues to have occasional hallucinations for several months. What is the most likely diagnosis in this patient?

a. Major depressive disorder
b. Depression with psychotic features
c. Schizophrenia
d. Schizoaffective disorder
e. Bipolar disorder

70. An 83-year-old man with moderate Alzheimer's disease is brought to his neurologist by his daughter. She reports he has been waking up at night and trying to leave the house. He has been very agitated at night, and once claimed that there were burglars digging a tunnel under his house, and began searching for his rifle so that he could protect his family. A few times, he has become so agitated that he pushed his daughter, and once mistook his wife for an intruder and hit her. During the day, he is less agitated, but does have hallucinations that seem to frighten him tremendously. The family wants to keep the man at home, despite the difficulties in his care. The neurologist discusses with the family therapeutic options, including an atypical antipsychotic agent. Which of the following statements is incorrect regarding use of atypical antipsychotic agents in patients with dementia?

a. There is an increased risk of mortality in patients with dementia being treated with atypical antipsychotic agents
b. There is an increased risk of stroke in patients with dementia being treated with atypical antipsychotic agents

    c. Atypical antipsychotic agents can be effective in the treatment of agitation or hallucinations and other behavioral and psychotic symptoms in dementia

    d. There is an increased risk of thromboembolic events in patients with dementia treated with atypical antipsychotic agents

    e. Because of the risks associated with atypical antipsychotics in patients with dementia, they are absolutely contraindicated in this patient population

71. A 62-year-old man with a history of depression presents to the psychiatrist with his first episode of major depression. He has not been sleeping well, and has had significant weight loss. He is suffering from erectile dysfunction, and complains of poor memory. Which of the following is incorrect regarding management of this patient?

    a. Optimal treatment for depression involves both pharmacologic therapy and psychotherapy

    b. Regardless of the antidepressant selected, a trial of 2 weeks of therapy is warranted before the medication is deemed ineffective

    c. Electroconvulsive therapy can be effective for both psychotic and nonpsychotic forms of depression, but side effects include cognitive impairment

    d. If a patient does not respond to the initial antidepressant chosen, he has an approximately 50% chance of response to an antidepressant from a different class

    e. In the treatment of depression, among the various antidepressants, clear superiority of one agent versus another has not been unequivocally demonstrated for the treatment of depression

Questions 72–74

72. Which of the following is correct regarding the second generation of antipsychotics, so-called atypical antipsychotics?

    a. They function primarily by antagonizing D_2 receptors

    b. They are more efficacious that the typical antipsychotics

    c. They do not lead to extrapyramidal side effects

    d. They differ from the typical antipsychotics in that they are antagonists at serotonergic $5\text{-}HT_{2A}$ receptors, and exert their action primarily at that receptor

    e. They are available only in oral or sublingual preparations

73. Regarding the adverse effects of atypical antipsychotic medications, which of the following is incorrect?

    a. Patients being treated with atypical antipsychotics should be regularly monitored for diabetes and dyslipidemia

    b. These medications can lead to arrhythmias

    c. The atypical antipsychotics have little activity at muscarinic and histaminic receptors

    d. Weight gain is a significant concern with these agents

    e. Amenorrhea can occur with exposure to atypical antipsychotics

74. Some of the individual antipsychotics are more likely to lead to specific side effects than others. Which of the following medication-side effect pair is least likely to be of concern in clinical practice?

    a. Clozapine and seizures

    b. Quetiapine and sedation

    c. Olanzapine and urinary retention

    d. Clozapine and agranulocytosis

    e. Aripiprazole and QT prolongation

75. A 33-year-old woman is brought to the emergency department after being found on the floor of her apartment with an empty bottle of oral diazepam on the floor next to her. She had filled the prescription the prior day, and there is a high suspicion that she had ingested more than 20 tablets in suicidal intent. On examination, she is comatose, and respiratory rate is 8. Which of the following medications should be administered in the treatment of this patient?

  a. Naloxone
  b. Naltrexone
  c. Flumazenil
  d. Thiamine
  e. Dextrose

76. Which of the following is incorrect regarding the neurotransmitters glutamate and aspartate?

  a. Overactivity at glutamate receptors leads to the phenomenon of excitotoxicity
  b. Glutamate and aspartate are the principle excitatory neurotransmitters in the CNS
  c. NMDA acts as an agonist at subtypes of glutamate receptors
  d. Memantine is an example of an NMDA agonist
  e. NMDA receptors are involved in the phenomenon of long-term potentiation

77. Which of the following psychotropic medications has been associated with an increased risk of seizures?

  a. Bupropion
  b. Clozapine
  c. Olanzapine
  d. Flumazenil
  e. All of the above

Questions 78–79

78. Which of the following medications is not used in the treatment of bipolar disorder?

  a. Lithium carbonate
  b. Valproic acid
  c. Lamotrigine
  d. Risperidone
  e. Levodopa

79. A 33-year-old woman is brought to a psychiatrist by her family for severe depressive symptoms, including insomnia, reduced appetite with weight loss, and anhedonia. By history, it is apparent that she has suffered several manic episodes in the past. She is started on an antidepressant as well as a mood-stabilizing agent. Her depressive symptoms improve somewhat, but she continues to have reduced appetite and reduced oral intake. On follow-up 6 weeks later, she has multiple complaints, an eruption of acne on her arms and face, and a tremor. On routine laboratory testing, her serum sodium is noted to be 155. Which of the following medications is she most likely being treated with?

  a. Lithium carbonate
  b. Sertraline
  c. Lamotrigine
  d. Risperidone
  e. Topiramate

Answer key

1. b	15. a	29. c	43. c	57. d	71. b
2. a	16. c	30. b	44. a	58. c	72. d
3. a	17. d	31. c	45. d	59. e	73. c
4. c	18. e	32. e	46. e	60. b	74. e
5. c	19. c	33. a	47. c	61. d	75. c
6. d	20. b	34. c	48. d	62. e	76. d
7. d	21. e	35. c	49. e	63. a	77. e
8. c	22. d	36. d	50. a	64. d	78. e
9. b	23. d	37. c	51. d	65. a	79. a
10. c	24. c	38. a	52. e	66. b	
11. a	25. b	39. b	53. e	67. c	
12. e	26. e	40. a	54. a	68. a	
13. e	27. b	41. e	55. b	69. d	
14. d	28. a	42. b	56. c	70. e	

Answers

1. b, 2. a

This woman's initial presentation is consistent with major depressive episode; following her second episode of depression 3 years later, a diagnosis of major depressive disorder can be made.

The diagnostic criteria for major depressive episode include the following (Diagnostic and Statistical Manual—Text Revision (DSM-IV-TR, 2000)):

A. Five or more of the following symptoms present over a 2-week period, nearly every day, that represent a change from previous function, with at least one symptom including either depressed mood or loss of pleasure:

   – Depressed mood for most of the day nearly every day, either subjective or as observed by others
   – Diminished interest or pleasure
   – Significant unintentional weight loss or weight gain
   – Insomnia or hypersomnia
   – Psychomotor agitation or retardation as observed by others
   – Fatigue or loss of energy
   – Feelings of worthlessness or excessive/inappropriate guilt
   – Diminished ability to think or concentrate
   – Recurrent thoughts of death, suicidal ideation, or suicide plan or attempt

B. Symptoms do not meet criteria for a mixed episode
C. Symptoms cause significant distress or functional, social, and/or occupational impairment
D. Symptoms are not due to a substance, medical condition, or bereavement

Major depressive disorder is diagnosed after the occurrence of two or more major depressive episodes that occurred at least 2 months apart. Dysthymic disorder is discussed in question 29 and bipolar disorder in questions 10 and 11. The DSM-IV no longer includes depressive personality disorder as a diagnosable personality disorder.

Diagnostic and Statistical Manual of Mental Disorders: DSM-IV-TR, 4th ed., text revision, Washington, DC: American Psychiatric Association; 2000.

Hales RE, Yudofsky SC, Gabbard GO (Eds). The American Psychiatric Publishing Textbook of
Psychiatry. Arlington, VA: American Psychiatric Publishing Inc; 2008.

Sadock BJ, Sadock VA, Ruiz P (Eds). Kaplan and Sadock's Comprehensive Textbook of Psychiatry,
9th ed. Philadelphia, PA: Lippincott Williams and Wilkins; 2009.

3. a

The occurrence of psychotic features does not preclude a diagnosis of major depressive episode.
Depression with psychotic symptoms, such as delusions and even hallucinations, may occur,
particularly in older adults, but the psychotic symptoms develop during the course of the
depression, and the diagnostic criteria for schizophrenia (discussed in questions 24 and 25)
or schizoaffective disorder are not met (discussed in question 69). The occurrence of psychotic symptoms in depression is a sign of higher severity of depression and a higher risk of
recurrence.

In older adults, depression may masquerade as cognitive impairment, what has also been
termed "pseudodementia." Diminished appetite and insomnia are the more common neuroveg-
etative symptoms in depression; with atypical depression, hyperphagia (excessive eating) and
hypersomnolence (excessive sleeping) occur. Up to 30% of patients with major depressive disorder have a seasonal pattern to their symptoms, with episodes of depression and remission
temporally related to specific seasons.

Hales RE, Yudofsky SC, Gabbard GO (Eds). The American Psychiatric Publishing Textbook of
Psychiatry. Arlington, VA: American Psychiatric Publishing Inc; 2008.

Sadock BJ, Sadock VA, Ruiz P (Eds). Kaplan and Sadock's Comprehensive Textbook of Psychiatry,
9th ed. Philadelphia, PA: Lippincott Williams and Wilkins; 2009.

4. c

There are no differences in the occurrence of depression among different races if social class,
education, and area of residence are controlled for. Depression is the most common mood
disorder. Depression carries with it significant morbidity, and is a common cause of disability.
It is approximately twice as common in females as compared to males across all age groups. Its
incidence peaks in the third and fourth decades of life, but it can occur at any age. It is more
common among lower socioeconomic populations and in those living in urban as compared to
rural areas.

Hales RE, Yudofsky SC, Gabbard GO (Eds). The American Psychiatric Publishing Textbook of
Psychiatry. Arlington, VA: American Psychiatric Publishing Inc; 2008.

Sadock BJ, Sadock VA, Ruiz P (Eds). Kaplan and Sadock's Comprehensive Textbook of Psychiatry,
9th ed. Philadelphia, PA: Lippincott Williams and Wilkins; 2009.

5. c

Genetic factors explain approximately 50% to 70% of the etiology of mood disorders, but environmental factors also play a large role. Mood disorders are familial, and both unipolar depression
and bipolar disorder are more common among family members of patients with mood disorders,
as is alcoholism. Linkage studies have identified several chromosomal regions linked to bipolar
disorder. Genes associated with mood disorders include the genes that encode for serotonin
and dopamine transporters, the gene for brain-derived neurotrophic factor, and the cyclic-AMP
response element-binding protein gene. Studies have found that patients with specific polymorphisms of a serotonin transporter have an increased chance of developing a mood disorder
following negative life events.

Sadock BJ, Sadock VA, Ruiz P (Eds). Kaplan and Sadock's Comprehensive Textbook of Psychiatry, 9th ed. Philadelphia, PA: Lippincott Williams and Wilkins; 2009.

6. d

The dorsolateral prefrontal cortex has been shown to be hypometabolic in patients with depression, whereas the orbitofrontal cortex is hypermetabolic, and pharmacologic therapies have been shown to reverse these changes. The pathophysiology of depression is clearly complex, and dysfunction of one specific brain area does not account for the occurrence of depression. Rather, depression results from alterations in neuronal function in many brain areas and their connections. The subcallosal cingulate gyrus is one of the potential targets for deep brain stimulation for the treatment of depression; it is a central component of the limbic system and the connections between frontal and subcortical circuits, and is metabolically overactive in depression. Other potential targets include the ventral portion of the anterior limb of the internal capsule. While gross hippocampal volume is likely preserved in depression, hippocampal abnormalities have been demonstrated, and these at least in part relate to abnormalities in the hypothalamic-pituitary-adrenal (HPA) axis and the effects of glucocorticoids on the hippocampus. Patients with depression have elevated levels of corticotrophin-releasing hormone and other abnormalities of the HPA axis.

Malone DA Jr, Dougherty DD, Rezai AR, et al. Deep brain stimulation of the ventral capsule/ventral striatum for treatment-resistant depression. Biol Psychiatry. 2009; 65:267–275.

Mayberg HS, Lozano AM, Voon V, et al. Deep brain stimulation for treatment-resistant depression. Neuron. 2005; 3(45):651–660.

Sadock BJ, Sadock VA, Ruiz P (Eds). Kaplan and Sadock's Comprehensive Textbook of Psychiatry, 9th ed. Philadelphia, PA: Lippincott Williams and Wilkins; 2009.

7. d, 8. c

The episodes described in question 7 are most consistent with panic attacks. Panic attacks are discrete episodes of symptoms that include a sense of intense fear associated with four or more of the following symptoms: palpitations, diaphoresis, trembling, dyspnea, feeling of choking, chest discomfort, nausea or abdominal pain, dizziness, derealization (a feeling of unreality) or depersonalization (a feeling of being detached from oneself), fear of losing control, fear of dying, paresthesias, and/or chills or hot flashes. Other types of panic attacks are cued, being situationally bound: occurring in relation to a specific internal or external trigger.

Panic disorder is diagnosed when recurrent panic attacks occur, associated with concern for having additional attacks, concern over the implications of these attacks, and changes in behavior as a result of the occurrence of these attacks. Panic disorder may occur in isolation or may be associated with agoraphobia. Agoraphobia is characterized by a fear of being in places or situations where escape would be difficult or embarrassing, or in which help would be difficult to obtain, as depicted in question 8. Agoraphobia may occur in isolation as well. The course of panic disorder is typically variable, with periods of exacerbations and remissions. Improvement occurs with age.

The differential diagnosis of panic disorder includes several medical conditions that need to be excluded on the basis of the history and examination, including but not limited to thyroid disorders, pheochromocytoma, and arrhythmias or other primary cardiac conditions.

Separation anxiety disorder is an anxiety disorder of childhood characterized by excessive and inappropriate fear of being away from home or from familiar figures such as parents or siblings. It usually presents around 6 months of age and declines by ages 2 to 3 years, but may persist and/or recur during ages 6 to 12 years.

Borderline personality disorder is discussed in questions 64 to 67, cyclothymic disorder in question 12, post-traumatic stress disorder in question 19, and generalized anxiety disorder in question 18.

Mayberg HS, Lozano AM, Voon V, et al. Deep brain stimulation for treatment-resistant depression. Neuron. 2005; 3(45):651–660.

Sadock BJ, Sadock VA, Ruiz P (Eds). Kaplan and Sadock's Comprehensive Textbook of Psychiatry, 9th ed. Philadelphia, PA: Lippincott Williams and Wilkins; 2009.

9. b

This man's history is consistent with dissociative amnesia. Dissociative amnesia is one of the dissociative disorders and is characterized by inability to recall a personal experience, with the amnesia being too extreme to be attributed to ordinary forgetfulness. The information forgotten usually relates to a stressful event. Some patients regain memory of the event, whereas others remain chronically amnestic for it.

Depersonalization disorder is another dissociative disorder in which there are intermittent or constant feelings of detachment from oneself as if a person is viewing him- or herself as an outside observer.

In another dissociative disorder, dissociative identity disorder (commonly known as "multiple personality disorder"), a person exists in two or more distinct identities or states, with these identities each unaware of the other and with each separately taking control of the person's behavior over different time periods.

Patients with dissociative fugue suddenly and unexpectedly travel away from their environment and are then unable to recall their past or their identity, and may assume a partial or completely new identity.

Post-traumatic stress disorder (PTSD) is discussed in question 19; patients with dissociative amnesia may subsequently develop PTSD.

Diagnostic and Statistical Manual of Mental Disorders: DSM-IV-TR, 4th ed., text revision, Washington, DC: American Psychiatric Association; 2000.

Sadock BJ, Sadock VA, Ruiz P (Eds). Kaplan and Sadock's Comprehensive Textbook of Psychiatry, 9th ed. Philadelphia, PA: Lippincott Williams and Wilkins; 2009.

10. c, 11. a

This man's presentation is consistent with an acute manic episode. The diagnostic criteria for acute manic episode include the following (Diagnostic and Statistical Manual—Text Revision (DSM-IV-TR, 2000)):

A. A distinct period of abnormally elevated or irritable mood of at least 1-week duration
B. During the mood disturbance, three or more of the following symptoms have been persistently present:

- Inflated self-esteem or grandiosity
- Decreased need for sleep
- Increased talkativeness and pressured speech
- Flight of ideas or racing thoughts
- distractibility
- Increased goal-directed behavior
- Excessive involvement in pleasurable activities with the potential for negative consequences

C. Symptoms do not meet criteria for a mixed episode (see below)
D. The mood disturbance is severe enough to cause marked functional impairment or require hospitalization
E. The mood disturbance is not due to a substance or general medical condition

In a mixed episode, criteria for both an acute manic episode and an acute depressive episode are met over at least a 7-day period, with rapid shifts between or combinations of manic symptoms, psychotic symptoms, and/or depressive symptoms.

In acute hypomanic episode, there is a persistently elevated mood for at least 4 days, in addition to the symptoms of mania described above under diagnostic criterion A, but in contrast to an acute manic episode, symptoms are milder and the patient characteristically has insight, without significant functional impairment.

Bipolar I and II disorders are diagnosed when one manic or hypomanic episode have occurred, respectively. A prior history of depression is not required for the diagnosis. However, in a patient with a depressive episode, a diagnosis of bipolar disorder is not made unless there is a history of symptoms meeting diagnostic criteria for acute manic or hypomanic episode as well.

Bipolar disorder is equally common in males and females. The first episode of either mania or depression typically occurs in young adulthood.

Borderline personality disorder is discussed in question 64 to 67 and cyclothymic disorder in question 12.

Hales RE, Yudofsky SC, Gabbard GO (Eds). The American Psychiatric Publishing Textbook of Psychiatry. Arlington, VA: American Psychiatric Publishing Inc; 2008.

Sadock BJ, Sadock VA, Ruiz P (Eds). Kaplan and Sadock's Comprehensive Textbook of Psychiatry, 9th ed. Philadelphia, PA: Lippincott Williams and Wilkins; 2009.

12. e

This man's history is consistent with cyclothymic disorder. This disorder can be thought of as a clinically attenuated form of bipolar disorder with symptoms spanning over several years. It is a disorder characterized by periods of hypomania and separate periods of depressive symptoms (which do not meet criteria for major depressive disorder) that have been occurring for at least 2 years. There are infrequent intervening periods of euthymia (normal mood). These patients often have pervasive conflicts in interpersonal relations. Bipolar I and II disorders are discussed in questions 10 and 11; borderline personality disorder is discussed in questions 64 to 67.

Diagnostic and Statistical Manual of Mental Disorders: DSM-IV-TR, 4th ed., text revision, Washington, DC: American Psychiatric Association; 2000.

Kaplan and Sadock's Comprehensive Textbook of Psychiatry, 9th ed. Sadock BJ, Sadock VA (Eds), Philadelphia, PA: Lippincott Williams and Wilkins; 2009.

13. e, 14. d

These patients' histories are consistent with phobias, which are classified under anxiety disorders. A phobia is an excessive fear of an object or situation. The phobias include agoraphobia (discussed in question 8), social phobia, and specific phobia.

The main features of phobias include a fear of a clearly identifiable object or situation, with exposure invariably leading to an anxiety response (which may or may not meet diagnostic criteria for panic attack). The phobia is severe enough to affect function and active avoidance of the object or situation occurs.

There are five types of specific phobias: (i) animal type (phobia of animals in general or a specific animal, such as a dog, or spiders (arachnophobia); (ii) natural environmental type (phobia for specific environmental or natural occurrences such as heights (acrophobia), thunderstorms, or water (hydrophobia)); (iii) blood-injury type (fear of blood (hemophobia) or of a bloody injury, or fear of needles (such as fear of venipuncture)); (iv) situational type (fear of specific situations or experiences such as fear of being in a closed space (claustrophobia) or transportation on airplanes or trains); and (5) residual type (when the phobia does not fit into the latter four categories).

Social phobia is characterized by fear of social or performance situations, such as fear of speaking in front of an audience or fear of eating in front of others. There is often a fear of potential embarrassment. The anxiety or fear is severe enough to affect function. Patients with social phobias may force themselves into the phobic situation but experience significant symptoms during that time.

Phobias are among the most common psychiatric disorders. They are more common in females. Adults with phobias often recognize their phobias as being excessive or unreasonable, though children with phobias may not. Fear of blood is often familial, and may be associated with recurrent vasovagal attacks on exposure to blood. Comorbid anxiety disorders often occur. Situational phobias may also be familial, and are epidemiologically similar to panic disorder with agoraphobia.

Generalized anxiety disorder is discussed in question 18. Panic disorder and agoraphobia are discussed in questions 7 and 8. Agoraphobia is a type of phobia, but differs from social phobia in that agoraphobia is fear of being in a social situation in which escape would be difficult, whereas social phobia is a fear of the social situation itself and its implications.

Diagnostic and Statistical Manual of Mental Disorders: DSM-IV-TR, 4th ed., text revision, Washington, DC: American Psychiatric Association; 2000.

Sadock BJ, Sadock VA, Ruiz P (Eds). Kaplan and Sadock's Comprehensive Textbook of Psychiatry, 9th ed. Philadelphia, PA: Lippincott Williams and Wilkins; 2009.

15. a

Serum concentrations of a medication do not necessarily reflect brain concentrations. This is in large part related to the blood-brain barrier (BBB) and blood-CSF barrier, which are selectively permeable barriers to diffusion or transport of substances from the bloodstream into the CNS. The BBB is formed from continuous tight junctions between brain capillary endothelial cells and also results from unique characteristics of pericapillary glial cells. The blood-CSF barrier is formed from tight junctions between epithelial cells in the choroid plexus. When intact, the BBB limits diffusion of most macromolecules and allows selective permeation of some small charged molecules (including neurotransmitter precursors and metabolites, and some drugs) through specific transport systems. Nonionized molecules and lipophilic (lipid-soluble) drugs have higher penetration into the CNS. Transport systems may also allow penetration of drugs into the CNS. The BBB also contains transport systems that allow efflux of substances out of the CNS. Metabolites of neurotransmitters are cleared through an acid transport system in the choroid plexus. The BBB does not exist in the peripheral nervous system, and is absent or less prominent in the circumventricular organs: the median eminence, area postrema, pineal gland, subfornical organ, and subcommissural organ. The BBB is disrupted by ischemia and inflammation, or can be intentionally disrupted with drugs such as mannitol, allowing access of substances that would not normally penetrate into the brain.

Brunton LL, Lazo JS, Parker KL (Eds). Goodman and Gilmans' Pharmacological Basis of Therapeutics, 11th ed. New York: McGraw-Hill; 2005.

16. c

This woman's history and examination are consistent with schizophreniform disorder: she exhibits multiple positive symptoms, including auditory hallucinations, grandiose delusions, disorganized thoughts, neologisms, and poor hygiene. Schizophreniform disorder is diagnosed when diagnostic criteria A, D, and E of schizophrenia are met (discussed in questions 24 and 25), but when symptom duration is more than 1 month and less than 6 months. These patients are managed similar to those with schizophrenia. Of patients with schizophreniform disorder, two-thirds eventually meet diagnostic criteria for schizophrenia and one-third recover within 6 months of symptom onset. Predictors of good prognosis include occurrence of psychotic symptoms within 4 weeks of change in behavior or functioning, presence of prominent positive symptoms, disorganization of thought, confusion, and good premorbid function.

Symptom duration distinguishes brief psychotic disorder (<1 month of symptoms) from schizophreniform disorder. Schizoid personality disorder is discussed in questions 41 to 43; the symptoms are more pervasive than in schizophreniform disorder. Schizoaffective disorder, characterized by both psychotic and affective symptoms, is discussed in question 69.

Sadock BJ, Sadock VA, Ruiz P (Eds). Kaplan and Sadock's Comprehensive Textbook of Psychiatry, 9th ed. Philadelphia, PA: Lippincott Williams and Wilkins; 2009.

17. d

Obsessive-compulsive disorder (OCD) is one of the anxiety disorders, and the main features of it are obsessions and compulsions. Obsessions are persistent ideas, thoughts, or impulses that provoke significant anxiety and distress. Compulsions are repetitive physical or mental acts that are meant to counteract the distress caused by an obsession. In order for a patient to meet diagnostic criteria for OCD, the individual (if an adult) must have recognized that these obsessions or compulsions are unreasonable or excessive, and the obsessions or compulsions must cause significant distress, be time consuming (more than 1 hour a day), and/or significantly affect function.

OCD typically begins in adolescence or early adulthood, but can begin in childhood. It is equally common in males and females, though males have an earlier age of onset. Other psychiatric conditions that are frequently comorbid with OCD include depression, attention deficit hyperactivity disorder, and eating disorders. Approximately 50% of patients with Tourette's syndrome also suffer from OCD. Deep brain stimulation of the ventral portion of the anterior limb of the internal capsule for the treatment of OCD is being studied with promising results.

Generalized anxiety disorder is discussed in question 18, post-traumatic stress disorder in question 19, obsessive-compulsive personality disorder in questions 46 to 48, and bipolar disorder in questions 10 and 11.

Diagnostic and Statistical Manual of Mental Disorders: DSM-IV-TR, 4th ed., text revision, Washington, DC: American Psychiatric Association; 2000.

Greenberg BD, Gabriels LA, Malone DA, et al. Deep brain stimulation of the ventral internal capsule/ventral striatum for obsessive-compulsive disorder: Worldwide experience. Mol Psychiatry. 2010; 15:64–79.

Sadock BJ, Sadock VA, Ruiz P (Eds). Kaplan and Sadock's Comprehensive Textbook of Psychiatry, 9th ed. Philadelphia, PA: Lippincott Williams and Wilkins; 2009.

18. e

This patient suffers from generalized anxiety disorder. The diagnostic criteria for this disorder include the following (Diagnostic and Statistical Manual—Text Revision (DSM-IV-TR, 2000)):

A. Excessive anxiety and worry occurring on most days for at least 6 months about various issues
B. Difficulty controlling the worry
C. Anxiety is associated with at least three of the following symptoms

- Restlessness or feeling keyed up or on edge
- Easy fatigability
- Difficulty concentrating
- Irritability
- Muscle tension
- Sleep disturbance

D. The focus of the anxiety is not related to another psychiatric disorder (such as worry about having a panic attack or worry about weight gain in patients with anorexia nervosa)
E. and F. The symptoms lead to functional impairments and are not due to substances or a medical condition

Generalized anxiety disorder is more common in females as compared to males, and usually begins in adolescence or young adulthood. Unlike panic disorder, which often improves with age, anxiety is significant during adulthood and older age.

Post-traumatic stress disorder is discussed in question 19, hypochondriasis in questions 20 to 22, social phobia in questions 13 and 14, and panic disorder in questions 7 and 8.

Diagnostic and Statistical Manual of Mental Disorders: DSM-IV-TR, 4th ed., text revision, Washington, DC: American Psychiatric Association; 2000.

Hales RE, Yudofsky SC, Gabbard GO (Eds). The American Psychiatric Publishing Textbook of Psychiatry. Arlington, VA: American Psychiatric Publishing Inc; 2008.

Sadock BJ, Sadock VA, Ruiz P (Eds). Kaplan and Sadock's Comprehensive Textbook of Psychiatry, 9th ed. Philadelphia, PA: Lippincott Williams and Wilkins; 2009.

19. c

Post-traumatic stress disorder (PTSD) is an anxiety disorder characterized by the occurrence of specific symptoms after experiencing a traumatic event involving threat of death or injury to oneself or others, resulting in intense fear or horror. These symptoms include re-experiencing the traumatic event (such as through nightmares or flashbacks), avoiding any stimuli associated with the event, and experiencing symptoms of autonomic arousal (such as increased startle reflex, insomnia, hypervigilance, and irritability). A diagnosis of PTSD is made only after symptoms have been occurring for more than 1 month; within a 1-month period of symptom onset, a diagnosis of acute stress reaction is made. The majority of patients with PTSD develop complete remission; however, up to a fourth of patients develop a chronic disorder.

Generalized anxiety disorder is discussed in question 18, panic disorder in questions 7 and 8, and night terrors in Chapter 5.

Diagnostic and Statistical Manual of Mental Disorders: DSM-IV-TR, 4th ed., text revision, Washington, DC: American Psychiatric Association; 2000.

Sadock BJ, Sadock VA, Ruiz P (Eds). Kaplan and Sadock's Comprehensive Textbook of Psychiatry, 9th ed. Philadelphia, PA: Lippincott Williams and Wilkins; 2009.

20. b, 21. e, 22. d

The somatoform disorders encompass disorders in which psychologic stresses manifest as physical symptoms. The somatoform disorders include somatization disorder, conversion disorder, pain disorder, hypochondriasis, and body dysmorphic disorder.

As with the patient in question 20, somatization disorder is characterized by the occurrence of multiple recurrent somatic complaints that cannot be explained by a general medical condition or substance. This disorder typically begins prior to the age of 30, results in excessive nondiagnostic testing and unnecessary medical treatments, and/or significantly affects function. The symptoms must include pain related to at least four different sites (such as head, abdomen, joints, or chest) or functions (such as menstruation, sexual intercourse, urination, or sleep), at least one sexual or reproductive system complaint other than pain (such as irregular menses or erectile dysfunction), in addition to two gastrointestinal symptoms besides pain (such as nausea and bloating). In order for the diagnosis to be made, there must also be history of at least one symptom other than pain that is suggestive of a neurologic condition (such as weakness, dysphagia, urinary retention, paresthesias, or loss of consciousness). An undifferentiated form of somatization disorder, in which only one or more symptoms are present that cannot be fully explained by a medical condition, has also been defined.

As with the patient depicted in question 21, conversion disorder is characterized by acute loss of motor or sensory function that cannot be explained by a neurologic or other medical condition. The symptoms often resemble neurologic syndromes, such as hemiparesis, cerebellar ataxia, or seizures. Nonneurologic symptoms such as blindness, deafness, or false pregnancy (pseudocyesis) also occur. Conversion disorder is also classified as a dissociative disorder in some texts.

Pain disorder is diagnosed when there is the presence of pain as the most prominent symptom and the pain cannot be explained by an identifiable medical condition.

In hypochondriasis, there is pervasive preoccupation with physical symptoms and fear of having a serious disease for at least 6 months, often resulting from misinterpretation of physical symptoms, even after diagnostic testing and exclusion of the condition of concern or any other identifiable medical condition.

As with the patient in question 22, patients with body dysmorphic disorder experience an intense preoccupation with a perceived defect of appearance or overconcern with minor physical abnormalities, with symptoms present for at least 6 months. Such patients often seek unnecessary and repeated surgical procedures to correct their perceived deformity.

Somatoform disorders are more frequent in women. Patients with somatoform disorders often have a history of physical and/or emotional abuse and neglect. They frequently have comorbid psychiatric disorders, including mood and anxiety disorders, personality disorders, and substance abuse. For example, one-third of patients with conversion disorder suffer from a mood or anxiety disorder, and half from a personality disorder.

The key point distinguishing somatoform disorders from factitious disorder is that with somatoform disorders, symptoms are not intentionally feigned, whereas with factitious disorder, symptoms are voluntarily feigned for secondary gain. Factitious disorder, including Munchausen's syndrome, is discussed further in question 44.

Diagnostic and Statistical Manual of Mental Disorders: DSM-IV-TR, 4th ed., text revision, Washington, DC: American Psychiatric Association; 2000.

Sadock BJ, Sadock VA, Ruiz P (Eds). Kaplan and Sadock's Comprehensive Textbook of Psychiatry, 9th ed. Philadelphia, PA: Lippincott Williams and Wilkins; 2009.

23. d

The monoamine hypothesis of depression postulates that deficiencies or dysfunctions in the monoamines serotonin, dopamine, and norepinephrine are implicated in the pathogenesis of depression. Although there is evidence to support this hypothesis, this is yet to be unequivocally proved, and some studies have not found alterations in monoamines in depressed patients. Evidence to support the monoamine hypothesis includes the induction of depression by reserpine, which depletes monoamines, increased risk for depression in carriers of specific serotonin transporter promoter gene polymorphisms, and response of depression to medications that increase levels of monoamines. However, another theory of depression pathogenesis, the neurotrophic hypothesis, holds that depression results from loss of neurotrophic support by nerve growth factors such as brain-derived growth factor.

Katzung BG. Basic and Clinical Pharmacology, 11th ed. New York: McGraw-Hill; 2009.

Sadock BJ, Sadock VA, Ruiz P (Eds). Kaplan and Sadock's Comprehensive Textbook of Psychiatry, 9th ed. Philadelphia, PA: Lippincott Williams and Wilkins; 2009.

24. c, 25. b

This patient's history is consistent with schizophrenia. Schizophrenia is a psychotic disorder characterized by both positive symptoms, such as hallucinations, delusions, and disorganized thought, and negative symptoms, such as emotional blunting, alogia (empty speech), apathy, and reduced communicativeness. The diagnostic criteria for schizophrenia include the following (Diagnostic and Statistical Manual—Text Revision (DSM-IV-TR, 2000)):

A. Two (or more) of the following present for a significant portion of time over a 1-month period:

   – Delusions
   – Hallucinations
   – Disorganized speech (e.g., frequent derailment or incoherence)
   – Grossly disorganized or catatonic behavior
   – Negative symptoms, i.e., affective flattening, alogia (empty speech), or avolition
     (or only one of five if the delusions are bizarre and auditory hallucinations consist of a running commentary or a conversation between two or more voices)
B. Social and occupational dysfunction in work, interpersonal relations, or self-care since onset of the symptoms
C. Continuous symptoms for at least 6 months
D. D and E. Schizoaffective disorder, mood disorder, and disturbance due to substance or general medication condition have been excluded as the cause
E. In patients with a prior history of pervasive developmental disorder, prominent delusions and hallucinations of at least 6 months' duration must be present

Schizophrenia affects 1% of the world's population. It is more prevalent in lower socioeconomic populations, but the relationship between schizophrenia and socioeconomic status is complex. Low socioeconomic status is likely an effect rather than a cause of schizophrenia, relating to the "downward drift" effect, in which during the prodromal phase of schizophrenia an individual drifts down into a lower socioeconomic class. Schizophrenia is equally common in males and females, though males typically have a younger age of onset. Schizophrenia typically manifests in adolescence and early adulthood, though late-onset forms, with symptom onset after the age of 45, have also been described. Premorbidly (prior to the onset of positive symptoms), 25% of patients have abnormalities in social or cognitive function, with some features of schizoid personality disorder (discussed in question 42). Positive symptoms predominate in the earlier stages of the illness and may diminish overtime; positive symptoms are more responsive to typical antipsychotics compared to negative symptoms.

Delusional disorder is discussed in question 31, brief psychotic episode in question 62, schizoaffective disorder in question 69, and schizoid personality disorder in question 42.

Diagnostic and Statistical Manual of Mental Disorders: DSM-IV-TR, 4th ed., text revision, Washington, DC: American Psychiatric Association; 2000.

Hales RE, Yudofsky SC, Gabbard GO (Eds). The American Psychiatric Publishing Textbook of Psychiatry. Arlington, VA: American Psychiatric Publishing Inc; 2008.

Kirkbride JB, Barker D, Cowden F, et al. Psychoses, ethnicity and socio-economic status. Br J Psychiatry. 2008; 193:18–24.

Sadock BJ, Sadock VA, Ruiz P (Eds). Kaplan and Sadock's Comprehensive Textbook of Psychiatry, 9th ed. Philadelphia, PA: Lippincott Williams and Wilkins; 2009.

26. e

In older adults, selection of antidepressant medication should be done with various considerations in mind, most notably side effects and risk of drug-drug interactions. The tricyclic antidepressants (TCAs), as discussed on question 50, have various side effects including cardiac conduction abnormalities and drug-drug interactions that make them undesirable for the treatment of depression in older adults. A selective serotonin reuptake inhibitor is more favorable than a TCA in this patient. Fluvoxamine has a high risk for drug-drug interactions, whereas escitalopram does not. Fluvoxamine also has high protein binding, and can therefore interact with anticoagulant medications, such a warfarin. Therefore, of the medications listed, escitalopram is the most appropriate in this patient. In older adults, psychotropic medications should be started at a low dose and titrated up slowly to the lowest effective dose.

Brunton LL, Lazo JS, Parker KL (Eds). Goodman and Gilmans' Pharmacological Basis of Therapeutics, 11th ed. New York: McGraw-Hill; 2005.

27. b, 28. a

The disruptive behavior disorders include conduct disorder and oppositional defiant disorder. Question 27 depicts conduct disorder, which is characterized by a pervasive violation of rules, of others' rights, and age-appropriate societal norms for at least 12 months, including aggression to people or animals, destruction of property, deceitfulness or theft, and serious violation of rules. Individuals with this disorder show little empathy or remorse. Conduct disorder is more common in males. Risk factors for conduct disorder include psychopathology in parents, dysfunctional family environment and poor parenting practices, exposure to physical, sexual, or emotional abuse or neglect, and exposure to violence. A diagnosis of antisocial personality disorder, discussed in questions 64 to 67, cannot be given to those younger than 18 years of age; some individuals with conduct disorder go on to meet criteria for antisocial personality disorder in adulthood, whereas in others, the conduct disorder remits and they are able to achieve adequate social and occupational adjustment. Management of conduct disorder centers primarily around institution of early multimodal psychosocial interventions to prevent conduct disorder when there are early signs of aggression or deviance in a child.

Question 28 depicts oppositional defiant disorder, in which there is a pattern of hostile and defiant behavior present for at least 6 months, not occurring as part of a mood or psychotic disorder, affecting function, and including at least four or more of the following: frequent loss of temper, frequent arguing with adults and defying or refusing to comply with adults' requests or rules, deliberately annoying others, blaming others for mistakes or misbehaviors, angry and resentful behavior, oversensitivity, and spiteful or vindictive behavior. Oppositional defiant disorder most frequently emerges between ages 6 and 8, and is more common in males and those of lower socioeconomic status and in urban dwellers.

Acute manic episode is discussed in questions 10 and 11, borderline personality disorder in questions 64 to 67 (*note:* personality disorder cannot be made in individuals younger than 18 years of age), and antisocial personality disorder in questions 64 to 67.

Diagnostic and Statistical Manual of Mental Disorders: DSM-IV-TR, 4th ed., text revision, Washington, DC: American Psychiatric Association; 2000.

Sadock BJ, Sadock VA, Ruiz P (Eds). Kaplan and Sadock's Comprehensive Textbook of Psychiatry, 9th ed. Philadelphia, PA: Lippincott Williams and Wilkins; 2009.

29. c

Dysthymic disorder is a mood disorder characterized by insidious and chronic symptoms of depression that have been present for at least 22 months over a 2-year period. It is different from major depressive episode and chronic depressive disorder. In the former, there is a clear-cut episode of depression with a relatively clear time of onset, and in the latter, there are persistent residual symptoms of depression after onset of a clear-cut major depressive episode. Rather, dysthymic patients often report they have always been depressed and express significant symptoms of depression, including hopelessness and anhedonia. Suicidal ideation, however, is not a common occurrence in dysthymic disorder, being much more common in severe depression. Dysthymic disorder is chronic and often difficult to treat pharmacologically. Depressive personality disorder is not a diagnosis on the basis of Diagnostic and Statistical Manual IV. Cyclothymic disorder is discussed in question 12.

Diagnostic and Statistical Manual of Mental Disorders: DSM-IV-TR, 4th ed., text revision, Washington, DC: American Psychiatric Association; 2000.

Hales RE, Yudofsky SC, Gabbard GO (Eds). The American Psychiatric Publishing Textbook of Psychiatry. Arlington, VA: American Psychiatric Publishing Inc; 2008.

Sadock BJ, Sadock VA, Ruiz P (Eds). Kaplan and Sadock's Comprehensive Textbook of Psychiatry, 9th ed. Philadelphia, PA: Lippincott Williams and Wilkins; 2009.

30. b

Serotonin, or 5-hydroxytryptamine (5-HT), is synthesized in a two-step process. The first step is catalyzed by tryptophan hydroxylase, which converts the essential amino acid tryptophan into an intermediate that is subsequently converted into serotonin by action of the enzyme aromatic L-amino acid decarboxylase. Serotonin is metabolized by action of monoamine oxidase (MAO), predominantly the MAO-A isoform. MAO-B, along with MAO-A, metabolizes dopamine and tryptamine; low-dose selegiline is a selective inhibitor of MAO-B. There are at least seven classes and fourteen subtypes of 5-HT receptors. The $5-HT_1$, $5-HT_2$, and $5-HT_4$ subtypes are coupled to G-proteins (which either inhibit or activate adenylyl cyclase, depending on the subtype). The $5-HT_3$ receptor is a ligand-gated ion channel.

In the CNS, the principle site of serotonergic neuronal cell bodies is in the raphe nuclei of the brain stem, with diffuse projections to the brain and spinal cord. Serotonin has various actions both in the CNS and systemically. In the CNS, serotonin has a role to play in the sleep-wake cycle; serotonin deficiency leads to insomnia, and tryptophan (a serotonin precursor) promotes sleep. Serotonin has also been implicated in violent behavior; low CSF levels of the serotonin metabolite 5-hydroxyindole acetic acid (5-HIAA) have been associated with aggressiveness and violent impulsivity. Serotonin deficiency has also been implicated in both anxiety and depression. Regarding the nonpsychotropic effects of serotonin, the $5-HT_{1B}$ receptors elicit vasoconstriction and the $5-HT_{1D}$ receptors inhibit neuronal transmission and trigeminal neurogenic inflammatory peptide release. Triptan medications such as sumatriptan are agonists at these latter receptors.

Action of serotonin at 5-HT$_{2A}$ receptors leads to platelet aggregation. Serotonin acts at 5-HT$_3$ in the area postrema and the antiemetic ondansetron is an antagonist at this receptor. Serotonin is released by enterochromaffin cells in the intestines where it increases intestinal motility. It also induces bronchoconstriction, and patients with malignant carcinoid syndrome, in which there is excessive production of serotonin, manifest many of the symptoms of a hyperserotonergic state, including wheezing and diarrhea.

Brunton LL, Lazo JS, Parker KL (Eds). Goodman and Gilmans' Pharmacological Basis of Therapeutics, 11th ed. New York: McGraw-Hill; 2005.

Katzung BG. Basic and Clinical Pharmacology, 11th ed. New York: McGraw-Hill; 2009.

31. c

This gentleman has had a fixed delusion of greater than 1-month duration, without any other psychotic symptoms. The most likely diagnosis is delusional disorder. The diagnostic criteria for delusional disorder include the following (Diagnostic and Statistical Manual—Text Revision (DSM-IV-TR, 2000)):

A. Nonbizarre delusions of at least 1-month duration
B. Criterion A for schizophrenia has never been met (see questions 24 and 25)
C. Apart from the impact of the delusion or its ramifications, functioning is not markedly impaired and behavior is not obviously odd or bizarre
D. If mood episodes have occurred concurrently with delusions, their total duration has been brief relative to the duration of the delusional periods
E. The disturbance is not due to the direct physiologic effects of a substance or a general medical condition

This man is convinced that a famous personality is in love with him. His delusional disorder can therefore be classified as the erotomanic type. Other types of delusional disorder include the following:

– Grandiose type, in which there are delusions of inflated worth, power, knowledge, or identity
– Jealous type, in which there are delusions that an individual's significant other is unfaithful
– Persecutory type, in which the delusion is one of being persecuted by someone
– Somatic type, delusions of having a physical defect or medical problem of some sort

The absence of psychotic features such as hallucinations, bizarre delusions, changes in affect, and changes in function distinguish delusional disorder from other psychotic disorders such as brief psychotic episode (discussed in question 62) and schizophrenia (discussed in questions 24 and 25). Schizoaffective disorder is discussed in question 69 and atypical depression in question 3.

Diagnostic and Statistical Manual of Mental Disorders: DSM-IV-TR, 4th ed., text revision, Washington, DC: American Psychiatric Association; 2000.

Sadock BJ, Sadock VA, Ruiz P (Eds). Kaplan and Sadock's Comprehensive Textbook of Psychiatry, 9th ed. Philadelphia, PA: Lippincott Williams and Wilkins; 2009.

32. e

Suicide is unfortunately a common cause of death worldwide. It is a more common cause of death in males, though females attempt suicide more often than males. The rate of suicide increases with increasing age among Caucasians; in African-Americans beyond the fourth decade, the rate of suicide decreases. Caucasians have a higher rate of suicide as compared to African-Americans. Native Americans have the highest rate of suicide among all ethnicities in the United States. Approximately 60% to 70% of patients who have committed suicide were suffering from a mood disorder; patients with schizophrenia are also at an increased risk of suicide. Substance abuse and panic disorder are frequent comorbidities in patients who commit suicide. Among patients with personality disorders, those with borderline personality disorder (discussed in question 66) are most likely to attempt suicide.

Sadock BJ, Sadock VA, Ruiz P (Eds). Kaplan and Sadock's Comprehensive Textbook of Psychiatry, 9th ed. Philadelphia, PA: Lippincott Williams and Wilkins; 2009.

33. a

The selective serotonin reuptake inhibitors (SSRIs) have various systemic side effects related to action of serotonin at various receptor subtypes. The SSRIs include fluoxetine, fluvoxamine, sertraline, paroxetine, citalopram, and escitalopram. They inhibit reuptake of serotonin through inhibition of the serotonin transporter, leading to increased availability of serotonin at the postsynaptic membrane. The antidepressant and/or anxiolytic effect of SSRIs may not become apparent for several days to weeks because their mechanism of action involves pre- and postsynaptic receptor changes that are not immediate.

They lead to various systemic effects due to the action of serotonin at various receptor subtypes (see question 30). They are used to treat mood disorders, including depression, premenstrual dysphoric disorder, and seasonal affective disorder; a variety of anxiety disorders, including generalized anxiety disorder, post-traumatic stress disorder, obsessive-compulsive disorder, and eating disorders, such as bulimia. The SSRIs are metabolized by the hepatic cytochrome P450 system and have various drug-drug interactions, with the extent varying with each of the SSRIs. Citalopram and escitalopram have the least potential for drug-drug interactions. At the time of this publication, the SSRIs were available only in oral formulation in the United States.

Katzung BG. Basic and Clinical Pharmacology, 11th ed. New York: McGraw-Hill; 2009.

Sadock BJ, Sadock VA, Ruiz P (Eds). Kaplan and Sadock's Comprehensive Textbook of Psychiatry, 9th ed. Philadelphia, PA: Lippincott Williams and Wilkins; 2009.

34. c

Schizophrenia (discussed in questions 24 and 25) and other psychotic disorders are thought to result, at least in part, from overactivity in dopaminergic pathways. Dopaminergic pathways include the mesolimbic and mesocortical pathways (which project from the midbrain to the limbic system and neocortex), nigrostriatal pathway (which consists of neurons projecting from the substantia nigra to the dorsal striatum, including the caudate and putamen), and tuberoinfundibular system (which arises from the hypothalamus and projects to the pituitary; dopamine released by these neurons inhibits prolactin release from the pituitary). It is the limbic and cortical-subcortical pathways (mesolimbic and mesocortical pathways) that are thought to be overactive in psychosis, rather than the nigrostriatal and tuberoinfundibular pathways.

There are five dopamine receptors identified, D_1 to D_5. It is mainly the D_2 receptor that is implicated in the dopamine hypothesis of schizophrenia. Support for the dopamine hypothesis comes from evidence that there is increased dopamine receptor density in the brains of schizophrenics postmortem and increased D_2 receptor occupancy in the brains of schizophrenics on functional imaging. Improvement of psychosis with D_2 antagonism and worsening of psychosis with dopaminergic agonists such as levodopa, amphetamines, and dopamine agonists further lend support to this theory. However, the dopamine hypothesis only partially explains the many features of schizophrenia and other psychotic disorders. For example, reduced dopaminergic activity in specific cortical areas including the medial temporal lobe and dorsolateral prefrontal cortex as well as the hippocampus is thought to underlie the negative symptoms of schizophrenia. The serotonin hypothesis of schizophrenia postulates a role for excessive serotonergic activity, particularly at serotonergic 5-HT$_{2A}$ receptors, in the pathogenesis of hallucinations and other symptoms of psychosis. The occurrence of hallucinations with exposure to lysergic acid diethylamide (discussed in Chapter 17), a serotonin agonist, lends support to this theory, as does the efficacy of atypical antipsychotics, which have serotonergic antagonism in addition to antidopaminergic activity. Underactivity of glutamate pathways, which normally excite inhibitory GABA pathways, has also been implicated in the pathogenesis of schizophrenia and other psychotic disorders, as evidenced by the ability of phencyclidine and ketamine (noncompetitive NMDA receptor antagonists, discussed in Chapter 17) to exacerbate cognitive dysfunction and psychosis in patients with schizophrenia.

Katzung BG. Basic and Clinical Pharmacology, 11th ed. New York: McGraw-Hill; 2009.

35. c

This patient's history is consistent with intermittent explosive disorder (IED), an impulse control disorder characterized by several episodes of verbal or physical aggression that is out of proportion to an instigating event. In between episodes, patients may express remorse or regret for their actions. IED typically starts in adolescence or early adulthood and is more common in men. Treatment of IED includes psychotherapy, as well as pharmacotherapy with mood stabilizers (discussed in questions 78 and 79), antipsychotics (discussed in questions 53–55 and 72–74), or selective serotonin reuptake inhibitors (discussed in questions 33).

Oppositional defiant disorder is a disorder of childhood and is discussed in question 28; antisocial personality disorder and borderline personality disorder are discussed in questions 65 and 66.

Diagnostic and Statistical Manual of Mental Disorders: DSM-IV-TR, 4th ed., text revision, Washington, DC: American Psychiatric Association; 2000.

Sadock BJ, Sadock VA, Ruiz P (Eds). Kaplan and Sadock's Comprehensive Textbook of Psychiatry, 9th ed. Philadelphia, PA: Lippincott Williams and Wilkins; 2009.

36. d

Kleptomania is an impulse control disorders and is defined as recurrent impulses to steal objects because of a sense of pleasure or gratification from the act of stealing, with the object being of little personal use or value. Kleptomania typically begins in adolescence, and is more common in women.

Other impulse control disorders include trichotillomania (recurrent pulling of one's hair resulting in hair loss and a sense of pleasure or gratification), pyromania (deliberate setting of fires, a fascination with fire, and pleasure or gratification when setting fires or observing their aftermath), and pathologic gambling. Borderline personality disorder and antisocial personality disorder are discussed in questions 64 to 67; kleptomania or pyromania can occur as part of these personality disorders, but other features of these personality disorders are not depicted in question 36.

Diagnostic and Statistical Manual of Mental Disorders: DSM-IV-TR, 4th ed., text revision, Washington, DC: American Psychiatric Association; 2000.

Sadock BJ, Sadock VA, Ruiz P (Eds). Kaplan and Sadock's Comprehensive Textbook of Psychiatry, 9th ed. Philadelphia, PA: Lippincott Williams and Wilkins; 2009.

548   Chapter 13

37. c, 38. a

The eating disorders include anorexia nervosa, bulimia nervosa, and eating disorder not otherwise specified. The case in question 37 depicts anorexia nervosa, a disorder characterized by intentional maintenance of body weight below 85% of expected, an intense fear of gaining weight, an impaired self-perception of weight (such as denial of the seriousness of low body weight), and amenorrhea. Anorexia nervosa is of two types: The first is a restricting type, which occurs in approximately 50% of patients, in which there is self-induced starvation and often compulsive exercising without binge eating or purging behaviors. The second type is a binge eating/purging type, in which the patient regularly engages in binge eating followed by purging. Anorexia nervosa is treated at least initially in the inpatient setting to allow for medical stabilization and initiation of nutrition under close supervision. Later, outpatient therapy revolves mainly around psychotherapy, with pharmacologic management of comorbid mood or anxiety disorders.

In bulimia nervosa, depicted in question 38, patients binge eat over a discrete period of time at least twice a week for 3 months, with a sense of lack of control over the extent of food intake during that time period, and subsequently partake in compensatory behaviors to prevent weight gain such as excessive exercise, induction of emesis or misuse of laxatives, diuretics, or other medications. Treatment of bulimia nervosa involves psychotherapy combined in some cases with selective serotonin reuptake inhibitors (discussed in question 33). Bulimia nervosa is a common comorbidity seen in persons with borderline personality disorder (discussed in question 66).

In patients with eating disorder not otherwise specified, patients may avoid food, binge with or without purging or participating excessively in exercise, and partake in other methods of minimizing weight loss, but the patient's weight is maintained within the normal range, the episodes of binging occur less than twice per week for 3 months, and menstruation remains regular. The binge eating form of eating disorder not otherwise specified is the most common eating disorder, followed by bulimia and anorexia nervosa.

Peak onset of eating disorders is in the teenage years, though they may begin at any age. Eating disorders are more common in females than in males, with a 3:1 ratio, though males are likely underdiagnosed. The pathophysiology relates to be both environmental and genetic factors; there is a 50% to 80% concordance rate among monozygotic twins. Comorbid mood, anxiety, and personality disorders are common among patients with eating disorders.

The impulse control disorders are discussed in questions 35 and 36.

bibDiagnostic and Statistical Manual of Mental Disorders: DSM-IV-TR, 4th ed., text revision, Washington, DC: American Psychiatric Association; 2000.

Sadock BJ, Sadock VA, Ruiz P (Eds). Kaplan and Sadock's Comprehensive Textbook of Psychiatry, 9th ed. Philadelphia, PA: Lippincott Williams and Wilkins; 2009.

39. b

The tricyclic antidepressants (TCAs) are among the oldest antidepressants and are still commonly used to treat depression. The TCAs with a tertiary amine side chain such as amitriptyline, doxepin, and imipramine inhibit reuptake of both serotonin and norepinephrine, whereas some such as clomipramine predominantly inhibit reuptake of serotonin. The TCAs do not directly inhibit reuptake of dopamine, though they may indirectly facilitate the effects of dopamine. All TCAs have some activity at muscarinic, histaminergic, and α-adrenergic receptors, though to varying degrees. Because of these effects at noncatecholaminergic receptors, they are used for various disorders not limited to depression and anxiety, including urinary retention and neuropathy. TCAs are also useful in the treatment of neuropathic pain.

Brunton LL, Lazo JS, Parker KL (Eds). Goodman and Gilmans' Pharmacological Basis of Therapeutics, 11th ed. New York: McGraw-Hill; 2005.

40. a

This boy exhibits features of reading disorder. The learning disorders include reading disorder,
mathematics disorder, and disorder of written expression. In reading disorder, there is difficulty
with learning to read (as opposed to loss of previously acquired reading skills), with reading
achievement as measured by standardized tests being lower than would be expected for an
individual's age and measured intelligence.

In mathematics disorder, an individual's mathematical abilities, as measured by standardized
tests, are below that expected (and are manifested, for example, by impairments in rapid retrieval
of number facts such as multiplication tables), whereas in disorder of written expression, performance in written expression is impaired (such as avoidance of writing, writing incomplete
sentences, limited use of vocabulary, improper punctuation, and misspelling).

In individuals with specific learning disorders, capabilities in other domains are typically
average or may be above average, though the various learning disabilities frequently co-occur.
Mental retardation is defined by significantly subaverage general intellectual functioning, in
more than one domain, as assessed by standardized tests. Mild mental retardation is defined by
an intelligence quotient (IQ) of 55 to 70, moderate mental retardation by an IQ of 35 to 55,
severe mental retardation by an IQ of 20 to 35, and profound mental retardation by an IQ of less
than 20 (see also Chapter 14). Acquired dyslexia is a loss of language skills that were previously
acquired, as may occur in patients with traumatic brain injury.

Diagnostic and Statistical Manual of Mental Disorders: DSM-IV-TR, 4th ed., text revision, Washington, DC: American Psychiatric Association; 2000.

Sadock BJ, Sadock VA, Ruiz P (Eds). Kaplan and Sadock's Comprehensive Textbook of Psychiatry,
9th ed. Philadelphia, PA: Lippincott Williams and Wilkins; 2009.

41. e, 42. b, 43. c

The personality disorders consist of 10 distinct entities that share in common a pervasive and
inflexible pattern of inner experiences, thoughts, and behaviors. They affect the domains of
cognition, impulse control, affectivity, and interpersonal functioning. Features are present in
adolescence or early adulthood and persist over time. They deviate from accepted societal culture
and norms and lead to distress or impairment. The caveat to the diagnosis of personality disorders
is that the features do not occur in the context of signs or symptoms that are part of a mood,
anxiety, impulse control, or psychotic disorder, or any other psychiatric disorder as the primarily
underlying illness. Personality traits are patterns of behavior or thinking about oneself and the
environment that are relatively consistent over time, but they do not lead to a diagnosis of
personality disorder unless they are maladaptive or cause functional impairment or distress. The
personality disorders are categorized into clusters A, B, and C. Different personality disorders
may co-occur in the same individual.

Questions 41 to 43 depict people that would be classified under cluster A of the personality disorders. This cluster includes paranoid, schizoid, and schizotypal personality disorders.
Paranoid personality disorder, depicted in question 41, is marked by a pervasive distrust and
suspiciousness of others, with convictions that others intend to exploit or harm, preoccupation
with paranoid thoughts, distrust of others' intentions, and interpretation of benign actions or
remarks as criticism or harm. Persons with paranoid personality disorders have an increased risk
of comorbid major depressive disorder (discussed in questions 1 and 2), substance abuse, and

agoraphobia (discussed in question 8). Paranoid personality disorder is more common in males and may be an antecedent to paranoid type of delusional disorder (discussed in question 31).

Schizoid personality disorder, depicted in question 42, is marked by a blunted range of affect and emotions, and a lack of interest in social relationships and little pleasure in social activities, with a preference for solitude, and lack of close friends outside of the immediate family. Schizoid personality disorder is more common in males, and may appear as an antecedent to delusional disorder (discussed in question 31) or schizophrenia (discussed in questions 24 and 25).

Schizotypal personality disorder, depicted in question 43, is marked by a pervasive pattern of discomfort with and inability to participate in close relationships, and odd, peculiar, and eccentric ideas, beliefs, and/or behaviors such as magical thinking (such as superstitiousness or belief in clairvoyance or telepathy), paranoid ideation, constricted affect, lack of close friends outside of immediate family members, and social anxiety. Patients with schizotypal personality disorder have comorbid major depression in 30% to 50% of cases.

See the last paragraph to the discussion to questions 64 to 67 for a brief overview of the treatment of personality disorders.

Diagnostic and Statistical Manual of Mental Disorders: DSM-IV-TR, 4th ed., text revision, Washington, DC: American Psychiatric Association; 2000.

Sadock BJ, Sadock VA, Ruiz P (Eds). Kaplan and Sadock's Comprehensive Textbook of Psychiatry, 9th ed. Philadelphia, PA: Lippincott Williams and Wilkins; 2009.

44. a

In factitious disorders, symptoms or signs are intentionally feigned, motivated by an intention to assume the role of the patient. The key feature is fabrication of subjective complaints, such as abdominal pain, or falsification of signs, such as intentional heating of a thermometer such that it shows an elevated reading. Munchausen's syndrome is a chronic, severe form of factitious disorder in which extensive deceptive means are often employed in feigning physical signs, resulting in recurrent hospitalizations in various geographic locations. In factitious disorder by proxy (also called Munchausen's syndrome by proxy), physical signs or symptoms are intentionally produced in another individual who is under the direct care of the perpetrator.

In malingering, the secondary gain is an external incentive (such as money). In comparison, the secondary gain in factitious disorder is assumption of the role of a patient.

Diagnostic and Statistical Manual of Mental Disorders: DSM-IV-TR, 4th ed., text revision, Washington, DC: American Psychiatric Association; 2000.

Sadock BJ, Sadock VA, Ruiz P (Eds). Kaplan and Sadock's Comprehensive Textbook of Psychiatry, 9th ed. Philadelphia, PA: Lippincott Williams and Wilkins; 2009.

45. d

Five subtypes of schizophrenia have been defined: catatonic, residual, disorganized, paranoid, and undifferentiated. Diagnostic criteria for schizophrenia are discussed in questions 24 and 25.

Catatonia is defined as an extreme motor state, whether it be lack of movement or excessive movement. Patients with the stuporous catatonic subtype of schizophrenia show reduced movements and reduced communicativeness with mutism or even stupor occurring in severe cases. However, they may also exhibit outbursts and sometimes unprovoked violent behavior. Patients with the catatonic subtype also exhibit echolalia (echoing the words of others) and echopraxia (imitation of the gestures of others). In some cases, waxy flexibility is present. There is also a less common excited form of catatonia, marked by psychomotor agitation and sometimes continuous speaking.

The residual subtype of schizophrenia is diagnosed when the patient once met all criteria for schizophrenia, but when there continues to be only some symptoms, such as mild hallucinations, blunting of affect, or social withdrawal, which no longer meet diagnostic criteria.

Disorganized schizophrenia is characterized by prominent disorganization in thought, behavior, and speech, and with a blunted or inappropriate affect, whereas delusions and hallucinations are less prominent.

Patients with paranoid-type schizophrenia exhibit prominent delusions, frequently persecutory or grandiose. They also have prominent auditory hallucinations and are paranoid, but with relative preservation of cognitive function and affect.

In undifferentiated schizophrenia, the patient meets all diagnostic criteria for schizophrenia, but cannot be categorized into any of the specific subtypes.

Hales RE, Yudofsky SC, Gabbard GO (Eds). The American Psychiatric Publishing Textbook of Psychiatry. Arlington, VA: American Psychiatric Publishing Inc; 2008.

Sadock BJ, Sadock VA, Ruiz P (Eds). Kaplan and Sadock's Comprehensive Textbook of Psychiatry, 9th ed. Philadelphia, PA: Lippincott Williams and Wilkins; 2009.

46. e, 47. c, 48. d

See the first paragraph of the discussion for questions 41 to 43 for the definition of personality disorders. Questions 46 to 48 depict people that would be classified under cluster C of the personality disorders. This cluster includes avoidant, dependent, and obsessive-compulsive personality disorders.

Avoidant personality disorder, depicted in question 46, is marked by hypersensitivity to criticism, feelings of inadequacy, and social inhibition, including avoidance of any occupation or other activity that will involve contact with others because of fear of criticism or rejection, restraint in personal relationships because of fear of being ridiculed, willingness to get involved with people only if certain of being liked, and viewing self as socially inept and inferior to others. Unlike persons with schizoid personality disorder (depicted in question 42), those with avoidant personality disorder want relationships but avoid them because of fear of criticism, whereas those with schizoid personality disorder prefer social isolation. Avoidant personality disorder shares features with panic disorder with agoraphobia (discussed in questions 7 and 8) but in the latter condition, avoidance is of specific social situations that lead to panic attacks. Avoidant personality disorder begins at an early age, without clear precipitants, and is stable over time. Social phobia (discussed in questions 13 and 14) and avoidant personality disorder may co-occur.

Dependent personality disorder, depicted in question 47, is marked by an excessive need to be taken care of, leading to clingy, submissive behavior and intense fear of separation, including difficulty making day-to-day decisions without advice and reassurance from others, a need for others to assume responsibility for major areas of life, avoidance of disagreement with others for fear of loss of approval, lack of self-confidence leading to avoidance of initiating projects or doing things independently, excessive need for support and nurturance by others, even if this entails doing or bearing unpleasant things, helplessness when alone because of fear of being unable to care for self, and urgent seeking of one relationship as a source of care if another relationship ends. Dependent personality disorder is equally common in males and females, and is one of the most common personality disorders.

Obsessive-compulsive personality disorder, depicted in question 48, is marked by a dysfunctional preoccupation with orderliness, perfection, and control at the expense of flexibility and efficiency, including preoccupation with details, rules, order, and schedules, to the point that the major purpose of an activity is lost. Other features include perfectionism that interferes with task completion, excessive devotion to work at the expense of leisure activities or friendship, inflexibility about moral matters and ethics, inability to discard worthless objects (to the extent of hoarding in some cases), reluctance to delegate tasks to others, frugal spending habits (money is seen as being something to hoard for future catastrophes), rigidity, and stubbornness. Although obsessive-compulsive disorder (discussed in question 17) may coexist with obsessive-compulsive personality disorder, distinct and definable obsessions and compulsions are absent in the latter, distinguishing the two.

See the last paragraph to the discussion to questions 64 to 67 for a brief overview of the treatment of personality disorders.

Diagnostic and Statistical Manual of Mental Disorders: DSM-IV-TR, 4th ed., text revision, Washington, DC: American Psychiatric Association; 2000.

Sadock BJ, Sadock VA, Ruiz P (Eds). Kaplan and Sadock's Comprehensive Textbook of Psychiatry, 9th ed. Philadelphia, PA: Lippincott Williams and Wilkins; 2009.

49. e

This couple suffers from shared psychotic disorder, or folie à deux, a type of disorder in which a psychotic belief develops in an individual that is similar to that held by a close relation. The diagnostic criteria for schizophrenia are discussed in questions 24 and 25; on the basis of the history provided, a diagnosis of schizophrenia cannot be made in this man and woman. The features of somatoform disorder (discussed in questions 20-22) are not present in this case; it is not contagious. Histrionic personality disorder is discussed in questions 64 to 67; there is no evidence in the history to suggest that this man and woman have this type of personality disorder.

Sadock BJ, Sadock VA, Ruiz P (Eds). Kaplan and Sadock's Comprehensive Textbook of Psychiatry, 9th ed. Philadelphia, PA: Lippincott Williams and Wilkins; 2009.

50. a

Tricyclic antidepressants (TCAs) lead to urinary retention due to inhibition of detrusor function, rather than bladder overactivity. Because the TCAs all have, to varying degrees, activity at muscarinic, histaminergic, and α_1-adrenergic receptors, they have various side effects. Antagonism at histamine receptors leads to sedation, xerostomia, and weight gain. Antimuscarinic activity leads to constipation, tachycardia, blurred vision (with increased risk of glaucoma), and urinary retention, and hence imipramine is used to treat overactive bladder and enuresis. α_1-adrenergic antagonism can lead to postural hypotension, which can be particularly detrimental in older adults. Of the commonly used TCAs, amitriptyline has the highest anti-muscarinic activity and α_1-adrenergic activity. Nortriptyline has the least α_1-adrenergic antagonism and is therefore less likely to cause orthostatic hypotension. Doxepin has the highest anti-histamine activity, and is therefore the most sedating. At toxic doses, TCAs can cause confusion, seizures, and arrhythmias. TCAs are metabolized through oxidation by various cytochrome P450 isozymes and subsequently undergo glucuronidation. Because their metabolism is strongly dependent on cytochrome P450 enzymes, they have various drug-drug interactions.

Brunton LL, Lazo JS, Parker KL (Eds). Goodman and Gilmans' Pharmacological Basis of Therapeutics, 11th ed. New York: McGraw-Hill; 2005.

51. d

Matt and Tom, the boys depicted in question 51, exhibit the features of attention-deficit/hyperactivity disorder (ADHD). ADHD includes a predominantly inattentive type, as in Matt; a predominantly hyperactive type, as in Tom; or a combined type.

The diagnostic criteria for the inattentive type include six or more symptoms of inattention that have been present for the prior 6 months with at least some symptoms occurring before age 7 years that are leading to functional impairment and are not consistent with developmental level and include failure to pay attention to details in schoolwork or other activities, difficulty sustaining attention on a task or activity, not listening when spoken to and not following instructions, difficulty with organization, avoidance or dislike of tasks that require sustained mental activity, loss of objects necessary for tasks or activities, easy distractibility, and forgetfulness in daily activities.

The diagnostic criteria for the hyperactive type include six or more symptoms of hyperactivity and impulsivity that have been present for the prior 6 months with at least some symptoms occurring before age 7 years that are leading to functional impairment and are not consistent with the developmental level and include frequent fidgeting or squirming, leaving a seat in situations when remaining seated is expected, running about or climbing excessively in inappropriate situations, or feelings of restlessness, difficulty engaging quietly in leisurely activities, talking excessively, blurting out of answers, difficulty awaiting a turn, and interruption of others.

Although the etiology of ADHD is not clear, dysfunction in frontal-subcortical circuits has been implicated. Genetic studies have suggested involvement of genes involved in dopamine action or metabolism, though environmental factors play a role as well. Children of parents with ADHD and siblings of children with ADHD are more likely to be affected with ADHD than the general population.

Oppositional defiant disorder (discussed in question 28) is a distinct entity from ADHD, but the two are often comorbid. Similarly, generalized anxiety disorder, discussed in question 18, is also comorbid with ADHD, as are the disruptive behavior disorders (discussed in questions 27 and 28). Tic disorder also frequently occurs with ADHD. In childhood, academic failure and peer rejection are the major consequences of ADHD, whereas in adolescence, there is a threefold increase in substance use and abuse. Approximately 60% of patients with ADHD in childhood continue to be impaired in adult life; ADHD may also not be recognized until adulthood. Adults with ADHD typically show instability with employment and relationships.

The first line of treatment for ADHD are psychostimulants, including amphetamines and methylphenidates, of which there are various oral preparations. Common side effects include reduced appetite, weight loss, insomnia, and headaches. An electrocardiogram prior to initiation of stimulant medications is recommended to exclude underlying structural or conduction problems. Other medications used to treat ADHD include the nonstimulant atomoxetine, tricyclic antidepressants, antipsychotics, mood stabilizers, and the α_2-agonist clonidine. Psychosocial treatment is also an important part of managing ADHD.

Diagnostic and Statistical Manual of Mental Disorders: DSM-IV-TR, 4th ed., text revision, Washington, DC: American Psychiatric Association; 2000.

Sadock BJ, Sadock VA, Ruiz P (Eds). Kaplan and Sadock's Comprehensive Textbook of Psychiatry, 9th ed. Philadelphia, PA: Lippincott Williams and Wilkins; 2009.

52. e

The selective serotonin reuptake inhibitors (SSRIs) have various side effects. Gastrointestinal side effects, including nausea, result in part from action of serotonin at $5HT_3$ receptors in the area postrema, but also from increased serotonin at the level of the enteric nervous system. Tolerance to this side effect typically develops after a few days of therapy. SSRIs cause sexual dysfunction, particularly leading to erectile dysfunction in men. They can lead to irritability and increased suicidal thoughts, particularly in younger age groups. Some of the SSRIs can lead to insomnia, whereas others are more sedating. Sertraline is one of the least sedating SSRIs. Paroxetine has the highest anticholinergic activity and therefore causes several anticholinergic side effects, including xerostomia and urinary retention.

Brunton LL, Lazo JS, Parker KL (Eds). Goodman and Gilmans' Pharmacological Basis of Therapeutics, 11th ed. New York: McGraw-Hill; 2005.

Katzung BG. Basic and Clinical Pharmacology, 11th ed. New York: McGraw-Hill; 2009.

53. e, 54. a, 55. b

Despite the development of newer antipsychotic agents (see questions 72-74), the typical antipsychotics are still commonly used; randomized controlled trials have shown the typical antipsychotics to be efficacious and cost-effective. The antipsychotics are first-line agents in the treatment of schizophrenia, schizoaffective disorder, and other psychotic disorders, including depression with psychotic features. Antipsychotics are also used as augmentation therapy in major depressive disorder and in the treatment of delirium, Tourette's syndrome (see Chapter 6), and behavioral and psychotic symptoms of dementia (discussed in question 70).

The typical antipsychotics, first brought into clinical use in the 1950s, include chlorpro-mazine and thioridazine, which have low potency at D_2 (dopamine) receptors and higher antag-onism at muscarinic, adrenergic, and histaminergic receptors. They are therefore more likely to cause side effects related to antagonism at these receptors, such as dry mouth, orthostasis, and sedation, respectively.

Those with higher potency at D_2 receptors, such as haloperidol and fluphenazine, have activity at muscarinic, adrenergic, and histaminergic receptors as well and can lead to similar side effects, but are less likely to do so. On the other hand, they are more likely to lead to extrapyramidal side effects (EPS), which result from D_2-antagonism in the nigrostriatal pathway. The EPS can be divided into acute reactions such as acute dystonia, which are in general reversible with treatment with anti-muscarinic agents such as benztropine, and tardive dyskinesia (such as the orolingual dyskinesias depicted in question 55, or tardive cervical dystonia), which are in general irreversible but may be treatable with botulinum toxin or deep brain stimulation to the globus pallidus interna (see Chapter 6).

Many of the typical antipsychotic agents can be administered orally, intravenous, or intra-muscularly, making them convenient in the treatment of psychotic patients for whom oral admin-istration is difficult. Prochlorperazine is an anti-dopaminergic agent used predominantly in the treatment of nausea.

Brunton LL, Lazo JS, Parker KL (Eds). Goodman and Gilmans' Pharmacological Basis of Therapeutics, 11th ed. New York: McGraw-Hill; 2005.

Katzung BG. Basic and Clinical Pharmacology, 11th ed. New York: McGraw-Hill; 2009.

56. c

This patient exhibits the features of adjustment disorder, which is a constellation of emotional and behavioral symptoms in response to a stressor that occurred within 3 months of symptom onset. This disorder is marked by distress that is in excess to what would be expected from the stressor, with impairment in social and occupational functioning, but that do not meet criteria for another disorder such as major depression (discussed in questions 1 and 2), and symptoms do not persist beyond 6 months of the stressor. Adjustment disorder may be further qualified as being accompanied by depressed mood, as in the patient depicted in question 56, or by anxiety.

Bereavement is a diagnosis that is made when an expectable response occurs in reaction to the death of a loved one. Adjustment disorder may subsequently be diagnosed if the bereavement reaction is more prolonged than would be expected (longer than 2 months) or more excessive than would be expected.

Diagnostic and Statistical Manual of Mental Disorders: DSM-IV-TR, 4th ed., text revision, Washington, DC: American Psychiatric Association; 2000.

Sadock BJ, Sadock VA, Ruiz P (Eds). Kaplan and Sadock's Comprehensive Textbook of Psychiatry, 9th ed. Philadelphia, PA: Lippincott Williams and Wilkins; 2009.

57. d

The benzodiazepines belong to a class of medications known as the sedative-hypnotics by nature of their ability to induce an anxiolytic calming effect and sleep. They include alprazolam, midazolam, chlordiazepoxide, temazepam, triazolam, flurazepam, clorazepate, oxazepam, and diazepam. They act at $GABA_A$ receptors, facilitating the action of GABA and increasing chloride conductance.

The benzodiazepines may be used in the treatment of acute anxiety, as is seen in generalized anxiety disorder (discussed in question 18), panic disorder, and agoraphobia (discussed in questions 7 and 8). However, chronic use leads to tolerance (decreased response to a specific dose after repeated exposure) as well as physiologic dependence. Other adverse effects include memory disturbance, sedation, and respiratory depression in overdose (or even at therapeutic doses in those with pulmonary disease). Chronic therapy for anxiety disorders therefore includes medications such as the selective serotonin reuptake inhibitors, tricyclic antidepressants, and serotonin-norepinephrine reuptake inhibitors. The latter medications do not have acute effects on anxiety, and in the initial weeks of therapy, benzodiazepines are often used as adjuncts until the anxiolysis takes effect. Of the benzodiazepines, flurazepam and clorazepate have the longest half-lives. Triazolam has a rapid onset and short duration of action.

Besides the treatment of acute anxiety, benzodiazepines are also used in the treatment of seizures, alcohol withdrawal, spasticity and movement disorders, and insomnia. Benzodiazepines are available in various oral, sublingual, intravenous, and intramuscular formulations, making them useful in the treatment of emergencies such as status epilepticus, as well as in anesthesia.

Buspirone is an anxiolytic agent without sedative-hypnotic activity. Its mechanism of action includes partial agonism at serotonergic ($5-HT_{1A}$) receptors as well as activity at dopaminergic D_2 receptors.

Katzung BG. Basic and Clinical Pharmacology, 11th ed. New York: McGraw-Hill; 2009.

58. c

Whole-brain and CSF volume studies in patients with schizophrenia have shown reduced brain volumes and higher CSF volumes compared to normal controls. There is evidence of ventricular enlargement, particularly of the third and lateral ventricles, with sulcal widening. There is atrophy of areas of the frontal and temporal lobes, as well as the hippocampus and thalamus. PET studies have shown hypometabolism of the dorsolateral prefrontal cortex during activation tasks. PET studies have not shown resting regional cerebral blood flow abnormalities in patients with schizophrenia compared to controls. Bilateral caudate head atrophy occurs in Huntington's disease, not schizophrenia.

Hales RE, Yudofsky SC, Gabbard GO (Eds). The American Psychiatric Publishing Textbook of
Psychiatry. Arlington, VA: American Psychiatric Publishing Inc; 2008.

Sadock BJ, Sadock VA, Ruiz P (Eds). Kaplan and Sadock's Comprehensive Textbook of Psychiatry,
9th ed. Philadelphia, PA: Lippincott Williams and Wilkins; 2009.

59. e

Hyponatremia is an established side effect of therapy with selective serotonin reuptake inhibitors
(SSRIs). Risk factors include older age, female sex, and concomitant use of diuretics. Hyponatremia resulting from SSRIs typically occurs within the first month of therapy, but may not occur
until several months after initiation of therapy. Among the SSRIs, fluoxetine and paroxetine
are more likely to lead to hyponatremia. The pathophysiology of SSRI-induced hyponatremia
is thought to at least in part be related to the syndrome of inappropriate antidiuretic hormone,
resulting from excessive release of antidiuretic hormone mediated by activation of serotonergic
receptors. Although there are no definitive data to support routine monitoring of serum sodium
in patients started on an SSRI, any change in mentation or other symptoms potentially suggesting hyponatremia should prompt a laboratory evaluation for this complication. In isovolemic
hyponatremia due to SSRIs, the treatment is discontinuation of the SSRI along with fluid restriction. In more severe symptomatic hyponatremia, treatment with intravenous sodium chloride
may be indicated. Rechallenge with SSRIs may not necessarily lead to recurrent hyponatremia,
though it can.

Jacob S, Spinler SA. Hyponatremia associated with selective serotonin-reuptake inhibitors in
older adults. Ann Pharmacother. 2006; 40:1618–1622.

60. b

Schizophrenia (discussed also in questions 24 and 25) is not thought to be a monogenic disorder; its genetics are thought to be more complex than simple Mendelian disorders, and it is
not transmitted in an autosomal dominant fashion. Schizophrenia aggregates in families, and
the results of epidemiologic studies, twin studies, adoption studies, and genetic linkage and
association studies suggest that schizophrenia is a genetic disorder, with phenotypic expression
of the disorder being influenced by a variety of environmental factors. The concordance rate
(the rate of twins that are each affected) for schizophrenia is higher among monozygotic compared to dizygotic twins. Several schizophrenia susceptibility loci have been mapped to various
chromosomes, with candidate genes including dysbindin on chromosome 6 and neuregulin-1
on chromosome 8. Other genetic abnormalities detected in schizophrenia include chromosomal
deletions, trinucleotide repeat expansions, and copy number variants. As of 2009, genome-wide
association studies have not identified single-nucleotide polymorphisms significantly associated
with schizophrenia at a genome-wide level.

Hales RE, Yudofsky SC, Gabbard GO (Eds). The American Psychiatric Publishing Textbook of
Psychiatry. Arlington, VA: American Psychiatric Publishing Inc; 2008.

Sadock BJ, Sadock VA, Ruiz P (Eds). Kaplan and Sadock's Comprehensive Textbook of Psychiatry,
9th ed. Philadelphia, PA: Lippincott Williams and Wilkins; 2009.

61. d

This patient's history and examination are consistent with serotonin syndrome. Serotonin syndrome results from overstimulation of brain stem serotonin receptors. Symptoms
include encephalopathy, autonomic hyperactivity manifesting as hypertension, tachycardia, and
diaphoresis, and myoclonus, hyperreflexia, and tremor. Serotonin syndrome can occur with any

agent that increases serotonin, and has even been reported with monotherapy, but is more likely to occur with a combination of therapies that increase serotonin, and particularly with concomitant use of nonselective monoamine oxidase inhibitors. Treatment generally includes supportive care and withdrawal of the offending agent.

Serotonin withdrawal syndrome can occur with abrupt discontinuation of serotonergic medications such as selective serotonin reuptake inhibitors. Symptoms include dizziness, paresthesias, dysphoria, and in some cases encephalopathy. Therefore, gradual tapering of such medications is generally recommended.

Thyroid storm can lead to similar symptoms as in this patient, but given the history presented, serotonin syndrome is more likely.

Katzung BG. Basic and Clinical Pharmacology, 11th ed. New York: McGraw-Hill; 2009.

62. e

This man's history is consistent with brief psychotic disorder. His symptoms started following a significant stressor and consisted of hallucinations, delusions, and disorganized speech, similar to the symptoms of schizophrenia. However, symptoms lasted less than 1 month, and did not recur, with a return to baseline. Brief psychotic disorder can also occur in the absence of an acute stressor, and can also occur postpartum.

The diagnostic criteria for brief psychotic disorder include the following (Diagnostic and Statistical Manual—Text Revision (DSM-IV-TR, 2000)):

A. Presence of one or more of the following: delusions, hallucinations, disorganized speech, and/or grossly disorganized or catatonic behavior
B. Duration of the episode is at least 1 day but less than 1 month, with eventual return to full premorbid function
C. Disturbance is not accounted for by other mood or psychotic disorders, and is not due to a substance or general medical condition

The duration of symptoms distinguishes brief psychotic disorder from the other choices listed. Schizophreniform disorder is discussed in question 16, schizophrenia in questions 24 and 25, delusional disorder in question 31, and schizoaffective disorder in question 69.

Sadock BJ, Sadock VA, Ruiz P (Eds). Kaplan and Sadock's Comprehensive Textbook of Psychiatry, 9th ed. Philadelphia, PA: Lippincott Williams and Wilkins; 2009.

63. a

GABA is an amino acid and the major inhibitory neurotransmitter in the CNS. Glycine is also an inhibitory amino acid neurotransmitter and plays a prominent role in the brain and spinal cord. GABA is synthesized from glutamic acid by action of the enzyme glutamic acid decarboxylase. Disorders of this enzyme lead to a deficiency in GABA and subsequently over-activation in the CNS, as is seen in stiff-person syndrome. The $GABA_A$ receptor is an example of an ionotropic receptor, activation of which leads to opening of chloride channels. The $GABA_B$ receptor is an example of a metabotropic receptor, which is coupled to an inhibitory G protein, inhibiting adenylyl cyclase. Baclofen is an example of a selective $GABA_B$ receptor agonist; benzodiazepines act at $GABA_A$ receptors.

Brunton LL, Lazo JS, Parker KL (Eds). Goodman and Gilmans' Pharmacological Basis of Therapeutics, 11th ed. New York: McGraw-Hill; 2005.

64. d, 65. a, 66. b, 67. c

See the first paragraph of the discussion for questions 41 to 43 for the definition of personality disorders. Questions 64 to 67 depict people that would be classified under cluster B of the personality disorders. This cluster includes narcissistic, antisocial, borderline, and histrionic personality disorders.

Narcissistic personality disorder, depicted in question 64, is marked by pervasive grandiosity, demand for admiration, and a lack of empathy, including a sense of self-importance, preoccupation with perceived positive attributes such as success or beauty, a conviction of superiority over others, a sense of self-entitlement, manipulation of others to achieve ends, a lack of empathy, envy or beliefs that others are envious, fear of having flaws revealed, and arrogance. Narcissistic personality disorder is more common in males, and major depression (discussed in questions 1 and 2) and substance abuse are common comorbidities.

Antisocial personality disorder, depicted in question 65, is marked by a disregard for and violation of others since age 15, and includes disrespect of others and the law, deceptiveness, impulsivity, aggressiveness, recklessness, irresponsibility (in the workplace, financially, etc.), and lack of remorse, with indifference to harming others. Conduct disorder (discussed in question 27) is a prerequisite for the diagnosis of antisocial personality disorder; antisocial personality disorder cannot be diagnosed in those younger than 18. Impulse control disorder (discussed in questions 35 and 36) may occur in persons with antisocial personality disorder, but the other features of antisocial personality disorder discussed distinguish the two. Antisocial personality disorder is three times more common in males as compared to females.

Borderline personality disorder, depicted in question 66, is marked by pervasive impulsivity, instability in relationships, self-image, and affect, including dramatic efforts to avoid abandonment, unstable interpersonal relationships with alternations between idealization and devaluation (so-called *splitting*), unstable self-image, potentially self-damaging impulsivity (such as excessive spending, sexual promiscuity, or binge eating), recurrent suicidal gesture or threats or self-mutilation, marked reactivity of mood, feelings of emptiness, difficulty with control of anger, and self-related paranoia or dissociative symptoms. Borderline personality disorder is more common in females. Frequent comorbidities include major depression, eating disorder (particularly bulimia; discussed in question 38), and substance abuse.

Histrionic personality disorder, depicted in question 67, is marked by pervasive excessive emotionality and attention-seeking behavior, including constant need to be the center of attention, inappropriately seductive or provocative behavior, shallow and rapidly shifting emotions, use of physical appearance to draw attention to self, impressionistic and vague style of speech, theatricals and self-dramatization, with exaggerated expression of emotions, suggestibility, and consideration of relationships as being more intimate than they are. Histrionic personality disorder is more common in females, and common comorbidities include major depression, conversion disorder, and somatization disorder.

Patients with personality disorders lack insight into their pathology, but may be asked to seek care from a psychiatrist by family members or others in the setting of dysfunction in relationships, occupation, or otherwise. Treatment includes a combination of psychotherapy combined with pharmacotherapy aimed at the most prominent psychiatric symptoms (such as anxiolytics if anxiety is the main symptom, or mood stabilizers or antipsychotics if lability, aggression, or impulsivity are the most prominent symptoms).

Diagnostic and Statistical Manual of Mental Disorders: DSM-IV-TR, 4th ed., text revision, Washington, DC: American Psychiatric Association; 2000.

Sadock BJ, Sadock VA, Ruiz P (Eds). Kaplan and Sadock's Comprehensive Textbook of Psychiatry, 9th ed. Philadelphia, PA: Lippincott Williams and Wilkins; 2009.

68. a

Duloxetine and venlafaxine are selective serotonin-norepinephrine reuptake inhibitors (SNRIs): they inhibit reuptake of both serotonin and norepinephrine by inhibiting serotonin and norepinephrine transporters, respectively. The SNRIs and tricyclic antidepressants (TCAs), because they increase both norepinephrine and serotonin, are useful in the treatment of pain disorders. Unlike the TCAs, the SNRIs are selective and have little activity at muscarinic, histaminergic, and α-adrenergic receptors.

Mirtazapine has complex pharmacology; it acts as an antagonist at presynaptic α_2-autoreceptors, increasing release of norepinephrine and serotonin, and also acts as an antagonist at 5-HT$_2$ and 5-HT$_3$ receptors. Its potent antagonism at histamine receptors accounts for its sedating effects. The mechanism of action of bupropion is not well understood, but animal studies have shown that it inhibits reuptake of norepinephrine and dopamine and increases presynaptic release of these neurotransmitters, without direct effects on the serotonin system. At high doses, bupropion increases risk of seizures. Bupropion, in addition to its use as an antidepressant, is used in smoking cessation. Trazodone and nefazodone act primarily by antagonism at the 5-HT$_2$ receptor; trazodone was initially used as an antidepressant, but its primary use today is as a hypnotic (sedative) because it is highly sedating and little tolerance develops to its sedating effect over time. An adverse effect that may occur with trazodone therapy is priapism or prolonged painful erection. Phenelzine and isocarboxazid are monoamine oxidase inhibitors (MAOIs) and are among the oldest antidepressants that are rarely used in clinical practice today due to their side-effect profile. Because nonselective MAOIs block metabolism of tyramine, found in certain foods such as cheese and wine, a lethal reaction resulting from hyperadrenergic state can occur with use of MAOIs, particularly when taken with other agents that increase serotonin.

Katzung BG. Basic and Clinical Pharmacology, 11th ed. New York: McGraw-Hill; 2009.

69. d

Schizoaffective disorder is a psychotic disorder with a concomitant mood disorder. The main feature of this disorder is the occurrence of a depressive episode, manic episode, or mixed episode, concurrent with symptoms that meet criterion A for schizophrenia (see questions 24 and 25), all within an uninterrupted period of time. In addition, there must be delusions or hallucinations for at least 2 weeks in the absence of prominent mood symptoms. The time of onset of the mood and psychotic symptoms must be clearly discernable.

Schizoaffective disorder is distinguished from depression (discussed in questions 1 and 2) or mania (discussed in questions 10 and 11) with psychotic features in that in schizoaffective disorder, there must be at least a 2-week period during which psychotic symptoms are present without prominent symptoms of a mood disorder.

The diagnostic criteria for schizoaffective disorder include the following (Diagnostic and Statistical Manual—Text Revision (DSM-IV-TR, 2000)):

A. An uninterrupted period of illness during which at some time there is either a major depressive, manic, or mixed episode concurrent with symptoms that meet criterion A for schizophrenia (see questions 24 and 25).
B. During the same period of illness, there are delusions or hallucinations present for at least 2 weeks in the absence of prominent mood symptoms.
C. Symptoms that meet criteria for a mood episode are present for a significant portion of the total duration of the active and residual periods of the illness.
D. The disturbance is not explained by a general medical condition or a substance.

Diagnostic and Statistical Manual of Mental Disorders: DSM-IV-TR, 4th ed., text revision, Washington, DC: American Psychiatric Association; 2000.

Sadock BJ, Sadock VA, Ruiz P (Eds). Kaplan and Sadock's Comprehensive Textbook of Psychiatry, 9th ed. Philadelphia, PA: Lippincott Williams and Wilkins; 2009.

70. e

Atypical antipsychotic agents (discussed in questions 72-74) can be efficacious in the treatment of behavioral and psychotic symptoms of dementia (BPSD), which include agitation and hallucinations. In this patient population, they carry significant risks, including increased mortality and increased risk of stroke and thromboembolic events. Despite these risks, in some patients, when BPSD poses a significant risk to the patient and his or her caregivers, as depicted in this case, their use may be indicated. Nonpharmacologic measures and medications besides atypical antipsychotic agents should be tried when feasible, though data regarding use of the latter in the treatment of BPSD are not robust. When necessary, atypical antipsychotic agents should be started at the lowest possible dose, and need for them should be reassessed regularly.

Salzman C, Jeste DV, Meyer RE, et al. Elderly patients with dementia-related symptoms of severe agitation and aggression: Consensus statement on treatment options, clinical trials methodology, and policy. J Clin Psychiatry. 2008; 69:889–898.

71. b

Before an antidepressant is deemed ineffective, a trial of at least 6 weeks of therapy is warranted.

The treatment of major depressive episode includes both pharmacologic therapy and nonpharmacologic therapy, the latter mainly including psychotherapy. Electroconvulsive therapy can be effective after 8 to 12 sessions, but is often reserved for medication-resistant depression because of cognitive side effects.

Clear superiority of one antidepressant over another has not been demonstrated in meta-analyses, and choice of antidepressant may depend more on side-effect profile, risk of drug-drug interactions, cost, and other such factors unrelated to efficacy. For example, in the patient presented in question 71, a selective serotonin reuptake inhibitor may be undesirable because of the risk of erectile dysfunction; alternative antidepressants with less risk of sexual side effects include bupropion and venlafaxine. A sedating agent such as a tricyclic antidepressant or mirtazapine may help with his poor sleep. Venlafaxine can cause a dose-dependent increase in blood pressure, and may be best avoided in a patient with known hypertension.

Less than 50% of patients respond to the initial antidepressant selected, and augmentation with another agent or discontinuation with switching to an agent from another class is often necessary. Several algorithms have been developed to aid physicians in selection of the most appropriate antidepressant. The duration of therapy depends on the patient's psychiatric history, response to treatment, and relapse rate. More than 80% of patients with an episode of major depression have at least one recurrence during their lifetime, and sometimes long-term and even life-long maintenance therapy with an antidepressant is required.

Katzung BG. Basic and Clinical Pharmacology, 11th ed. New York: McGraw-Hill; 2009.

Sadock BJ, Sadock VA, Ruiz P (Eds). Kaplan and Sadock's Comprehensive Textbook of Psychiatry, 9th ed. Philadelphia, PA: Lippincott Williams and Wilkins; 2009.

72. d, 73. c, 74. e

The second generation of antipsychotics, so-called atypical antipsychotics, includes clozapine, olanzapine, quetiapine, risperidone, ziprasidone, and aripiprazole. These agents do have antagonistic activity at D_2 (dopamine) receptors. However, their clinical antipsychotic effect results in large part from antagonism at serotonergic 5-HT$_{2A}$ receptors. Studies to date have not shown overall superior efficacy of the atypical antipsychotics over the typical ones, though atypical antipsychotics may be more effective at treating some of the negative symptoms of schizophrenia. Because they have less antagonism at D_2 receptors, they are less likely to cause extrapyramidal side effects (EPS), but certainly can. As a class, the atypical antipsychotics carry with them an increased risk of weight gain, diabetes, and dyslipidemia. Patients being treated with these medications should therefore periodically be assessed for such side effects. Clozapine and olanzapine are most likely to lead to weight gain. Ziprasidone and aripiprazole are less likely to cause weight gain than the others.

Some of the typical and atypical antipsychotics including thioridazine, haloperidol, ziprasidone, and quetiapine have negative ionotropic action on the heart and a quinidine-like effect, leading to QT prolongation with the potential for arrhythmias. Aripiprazole is least likely to do so. Other cardiac side effects include myocarditis, which can rarely be seen with clozapine. The atypical antipsychotics also have activity at muscarinic, adrenergic, and histaminergic receptors, and several side effects result from activity at these sites. Clozapine can lead to agranulocytosis in 1% to 2% of patients, and patients being treated with this medication are required to have periodic complete blood counts checked. Clozapine also leads to a dose-dependent increased risk of seizures. Clozapine is least likely of all the atypical antipsychotics to lead to EPS. Because of the side-effect profile of clozapine, its use is usually limited to treatment of patients who have failed trials of other typical and atypical antipsychotics. Among the atypical antipsychotics, olanzapine has the highest antimuscarinic activity, and side effects resulting from this include dry mouth, urinary retention, confusion, and constipation. Clozapine also has significant antimuscarinic activity. Quetiapine has significant anti-histaminergic activity, and along with olanzapine, is the most likely to lead to sedation.

Dopamine inhibits prolactin release, and treatment with both typical and atypical antipsychotics can lead to hyperprolactinemia and amenorrhea resulting from dopaminergic antagonism in the tuberoinfundibular pathway. Some of the atypical antipsychotics are available in injectable forms, including long-acting depot formulations.

Brunton LL, Lazo JS, Parker KL (Eds). Goodman and Gilmans' Pharmacological Basis of Therapeutics, 11th ed. New York: McGraw-Hill; 2005.

Katzung BG. Basic and Clinical Pharmacology, 11th ed. New York: McGraw-Hill; 2009.

75. c

Flumazenil is an antagonist of benzodiazepines and other sedative-hypnotic agents such as zolpidem and eszopiclone (the latter two agents are used in the treatment of insomnia). Flumazenil does not however antagonize the action of barbiturates. Naloxone and naltrexone are used in the treatment of opioid overdose. Thiamine and dextrose are used in the treatment of thiamine deficiency and hypoglycemia as is seen in alcoholics or other chronic states of malnourishment (see Chapter 17).

Katzung BG. Basic and Clinical Pharmacology, 11th ed. New York: McGraw-Hill; 2009.

76. d

Glutamate and aspartate are excitatory neurotransmitters. The glutamate receptors are divided into NMDA receptors, those at which NMDA acts as an agonist, and non-NMDA receptors, which include AMPA and kainic acid receptors, named according to the substances that act as agonists at these receptors. Specific patterns of activation of NMDA receptors can lead to induction of long-term potentiation, which is a prolonged increase in a postsynaptic response resulting from a finite presynaptic stimulus and is thought to be involved in memory formation. High concentrations of glutamate lead to neuronal cell death triggered by excessive glutamate receptor activation, with excessive calcium influx into cells. Glutamate excitotoxicity has been implicated in neuronal damage seen in ischemia and hypoglycemia. Memantine is an NMDA antagonist used in the treatment of dementia.

Brunton LL, Lazo JS, Parker KL (Eds). Goodman and Gilmans' Pharmacological Basis of Therapeutics, 11th ed. New York: McGraw-Hill; 2005.

77. e

Both bupropion (discussed in question 68) and clozapine (discussed in questions 72–74) have been associated with increased risk of seizure at higher dosages. Olanzapine (discussed in questions 72–74) is less likely to cause seizures, but can do so; other atypical antipsychotics rarely cause seizures. On the other hand, amitriptyline, which is a tricyclic antidepressant (discussed in question 39) is associated with increased seizure risk with acute toxicity. Flumazenil, by inducing a state of benzodiazepine withdrawal, can lead to increased risk of seizures, particularly in patients with a prior history of seizures.

Katzung BG. Basic and Clinical Pharmacology, 11th ed. New York: McGraw-Hill; 2009.

78. e, 79. a

Levodopa is a dopaminergic agent used in the treatment of Parkinson's disease and other movement disorders (see Chapter 6), and is not used in the treatment of mood disorders. Mood-stabilizing agents used to treat bipolar disorder include lithium carbonate, as well as the anticonvulsants including valproic acid and lamotrigine. Antipsychotic agents including risperidone are used as adjuncts in the treatment of acute mania. The depressive phase of bipolar disorder often warrants concurrent antidepressant therapy. Mood-stabilizing agents are also used in the treatment of schizoaffective disorder.

The mechanism of action of lithium carbonate is not clear, but does include inhibition of the inositol and glycogen synthase kinase 3 signal pathways and downstream enzyme activity. Valproic acid may similarly exert its effects. Serum levels of lithium should be monitored periodically. Common adverse effects of lithium include tremor, thyroid dysfunction, acne, and nephrogenic diabetes insipidus, which can lead to hypernatremia if there is not adequate oral intake of fluids, as in the case depicted in question 79. Lithium is contraindicated in patients with sick sinus syndrome because it has a negative chronotropic effect. The side effects of valproic acid, lamotrigine, and other anticonvulsants are discussed in Chapter 5.

Katzung BG. Basic and Clinical Pharmacology, 11th ed. New York: McGraw-Hill; 2009.

Buzz Phrase	Key Points
Duration of symptoms distinguishing schizophrenia, schizophreniform disorder, and brief psychotic disorder	Brief psychotic disorder: ≤ 1 month
	Schizophreniform disorder: >1 to <6 months
	Schizophrenia: ≥ 6 months
Secondary gain in factitious disorder	Assumption of role of patient
Secondary gain in malingering	External incentive such as money
Duration of symptoms distinguishing acute stress reaction from post-traumatic stress disorder (PTSD)	Acute stress reaction: <1 month
	PTSD: ≥ 1 month
Pathologic stealing	Kleptomania
Pathologic impulse to set fires	Pyromania
Cluster A personality disorders	Paranoid: paranoid, distrustful
	Schizoid: loner, unsociable
	Schizotypal: weird, odd, eccentric
Cluster B personality disorders	Narcissistic: conceited, grandiose
	Antisocial: cruel, reckless, unremorseful
	Borderline: unstable relationships, self-injurious behavior, splitting
	Histrionic: dramatic, emotional, attention-seeking
Cluster C personality disorders	Avoidant: hypersensitivity to criticism, feelings of inadequacy
	Dependent: clingy, submissive
	Obsessive-compulsive: perfectionist, too organized but not necessarily productive, rigid
Antidepressants leading to convulsions, coma, cardiac arrhythmias (three Cs) in toxicity	Tricyclic antidepressants
Antidepressants that lead to hyponatremia	Selective serotonin reuptake inhibitors
Antipsychotic that causes agranulocytosis	Clozapine
Mechanism of action of haloperidol and other typical antipsychotics	Antagonists at D_2 (dopamine) receptors
Mechanism of action of risperidone and other atypical antipsychotics	Antagonists at D_2 receptors and 5-HT_{2A} receptors
Mood-stabilizing agent that leads to thyroid dysfunction, tremor, and hypernatremia	Lithium carbonate
Benzodiazepine antagonist	Flumazenil

Chapter 14

Child Neurology

Questions

Questions 1–3

1. Regarding embryonal nervous system development, which of the following statements is correct?
   a. The main embryonal layer giving rise to the nervous system is the endoderm
   b. The notochord is the main structure giving rise to the CNS
   c. The neural plate, through a process called neurulation, forms the neural tube
   d. The neural plate fuses to form the neural tube in all areas at once, simultaneously
   e. The notochord consists of ectodermal cells

2. Regarding embryonal nervous system development, which of the following statements is correct?
   a. The rhombencephalon gives rise to the cerebral hemispheres
   b. The mesencephalon gives rise to the hypothalamus and thalamus
   c. The prosencephalon gives rise to the telencephalon, which ultimately forms the cerebral hemispheres
   d. The diencephalon gives rise to the midbrain
   e. The prosencephalon gives rise to the telencephalon, which ultimately forms the brain stem

3. Regarding embryonal nervous system development, which of the following statements is correct?
   a. Vertebral bodies arise from ectodermal cells of the neural plate
   b. Neural crest cells give rise to the peripheral nervous system
   c. Failure of fusion of the posterior neuropore leads to disorders such as anencephaly
   d. Failure of fusion of the anterior neuropore leads to disorders such as spina bifida
   e. The notochord gives rise to chromaffin cells of the adrenal medulla

4. A 7-day-old baby boy is brought to the hospital because of persistent vomiting and diarrhea, predominantly after being fed. He is noted to be jaundiced, and examination demonstrates hypotonia and hepatosplenomegaly. Reducing substances are detected in the urine. A presumptive diagnosis of galactosemia is made. Which of the following is incorrect regarding this disorder?
   a. Galactose-1-phosphate uridyltransferase deficiency is the only defect associated with galactosemia

564

b. Galactitol accumulation produces cataracts that are reversible

c. It is autosomal recessive

d. The treatment is removal of lactose and galactose from the diet

e. Patients with this disorder may develop ataxia and tremor despite treatment

5. An 8-month-old baby is brought for evaluation. He has hypotonia, growth retardation and poor psychomotor development. He also has a history of episodes of incoordination, especially with high-carbohydrate meals and during systemic infections. On laboratory evaluation, he is found to have elevated levels of lactate and pyruvate, with a low lactate:pyruvate ratio. Deficiency of the enzyme pyruvate dehydrogenase (PDH) is detected. Which of the following is incorrect regarding this condition?

   a. PDH is responsible for oxidative decarboxylation of pyruvate to carbon dioxide and acetyl coenzyme A

   b. Only inherited in an autosomal recessive fashion

   c. Can present with severe neonatal acidosis

   d. High-carbohydrate diet can precipitate episodes of ataxia

   e. Ketogenic diet has been used to treat patients with this condition

6. Which of the following is not correct regarding neurofibromatosis type 1 (NF1)?

   a. Renal artery stenosis and pheochromocytoma are on the differential diagnosis of hypertension occurring in NF1 patients

   b. There is an association between NF1 and Moyamoya disease

   c. The majority of patients with NF1 have severe developmental delay

   d. Macrocephaly is the most common head size abnormality seen in NF1 patients and is independent of the extent of hydrocephalus

   e. NF1 patients have an increased risk of intracranial aneurysms

7. An infant with epileptic encephalopathy is brought for evaluation. He has microcephaly and prominent developmental delay. On CSF analysis, it was noticed that the level of glucose was 30 mg/dL, whereas the level of serum glucose was 112 mg/dL. Other CSF tests are normal. Which of the following is correct regarding the most likely condition in this patient?

   a. Brain MRI usually suggests the diagnosis

   b. It is caused by deficiency in the glucose transporter type 1

   c. Phenobarbital is the treatment of choice

   d. Ketogenic diet has been shown to be ineffective for seizure control

   e. It is inherited in an X-linked fashion

8. Regarding neural tube defects resulting from failure of fusion of the anterior neuropore, which of the following statements is correct?

   a. Failure of fusion of the anterior neuropore leads to spina bifida

   b. Failure of fusion of the anterior neuropore leads to anencephaly and encephalocele

   c. Anterior neuropore defects typically occur from insults in the last trimester of gestation

   d. Anencephaly may be occult and diagnosed in early childhood or even adolescence

   e. Encephalocele is incompatible with life

9. A 7-month-old baby boy is brought for evaluation of seizures. He and his parents recently immigrated from a developing country, and the baby did not undergo newborn screening at birth. He has significant developmental delay, is hypotonic, has failure to thrive, and is

microcephalic. His urine has a musty odor. Which of the following is incorrect regarding this condition?

   a. Phenylalanine transaminase deficiency is the cause of this condition

   b. Tetrahydrobiopterin is a cofactor in the conversion of phenylalanine to tyrosine

   c. Dietary restriction of phenylalanine is the treatment for this condition

   d. Cognitive impairment and seizures are common

   e. The musty odor in the urine and sweat is caused by phenylacetic acid

10. A 1-week-old baby was admitted in the hospital with altered sensorium, opisthotonic posture, and abnormal movements. He is now intubated, comatose, and began having seizures last night. The urine smells like maple syrup. Which of the following is correct regarding this condition?

   a. It is caused by the accumulation in blood of essential amino acids such as phenylalanine and tryptophan

   b. The classic form presents in late infancy

   c. It is caused by a deficiency of branched-chain α-ketoacid dehydrogenase complex

   d. It is X-linked

   e. There is no role for protein restriction in the diet as a therapeutic intervention

11. Which of the following definitions of neural tube defects is incorrect?

   a. Meningocele—isolated meningeal protrusion

   b. Myelomeningocele—protrusion of spinal cord and meninges

   c. Diastematomyelia—splitting of the spinal cord into two portions by a midline septum

   d. Diplomyelia—duplication of the spinal cord

   e. Sacral agenesis—isolated absence of the sacral spinal cord

12. Which of the following statements is incorrect regarding the systemic manifestations of tuberous sclerosis complex (TSC)?

   a. Cardiac rhabdomyomas may occur and often regress over time

   b. Periodic echocardiography is indicated for patients with cardiac rhabdomyomas

   c. Renal angiomyolipomas are benign lesions

   d. Lymphangiomyomatosis is a benign disorder often occurring in TSC patients, particularly in male patients

   e. Retinal hamartomas are common and usually do not affect vision although they may in some cases

13. A newborn baby is being evaluated for encephalopathy in the setting of metabolic acidosis and hyperammonemia. There is also ketoacidosis, and elevated blood propionic acid and glycine levels with normal methylmalonic acid levels. You suspect propionic acidemia. Which of the following is correct regarding this condition?

   a. It is caused by deficiency of D-methylmalonyl-CoA mutase

   b. It is X-linked

   c. High-protein diet is recommended for these patients

   d. Hematologic disorders occur in this condition

   e. Propionyl-CoA carboxylase activity is increased

14. A 6-month-old baby is brought to the pediatrician for routine well-child visit. On examination, the infant is found to have a small, midline tuft of hair over the lower lumbar region. The child's physical examination is otherwise entirely normal. On annual follow-up at 3 years of age, the

child continues to have normal development and a normal neurologic examination. Which of the following statements regarding this child is correct?

a. On the basis of the finding of this tuft of hair, it can be concluded that he will eventually have significant cognitive delay, even if he has developed normally up until the age of 3 years

b. On the basis of the finding of this tuft of hair, it can be concluded that he will eventually have significant motor and cognitive delay even if he has developed normally up until the age of 3 years

c. This tuft of hair signifies a possible underlying defect in the posterior bony component of the vertebral column

d. This tuft of hair signifies the presence of a myelomeningocele

e. On the basis of the finding of this tuft of hair, it can be concluded that abnormalities in the spinal cord will definitely be seen on imaging

15. A 3-year-old boy is brought for follow-up evaluation. He has had developmental delay and mental retardation since early in life and has developed torticollis and spasticity in his limbs. He also has a history of seizures and aggressive behavior. His mother reports that he began biting himself to the point of bleeding and constantly self-inflicts injuries. He has had kidney stones and hyperuricemia. Which of the following is incorrect regarding this condition?

a. The genetic defect is in the gene HPRT1

b. It is autosomal recessive

c. Hypoxanthine guanine phosphoribosyltransferase is the deficient enzyme

d. It is caused by an enzymatic defect in the purine salvage pathway

e. Patients may have choreoathetotic movements

16. Which of the following is not a risk factor for the occurrence of neural tube defects?

a. Male gender

b. Folate deficiency

c. Exposure to retinoic acid

d. Exposure to valproic acid

e. Maternal diabetes

17. A 10-month-old baby is brought for follow-up. He has significant developmental delay with psychomotor retardation and failure to thrive. On examination, he also has a cherry-red spot on retinal examination and hepatosplenomegaly. Bone marrow specimen demonstrates foam cells. He carries a diagnosis of Niemann-Pick disease. Which of the following is correct regarding this diagnosis?

a. This patient has Niemann-Pick type A

b. This patient has Niemann-Pick type C

c. The activity of the enzyme acid sphingomyelinase is increased

d. The cause is a defect in intracellular cholesterol trafficking

e. Interstitial lung disease does not occur in any of the types of Niemann-Pick disease

18. A 6-year-old girl is evaluated for progressive neurologic deterioration, including vertical gaze apraxia, ataxia, and spasticity. A filipin test (which demonstrates impaired ability of cultured fibroblasts to esterify cholesterol) was abnormal. Which of the following is correct regarding this condition?

a. This patient has Niemann-Pick type A

b. This patient has Niemann-Pick type C

c. This condition is X-linked

d. The cause is acid sphingomyelinase deficiency

e. The deficient enzyme is hexosaminidase A

19. In the setting of a fetus with a neural tube defect (NTD), which of the following statements regarding prenatal diagnosis is incorrect?

    a. α-Fetoprotein level is elevated in maternal serum

    b. α-Fetoprotein level is elevated in amniotic fluid

    c. Acetylcholinesterase is elevated in amniotic fluid and increases sensitivity and specificity of NTD screening

    d. There is little utility in prenatal ultrasonography in the detection of NTDs

    e. When a NTD is detected prenatally, karyotyping to assess for trisomies and other genetic defects may be indicated

20. A 4-year-old boy presents with progressive neurologic deterioration. The onset of his symptoms was around the age of 1 year with hypotonia and inability to walk, with subsequent visual and hearing loss. He is now unable to walk and has generalized spasticity and cognitive regression. Brain MRI shows T2 hyperintense signal changes in the periventricular and subcortical white matter sparing the U fibers. Arylsulfatase A deficiency is detected on leukocyte analysis. Which of the following is the most likely diagnosis?

    a. Metachromatic leukodystrophy

    b. Niemann-Pick type C

    c. Niemann-Pick type A

    d. Krabbe disease

    e. Tay-Sachs disease

21. A 7-year-old girl is brought to the pediatric neurologist with gait abnormalities and headache. On examination, she has nystagmus, and truncal and limb ataxia. An image from her MRI is shown in Figure 14.1. Which of the following statements regarding this patient's disorder is incorrect?

    a. Chiari I malformations may be asymptomatic and do not necessarily require surgical intervention

    b. Myelomeningocele occurs in patients with Chiari II malformation

    c. Hydrocephalus is a complication of Chiari malformation

    d. Management of Chiari malformations may include suboccipital decompression

    e. Syringomyelia, which may occur in association with a Chiari I malformation, is an enlargement of the central canal of the spinal cord

22. Which of the following is correct regarding sialidosis?

    a. Sialidosis type I has infantile onset

    b. Sialidosis type II has adult onset

    c. A cherry-red spot is rarely seen in this condition

    d. Coarse facial features are almost never seen in sialidosis type II

    e. These patients have myoclonic epilepsy

23. A 2-year-old boy with developmental delay and ataxia presents for evaluation. He has extraocular muscle abnormalities, but visual acuity is unaffected and his irises appear normal. MRI of the brain is done, and an image is shown in Figure 14.2. What is the most likely diagnosis in this patient?

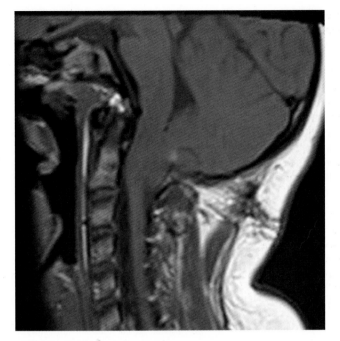

FIGURE 14.1   Sagittal T1-weighted MRI

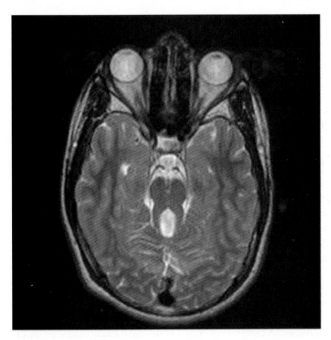

FIGURE 14.2   Axial T2-weighted MRI. Courtesy of Dr. Manikum Moodley and Dr. Gary Hsich

    a. Ataxia with oculomotor apraxia type I
    b. Ataxia with oculomotor apraxia type II
    c. Joubert syndrome
    d. Leber congenital amaurosis
    e. COACH syndrome

24. A 29-year-old man is admitted with an acute ischemic stroke. He has a cardiomyopathy of uncertain cause, severe hypertension, and end-stage renal disease. He reports that his initial symptoms consisted of a burning sensation in his feet. He has three brothers who died of end-stage renal disease. When he was being worked up for his renal disease, a biopsy was obtained and showed birefringent lipid deposits in the glomeruli, and electron microscopy showed membrane-bound lamellar deposits. Which of the following is the most likely diagnosis?
    a. Metachromatic leukodystrophy
    b. Fabry disease
    c. Niemann-Pick type A
    d. Gaucher disease
    e. GM1 gangliosidosis

25. Which of the following statements regarding holoprosencephaly is incorrect?
    a. It results from failure of the prosencephalon to ultimately generate separate cerebral hemispheres
    b. Variable degrees of division of the cerebral hemispheres, thalamus, and hypothalamus occur
    c. Endocrinologic disturbances are common
    d. The pathophysiology relates to abnormalities in the signaling molecule sonic hedgehog and to defective cholesterol metabolism
    e. All forms of holoprosencephaly are incompatible with life

26. A 5-year-old boy is brought for evaluation of seizures. He has had gradual vision loss and progressive psychomotor retardation. Neuronal ceroid lipofuscinosis (NCL) is within the differential diagnosis. Which of the following is correct regarding NCL?
    a. NCL occurs only in childhood
    b. It is autosomal dominant
    c. Myoclonic seizure is the least common type of seizure seen in these patients
    d. The infantile form is more common in Finnish people
    e. Electron microscopy is useless as there are no characteristic findings

27. Which of the following statements is incorrect regarding congenital aqueductal stenosis?
    a. It occurs in an X-linked form associated with pachygyria
    b. It is a disorder of neurulation
    c. It may occur in association with holoprosencephaly
    d. It may result from congenital infections such as cytomegalovirus
    e. It is stenosis of the connection between the lateral and third ventricle

28. A 5-month-old baby is being evaluated for seizures. He has multiple dysmorphic features and severe hypotonia, and MRI of the brain shows pachygyria. Skeletal radiographs show calcific stippling of the patella. Very long-chain fatty acid levels are elevated in plasma. Which of the following is incorrect regarding this condition?

a. This is a peroxisomal disorder
b. Liver cirrhosis occurs in these patients
c. Kidney cysts can be seen in these patients
d. White matter is not involved
e. Polymicrogyria may be seen in these patients

29. Which of the following statements is incorrect regarding disorders that involve the skin and CNS?
    a. Multiple intracranial arteriovenous malformations are a manifestation of hereditary hemorrhagic telangiectasia (Osler-Weber-Rendu syndrome)
    b. Patients with pseudoxanthoma elasticum are at increased risk of cerebral arterial occlusive disease
    c. Ehlers-Danlos syndrome is associated with increased risk of intracranial aneurysms and carotid dissection
    d. Xeroderma pigmentosa is associated with peripheral neuropathy, cognitive decline, ataxia, and hyperkinetic involuntary movements
    e. Fabry disease is a multiorgan disorder associated with neuropathy and cerebral artery ectasia and results from a defect in the enzyme sphingomyelinase

30. A 7-year-old boy has short stature due to growth hormone deficiency and is also being treated for hypothyroidism. His motor and cognitive development has been normal. He has reduced visual acuity. His MRI shows absence of the septum pellucidum and hypoplasia of the optic nerves and chiasm. The cortex and other areas appear normal. What is the most likely diagnosis in this patient?
    a. Holoprosencephaly
    b. Septo-optic dysplasia
    c. Lissencephaly
    d. Arrhinencephaly
    e. Cavum septum pellucidum

31. A 6-year-old boy began having behavioral problems with aggressiveness approximately 1 year ago. He has also had progressive cognitive deterioration and spasticity and visual loss. Plasma levels of very long-chain fatty acids are elevated, and MRI shows white matter T2 hyperintensities, which are symmetric, involving posterior regions, and sparing the U fibers. Which of the following is the most likely diagnosis?
    a. Canavan disease
    b. Adrenoleukodystrophy
    c. Alexander disease
    d. Zellweger syndrome
    e. Fabry disease

32. Which of the following options is correct regarding Leigh disease?
    a. It is a static encephalopathy
    b. It is due to mitochondrial abnormalities
    c. It is inherited in an autosomal recessive fashion
    d. Lactate levels are reduced during episodic exacerbations
    e. Clinical manifestations most commonly begin during late childhood

33. A 14-year-old boy is brought for evaluation of growth retardation, generalized weakness, and ataxia. On examination, he has bilateral ptosis and restricted gaze in all directions. An electro-cardiogram is obtained and shows complete heart block. Which of the following is the most likely diagnosis?

   a. Kearns-Sayre syndrome
   b. Mitochondrial encephalopathy, lactic acidosis, and strokes
   c. Myoclonic epilepsy with ragged red fibers
   d. Leigh disease
   e. Myasthenia gravis

34. A boy with developmental delay, hypotonia, and dysmorphic features is brought for evaluation. On examination, he has inverted nipples and prominent fat pads in the buttocks area. A diagnosis of a congenital disorder of glycosylation is suspected. Which of the following is incorrect regarding this condition?

   a. It affects multiple organ systems
   b. Analysis of transferrin glycoforms can help make the diagnosis
   c. Patients can present with stroke-like episodes
   d. Some patients may have hypogonadism
   e. It is inherited in an X-linked fashion

35. Which of the following statements is correct regarding disorders of corpus callosum development?

   a. They result from abnormalities in the third trimester of pregnancy
   b. Most commonly, complete agenesis of the corpus callosum occurs
   c. They result from abnormalities in the commissural plate
   d. Corpus callosum agenesis is most often seen in isolation
   e. Severe developmental delay is invariably present

36. Which of the following statements is incorrect regarding cortical development?

   a. The cerebral hemispheres form from a single layer of columnar epithelium located in the subependymal region known as the primary germinal zone
   b. Cells of the marginal zone proliferate and migrate along a scaffold formed by the processes of radial glia
   c. The most superficial cortical layers form from cells that migrate first (the cortex forms outside-in)
   d. Neuron types include pyramidal neurons, cortical granular or stellate neurons, and Betz cells
   e. Glial cell types include astrocytes, oligodendrocytes, ependyma, and microglia

37. Regarding the phakomatoses, which of the following features is not appropriately paired with the specified disorder?

   a. Hyperpigmented cutaneous lesions and leptomeningeal melanoma—neurocutaneous melanosis
   b. Hemifacial atrophy—Parry-Romberg syndrome
   c. Multiple endochondromas and secondary hemangiomas—Maffucci syndrome
   d. Hypopigmented streaks or patches that follow skin lines—incontinentia pigmenti
   e. Retinal, cerebellar, and spinal hemangioblastomas—von Hippel-Lindau disease

38. Which of the following malformations is not paired with the appropriate underlying mechanism?
   a. Focal cortical dysplasia—disorder of cell proliferation
   b. Lissencephaly—disorders of neuronal migration
   c. Polymicrogyria—disorder of cortical organization
   d. Periventricular nodular heterotopias—disorder of cell proliferation
   e. Schizencephaly—disorder of cortical organization

Questions 39–40

39. A 2-year-old child is brought to the pediatric neurology clinic by his parents with concerns about small head size noted by the child's pediatrician. The child's head size had been small at birth and the rate of growth had been below average over time. Which of the following statements is correct regarding microcephaly?
   a. It always implies an underlying neurologic disorder and developmental delay is invariably present
   b. Causes include infection, trauma, and hypoxic-ischemic insult
   c. Microcephaly is defined as a head circumference less than 1 standard deviation below the mean
   d. Seizures are infrequently seen in children with microcephaly
   e. Maternal exposure to AEDs has not been associated with microcephaly

40. Which of the following statements is incorrect regarding the abnormality depicted in Figure 14.3?

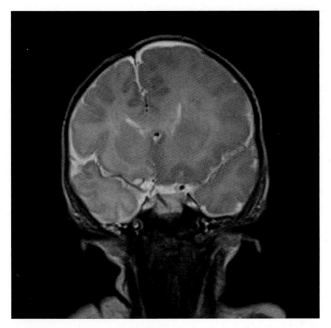

FIGURE 14.3   Coronal T2-weighted MRI

a. Hemimegalencephaly frequently presents with seizures

b. Macrocephaly may be due to hydrocephalus or megalencephaly

c. Hemimegalencephaly rarely leads to motor manifestations

d. Megalencephaly is an oversized brain, with brain weight greater than 2 standard deviations above the mean

e. Megalencephaly may be a benign finding in some cases

Questions 41–42

41. A 7-month-old boy is brought to the epileptologist for intractable seizures. On examination, he has a short small chin, thin upper lip, and low-set ears. He has spastic quadriparesis and requires a feeding tube because of recurrent aspirations. MRI of the brain shows essentially smooth frontal, parietal, and occipital lobes, with a thick cortex and without sulci or gyri. What is the most likely diagnosis?

a. Miller-Dieker syndrome

b. Lissencephaly type II

c. Subcortical band heterotopias

d. Cobblestone lissencephaly

e. Polymicrogyria

42. Which of the following statements is incorrect regarding the disorder depicted in question 41?

a. It results from abnormal neuronal migration

b. The cortex in this disorder consists of six layers

c. Associated malformations including corpus callosum agenesis may occur

d. LIS1 mutation disrupts microtubule-directed neuronal migration

e. Microcephaly and intractable seizures occur

43. A 6-month-old boy is seen in the outpatient pediatric neurology department. At birth, he was noted to have hypopigmented streaks on his skin that occurred in a V-shape on his back, and in a linear pattern on his legs, following the skin lines. He also had seizures. Ophthalmologic examination revealed cataracts. Head circumference was 2 standard deviations above the mean. What is the most likely diagnosis in this patient?

a. Neurocutaneous melanosis

b. Incontinentia pigmenti

c. Hypomelanosis of Ito

d. Sturge-Weber syndrome

e. Epidermal nevus syndrome

Questions 44–45

44. A 3-year-old girl with intractable seizures presents to the clinic for seizure management. On examination, she has spastic quadriparesis and requires a feeding tube because of recurrent aspirations. Images from her MRI are shown in Figure 14.4. What is the diagnosis in this patient?

a. Miller-Dieker syndrome

b. Lissencephaly type II

c. Subcortical band heterotopia

d. Cobblestone lissencephaly

e. Polymicrogyria

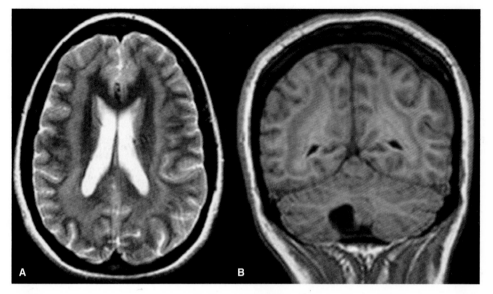

FIGURE 14.4   (**A**) Axial T2-weighted MRI (*left*); (**B**) Coronal T1-weighted MRI. Courtesy of Dr. Ajay Gupta and Dr. Joanna Fong

45. Which of the following statements is incorrect regarding the disorder depicted in Figure 14.4?
  a. It is a disorder of neuronal migration
  b. It results from abnormalities in a protein involved in microtubule organization and stabilization
  c. It is an X-linked disorder
  d. Mutations in the DCX gene lead to this disorder in females and lissencephaly in males
  e. This disorder is classically associated with muscular dystrophy

Questions 46–48

46. A 9-year-old boy presents to his general pediatrician for routine follow-up. On examination, he has more than six hyperpigmented lesions, as shown in Figure 14.5. What term best describes these lesions?
  a. Ashleaf spots
  b. Cutaneous neurofibromas
  c. Plexiform neurofibromas
  d. Shagreen patches
  e. Café au lait spots

47. The patient in question 46 also has the lesions shown in Figure 14.6 on his upper trunk, face, and extremities. What term best describes these lesions?
  a. Ashleaf spots
  b. Cutaneous neurofibromas
  c. Plexiform neurofibromas
  d. Shagreen patches
  e. Café au lait spots

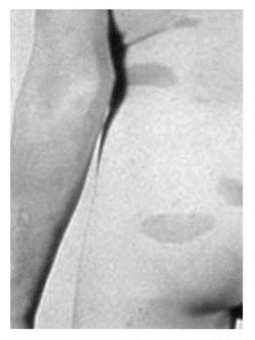

FIGURE 14.5 Courtesy of Dr. David Rothner. Shown also in color plates

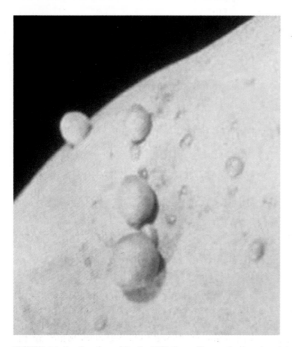

FIGURE 14.6 Courtesy of Dr. David Rothner. Shown also in color plates

48. The mother of the patient depicted in question 46 has axillary findings as shown in Figure 14.7. She also has three hyperpigmented lesions on her trunk (similar to those depicted in Figure 14.5), two on her arms, and one on each leg. What is the most likely diagnosis in this patient?

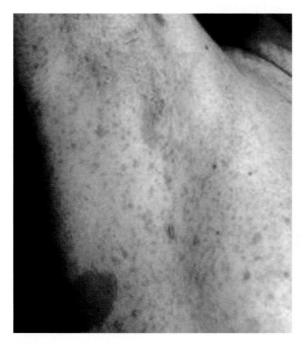

FIGURE 14.7   Courtesy of Dr. David Rothner. Shown also in color plates

    a. Tuberous sclerosis complex
    b. Neurofibromatosis type 1 (NF1)
    c. Neurofibromatosis type 2 (NF2)
    d. Sturge-Weber syndrome
    e. Epidermal nevus syndrome

49. Which of the following statements is incorrect regarding the syndromes of cobblestone lissencephaly?
    a. Muscle-eye-brain disease of Santavuori is most often seen in Finland
    b. Fukuyama muscular dystrophy is most often seen in Japan
    c. Muscular dystrophy is seen in all these syndromes
    d. Eye abnormalities seen include retinal hypoplasia and glaucoma
    e. They are autosomal dominant in inheritance

50. An 8-year-old boy with developmental delay and mental retardation is brought for evaluation of poor vision. He is tall, thin, with a marfanoid habitus with chest deformity, but no other features of Marfan syndrome. On examination, he is found to have ectopia lentis. Given the suspected diagnosis, plasma homocysteine levels are tested, and are found to be elevated. Which of the following is incorrect regarding this condition?

a. It is caused by cystathionine-β-synthase deficiency
b. Some cases are pyridoxine responsive
c. There is elevation of urine homocysteine
d. Thromboembolic events are common
e. Methionine levels are reduced in plasma and CSF

Questions 51–52

51. A 17-year-old girl presents to the clinic with complaints of headache. On examination, she has multiple hyperpigmented macules on various body parts. Ophthalmologic evaluation reveals the findings shown in Figure 14.8. What term best describes these lesions?

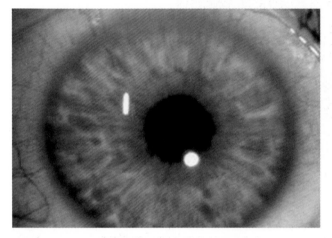

FIGURE 14.8 Courtesy of Dr. David Rothner. Shown also in color plates

a. Kayser-Fleischer rings
b. Brushfield spots
c. Lisch nodules
d. Iris coloboma
e. Iris mamillations

52. What is the most likely diagnosis of the patient depicted in question 51?
a. Tuberous sclerosis complex
b. Neurofibromatosis type 1 (NF1)
c. Neurofibromatosis type 2 (NF2)
d. Sturge-Weber syndrome
e. Epidermal nevus syndrome

53. Which of the following is incorrect regarding periventricular nodular heterotopia?
a. Heterotopias are clusters of defective neurons in an area of otherwise normal cortex
b. It is a disorder of neuronal migration
c. It is more common in females
d. It is most commonly X-linked
e. Seizures are a common clinical manifestation

54. Regarding the arm finding in a patient with neurofibromatosis type 1 depicted in Figure 14.9, which of the following statements is incorrect?

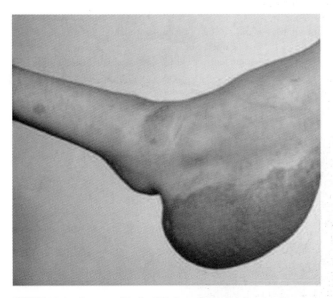

FIGURE 14.9   Courtesy of Dr. David Rothner. Shown also in color plates

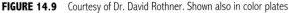

   a. It is a plexiform neurofibroma
   b. These types of neurofibromas can invade the skin, causing thickening and skin hypertrophy
   c. Plexiform neurofibromas consist of mainly Schwann cells and fibroblasts
   d. In a minority of cases, plexiform neurofibromas undergo malignant degeneration into malignant peripheral nerve tumors
   e. Plexiform neurofibromas typically regress with age, particularly when they first form at a younger age

55. A newborn patient is noticed to be lethargic with poor feeding. He rapidly becomes encephalopathic and develops seizures. His laboratory tests demonstrate hyperammonemia with respiratory alkalosis and normal anion gap. Eventually, the baby requires intubation and mechanical ventilation. A urea cycle disorder is suspected. Which of the following is correct regarding this group of disorders?
   a. This is a group of disorders that are all inherited in an X-linked fashion
   b. Ornithine transcarbamylase deficiency is the most common cause
   c. Hyperammonemia and organic acidemias are commonly found in patients with these disorders
   d. Arginase deficiency commonly presents in the newborn period
   e. High protein diet is indicated for their treatment

56. Which of the following statements is incorrect regarding polymicrogyria and schizencephaly?
   a. Polymicrogyria is characterized by excessive abnormal gyri that are small and separated by shallow sulci
   b. Schizencephaly is a deep cleft that extends from the pial surface to the ventricle and is lined with cortex

c. Polymicrogyria most often occurs in the perisylvian region
d. Porencephaly describes a type of schizencephaly
e. They are disorders of cortical organization

57. A 16-year-old boy with neurofibromatosis type 1 (NF1) presents with diplopia. An MRI of the brain is done and shows abnormalities in the left optic nerve and in the pons, shown in Figure 14.10. Which of the following statements is incorrect regarding these abnormalities?

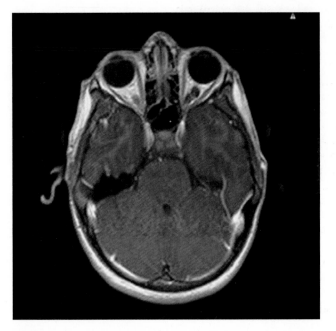

FIGURE 14.10 Axial T1-weighted postcontrast MRI. Courtesy of Dr. Manikum Moodley

a. He likely has an optic nerve glioma
b. Optic nerve gliomas are common in NF1
c. Schwannomas and ependymomas are the most common tumors occurring in NF1 patients
d. Optic nerve gliomas in patients with NF1 typically are low grade and often can be monitored for years without intervention
e. In NF1, optic gliomas can occur anywhere along the optic pathways, from the optic nerve to the optic radiations

58. A 3-year-old boy is brought to the pediatrician by his parents. They are concerned that he seems to be "emotionless" as compared with his affectionate siblings. He never quite makes eye contact. He does not like to be hugged or kissed and does not play with others. Rather, he prefers to sit alone in his room, playing with the miniature toy cars, although his parents have bought him several other toys. He often flaps his arms at his sides and sometimes when upset will repeatedly bang his forehead on the nearest piece of furniture or on a wall. He says a few words, but not nearly as many as his siblings did at his age. What is the most likely diagnosis in this patient?

a. Autism
b. Schizophrenia

c. Depression
d. Schizoid personality disorder
e. Avoidant personality disorder

59. A 4-year-old girl diagnosed prenatally with trisomy 21 is brought to the clinic for annual checkup. Which of the following statements is incorrect regarding this disorder?
   a. Mental retardation of varying degrees of severity may be present
   b. Patients with trisomy 21 are at increased risk of leukemia
   c. MRI of the brain would show hypertrophy of the frontal lobes, with macrocephaly
   d. There is increased risk of atlanto-axial dislocation
   e. Early dementia with Alzheimer type pathology is seen

60. A 3-year-old girl is brought to the clinic for evaluation. Her parents reported that early on, she seemed to be a very happy baby, she made eye contact and smiled and cooed all the time. She had met motor milestones similar to her siblings: holding her head up, crawling, and sitting unsupported. However, around the age of 1 year, she started to have difficulty sitting up and never developed any words. She later stopped smiling and laughing, and progressively lost use of her hands, constantly rubbing her hands against each other. Which of the following statements is correct regarding the most likely diagnosis in this patient?
   a. It is more common in males but can also be seen in females
   b. Macrocephaly is a common finding
   c. It results from a mutation in the gene encoding the MeCP2 protein
   d. It is autosomal dominant in inheritance
   e. It results from mutations in mitochondrial DNA

Questions 61–63

61. An 11-year-old boy presents to the clinic for evaluation of seizures. On examination, he has multiple hypopigmented lesions, as shown in Figure 14.11. What term best describes these lesions?
   a. Ashleaf spots
   b. Cutaneous neurofibromas
   c. Angiofibromas
   d. Shagreen patches
   e. Tinea corporis

62. The patient in question 61 also has lesions on his face as shown in Figure 14.12. What term best describes these lesions?
   a. Ashleaf spots
   b. Cutaneous neurofibromas
   c. Angiofibromas
   d. Shagreen patches
   e. Severe acne

63. What is the most likely diagnosis of the patient whose cutaneous lesions are shown in Figures 14.11 and 14.12?
   a. Tuberous sclerosis complex
   b. Neurofibromatosis type 1

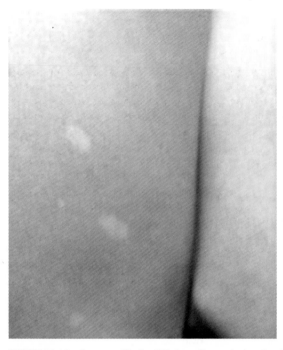

FIGURE 14.11   Courtesy of Dr. David Rothner. Shown also in color plates

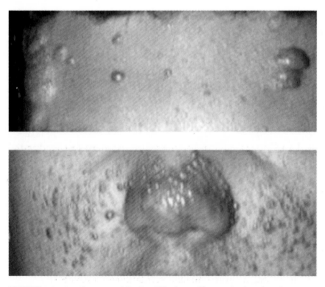

FIGURE 14.12   Courtesy of Dr. David Rothner. Shown also in color plates

c. Hypomelanosis of Ito
d. Sturge-Weber syndrome
e. Epidermal nevus syndrome

64. A 16-year-old boy is brought for evaluation in the clinic. He has a known history of mental retardation and a brother and two maternal cousins with mental retardation as well. Examination shows an elongated face, with a high forehead and elongated jaw, and protuberant ears. He has enlarged testes. Which of the following is incorrect regarding the most likely diagnosis in this patient?
    a. It is the most common inherited form of mental retardation
    b. Females may be affected, although to a lesser degree
    c. It results from expansion of the CGG repeat in the familial mental retardation 1 gene on chromosome X
    d. A family history of mental retardation may be present, but not necessarily
    e. Severe mental retardation is invariably present

65. A 16-year-old girl was noted to be hypotonic at birth. As she became older, various abnormalities were noticed, including developmental delay, a wide mouth, and small feet. She is obese and constantly eats when left to do so, to the point that locks have been placed on the refrigerator at home to control her eating. She has not had menarche yet. What is the most likely diagnosis in this patient?
    a. Fragile X syndrome
    b. Prader-Willi syndrome
    c. Angelman syndrome
    d. Cri-du-chat syndrome
    e. Rett syndrome

66. A newborn baby is being evaluated for encephalopathy in the setting of metabolic acidosis and hyperammonemia. There is also ketoacidosis and elevated methylmalonic acid levels. You suspect methylmalonic acidemia. Which of the following is incorrect regarding this condition?
    a. The deficient enzyme is D-methylmalonyl-CoA mutase
    b. Propionyl-CoA levels are not altered in this enzymatic disorder
    c. Adenosylcobalamin acts as cofactor in the involved enzymatic step
    d. Protein restriction in the diet is part of the treatment plan
    e. The enzyme affected participates in the conversion of L-methylmalonyl-CoA to succinyl-CoA

67. The skin lesion shown in Figure 14.13 is seen in a neurocutaneous disorder associated with seizures and hamartomas in multiple body parts. What is the most likely diagnosis in a patient with such a lesion?
    a. Tuberous sclerosis complex
    b. Neurofibromatosis type 1
    c. Hypomelanosis of Ito
    d. Sturge-Weber syndrome
    e. Epidermal nevus syndrome

68. Which of the following statements regarding acquired mental retardation are incorrect?
    a. Congenital infections such as cytomegalovirus or rubella are associated with mental retardation
    b. Mental retardation has been associated with exposure to radiation during the first trimester

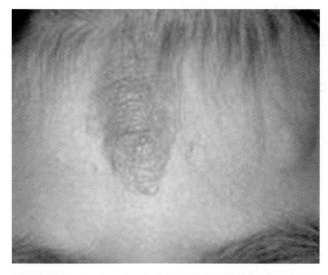

FIGURE 14.13 Courtesy of Dr. David Rothner. Shown also in color plates

    c. In utero exposure to AEDs can lead to varying degrees of mental retardation and other CNS abnormalities

    d. Maternal alcohol intake is a common cause of acquired mental retardation

    e. In utero exposure to alcohol does not lead to abnormalities outside of the CNS

69. The skin lesion shown in Figure 14.14 is seen in a neurocutaneous disorder associated with seizures and hamartomas in multiple body parts. What term best describe this lesion?

    a. Periungual hematoma

    b. Cutaneous neurofibromas

    c. Subungual fibroma

    d. Periungual fibroma

    e. Angiokeratoma

70. A 10-month-old boy with hypotonia, alopecia, and seizures is brought for evaluation. Laboratory studies show ketoacidosis, hyperammonemia, and elevated urine organic acid levels. Biotinidase deficiency is suspected. Which of the following is incorrect regarding this condition?

    a. Biotin levels are elevated in biotinidase deficiency and should not be supplemented

    b. Hearing and vision loss can occur

    c. Biotinidase cleaves biocytin and participates in biotin recycling

    d. Biotinidase participates in processing of dietary protein-bound biotin

    e. Patients have ketoacidosis, hyperammonemia, and organic aciduria

71. Which of the following statements is incorrect regarding Dandy-Walker malformation?

    a. It includes cerebellar vermis hypoplasia

    b. It includes fourth ventricle cystic dilatation

    c. Lateral and third ventricular hydrocephalus is common

    d. It may present in infancy with macrocephaly or may be asymptomatic into adulthood

    e. It is associated with the "molar tooth sign" on imaging

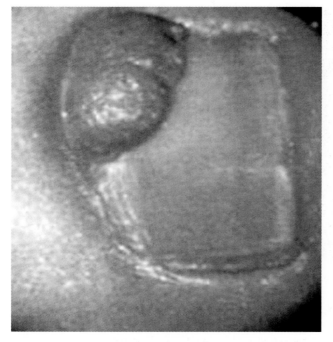

FIGURE 14.14   Courtesy of Dr. David Rothner. Shown also in color plates

72. An 8-year-old boy with seizures presents with headache. An MRI of the brain is obtained and an image shown in Figure 14.15. The lesion is resected and pathologic analysis is consistent with subependymal giant cell astrocytoma. What disorder does this patient most likely have?
   a. Tuberous sclerosis complex
   b. Neurofibromatosis type 1 (NF1)
   c. Neurofibromatosis type 2 (NF2)
   d. Sturge-Weber syndrome
   e. He probably does not have a neurocutaneous disorder; this tumor is most often seen sporadically

73. Regarding normal cerebral cortex architecture, which of the following statements is incorrect?
   a. Normal cerebral cortex has six layers
   b. Pyramidal cells are the most common type of cortical neurons
   c. Granular cells are found in higher numbers in sensory cortex
   d. Different cortical and subcortical areas project to and receive projections from specific cortical layers
   e. Betz cells function predominantly as interneurons and are found in secondary association cortices

74. A 10-year-old boy is brought for evaluation. He has developmental delay with psychomotor retardation, and on examination, there is limited horizontal gaze, ataxia, and generalized spasticity. He has hepatosplenomegaly as well. Enzymatic activity of glucocerebrosidase in leukocytes is depressed. Which of the following is correct regarding this condition?

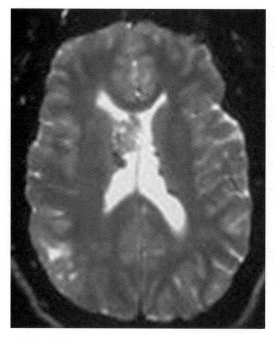

FIGURE 14.15   Axial T2-weighted MRI. Courtesy of Dr. Ajay Gupta

a. There is accumulation of lysosomal glucocerebrosides
b. Patients with type 1 of this disease have severe neurologic impairment by age 2
c. Type 3 has its onset before age 2 and progresses rapidly to death between age 2 and 4
d. Enzyme replacement therapy is not available for this condition
e. It is more prevalent in Asian populations than in Ashkenazi Jews

75. A 13-year-old boy recently diagnosed with tuberous sclerosis complex undergoes an MRI of the brain as part of routine surveillance, and an image from it is shown in Figure 14.16. Which of the following statements is incorrect regarding the findings on this MRI?
a. These are known as cortical tubers
b. These lesions are hamartomas
c. The burden of such lesions correlates with cognitive function
d. The burden of such lesions correlates with the occurrence and severity of seizures
e. These lesions are premalignant

Questions 76–77

76. A 6-month-old baby of Ashkenazi Jewish background is brought for evaluation of seizures. He has prominent startle response and developmental delay. He had reached some early developmental milestones but then began to regress. It is also noticed that he is macrocephalic and spastic, but there is no visceromegaly. A cherry-red spot is seen on ophthalmologic examination. There is suspicion for a GM2 gangliosidosis. Which of the following is correct regarding this patient's condition?
a. This patient has Sandhoff disease
b. Hexosaminidase A is the only cause

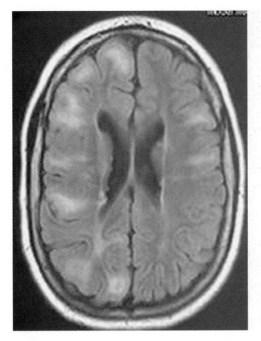

FIGURE 14.16   Axial FLAIR MRI. Courtesy of Dr. Ajay Gupta

    c. It is autosomal dominant

    d. It occurs only in Ashkenazi Jews

    e. β-Galactosidase deficiency is the most common cause

77. A 6-month-old baby is brought for evaluation of seizures. He has a prominent startle response and developmental delay. He had reached some developmental milestones but has started regressing now. It is also noticed that he is macrocephalic and spastic. A cherry-red spot is seen on ophthalmologic examination, and he also has prominent hepatosplenomegaly. There is suspicion for a GM2 gangliosidosis. Which of the following is correct regarding this patient's condition?

    a. Hexosaminidase A is the only enzyme affected

    b. Both hexosaminidases A and B are affected

    c. β-Galactosidase deficiency is the most common cause

    d. Sphingomyelinase deficiency is the cause

    e. This patient has Tay-Sachs disease

78. A brain CT scan is obtained in a patient with tuberous sclerosis complex (TSC), and it demonstrates hyperdensities, as shown in Figure 14.17. Which of the following statements is correct regarding these lesions?

    a. These are all malignant and should be resected

    b. This patient likely has, in addition to TSC, benign hereditary calcification of the basal ganglia (Fahr disease)

    c. The burden of these lesions correlates with the severity of mental retardation in TSC patients

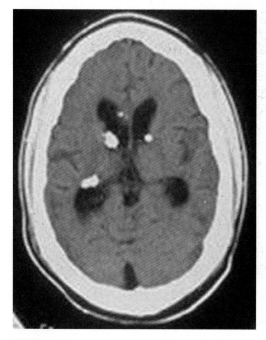

FIGURE 14.17 Axial CT. Courtesy of Dr. Ajay Gupta

    d. These are calcified subependymal nodules and are one of the major diagnostic criteria for TSC

    e. These are malignant subependymal giant cell astrocytomas

79. A 6-month-old baby is being evaluated for developmental delay and regression of already-achieved developmental milestones. She has poor fixation and does not track, and there is prominent hypotonia with inability to hold her head upright. MRI demonstrates diffuse symmetric white matter changes with involvement of the U fibers. MR spectroscopy demonstrates an increased peak of N-acetylaspartic acid. Which of the following is the most likely diagnosis?

    a. Canavan disease

    b. Adrenoleukodystrophy

    c. Alexander disease

    d. Zellweger syndrome

    e. Fabry disease

Questions 80–81

80. The findings shown in Figure 14.18 are consistent with which neurocutaneous syndrome?

    a. Neurocutaneous melanosis

    b. Incontinentia pigmenti

    c. Hypomelanosis of Ito

    d. Sturge-Weber syndrome

    e. Epidermal nevus syndrome

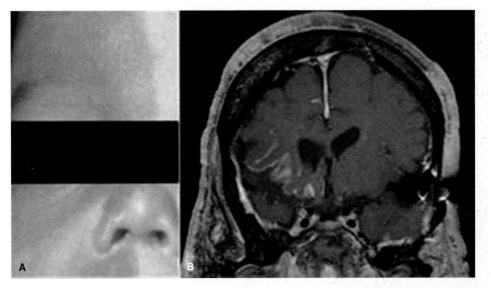

FIGURE 14.18   (**A**) Courtesy of Dr. David Rothner; (**B**) Coronal T1-weighted precontrast MRI. Shown also in color plates

81. Which of the following statements is correct regarding the disorder depicted in question 80 and Figure 14.18?
    a. It is invariably associated with mental retardation and seizures
    b. Cutaneous involvement in any area implies involvement of the CNS
    c. Cataracts are a common complication of this disorder
    d. Hemimegalencephaly is a common feature of this disorder
    e. The gyral calcifications seen result from angiomatosis of the leptomeninges and brain

82. Which of the following statements is incorrect regarding the genetics and molecular biology of neurofibromatosis type 1 (NF1, von Recklinghausen disease)?
    a. NF1 results from a mutation in the neurofibromin gene on chromosome 17
    b. Neurofibromin activates a GTPase that inhibits the ras proto-oncogene, a protein involved in cell proliferation
    c. Several mutations in the NF1 gene have been identified, but in general, strong phenotype-genotype correlations do not occur
    d. NF1 is an autosomal recessive disorder
    e. NF1 has complete penetrance but variable expressivity

83. A newborn is evaluated 48 hours after birth because of seizures. The mother reports that the baby refused feeding and seemed irritable in the first few hours of life. The patient subsequently developed respiratory failure and required intubation. An extensive workup is obtained, and a brain MRI is shown in Figure 14.19. A high glycine level in the CSF is also found. Which of the following is incorrect regarding this condition?
    a. This patient has a disturbance of glycine degradation
    b. Patients who survive the acute phase are left with mental retardation, spasticity, and epilepsy
    c. Treatment with sodium benzoate is effective and prevents progression of the disease
    d. It is autosomal recessive
    e. EEG may show burst suppression

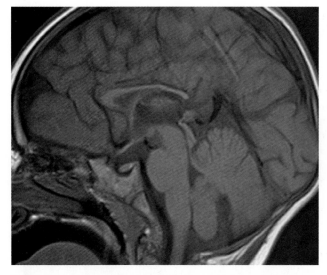

FIGURE 14.19 Sagittal T2-weighted MRI

84. A brain specimen obtained from an autopsy of an 11-month-old baby is shown in Figure 14.20. The patient initially presented with irritability and hypersensitivity to stimuli at 4 months of age. The baby was also blind and had prominent regression by age 6 months. He also had developed stiffness of all four limbs and later of the trunk to the point that he was in an opisthotonic posture. Which of the following is correct regarding this condition?

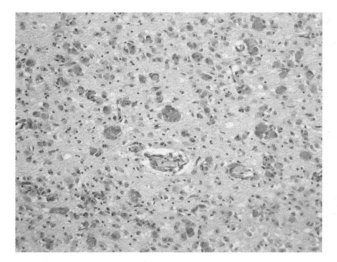

FIGURE 14.20 Brain specimen. Courtesy of Dr. Richard A. Prayson. Shown also in color plates

   a. It is autosomal dominant
   b. The deficient enzyme is β-glucosylceramidase
   c. There is demyelination with relative sparing of the U fibers

d. It is only seen in newborns, and all patients die by 1 year of age
e. The cause is deficiency of the enzyme α-galactosidase

Questions 85–86

85. A 52-year-old man presents for evaluation of right ear hearing loss with vertigo. His MRI shows bilateral vestibular schwannomas. He has a family history of bilateral vestibular schwannomas and multiple meningiomas in his mother. Which of the following is the most likely diagnosis?
   a. Neurofibromatosis type 1 (NF1)
   b. Neurofibromatosis type 2 (NF2)
   c. Tuberous sclerosis complex
   d. Gorlin syndrome
   e. Rubinstein-Taybi syndrome

86. Which of the following statements is incorrect regarding the disorder depicted in question 85?
   a. It is autosomal dominant in inheritance
   b. It results from a mutation in the merlin gene on chromosome 22
   c. Various CNS tumors including schwannomas, meningiomas, astrocytomas, and ependymomas can occur in this disorder
   d. Cutaneous findings such as neurofibromas and axillary freckling are common in this disorder
   e. Subcapsular cataracts are a feature of this disorder

87. A 10-month-old baby is brought for evaluation. Even though she had gained some developmental milestones, she began regressing by 7 months of age. She has coarse facial features, generalized spasticity, and motor impairment. A retinal picture is shown in Figure 14.21. Enzymatic analysis showed a β-galactosidase deficiency in leukocytes. Which of the following is correct?

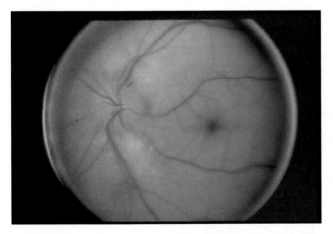

FIGURE 14.21   Courtesy of Dr. Gregory Kosmorsky. Shown also in color plates

   a. This patient has GM2 gangliosidosis
   b. Gangliosides accumulate in the brain and visceral organs
   c. Sandhoff disease is caused by this enzymatic deficiency
   d. Tay-Sachs disease is caused by this enzymatic deficiency
   e. Mucopolysacchariduria is common

88. An autopsy is performed on an 18-month-old boy who had a progressive neurologic disorder. He had macrocephaly, psychomotor retardation, spasticity and seizures. Figure 14.22 shows a histopathologic specimen obtained at autopsy. Which of the following is the most likely diagnosis?

FIGURE 14.22   Brain specimen. Courtesy of Dr. Richard A. Prayson. Shown also in color plates

a. Canavan disease
b. Adrenoleukodystrophy
c. Alexander disease
d. Zellweger syndrome
e. Fabry disease

89. Which of the following statements is incorrect regarding the genetics of tuberous sclerosis complex (TSC)?
    a. It is autosomal recessive with complete penetrance
    b. It is autosomal dominant with variable penetrance
    c. It can be caused by a mutation in the TSC1 gene that encodes for the protein tuberin
    d. It can be caused by a mutation in the TSC2 gene that encodes for the protein hamartin
    e. The presence of specific clinical features does not reliably distinguish between the different genetic mutations that can cause this condition

90. A 6-month-old baby boy is brought for evaluation of psychomotor retardation. After birth, he was noticed to have prominent nystagmus, abnormal eye movements, and prominent incoordination. MRI demonstrates diffuse white matter changes sparing the U fibers, with a "tigroid" appearance. Which of the following is correct regarding this condition?
    a. It is inherited in an autosomal recessive fashion
    b. The gene involved is PLP1
    c. Central and peripheral myelin are affected
    d. This patient has Alexander disease
    e. The mutation is in the gene for glial fibrillary acidic protein (GFAP)

Questions 91–92

91. A 5-year-old boy is brought for evaluation. He has coarse facial features, short stature with dysmorphic appearance, prominent psychomotor retardation, hepatosplenomegaly, and several nodular lesions that are ivory colored on his upper back. The activity of iduronate sulfatase in leukocytes is almost absent. Which of the following is correct regarding this condition?
 a. It is inherited in an X-linked fashion
 b. Corneal clouding is a prominent feature in this syndrome
 c. He has Hurler syndrome
 d. Heparan sulfate, but not dermatan sulfate, will be elevated in the urine
 e. This patient has mucopolysaccharidoses type I

92. Which of the following is incorrect regarding mucopolysaccharidoses (MPS)?
 a. There is accumulation of glucosaminoglycans, which are detected in urine
 b. Hurler syndrome is caused by α-L-iduronidase deficiency
 c. Sanfilippo syndrome is a group of MPS with accumulation of heparan but not dermatan sulfate
 d. Morquio syndrome manifests with prominent mental retardation
 e. Zebra bodies can be seen on electron microscopy

93. Which of the following statements is incorrect regarding epidermal nevus syndrome (ENS)?
 a. This syndrome is a manifestation of a heterogeneous group of disorders that share in common the presence of epidermal nevi
 b. Hemimegalencephaly may occur ipsilateral to a facial nevus
 c. The epidermal nevi in this disorder may undergo malignant transformation
 d. There is increased risk of astrocytoma and other tumors in patients with ENS
 e. Lisch nodules are a feature of ENS

94. A 17-year-old girl presents to the ED for severe abdominal pain, along with nausea, vomiting, fever, and tachycardia. She has been evaluated multiple times over the past year for similar symptoms and has undergone evaluation for appendicitis and other gynecologic causes, including exploratory laparoscopy in the past. There are no cutaneous manifestations. She has increased aminolevulinic acid and porphobilinogen (PBG) concentrations in the urine, with no increase in urinary or fecal coproporphyrin III. Which of the following is correct regarding this condition?
 a. The enzyme affected is PBG deaminase
 b. The enzyme affected is coproporphyrinogen oxidase
 c. The enzyme affected is protoporphyrinogen oxidase
 d. Seizures can occur and should be treated with phenobarbital
 e. A symmetric distal demyelinating polyneuropathy occurs predominantly in the lower limbs

95. A 12-year-old boy is found to have large orange-colored tonsils, hepatosplenomegaly, and sensory deficits in the upper limbs. Which of the following is correct regarding this condition?
 a. It is caused by deficiency of low-density lipoproteins
 b. It is autosomal dominant in inheritance
 c. Peripheral nerves are not involved
 d. It is caused by a mutation in the adenosine triphosphate cassette transporter protein
 e. Total cholesterol level in the serum is very elevated

96. A 2-month-old infant is being evaluated for developmental delay. MRI of the brain shows atrophy with bilateral subdural hematomas. Examination shows hypotonia, coarse, brittle hair, hyperelastic skin, and absent eyebrows. What is the most likely diagnosis in this patient?

a. Menkes disease
b. Wilson disease
c. Ehlers-Danlos syndrome
d. Nonaccidental injury (child abuse)
e. Hypomelanosis of Ito

97. A 15-year-old boy with growth and psychomotor retardation, sensorineural hearing loss, frequent headaches, and seizures presents for evaluation of multiple stroke-like episodes. Two MRIs from different time points are shown in Figure 14.23. Lactate level is found to be elevated. Which of the following is the most likely diagnosis?

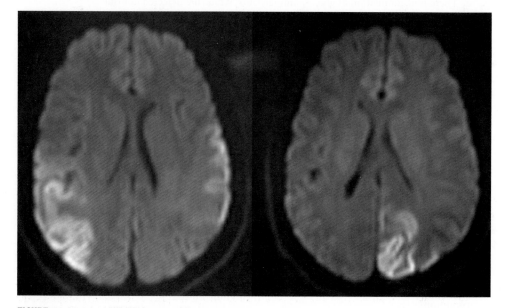

FIGURE 14.23 Axial DWI MRI from two different time points

a. Kearns-Sayre syndrome
b. Mitochondrial encephalopathy, lactic acidosis, and strokes
c. Myoclonic epilepsy with ragged red fibers
d. Leigh disease
e. Neuronal ceroid lipofuscinosis

98. Which of the following is incorrect regarding abetalipoproteinemia or Bassen-Kornzweig syndrome?

a. It is autosomal dominant
b. There is demyelination of the posterior columns of the spinal cord
c. There is demyelination of peripheral nerves
d. There is vitamin E deficiency
e. It is associated with fat malabsorption

Answer key

1. c	**18.** b	**35.** c	**52.** b	**69.** d	**86.** d
2. c	**19.** d	**36.** c	**53.** a	**70.** a	**87.** b
3. b	**20.** a	**37.** d	**54.** e	**71.** e	**88.** c
4. a	**21.** e	**38.** d	**55.** b	**72.** a	**89.** a
5. b	**22.** e	**39.** b	**56.** d	**73.** e	**90.** b
6. c	**23.** c	**40.** c	**57.** c	**74.** a	**91.** a
7. b	**24.** b	**41.** a	**58.** a	**75.** e	**92.** d
8. b	**25.** e	**42.** b	**59.** c	**76.** b	**93.** e
9. a	**26.** d	**43.** c	**60.** c	**77.** b	**94.** a
10. c	**27.** e	**44.** c	**61.** a	**78.** d	**95.** d
11. e	**28.** d	**45.** e	**62.** c	**79.** a	**96.** a
12. d	**29.** e	**46.** e	**63.** a	**80.** d	**97.** b
13. d	**30.** b	**47.** b	**64.** e	**81.** e	**98.** a
14. c	**31.** b	**48.** b	**65.** b	**82.** d	
15. b	**32.** b	**49.** e	**66.** b	**83.** c	
16. a	**33.** a	**50.** e	**67.** a	**84.** c	
17. a	**34.** e	**51.** c	**68.** e	**85.** b	

Answers

1. c, 2. c, 3. b

The main embryonal layer giving rise to the nervous system is the ectoderm. In early stages of nervous system development, a structure known as the neural plate forms. The notochord, a layer of mesodermal cells in contact with the ectoderm, induces formation of the neural plate from the ectoderm and later signals differentiation of various cell types mediated by inductive signals. The notochord later gives rise to the vertebral column.

The neural plate forms a structure known as the neural tube through a process called neurulation. Neurulation involves proliferation and migration of ectodermal cells and invagination, folding, and fusion of the neural plate in a specific pattern. An important step in neurulation includes the formation of a midline groove along which the lateral margins of the neural plate fold. These lateral margins start to fuse in the center, so that for a period of time, there are openings at each end, the anterior and posterior neuropore. Fusion then reaches the neuropores, the anterior one first, then the posterior one, and the neural tube is thus formed. The ventral and dorsal aspects of the neural tube each give rise to specific cell populations and ultimately specific parts of the nervous system. As mentioned, mesodermal cells of the notochord provide signals for differentiation to cells in the ventral aspect of the neural tube. These signals include sonic hedgehog protein and bone morphogenetic proteins, of which several types have been identified.

Neurulation occurs at 3 to 6 weeks' gestation, and failure of crucial processes at any stage leads to a variety of abnormalities, collectively known as neural tube defects. As mentioned earlier, the neural plate undergoes fusion to form the neural tube in different areas at different times, and failure to fuse at each site results in specific defects. Abnormal rostral fusion at the anterior neuropore leads to abnormalities such as encephalocele or anencephaly, whereas abnormal caudal fusion (at the posterior neuropore) leads to disorders such as spina bifida.

Following neurulation, the neural tube undergoes segmentation into three vesicles, in a process called specification, whereby different segments begin to acquire cell types and characteristics specific to the CNS structure that will eventually arise from them (malformations resulting from defects in this stage of development are discussed in subsequent questions). The three segments include the prosencephalon, mesencephalon, and rhombencephalon. The prosencephalon subsequently forms the telencephalon, which gives rise to the cerebral hemispheres, as well as the diencephalon, which forms the hypothalamus and thalamus. The rhombencephalon gives rise to the brain stem. Abnormalities during specification, which occurs at 5 to 6 weeks of gestation, lead to disorders such as septo-optic dysplasia (discussed in question 30). As the nervous system becomes more organized and specific areas more specialized, neuronal migration begins along specific routes, and abnormalities of neuronal proliferation and migration in turn lead to specific developmental abnormalities (discussed in subsequent questions).

The peripheral nervous system (including the autonomic ganglia) forms from neural crest cells that are derived from the neural tube after it fuses. In addition to peripheral nervous system structures, neural crest cells give rise to the chromaffin tissue of the adrenal medulla and melanocytes.

Swaiman KF, Ashwal S, Ferriero DM. Pediatric Neurology Principles and Practice, 4th ed. Philadelphia, PA: Mosby Elsevier; 2006.

4. a

Galactosemia is an autosomal recessive disorder that presents in newborns. There are three enzymatic defects that account for galactosemia: galactose-1-phosphate uridyltransferase deficiency, galactokinase deficiency, and uridine diphosphate galactose 4' epimerase deficiency. Galactose-1-phosphate uridyltransferase deficiency causes classic galactosemia and is the only type associated with mental retardation. Patients present in the first days of life with feeding difficulties, vomiting, diarrhea, and jaundice. They also have hepatomegaly, failure to thrive, lethargy, and hypotonia. Cataracts also occur and are caused by an accumulation of galactitol. Late neurologic sequelae include developmental delay, cognitive impairment, ataxia, and tremor, with brain MRI demonstrating white matter changes and cortical and cerebellar atrophy.

Prenatal diagnosis of galactosemia can be made, and newborn screening is available for this condition, thus allowing for treatment prior to the onset of symptoms. The diagnosis can be presumed in patients presenting with the clinical manifestations described, and the detection of reducing substances in the urine, especially after feeding. The enzymatic defect can be detected in plasma and/or erythrocytes.

Lactose and galactose should be immediately restricted from the diet. This intervention may reverse cataracts and hepatomegaly and may prevent progression of neurologic disease. However, despite this intervention, these patients may develop long-term neurologic sequelae, including learning disability, cognitive impairment, ataxia, and tremor.

Fenichel GM. Clinical Pediatric Neurology: A Signs and Symptoms Approach, 6th ed. Philadelphia, PA: Saunders Elsevier; 2009.

5. b

Pyruvate dehydrogenase (PDH) deficiency is caused by defects of the PDH complex, which is responsible for the oxidative decarboxylation of pyruvate to carbon dioxide and acetyl coenzyme A. This enzymatic complex has three main components called E1 (α and β subunits), E2, and E3. E1 deficiency is the most common and is inherited in an X-linked fashion, whereas the other defects are autosomal recessive.

Since the brain derives energy primarily from glucose oxidation, neurologic dysfunction is one of the main clinical features. The clinical presentation is variable, ranging from severe neonatal lactic acidosis with death in the neonatal period, to less severe forms that are manifested in infancy, in which patients have lactic and pyruvic acidosis, and episodic or progressive ataxia, nystagmus, dysarthria, lethargy, weakness with arreflexia, hypotonia, and psychomotor retardation, which can be profound. These patients have periodic exacerbations, which can be spontaneous or triggered by infections, stress, or high-carbohydrate meals. Some patients may have a presentation of Leigh disease (see question 32).

The diagnosis is suspected in children with clinical manifestations as described and with elevations of lactate and pyruvate levels, with a low lactate:pyruvate ratio. Enzyme analysis can be performed in leukocytes, cultured fibroblasts, muscle, or liver biopsy specimens. Pathologically, there may be cystic lesions in the white matter and basal ganglia, and certain cases of the neonatal form may have agenesis of the corpus callosum.

Management of PDH deficiency includes ketogenic diet (high fat with low carbohydrates) and thiamine supplementation. Carnitine, coenzyme Q10, and biotin supplementation may be given, but their efficacy is not well established. Acetazolamide may be used for the treatment of episodes of ataxia.

Fenichel GM. Clinical Pediatric Neurology: A Signs and Symptoms Approach, 6th ed. Philadelphia, PA: Saunders Elsevier; 2009.

6. c

The majority of patients with neurofibromatosis type 1 (NF1) have normal cognition or mild developmental delay. Other neuropsychiatric manifestations in NF1 include behavioral problems and learning disabilities, which may be present in approximately half of NF1 patients.

Renal artery stenosis due to renal artery dysplasia occurs in some patients with NF1 and can lead to hypertension. Pheochromocytoma has also been associated with NF1 and the latter two causes of hypertension should be considered in an NF1 patient with hypertension. Moyamoya disease and other cerebral artery abnormalities including intracranial aneurysms may occur in NF1 patients.

Macrocephaly is the most common head size abnormality seen in NF1 patients and occurs independent of hydrocephalus, although aqueductal stenosis may occur in NF1. Thinning of the cortex of long bones and other long bone dysplasias may lead to pathologic fractures and pseudoarthrosis. Other skeletal abnormalities in NF1 include scoliosis and sphenoid wing dysplasia. NF1 is further discussed in questions 46 to 48.

Bradley WG, Daroff RB, Fenichel GM, et al. Neurology in Clinical Practice, 5th ed. Philadelphia, PA: Elsevier; 2008.

Swaiman KF, Ashwal S, Ferriero DM. Pediatric Neurology Principles and Practice, 4th ed. Philadelphia, PA: Mosby Elsevier; 2006.

7. b

This patient has a glucose transporter type 1 (GLUT-1) deficiency.

The brain utilizes glucose as its primary source of energy. In fasting conditions, glycogen is exhausted within minutes, and since amino acids and fat cannot be used for the production of energy in the brain, ketones become the alternative fuel. Glucose crosses the blood brain barrier facilitated by GLUT-1, which is a membrane-bound protein encoded by the SLC2A1 gene on chromosome 1p35-31.3. GLUT-1 deficiency syndrome is inherited in an autosomal dominant fashion and causes a defect in glucose transport across the blood-brain barrier and into brain cells, manifesting as an epileptic encephalopathy with infantile-onset seizures, developmental delay, microcephaly, and complex movement disorders. CSF glucose level is low with a normal serum glucose level, and other CSF studies are normal, excluding other causes of hypoglycorrhachia (such as CNS infection). EEG may show 2.5 to 4 Hz spikes and waves and the interictal EEG findings may improve with glucose. Neuroimaging does not show specific abnormalities.

Later-onset forms with episodic movement disorders and ataxia, paroxysmal exertional dyskinesia, or early-onset atypical absence epilepsy have been described.

A ketogenic diet should be started as soon as the diagnosis is suspected, since this treatment option improves seizure control and the abnormal movements; however, it is less effective for the psychomotor impairment.

Klepper J. Glucose transporter deficiency syndrome (GLUT1DS) and the ketogenic diet. Epilepsia. 2008; 49:46–49.

8. b

The neural plate fuses to form the neural tube at different sites and at different times, and failure of fusion at these various sites leads to various neural tube defects. Failure of fusion rostrally, at the anterior neuropore, leads to anencephaly and encephalocele. The anterior neuropore fuses by day 26 of gestation, and abnormalities in neurulation leading to these disorders therefore likely occur at or prior to this time (weeks 1 to 4 gestation).

Anencephaly is the complete absence of both cerebral hemispheres. Because the underlying mesoderm also fails to properly differentiate, a large cranial vault defect (in skull, meninges, and skin) also occurs. This is most often not compatible with life, and most such infants are still born; in rare cases in which the infant is born alive, death occurs soon after birth.

Encephalocele is defined by herniation of neural tissues (hamartomatous brain tissue, without recognizable architecture) into a midline defect in the skull. Encephaloceles are most often located in the occipital area and less often in frontal areas. Clinically, they appear as round, protuberant, fluctuant masses covered by an opaque membrane or normal skin. They are compatible with life although they cause multiple complications. Associated clinical features include microcephaly, developmental delay (which is more severe in occipital as compared with frontal encephaloceles), and invariably hydrocephalus. Chromosomal aberrations commonly seen in patients with encephaloceles include trisomy 13 and trisomy 18. Occipital encephaloceles should be distinguished from cranial meningocele in which only leptomeninges and CSF are herniated through a skull defect.

Spina bifida results from failure of fusion of the posterior neuropore.

Bradley WG, Daroff RB, Fenichel GM, et al. Neurology in Clinical Practice, 5th ed. Philadelphia, PA: Elsevier; 2008.

Swaiman KF, Ashwal S, Ferriero DM. Pediatric Neurology Principles and Practice, 4th ed. Philadelphia, PA: Mosby Elsevier; 2006.

9. a

This patient has phenylketonuria (PKU). This is a disorder of phenylalanine metabolism, caused by a deficiency of phenylalanine hydroxylase. This enzyme converts phenylalanine to tyrosine, and its deficiency leads to accumulation of phenylalanine, which is then metabolized by phenylalanine transaminase to phenylpyruvic acid, which is subsequently oxidized to phenylacetic acid, responsible for the musty odor of the sweat and urine of these patients.

This condition is autosomal recessive. Patients with PKU are normal at birth, with a rise in the phenylalanine levels after initiation of feeding. These patients will have developmental delay, cognitive impairment, microcephaly, seizures, hypotonia, and severe behavioral disturbances. A musty odor, as described, is characteristic. These children are fair, with blond hair, blue eyes, and pale skin given the lack of tyrosine and melanin pigment production.

Newborn screening detects hyperphenylalaninemia, and the diagnosis is made on the basis of elevation of phenylalanine levels in blood. Tetrahydrobiopterin is a cofactor for phenylalanine hydroxylase, and its deficiency may also produce hyperphenylalaninemia (and PKU). A reduction of phenylalanine levels in blood and urine after a trial of tetrahydrobiopterin is used to make the diagnosis of this condition.

The treatment of PKU is dietary restriction of phenylalanine, and these patients should be placed on a low-protein diet and phenylalanine-free feeding formula as soon as possible after birth, which will prevent neurologic deterioration. Untreated patients have severe mental retardation. Despite treatment, some patients still have varying degrees of mild to moderate cognitive delays. Tetrahydrobiopterin is used as a treatment adjunct in select patients.

Fenichel GM. Clinical Pediatric Neurology: A Signs and Symptoms Approach, 6th ed. Philadelphia, PA: Saunders Elsevier; 2009.

10. c

This patient has maple syrup urine disease. This is an autosomal recessive condition caused by branched-chain α-ketoacid dehydrogenase complex deficiency, leading to the accumulation of branched amino acids and their ketoacids. The branched-chain amino acids are leucine, isoleucine, and valine, which are normally transaminated to α-ketoacids and subsequently catabolized by oxidative decarboxylation by branched-chain α-ketoacid dehydrogenase complex. Leucine, isoleucine, and valine are essential amino acids; accumulation of other essential amino acids does not play a role in this disease.

There are three main phenotypes of this condition: a classic, and intermittent, and an intermediate form. The classic type is the most severe and presents in the neonatal period with lethargy, poor feeding, and hypotonia after ingestion of protein. At 2 to 3 days of life, a progressive encephalopathy develops with opisthotonus and abnormal movements. At around 1 week, these patients may have coma and respiratory failure, with subsequent cerebral edema and seizures, and eventually death.

The intermediate form presents in late infancy with developmental delay, failure to thrive, ataxia, and seizures. There may be exacerbations with protein intake or intercurrent infections. Some cases are responsive to thiamine.

In the intermittent form, patients are normal in between episodes, and alteration of consciousness and ataxia occur during intercurrent illness or in the presence of other stressors.

These patients typically have urine with a maple syrup odor, which is more prominent during exacerbations. Diagnosis is made by detection of elevated levels of branched-chain amino acids and their ketoacids in blood and urine. Enzyme activity can be measured in fibroblasts and hepatocytes.

Treatment is a low-protein diet, more specifically a branched-chain amino acid–restricted diet, which should be started early in life (as soon as the diagnosis is suspected) to prevent cognitive decline. Thiamine should be provided, since some patients may be responsive to this vitamin. Orthotopic liver transplantation may be a therapy for these patients.

This condition is screened for by extended newborn screening, thus allowing for presymptomatic treatment in most patients with the classic or severe form of the disease.

Fenichel GM. Clinical Pediatric Neurology: A Signs and Symptoms Approach, 6th ed. Philadelphia, PA: Saunders Elsevier; 2009.

11. e

Sacral agenesis is absence of the sacrum, rather than absence of the sacral spinal cord, and is frequently associated with other malformations. The neural tube defects (NTDs) include meningocele, myelomeningocele, diastematomyelia, diplomyelia, and sacral agenesis. Caudal NTDs result from failure of fusion of the posterior neuropore at day 26 of gestation.

Meningocele is isolated protrusion of the meninges into a bony defect within the vertebral column. This protrusion is typically covered by skin. It is not usually associated with neurologic deficits, and if neurologic deficit is found, myelomeningocele should be suspected.

Myelomeningocele (also known as spinal dysraphism or rachischisis) is protrusion of potentially all layers of intraspinal contents through a bony defect: spinal cord, nerve roots, and meninges. Either the spinal cord may be exposed or a thin membrane may cover the protrusion. They most often occur in the lumbosacral region but can occur at any level. This is a clinically severe NTD associated with hydrocephalus, motor and sensory abnormalities of the legs, and bowel/bladder dysfunction. Myelomeningocele occurs in association with Chiari II malformations (discussed in question 21).

Diastematomyelia is splitting of the spinal cord into two portions by a midline septum. Diplomyelia is duplication of the spinal cord and is distinguished from diastematomyelia by the presence of two central canals each surrounded by gray and white matter as in a normal spinal cord.

Sacral agenesis, or absence of the whole (or in some cases parts of) the sacrum, classically occurs in association with a variety of other urogenital, gastrointestinal, and spinal cord abnormalities. It has been associated with maternal insulin-dependent diabetes. Autosomal dominant forms associated with homeobox gene mutations have been identified. Clinical manifestations range from mild motor deficits to severe sensory and motor deficits and bowel and bladder dysfunction.

Management of NTDs involves surgical approaches and management of complications including hydrocephalus and bowel and bladder dysfunction. A search for associated malformations in other organs (such as the heart or kidneys) should always occur.

Bradley WG, Daroff RB, Fenichel GM, et al. Neurology in Clinical Practice, 5th ed. Philadelphia, PA: Elsevier; 2008.

Swaiman KF, Ashwal S, Ferriero DM. Pediatric Neurology Principles and Practice, 4th ed. Philadelphia, PA: Mosby Elsevier; 2006.

12. d

Lymphangiomyomatosis is a rare, often fatal pulmonary disease occurring most often in female patients with tuberous sclerosis complex (TSC, discussed also in questions 61–63). It can lead to a variety of symptoms, including dyspnea, cough, and hemoptysis. Pneumothorax may develop in some. Treatment may include progesterone or the estrogen receptor modulator tamoxifen but this disease is often fatal a few years after onset. Patients with TSC, especially women, should undergo chest imaging if respiratory symptoms arise.

Single or multiple cardiac rhabdomyomas occur in more than half of TSC patients. The majority of them regress over time, and they are often clinically irrelevant over the long term. In other patients with cardiac rhabdomyomas, manifestations may include heart failure due to obstructive or ischemic cardiomyopathy, arrhythmias, and stroke from cerebral embolization. Surveillance with periodic echocardiograms should occur in TSC patients with rhabdomyomas to ensure lack of enlargement and regression. Medical management of arrhythmias, heart failure, or surgical removal is necessary in some patients.

Angiomyolipomas, benign tumors consisting of vessels, fat, and smooth muscle, occur in more than half of patients with TSC and are a minor criterion for diagnosis. They may be single or bilateral and multiple. Enlarging angiomyolipomas may need to be embolized endovascularly. Rapamycin may be useful in inhibiting their growth. Less commonly, renal cell carcinoma occurs. Renal cysts also occur in TSC and are another minor criterion; surveillance with periodic renal ultrasound is recommended.

In TSC patients, retinal hamartomas may occur, ranging from subtle to classic mulberry-like lesions near the optic disc to plaques or depigmented lesions. In some patients, when the lesion involves the macula, vision loss may occur. Other less common complications that may threaten vision in TSC patients include retinal detachment or hemorrhage into the vitreous.

Bradley WG, Daroff RB, Fenichel GM, et al. Neurology in Clinical Practice, 5th ed. Philadelphia, PA: Elsevier; 2008.

Swaiman KF, Ashwal S, Ferriero DM. Pediatric Neurology Principles and Practice, 4th ed. Philadelphia, PA: Mosby Elsevier; 2006.

13. d

This patient has propionic acidemia, in which hematologic manifestations such as pancytopenia and bleeding disorders may occur.

Propionic acidemia is an autosomal recessive disorder caused by a deficiency of propionyl-CoA carboxylase. This enzyme normally participates in the carboxylation of propionyl-CoA to D-methylmalonyl-CoA, a step that requires the coenzyme biotin. Children with propionic acidemia appear normal at birth but develop symptoms either in the early neonatal period, in infancy, or later in childhood. Patients present with feeding difficulty, lethargy, hypotonia, dehydration, and attacks of metabolic acidosis and hyperammonemia. They may progress to have seizures and coma. Other findings include hepatomegaly, pancytopenia, and bleeding disorders including intracranial hemorrhage. Patients who survive have mental retardation and basal ganglia abnormalities.

The diagnosis is suspected in newborn babies with ketoacidosis, with an anion gap, and elevated propionic acid levels in the blood and sometimes in the urine. Elevation of glycine levels in plasma and urine and of methylcitrate and β-hydroxypropionate in urine are also observed. Enzyme activity in leukocytes or fibroblasts is reduced.

Treatment involves restricting protein from the diet and providing parenteral fluids for hydration, as well as carnitine and biotin supplementation. Dialysis may be required in some patients. Antibiotics such as metronidazole may decrease the production of propionate by enteric bacteria.

D-methylmalonyl-CoA mutase deficiency causes methylmalonic acidemia (discussed in question 66).

Propionic acidemia is screened for by extended newborn screening, thus allowing for presymptomatic treatment in most patients with the classic or severe form of the disease.

Fenichel GM. Clinical Pediatric Neurology: A Signs and Symptoms Approach, 6th ed. Philadelphia, PA: Saunders Elsevier; 2009.

14. c

This patient's history and examination are consistent with spina bifida occulta. This is a defect in the bony components along the posterior aspect of the vertebral column. It can often be asymptomatic, but an abnormal conus medullaris and filum terminale are possible. The presence of a tuft of hair, implying underlying spina bifida occulta, does not necessarily imply impending cognitive or motor delay. In fact, when early neurologic development is normal, it will typically continue to be so. However, associated neurologic dysfunction may portend future neurologic impairment.

When there is associated neurologic dysfunction in a child with a tuft of hair over the lumbar region but with no other evidence of neural tube defect, the disorder is named occult spinal dysraphism. In occult spinal dysraphism, a variety of developmental abnormalities may be seen involving the spinal cord or roots and posterior fossa, and associated findings may include dermoid or epidermoid cysts, intraspinal or cutaneous lipomas, and tethered cord. Diastematomyelia, or splitting of the spinal cord, may also be seen. Rarely, a sinus tract connects the dura with the surface of the skin. In occult spinal dysraphism, neurologic manifestations vary widely and may range from minimal motor deficits and ankle hyporeflexia to bowel and bladder dysfunction, sensory loss, and paraparesis or paraplegia. Although patients may be initially asymptomatic, these neurological deficits can develop suddenly and be irreversible.

Swaiman KF, Ashwal S, Ferriero DM. Pediatric Neurology Principles and Practice, 4th ed. Philadelphia, PA: Mosby Elsevier; 2006.

Volpe JJ. Neurology of the Newborn, 4th ed. Philadelphia, PA: WB Saunders; 2001.

15. b

This patient has Lesch-Nyhan syndrome (LNS), which is inherited in an X-linked fashion and is caused by deficiency of the enzyme hypoxanthine guanine phosphoribosyltransferase (HGPRT), which participates in the salvage pathway of purines. HGPRT is encoded by the gene HPRT1 on chromosome Xq26, and deficiency of this enzyme leads to the accumulation of purines with their subsequent conversion to uric acid.

There is a spectrum of the disease, ranging from the classic LNS form to milder forms without neurologic manifestations. The classic LNS form may manifest in the newborn period with severe hypotonia. These children will have delayed motor development, progressive limb and neck rigidity with dystonia, choreoathetotic movements, facial grimacing, seizures, spasticity, and mental retardation. These patients have aggressive and severe self-mutilation behavior.

Milder forms include those with less severe neurologic disease, and those in which there are no neurologic manifestations, presenting with hyperuricemia, gout, and nephrolithiasis.

The clinical picture, including neurologic manifestations, self-mutilation behavior, and hyperuricemia suggests the diagnosis. HGPRT activity can be assessed in fibroblasts, and genetic testing can also be used.

Treatment includes purine-restricted diet, hydration to prevent kidney stones, allopurinol to decrease the production of uric acid, and supportive care to prevent self-inflicted injuries and control abnormal movements. Levodopa and tetrabenazine have been tried for the neuropsychiatric manifestations.

Fenichel GM. Clinical Pediatric Neurology: A Signs and Symptoms Approach, 6th ed. Philadelphia, PA: Saunders Elsevier; 2009.

Torres RJ, Puig JG. Hypoxanthine-guanine phosphoribosyltransferase (HPRT) deficiency: Lesch-Nyhan syndrome. Orphanet J Rare Dis. 2007; 2:48.

16. a

Several risk factors for neural tube defects (NTDs) have been identified. NTDs are more common in females. Folate is involved in various pathways of nucleic acid synthesis and DNA methylation reactions, and maternal folate deficiency is a well-established risk factor for NTD. Therefore, prenatal and perinatal maternal supplementation with 0.4 mg folic acid is recommended. Teratogens associated with NTDs include retinoic acid (vitamin A or the acidic form, tretinoin, found in acne medications). Other teratogens associated with NTDs include antiepileptics, particularly valproic acid and carbamazepine, which may lead to NTDs by affecting folate metabolism. Other risk factors for NTDs include maternal diabetes and history of a prior pregnancy resulting in an infant with an NTD.

Swaiman KF, Ashwal S, Ferriero DM. Pediatric Neurology Principles and Practice, 4th ed. Philadelphia, PA: Mosby Elsevier; 2006.

17. a

This patient has Niemann-Pick type A. Niemann-Pick types A and B are caused by acid sphingomyelinase deficiency, leading to accumulation of sphingomyelin. This disorder is autosomal recessive.

Type A involves the CNS and other viscera and manifests in infancy with feeding difficulty, failure to thrive, psychomotor retardation with regression, hypotonia, and failure to thrive. Cherry-red spot is commonly seen, and these patients have massive hepatosplenomegaly. Most children die by age 3.

Type B is purely visceral and does not affect the CNS, presenting with hepatosplenomegaly and interstitial lung disease.

In both types, bone marrow biopsy will demonstrate vacuolated histiocytes with lipid accumulation and foam cells, in which the sphingomyelin adopts the form of concentric lamellar bodies. The foamy histiocytes can be seen also in the spleen, lymph nodes, hepatic sinusoids, and pulmonary alveoli. The diagnosis is based on detecting deficient activity of acid sphingomyelinase.

Treatment is supportive. Niemann-Pick type C is discussed in question 18 and is caused by an intracellular cholesterol trafficking defect.

Fenichel GM. Clinical Pediatric Neurology: A Signs and Symptoms Approach, 6th ed. Philadelphia, PA: Saunders Elsevier; 2009.

Prayson RA, Goldblum JR. Neuropathology, 1st ed. Philadelphia, PA: Elsevier; 2005.

18. b

This patient has Niemann-Pick type C, which is an autosomal recessive disorder caused by defects in intracellular cholesterol circulation, resulting in lysosomal storage of phospholipids and glycolipids, with alteration in glycolipid metabolism. Normally, cholesterol is hydrolyzed in lysosomes and later transported to the plasma membrane; however, in Niemann-Pick type C, there is a problem in cholesterol transport, and it therefore accumulates in perinuclear lysosomes. The abnormal gene is NPC1 located on chromosome 18q11.

The onset of this disorder ranges from the neonatal period, through infancy, childhood, adolescence, and even adulthood. Patients with early-onset disease have visceromegaly and hepatic dysfunction in the first year of life and neurologic deterioration between 1 and 3 years of age, including ataxia, vertical gaze apraxia, and mental retardation. Patients with delayed-onset forms have normal initial development, subsequently manifesting ataxia, oculomotor abnormalities, especially vertical gaze apraxia, spasticity, seizures, and progressive neurologic deterioration with cognitive impairment. Later-onset disease has a much slower course.

Pathologically, there are visceral accumulation of lipids and foamy histiocytes with membrane-bound lamellar structures and lucent vacuoles. Neuronal ballooning is also seen, as well as meganeurites, and eventually neuronal loss associated with cerebral and cerebellar atrophy. Diagnosis is achieved with the filipin test, which demonstrates impaired ability of cultured fibroblasts to esterify cholesterol. Unesterified cholesterol accumulates in perinuclear lysosomes, and this is detected by the fluorescent stain filipin. Treatment is supportive.

Disorders associated with hexosaminidase A deficiency are discussed in questions 76 and 77. Disorders associated with acid sphingomyelinase deficiency are Niemann-Pick types A and B and are discussed in question 17.

Fenichel GM. Clinical Pediatric Neurology: A Signs and Symptoms Approach, 6th ed. Philadelphia, PA: Saunders Elsevier; 2009.

Prayson RA, Goldblum JR. Neuropathology, 1st ed. Philadelphia, PA: Elsevier; 2005.

19. d

Prenatal ultrasonography is used in detecting neural tube defects (NTDs) and characterizing them. Prenatally, in the setting of most NTDs, serum maternal α-fetoprotein level is elevated. α-Fetoprotein is a normal component of fetal CSF, and leakage into the amniotic fluid from an open neural tube leads to elevated amniotic α-fetoprotein level. The extent of elevation correlates with the severity of the NTD. Elevations in amniotic fluid acetylcholinesterase levels also occur, and combined with an elevated α-fetoprotein level, increase sensitivity and specificity in prenatal screening. Ultrasonography also can be used to detect NTDs and characterize them. Prenatal MRI is also used in some cases to assess the extent of the abnormality, aiding in prognostication of neurologic function in life. When an NTD is detected with screening, and/or other abnormalities are detected on ultrasonography, fetal karyotyping to assess for trisomy 13, 18, and others may be done to assist in management of the pregnancy.

Swaiman KF, Ashwal S, Ferriero DM. Pediatric Neurology Principles and Practice, 4th ed. Philadelphia, PA: Mosby Elsevier; 2006.

20. a

Metachromatic leukodystrophy is an autosomal recessive disorder caused by deficiency of the lysosomal enzyme arylsulfatase A with accumulation of sulfatide, resulting in demyelination of the central and peripheral nervous system. There are three forms: an infantile form with onset between 1 and 3 years of age, a juvenile form with onset in late childhood and early teens, and the adult form with onset in the 20s or 30s. The infantile form manifests with clumsiness, frequent falls, slurred speech, and is associated with weakness and hypotonia. With progression of the disease, these children are unable to stand, and their tone increases. They have loss of vision and hearing, peripheral neuropathy, and progressive deterioration of mental function to a vegetative state and death. The juvenile form has a slower progression. The adult form presents with behavioral changes, psychosis, and dementia.

MRI demonstrates T2 hyperintense signal changes in periventricular and subcortical white matter, sparing the U fibers. Cerebellar white matter is also involved. Pathologically, there are confluent symmetric lesions in the white matter and later atrophy. Central and peripheral demyelination is seen, with accumulation of metachromatic material in macrophages. Nerve conduction velocities are initially normal, but slowing is seen later in the course.

The diagnosis is suspected on the basis of typical MRI findings and confirmed by demonstrating deficiency of arylsulfatase A in leukocytes and/or fibroblasts. Treatment is supportive.

Niemann-Pick type C is a disorder of intracellular cholesterol trafficking and is discussed in question 18. Niemann-Pick type A is caused by acid sphingomyelinase deficiency and is discussed in question 17. Krabbe disease is caused by deficiency of galactosylceramidase and is discussed in question 84. Tay-Sachs disease is caused by hexosaminidase A deficiency and is discussed in questions 76 and 77.

Fenichel GM. Clinical Pediatric Neurology: A Signs and Symptoms Approach, 6th ed. Philadelphia, PA: Saunders Elsevier; 2009.

Prayson RA, Goldblum JR. Neuropathology, 1st ed. Philadelphia, PA: Elsevier; 2005.

21. e

While syringomyelia and hydromyelia are erroneously used interchangeably by some, the two are distinct by definition. Syringomyelia is a fluid-filled cavity within the spinal cord that is separate from the central canal; hydromyelia is the termed used to describe an enlargement in the central canal itself.

Chiari I malformation is defined as displacement of the cerebellum and cerebellar tonsils downward through the foramen magnum. Figure 14.1 depicts a Chiari I malformation with 1.3 cm downward displacement of the cerebellar tonsils. In minor downward displacement of less than 1 cm, the patient may be asymptomatic and care should be taken in attributing nonspecific neurologic symptoms to the Chiari malformation. In more severe downward displacement, as in this case, headache, cranial nerve abnormalities, and other brain stem symptoms, nystagmus, and ataxia may occur. Associated findings include syringomyelia. The pathophysiology of Chiari I malformation may relate to posterior fossa overcrowding due to posterior fossa hypoplasia. In symptomatic cases, treatment includes posterior fossa decompression and duraplasty.

Chiari II malformation, also known as Arnold-Chiari malformation, includes displacement of the cerebellar vermis and tonsils in association with a myelomeningocele. Brain stem dysfunction is often prominent, including prominent cranial nerve abnormalities, stridor, apnea, and feeding difficulties. Fourth ventricle compression leads to hydrocephalus. Pathophysiologically, Chiari II malformation is thought to be secondary to the presence of the caudal myelomeningocele, producing downward traction and hence herniation of the brain stem and cerebellum through the foramen magnum. Management of Chiari II malformation includes shunting for hydrocephalus and surgical intervention for myelomeningocele and may include posterior fossa decompression through suboccipital craniectomy. Management of complications including seizures, feeding difficulties, and bowel and bladder dysfunction is also necessary.

Chiari III malformation is cerebellar herniation into a cervical encephalocele. Chiari IV malformation is the term previously used to describe cerebellar hypoplasia but is no longer used.

Swaiman KF, Ashwal S, Ferriero DM. Pediatric Neurology Principles and Practice, 4th ed. Philadelphia, PA: Mosby Elsevier; 2006.

22. e

Sialidosis belongs to the group of glycoproteinoses, and myoclonic epilepsy is seen in these patients.

Glycoproteinoses are a group of lysosomal storage disorders of autosomal recessive inheritance, in which the enzymatic defect leads to accumulation of oligosaccharides, glycopeptides, and glycolipids. Accumulation in the brain and viscera leads to vacuolization of multiple cell types. There are multiple phenotypes depending on the enzyme affected. In general, these patients have coarse facial features, skeletal abnormalities, and psychomotor retardation.

Sialidosis is caused by deficiency of lysosomal α-neuraminidase (sialidase), leading to increased urinary excretion of sialic acid-containing oligosaccharides. Type I sialidosis (cherry-red spot myoclonus syndrome) has its onset in adolescence to adulthood and manifests with myoclonic epilepsy, visual deterioration, and cherry-red spots without dysmorphism. Type II is the childhood form, and these patients have not only myoclonic epilepsy and cherry-red spots in the retina but also severe neurologic abnormalities, coarse facial features, severe dysostosis, and psychomotor retardation. The neonatal form is characterized by hydrops fetalis, nephrotic syndrome, and early death.

Other glycoproteinoses include α-mannosidosis caused by α-mannosidosidase deficiency, β-mannosidosis caused by β-mannosidosidase deficiency, fucosidosis caused by α-fucosidase deficiency, aspartylglucosaminuria caused by aspartylglucosaminidase deficiency, and Schindler disease caused by α-N-acetylgalactosaminidase deficiency.

Abnormal urinary excretion of oligosaccharides and glycopeptides, as well as vacuolated lymphocytes with membrane-bound vacuoles, can be seen. Definitive diagnosis is made with analysis of enzyme activity.

Bradley WG, Daroff RB, Fenichel GM, et al. Neurology in Clinical Practice, 5th ed. Philadelphia, PA: Elsevier; 2008.

Prayson RA, Goldblum JR. Neuropathology, 1st ed. Philadelphia, PA: Elsevier; 2005.

23. c

Figure 14.2 shows the molar tooth sign, which results from cerebellar vermis hypoplasia with fourth ventricular enlargement, a large interpeduncular fossa, and abnormal superior cerebellar peduncles. It is seen in a variety of conditions associated with cerebellar hypoplasia, including Joubert syndrome, which is depicted in this question. Joubert syndrome is an autosomal recessive disorder characterized clinically by developmental delay, ataxia, oculomotor abnormalities, and respiratory difficulties. The molar tooth sign is also seen in COACH syndrome (cerebellar vermis hypoplasia, oligophrenia, congenital ataxia, coloboma, and hepatic fibrosis), features of which are not present in the patient depicted. It is also seen in Leber congenital amaurosis, in which vision loss occurs due to rod and cone dystrophy. The molar tooth sign has not been associated with ataxia with oculomotor apraxia types I and II (see Chapter 6).

Swaiman KF, Ashwal S, Ferriero DM. Pediatric Neurology Principles and Practice, 4th ed. Philadelphia, PA: Mosby Elsevier; 2006.

24. b

This patient has Fabry disease. Fabry disease is an X-linked disorder caused by deficiency of the enzyme α-galactosidase, resulting in accumulation of ceramide trihexoside in epithelial, mesenchymal, and neural cells.

The initial manifestations begin in childhood or adolescence, presenting with dysesthesias, lancinating pain and episodes of burning sensation from small fiber neuropathy, which also may be associated with autonomic dysfunction. Dermatologic manifestations include the characteristic angiokeratomas, which are more prominent in the lower abdomen and legs, especially in the groins, hips, and periumbilical regions, and consist of cutaneous telangiectasias. Cardiac involvement manifests with valvular disease, arrhythmias, cardiomyopathy, and ischemic heart disease. There is also renal involvement from endothelial and glomerular damage, causing acute renal failure and eventually chronic renal disease leading to hypertension and uremia. Vascular compromise arises from endothelial and vascular smooth muscle involvement and is associated with ischemic stroke. Another frequent clinical finding is corneal opacity.

Pathologically, there is lysosomal storage of birefringent lipids, with membrane-bound lamellar deposits on electron microscopy. Treatment includes enzyme replacement therapy.

Metachromatic leukodystrophy is caused by deficiency of arylsulfatase A and is discussed in question 20. Niemann-Pick type A is caused by acid sphingomyelinase deficiency and is discussed in question 17. Gaucher disease is caused by deficiency of the enzyme glucocerebrosidase, and this condition is discussed in question 74. GM1 gangliosidosis is caused β-galactosidase deficiency, and this is discussed in question 87.

Prayson RA, Goldblum JR. Neuropathology, 1st ed. Philadelphia, PA: Elsevier; 2005.

Ropper AH, Samuels MA. Adams and Victor's Principles of Neurology, 9th ed. New York, NY: McGraw-Hill; 2009.

25. e

The less severe forms of holoprosencephaly may be compatible with life with few neurologic deficits.

During embryologic development, after fusion of the anterior neuropore, vesicles form and ultimately give rise to different brain structures. The prosencephalon vesicle gives rise to the telencephalon. The telencephalon divides to give the two cerebral hemispheres and the basal ganglia. The prosencephalon also gives rise to the diencephalon, which in turn gives rise to the thalamus and hypothalamus. The mesoderm of the notochord provides signals for this differentiation; one such signaling molecule is the sonic hedgehog protein. Abnormalities of this stage of development, which typically occurs around weeks 4 to 8 of gestation, lead to a variety of midline brain and face malformations.

Failure of the prosencephalon to form the telencephalon and diencephalon, and failure of formation of two distinct cerebral hemispheres, results in the malformation known as holoprosencephaly. In alobar holoprosencephaly, the cerebral hemispheres are almost completely fused, with absence of the interhemispheric fissure and corpus callosum. There is a single midline ventricle. Variable dysgenesis and fusion of the thalamus, hypothalamus, and basal ganglia is present. In semilobar holoprosencephaly, parts of the posterior hemispheres may be separated by a fissure. In lobar holoprosencephaly, only the most anterior portions of the hemispheres are not separated, and there is partial agenesis of the corpus callosum, but the splenium and genu are present.

The olfactory bulb and tracts develop from the prosencephalon a few days after the hemispheres divide. In severe forms of holoprosencephaly, arrhinencephaly (agenesis of only the olfactory bulb and tract) invariably occurs. However, in less severe forms of holoprosencephaly, arrhinencephaly may occur in isolation. Kallmann syndrome, an X-linked dominant disorder, is characterized by anosmia (due to arrhinencephaly) and hypogonadism.

In infants with alobar holoprosencephaly, associated midline facial defects, such as cyclopia (single midline eye) and proboscis (single-nostril nose), often occur, and these more severely affected individuals are usually stillborn or do not survive long after birth. If death does not occur in utero, the clinical picture includes severe cognitive and motor delay, feeding difficulties, and seizures. Endocrinologic problems including diabetes insipidus and panhypopituitarism are frequent. Hydrocephalus is a frequent complication.

In less severe forms such as arrhinencephaly, little neurologic dysfunction may be clinically apparent.

Chromosomal aberrations associated with holoprosencephaly include trisomy 13 and trisomy 18. Autosomal recessive and dominant forms, due to mutations in the sonic hedgehog gene and other genes, exist. In addition to a variety of genetic and environmental mechanisms, the pathophysiology of holoprosencephaly also relates to abnormal cholesterol metabolism, as cholesterol influences sonic hedgehog protein function. Hence, holoprosencephaly has an association with the cholesterol synthesis disorder Smith-Lemli-Opitz, which results from a defect in 7-dehydrocholesterol reductase, the enzyme that catalyzes the final step in cholesterol synthesis.

Bradley WG, Daroff RB, Fenichel GM, et al. Neurology in Clinical Practice, 5th ed. Philadelphia, PA: Elsevier; 2008.

Swaiman KF, Ashwal S, Ferriero DM. Pediatric Neurology Principles and Practice, 4th ed. Philadelphia, PA: Mosby Elsevier; 2006.

26. d

Neuronal ceroid lipofuscinosis is a group of autosomal recessive disorders characterized by progressive psychomotor retardation, seizures, and blindness, which can present in infantile, late infantile, juvenile, and adult forms.

Mutations in eight genes causing the disorder (CLN1 through CLN8) have been described. The most commonly involved genes are CLN1 and CLN2. CLN1 encodes for palmitoyl protein thioesterase 1 (PPT1), and CLN2 encodes for tripeptidyl peptidase 1 (TPP1). The storage products are saposins A and D in the infantile forms and subunit C of ATP synthase in the other forms.

The infantile form is most common in Finland and is associated with CLN1 gene mutations. These patients are normal at birth, with onset of symptoms between 6 and 24 months, including microcephaly, hypotonia, myoclonus, seizures, ataxia, progressive psychomotor retardation, and blindness. Neurons accumulate membrane-bound osmophilic deposits (seen on electron microscopy) and neuronal loss with cortical atrophy will ensue.

The late-infantile form presents between 2 and 4 years of age and is associated with CLN2 mutations, and these patients develop seizures, myoclonus, ataxia, involuntary movements, blindness, and psychomotor retardation. Neurons accumulate curvilinear bodies, which are seen on electron microscopy.

The juvenile form begins between 4 and 10 years of age and is associated with CLN3 mutation, and these patients develop visual loss, seizures, myoclonus, psychomotor retardation, and focal neurologic deficits. The storage product consists of fingerprint bodies, which are seen on electron microscopy.

The adult form is evident at approximately 30 years of age and is characterized by myoclonus, ataxia, behavioral abnormalities, and dementia. The storage material consists of a combination of fingerprint bodies, granular osmiophilic deposits, and rectilinear profiles.

The diagnosis is based on the clinical presentation and supported with electron microscopic examination of lymphocytes or cells from other tissues. Enzyme activity studies for PPT1 and TPP1 are also available, as is genetic testing for all of the identified CLN genes. The treatment is symptomatic.

Prayson RA, Goldblum JR. Neuropathology, 1st ed. Philadelphia, PA: Elsevier; 2005.

Ropper AH, Samuels MA. Adams and Victor's Principles of Neurology, 9th ed. New York, NY: McGraw-Hill; 2009.

27. e

The foramen of Monroe connects the lateral ventricle with the third ventricle. The cerebral aqueduct connects the third ventricle with the fourth ventricle. Congenital aqueductal stenosis, or narrowing of the cerebral aqueduct that connects the third and fourth ventricle, is a disorder of neurulation, resulting from abnormal septation of the dorsomedial septum of the midbrain.

There are various causes of congenital aqueductal stenosis, including presumed genetic or acquired causes. There is an X-linked form associated with pachygyria. It may occur in association with holoprosencephaly or Chiari II malformation. Acquired causes include congenital infections such as cytomegalovirus or mumps virus, or a variety of tumors such as ependymomas or hamartomas. Tumors of the midbrain region that compress the aqueduct may also lead to secondary congenital aqueductal stenosis. Symptoms are related to hydrocephalus and include macrocephaly and sundowning of the eyes (downward rotation of the eyes). In those presenting after fusion of the cranial sutures; headache, projectile vomiting, and altered mental status may occur. Management is directed at relieving the hydrocephalus with shunts or ventriculostomies.

Bradley WG, Daroff RB, Fenichel GM, et al. Neurology in Clinical Practice, 5th ed. Philadelphia, PA: Elsevier; 2008.

28. d

This patient has Zellweger syndrome, a peroxisomal disorder in which the white matter is involved.

Peroxisomes are organelles involved in the biosynthesis of ether phospholipids and bile acids, oxidation of very long-chain fatty acid, prostaglandins, and unsaturated long-chain fatty acids, and the catabolism of phytanate, pipecolate, and glycolate. The infantile syndromes of peroxisomal dysfunction include Zellweger syndrome, neonatal adrenoleukodystrophy, and infantile Refsum disease. Zellweger is the most severe form and is caused by mutations in the PEX genes, the majority with PEX1 resulting in abnormal peroxisomal biogenesis.

Zellweger syndrome, or "cerebrohepatorenal syndrome", is characterized by dysmorphic features such as a high forehead, large fontanelles, flat supraorbital ridges, hypertelorism, epicanthal folds, broad nasal bridge, micrognathia, and flat occiput. These children have cataracts, retinal dystrophy, sensorineural hearing loss, severe hypotonia, decreased sucking and crying, hyporeflexia, deformities in flexion of the lower limbs with arthrogryposis, profound mental retardation, and seizures. The brain demonstrates white matter changes and abnormalities in neuronal migration. There is liver dysfunction with cirrhosis and polycystic kidney disease. A very typical feature is chondrodysplasia punctata with bony stippling of the patella. Other congenital abnormalities have been reported, such as ventricular septal defects and other cardiac abnormalities.

Diagnostic workup demonstrates increased plasma very long-chain fatty acids, decreased red blood cell plasmalogens, and decreased or absent hepatic peroxisomes. Pathologically, the brain may be enlarged, and there is evidence of neuronal migration abnormality, white matter changes with lipid accumulation, and sometimes pachygyria and/or polymicrogyria. The treatment of Zellweger syndrome is symptomatic. Most of these patients die early.

The other peroxisomal abnormalities are much milder. Neonatal adrenoleukodystrophy patients have liver cirrhosis, adrenocortical atrophy, and brain abnormalities such as polymicrogyria, subcortical heterotopia, and cerebellar dysplasia but no pachygyria.

Infantile Refsum disease manifests with psychomotor retardation, sensorineural hearing loss, retinal degeneration, anosmia, and mild dysmorphic features and there may be cirrhosis and adrenal atrophy. In Refsum disease, phytanic acid levels are elevated and peroxisomes are reduced or absent. These patients may survive into adulthood.

Fenichel GM. Clinical Pediatric Neurology: A Signs and Symptoms Approach, 6th ed. Philadelphia, PA: Saunders Elsevier; 2009.

Prayson RA, Goldblum JR. Neuropathology, 1st ed. Philadelphia, PA: Elsevier; 2005.

29. e

Fabry disease is an X-linked disorder that results from a mutation in the gene encoding the lysosomal enzyme α-galactosidase. Multiple organs are involved; renal involvement leads to renal failure and cardiac involvement to cardiomyopathy. Cutaneous manifestations in Fabry disease include purplish angiokeratomas often occurring in the groin. Neurologic manifestations involve both the peripheral nervous system (including small fiber neuropathy with attacks of cold-induced painful paresthesias in the extremities, acroparesthesias) and the CNS. CNS manifestations include stroke and other vascular events related to vascular ectasia, with often marked dolichoectatic enlargement of the basilar artery. Fabry's disease is also discussed in question 24.

Hereditary hemorrhagic telangiectasia, or Osler-Weber-Rendu syndrome, is an autosomal dominant disorder in which telangiectasia occurs in the skin, mucous membranes, and several organs including the retina and gastrointestinal tract. Recurrent epistaxis is a common manifestation. CNS involvement results from single or multiple arteriovenous malformations (AVMs) or cerebral embolization from pulmonary AVMs. It results from a mutation in the HHT1 gene on chromosome 9 that encodes for endoglin, a protein that binds transforming growth factor-β (TGF-β), or from a mutation in the HHT2 gene on chromosome 12. Wyburn-Mason syndrome is another neurocutaneous disorder in which multiple AVMs occur on the face, in the retina, and intracranially.

In pseudoxanthoma elasticum (Gronblad-Strandberg syndrome), a connective tissue disorder that may be autosomal dominant or recessive, yellowish xanthomas occur in various skin regions, on mucous membranes, and in the retina. Neurological manifestations relate to vascular occlusions and intracranial carotid artery aneurysms.

Ehlers-Danlos syndrome exists in 10 subtypes, with types I, II, and III being the most common. These subtypes share the occurrence of hyperelastic skin, hyperextensible joints, and vascular lesions. This syndrome results from mutations in various genes encoding for different types of collagen. The main neurologic significance of this disorder is the increased risk of intracranial aneurysms, carotid-cavernous fistulas (that may be spontaneous or due to mild trauma), and arterial dissection.

Xeroderma pigmentosum (XP) is a neurocutaneous disorder marked by sensitivity to ultraviolet light that predisposes affected individuals to skin freckling and multiple cutaneous malignancies including melanoma, basal cell carcinoma, and squamous cell carcinoma as well as other cutaneous and systemic tumors. Neurologic abnormalities include progressive cognitive dysfunction, hearing loss, tremor, chorea, and ataxia as well as peripheral neuropathy. XP is autosomal recessive and results from mutations on chromosome 9 that result in abnormal DNA repair. Cockayne syndrome is a related disorder. Another disorder of DNA repair associated with neurologic features is ataxia telangiectasia (discussed in Chapter 6).

Bradley WG, Daroff RB, Fenichel GM, et al. Neurology in Clinical Practice, 5th ed. Philadelphia, PA: Elsevier; 2008.

Swaiman KF, Ashwal S, Ferriero DM. Pediatric Neurology Principles and Practice, 4th ed. Philadelphia, PA: Mosby Elsevier; 2006.

30. **b**

This patient's history and imaging findings are consistent with septo-optic dysplasia, a group of malformations that include hypoplasia or absence of the septum pellucidum, optic nerve and optic chiasm hypoplasia, dysgenesis of the corpus callosum and anterior commissure, and fornix detachment from the corpus callosum. Arrhinencephaly (agenesis of only the olfactory bulb and tract) and/or hypothalamic hamartomas may be associated features. Other less commonly associated abnormalities include cerebellar vermis defects and hydrocephalus. Septo-optic dysplasia can also be associated with lobar holoprosencephaly and other malformations of cortical development.

Clinical manifestations include vision loss, ataxia when the cerebellum is involved, symptoms of hydrocephalus when it is present, and endocrinologic disturbances. Endocrinologic disturbances can range from panhypopituitarism (with deficiencies in both anterior and posterior pituitary hormones) to isolated hormone deficiencies. Mutations in the transcription factors HESX1, a homeobox gene, and SOX may be implicated in this disorder.

Cavum septum pellucidum, in which the septum pellucidum is not fused but rather exists in two separate pieces of tissue, is considered nonpathologic, with little clinical implications. The presence of normal cortex excludes holoprosencephaly, and lissencephaly. This patient has several features making septo-optic dysplasia the likely diagnosis rather than arrhinencephaly.

Bradley WG, Daroff RB, Fenichel GM, et al. Neurology in Clinical Practice, 5th ed. Philadelphia, PA: Elsevier; 2008.

Volpe P, Campobasso V, De Robertis V, et al. Disorders of prosencephalic development. Prenat Diagn. 2009; 29:340–354.

31. b

Adrenoleukodystrophy is an X-linked disorder caused by a deficiency of the peroxisomal enzyme acyl coenzyme A synthetase, leading to the impaired ability to oxidize very long-chain fatty acids, with subsequent accumulation in tissues and plasma. There are four phenotypes: childhood cerebral type, adrenomyeloneuropathy, pure adrenal insufficiency, or asymptomatic. Female carriers may have mild symptoms of adrenomyeloneuropathy.

The cerebral type has an onset between 4 and 8 years of age, with behavioral changes progressing to cognitive impairment, spasticity, disturbances of gait and coordination, and vision and hearing loss. The prognosis is poor, and these patients die early. MRI demonstrates confluent T2 hyperintensity in the white matter affecting more predominantly the parieto-occipital regions and the posterior corpus callosum. Pathologically, there is symmetric and confluent demyelination affecting initially the posterior regions and sparing the U fibers. There is involvement of other tissues, including the adrenal cortex and Leydig cells of the testis. Histopathologically, cerebral lesions are characterized by the presence of perivascular cuffing, with predominance of T cells.

Adrenomyeloneuropathy is the most common phenotype and manifests with paraparesis that begins after age 20, and is slowly progressive into adulthood. There is also a sensory neuropathy in these patients. Some degree of cognitive impairment and adrenal insufficiency may be seen. Pathologically, there is long tract degeneration with axon and myelin loss. Peripheral nerve demyelination without inflammation also occurs. Patients with adrenoleukodystrophy have increased plasma levels of very long-chain fatty acids, and ACTH is increased secondary to adrenal insufficiency.

Treatment involves supportive care with steroid replacement therapy for adrenal insufficiency. "Lorenzo's oil", which consists of 4:1 glyceryl trioleate-glyceryl trierucate, has been shown to reduce levels of very long-chain fatty acids in plasma. Dietary use of Lorenzo's oil may be beneficial in young asymptomatic patients but not in patients with neurologic deficits. Bone marrow transplantation may have a role in early stages of the disease.

Canavan disease is discussed in question 79. Alexander disease is discussed in question 88. Zellweger syndrome is discussed in question 28. Fabry disease is discussed in questions 24 and 29.

Fenichel GM. Clinical Pediatric Neurology: A Signs and Symptoms Approach, 6th ed. Philadelphia, PA: Saunders Elsevier; 2009.

Moser HW, Raymond GV, Lu SE, et al. Follow-up of 89 asymptomatic patients with adrenoleukodystrophy treated with Lorenzo's oil. Arch Neurol. 2005; 62:1073–1080.

Prayson RA, Goldblum JR. Neuropathology, 1st ed. Philadelphia, PA: Elsevier; 2005.

32. b

Leigh disease or acute necrotizing encephalomyelopathy is a manifestation of mitochondrial disorders that can be sporadic or familial, with only some cases with the typical maternal inheritance pattern. This condition affects neurons of the brain stem, thalamus, basal ganglia, and cerebellum. Most of the affected patients have onset of neurologic manifestations in the first year of life, but there are forms with late onset. Clinical features manifest with decompensation associated with intercurrent illnesses.

In infancy, patients present with hypotonia, loss of head control, poor sucking, vomiting, irritability, seizures, and myoclonic jerks. If the onset is beyond the first year, patients present with gait disturbance, cerebellar ataxia, dysarthria, psychomotor retardation, spasticity, external ophthalmoplegia, nystagmus, abnormal movements with chorea or dystonias, and peripheral neuropathy in some cases with autonomic failure. The disorder is progressive with episodic deterioration.

Lactate level is increased in blood and CSF. Lactate and pyruvate levels in blood are elevated during exacerbations. MRI of the brain demonstrates bilateral symmetric hyperintense T2 signal abnormalities in the brain stem and/or basal ganglia, and in some cases in the spinal cord. Treatment is supportive and symptomatic.

Fenichel GM. Clinical Pediatric Neurology: A Signs and Symptoms Approach, 6th ed. Philadelphia, PA: Saunders Elsevier; 2009.

Ropper AH, Samuels MA. Adams and Victor's Principles of Neurology, 9th ed. New York, NY: McGraw-Hill; 2009.

33. a

This patient has Kearns-Sayre syndrome, which is a disorder caused by multiple mtDNA deletions. The diagnosis is made with the triad of progressive external ophthalmoplegia, onset before the age of 20 years, and at least one of the following: short stature, retinitis pigmentosa, cerebellar ataxia, heart block, and increased CSF protein (>100 mg/dL). Chronic progressive external ophthalmoplegia may be an isolated finding seen in some patients.

Patients with Kearns-Sayre syndrome have a gradual progression of symptoms and most will have cognitive regression by third or fourth decade of life. Most cases are sporadic.

An electrocardiogram is required to diagnose heart block, in which case, a pacemaker is needed. Pathologically, patients may have muscles with ragged red fibers and white matter showing spongy myelinopathy without gliosis or macrophage reactions.

Mitochondrial encephalopathy, lactic acidosis, and strokes is discussed in question 97. Myoclonic epilepsy with ragged red fibers is discussed in Chapter 5. Leigh disease is discussed in question 32. Myasthenia gravis is discussed in Chapter 10.

Fenichel GM. Clinical Pediatric Neurology: A Signs and Symptoms Approach, 6th ed. Philadelphia, PA: Saunders Elsevier; 2009.

Prayson RA, Goldblum JR. Neuropathology, 1st ed. Philadelphia, PA: Elsevier; 2005.

34. e

Congenital disorders of glycosylation (CDG), previously known as carbohydrate-deficient glycoprotein syndrome, are a group of genetic disorders inherited in an autosomal recessive fashion. These disorders affect multiple organ systems, especially the CNS. The defect is abnormal synthesis, transport, modification, and/or processing of the carbohydrate moieties or glycans of glycoproteins, therefore affecting protein components in many tissues.

Type I CDGs are caused by abnormal synthesis of these glycans. Clinical manifestations are widely variable, with multiple subtypes, including combinations of failure to thrive, developmental delay, dysmorphic features, hypotonia, ataxia, weakness, retinitis pigmentosa, short stature with skeletal abnormalities, polyneuropathy, stroke-like episodes, liver dysfunction, hypogonadism, and multisystem involvement. Lipodystrophy with prominent fat pads in the buttocks and suprapubic area and inverted nipples are distinctive features.

Type II CDGs are caused by abnormal processing and modification of glycans and lead to profound mental retardation but no cerebellar ataxia or peripheral neuropathy.

CDGs are characterized by the presence of a carbohydrate-deficient transferrin in the serum and CSF, and the analysis of the glycoforms of this protein is a diagnostic test. Genetic confirmation is available. Treatment is supportive.

Fenichel GM. Clinical Pediatric Neurology: A Signs and Symptoms Approach, 6th ed. Philadelphia, PA: Saunders Elsevier; 2009.

Kliegman RM, Behrman RE, Jenson HB, et al. Nelson Textbook of Pediatrics, 18th ed. Philadelphia, PA: Saunders Elsevier; 2007.

35. c

During the fifth week of gestation, within the lamina terminalis, the commissural plate develops and serves as a bridge over which axonal processes decussate. The corpus callosum is fully developed by week 17th of gestation. Abnormalities in the commissural plate lead to agenesis or dysgenesis of the corpus callosum. Agenesis of the corpus callosum may be complete or more commonly partial and may occur in isolation or more commonly is associated with dysplasias of other prosencephalon derivatives and aplasia of the cerebellar vermis. It may also be seen in a variety of syndromes, including Aicardi syndrome, or may be associated with metabolic disorders such as nonketotic hyperglycinemia. Clinical manifestations may be absent, or there may be subtle cognitive or perceptual abnormalities; developmental delay and seizures may also occur. Hypertelorism is seen in many. Coronal MRI shows vertically oriented lateral ventricles ("steer horn sign," or "racing car sign" on axial images).

Bradley WG, Daroff RB, Fenichel GM, et al. Neurology in Clinical Practice, 5th ed. Philadelphia, PA: Elsevier; 2008.

Prayson RA, Goldblum JR. Neuropathology, 1st ed. Philadelphia, PA: Elsevier; 2005.

36. c

The cortex forms inside-out: cells that migrate out first form deeper layers, whereas cells that migrate later form more superficial structures.

The cerebral hemispheres form from an initially single layer of columnar epithelium located in the subependymal region known as the ventricular zone (or primary germinal zone). Cells in this layer are pluripotential and frequently divide. Another layer, the subventricular zone, consists of cells known as radial glia, which send out processes that extend all the way to the pial membrane at the cortical surface. Yet another, more superficial layer, the marginal zone, forms by the fifth week of gestation. Cells leave the marginal zone and migrate along the radial glial processes in two waves, one at approximately 6 weeks' gestation and the other at 11 weeks' gestation, peaking at weeks 12 to 14. Cells destined to form layers 2 to 6 of the cortex originate in this second wave. The cortex develops inside-out, such that cells in the earliest portion of migration form deeper layers, whereas cells that migrate later form more superficial structures.

Several factors influence neurogenesis (formation of neurons, including pyramidal neurons, cortical granular or stellate neurons, Betz cells, and others) and gliogenesis (formation of glia, including astrocytes, oligodendrocytes, ependyma, and microglia), as well as cell migration. These include regulatory proteins, transcription factors, and neurotransmitters, each varying with the stage of development. Cajal-Retzius cells are a group of stellate neurons found in the cortex prior to arrival of the first wave of cells. These cells secrete GABA and acetylcholine and express several products including LIS1 and Reelin, genes necessary for neuronal migration along radial glia. All six layers of the cortex are identifiable by 27 weeks' gestation.

Bradley WG, Daroff RB, Fenichel GM, et al. Neurology in Clinical Practice, 5th ed. Philadelphia, PA: Elsevier; 2008.

Swaiman KF, Ashwal S, Ferriero DM. Pediatric Neurology Principles and Practice, 4th ed. Philadelphia, PA: Mosby Elsevier; 2006.

37. d

Hypopigmented streaks or patches that follow skin lines occur in Hypomelanosis of Ito (HI, discussed in question 43), not in incontinentia pigmenti.

The phakomatoses are a group of disorders that share in common the occurrence of dysplastic lesions and the tendency for tumor formation. They include neurofibromatosis, tuberous sclerosis, Sturge-Weber syndrome, epidermal nevus syndrome, and HI, in addition to a variety of other rare disorders, some of which are discussed briefly later.

In incontinentia pigmenti, skin involvement occurs in stages including vesiculobullous lesions present at birth, verrucous lesions that appear at approximately 6 weeks of age, then hyperpigmented lesions that appear "splashed-on." Some patients have normal cognition and no evidence of neurologic dysfunction; neurologic manifestations include mental retardation, pyramidal tract findings, and ocular abnormalities. It is X-linked dominant in inheritance and affects only females; it is thought to be lethal in males. It results from a mutation in the NEMO gene, which encodes a protein involved in the nuclear factor κ B pathway.

Neurocutaneous melanosis is characterized by the presence of various types of congenital cutaneous lesions that are abnormally pigmented (such as giant hair pigmented nevi and congenital melanocytic nevi) in association with leptomeningeal melanoma. The leptomeningeal areas most often affected include those around the base of the brain, brain stem, and cerebellum. The pathophysiology of this disorder is not well defined; the cells of origin of the leptomeningeal melanomas are thought to be melanoblasts, pigmented cells normally found in the pia mater.

Parry-Romberg syndrome is marked by the occurrence of facial atrophy, which involves atrophy of facial bone, cartilage, and soft tissue, often with ipsilateral loss of eyelashes, eyebrows, and scalp hair. This begins typically after birth or in early childhood and the atrophy ceases by the third decade of life. Neurologic manifestations include headaches, Horner syndrome, seizures, and hemiparesis. Patients with Parry-Romberg syndrome are at increased risk for a variety of benign tumors.

In Maffucci syndrome, multiple endochondromas (tumors of cartilage) occur, in association with secondary hemangioma formation, and various skin findings including vitiligo and café au lait spots. These endochondromas grow over time, leading to disfigurement and skeletal abnormalities. Neurologic manifestations result from the association of this syndrome with various CNS tumors, including CNS teratomas and pituitary adenomas, as well as compression of nervous system structures by the endochondromas, such as cerebral compression by calvarial endochondromas.

In von Hippel-Lindau disease, multiple retinal, cerebellar, and spinal hemangioblastomas occur. Benign hemangiomas and cysts in various body parts can also occur. Cutaneous manifestations are not a feature of this disorder. This disorder is autosomal dominant and results from a mutation in a gene on chromosome 3 that encodes for a tumor suppressor protein.

Bradley WG, Daroff RB, Fenichel GM, et al. Neurology in Clinical Practice, 5th ed. Philadelphia, PA: Elsevier; 2008.

Swaiman KF, Ashwal S, Ferriero DM. Pediatric Neurology Principles and Practice, 4th ed. Philadelphia, PA: Mosby Elsevier; 2006.

38. d

Periventricular nodular heterotopia is a disorder of neuronal migration.

Malformations of cortical development are divided into three categories based on the underlying cause: disorders of cell proliferation, migration, or cortical organization. Disorders of neuronal proliferation include some forms of megalencephaly (see questions 39 and 40) and focal cortical dysplasia. Disorders of neuronal migration include lissencephaly, periventricular nodular heterotopias, and others. Disorders of cortical organization include polymicrogyria and schizencephaly.

Focal cortical dysplasia may be seen in isolation or in the setting of tuberous sclerosis. One type of focal cortical dysplasia is characterized pathologically by the presence of balloon cells, which result from proliferation of abnormal cells within the germinal matrix. This is a common pathology in focal epilepsy, with the seizures often being intractable to medical therapy.

Swaiman KF, Ashwal S, Ferriero DM. Pediatric Neurology Principles and Practice, 4th ed. Philadelphia, PA: Mosby Elsevier; 2006.

39. b, 40. c

Figure 14.3 shows left hemispheric hemimegalencephaly, which frequently leads to contralateral hemiparesis.

Microcephaly is defined as a head circumference less than 2 standard deviations below the mean. A variety of causes of microcephaly exist. It can be a normal variant that is often hereditary, without clinical implications. When pathologic, causes include in utero infections, toxin exposure (such as alcohol, tobacco, and prescription drugs such as chemotherapeutic agents and antiepileptics), hypoxic-ischemic injury, birth trauma, and metabolic disorders such as prolonged hypoglycemia. A wide variety of hereditary disorders including enzyme deficiencies can lead to microcephaly, as can chromosomal abnormalities. Clinical manifestations depend on the underlying cause and can range from none (asymptomatic microcephaly) to severe developmental delay and seizures.

Macrocephaly is defined as a head circumference greater than 2 standard deviations above the mean. Macrocephaly may be a normal variant that is often hereditary, may result from increased CSF, as in hydrocephalus due to a variety of causes, from mass lesions such as tumors or subdural hematomas, or may result from megalencephaly, an oversized brain (brain weight greater than 2 standard deviations above the mean). Causes of megalencephaly include storage diseases such as mucopolysaccharidoses or Tay-Sachs disease, Canavan disease, Alexander disease, genetic disorders including Sotos syndrome, and others. In the latter disorders, eventual cell loss with subsequent atrophy typically occurs. Megalencephaly may also be a benign familial finding. Clinical manifestations depend on the underlying cause. Neurologic deficits may be absent in the benign familial form. Hemimegalencephaly, or enlargement of only one brain hemisphere, as depicted in Figure 14.3, invariably presents with seizures and hemiparesis. Hemimegalencephaly is associated with various genetic disorders, including Beckwith-Wiedemann syndrome, which is characterized by gigantism, macroglossia, and midline abdominal wall defects.

Swaiman KF, Ashwal S, Ferriero DM. Pediatric Neurology Principles and Practice, 4th ed. Philadelphia, PA: Mosby Elsevier; 2006.

41. a, 42. b

The history and imaging findings depicted in question 41 are consistent with Miller-Dieker syndrome, a form of lissencephaly type I. In lissencephaly type I (classic lissencephaly), the cortex is thick but consists of only four layers or less.

Lissencephaly is a malformation of cortical development resulting from abnormal neuronal migration resulting in impaired formation of gyri. It is characterized by the presence of reduced cortical gyration and, in the most severe form, no gyri, or agyria, resulting in a smooth brain.

In classic lissencephaly, or lissencephaly type I, the cortex is thick but consists of only four layers (or less often two or three layers, as opposed to the normal six neocortical layers). Associated malformations may include agenesis of the corpus callosum or hypoplasia of the cerebellum, with sparing of the thalamus and basal ganglia.

Miller-Dieker syndrome (MDS), one form of lissencephaly type I, is characterized by lissencephaly associated with microcephaly, typical facies including micrognathia (small jaw), low-set ears, thin upper lip, and other features. Clinical manifestations include global developmental delay, hypotonia and later spasticity, and intractable seizures. Life expectancy is often not beyond 1 year. MDS has been associated with microdeletions on chromosome 17 in the LIS1 gene. LIS1 gene encodes a protein involved in regulation of microtubules and dynein function, and mutations interfere with microtubule-directed migration of neurons from the ventricular zone. Mutations in LIS1 gene can also lead to isolated lissencephaly (so-called isolated lissencephaly sequence, without other features of MDS).

X-linked lissencephaly is another form that results from mutations in the DCX gene on chromosome X when occurring in males. This gene encodes for the protein doublecortin, which is involved in microtubule organization and stabilization. In another form of lissencephaly that results from mutations in the gene ARX, which encodes for a transcription factor involved in nonradial migration of cortical interneurons, the basal ganglia are abnormal in addition to the cortex and corpus callosum. In some forms of lissencephaly, there may be an anterior to posterior (or vice versa) gradient of gyral formation (e.g., with some gyral formation in the anterior or posterior aspects of the brain).

Cobblestone lissencephaly, also known as lissencephaly type II, is seen in several disorders including Walker-Warburg syndrome, Fukuyama muscular dystrophy, and muscle-eye-brain disease of Santavuori. In polymicrogyria, there are excess, abnormal gyri. Subcortical band heterotopia is discussed in questions 44 and 45.

Bradley WG, Daroff RB, Fenichel GM, et al. Neurology in Clinical Practice, 5th ed. Philadelphia, PA: Elsevier; 2008.

Spalice A, Parisi P, Nicita F, et al. Neuronal migration disorders: clinical, neuroradiologic and genetic aspects. Acta Paediatr. 2009; 98:421–433.

Swaiman KF, Ashwal S, Ferriero DM. Pediatric Neurology Principles and Practice, 4th ed. Philadelphia, PA: Mosby Elsevier; 2006.

43. C

Hypomelanosis of Ito (HI) is a neurocutaneous disorder that involves multiple organ systems including the skin, eyes, brain, and skeleton. The cutaneous features of HI include multiple hypopigmented streaks or patches that are present at birth and in some follow Blaschko lines (skin lines that form specific patterns over the trunk and extremities, such as a V shape over the back and linear lines over the limbs). These lesions are either present at birth or emerge in infancy and are best detected under ultraviolet light in light-skinned children. The extent of the skin lesions does not correlate strongly with neurologic involvement.

Neurologic manifestations include mental retardation that is seen in some but not all patients, and may be severe in some cases. Seizures are the other main neurologic manifestation. Macrocephaly or microcephaly may be seen, with the former being more common. Cerebral and cerebellar hypoplasia are also often seen, although various malformations of cortical development may occur in patients with HI, including hemimegalencephaly, lissencephaly, and polymicrogyria.

Other manifestations of HI include eye involvement (commonly, with a variety of findings including microphthalmia, cataracts, optic atrophy, and retinal detachment), skeletal hemihypertrophy, cleft lip and palate, and congenital heart disease such as tetralogy of Fallot.

Various karyotype abnormalities have been found in patients with HI, including autosomal mosaicism for aneuploidy or unbalanced translocations, mosaic trisomy 18, ring chromosome 22, and translocations involving the X chromosome. There is not a clear genotypic-phenotypic correlation.

The other options listed are also neurocutaneous syndromes but each with distinct cutaneous and other neurologic findings. Neurocutaneous melanosis and incontinentia pigmenti are discussed in question 37, Sturge-Weber syndrome in questions 80 and 81, and epidermal nevus syndrome in question 93.

Bradley WG, Daroff RB, Fenichel GM, et al. Neurology in Clinical Practice, 5th ed. Philadelphia, PA: Elsevier; 2008.

Swaiman KF, Ashwal S, Ferriero DM. Pediatric Neurology Principles and Practice, 4th ed. Philadelphia, PA: Mosby Elsevier; 2006.

44. c, 45. e

The disorder depicted is subcortical band heterotopia. The neuronal migration disorder associated with muscular dystrophy is cobblestone lissencephaly (lissencephaly type II, discussed in question 49).

The lissencephaly syndromes result from neuronal migration abnormalities and include subcortical band heterotopia, or double cortex, in which there is relatively normal cortex with an underlying band of white matter, underneath which is a band of gray matter (as shown in Figure 14.4). This disorder results from a mutation in the DCX gene on chromosome X, which encodes for the protein doublecortin, which is involved in microtubule organization and stabilization. The same mutation can lead to classic lissencephaly (smooth brain, agyria, or pachygyria) when occurring in males. This difference in manifestations in females as compared with males is thought to result from lyonization (random X inactivation) in females, such that in neurons in which the mutated gene is inactivated, normal migration occurs. Clinical features include intractable seizures, microcephaly, hypotonia, spastic quadriparesis, recurrent aspirations necessitating feeding tube, and shortened life expectancy.

Lissencephaly type I is discussed in questions 41 and 42; it is characterized by agyria or pachygyria rather than the presence of two bands of gray matter separated by a band of white matter.

Cobblestone lissencephaly (rather than subcortical band heterotopia), or lissencephaly type II, is seen in several disorders, including Walker-Warburg syndrome, Fukuyama muscular dystrophy, and muscle-eye-brain disease of Santavuori. In polymicrogyria, there are excess, abnormal gyri (discussed in question 56).

Bradley WG, Daroff RB, Fenichel GM, et al. Neurology in Clinical Practice, 5th ed. Philadelphia, PA: Elsevier; 2008.

Spalice A, Parisi P, Nicita F, et al. Neuronal migration disorders: clinical, neuroradiologic, and genetic aspects. Acta Paediatr. 2009; 98:421–433.

Swaiman KF, Ashwal S, Ferriero DM. Pediatric Neurology Principles and Practice, 4th ed. Philadelphia, PA: Mosby Elsevier; 2006.

46. e, 47. b, 48. b

The cutaneous findings shown in Figures 14.5, 14.6, and 14.7 are seen in neurofibromatosis type 1 (NF1), or von Recklinghausen disease. NF1 is a neurocutaneous disorder that involves multiple organs including the skin, brain, eyes, and bones. Figure 14.5 depicts hyperpigmented macules known as café au lait spots. Figure 14.6 depicts cutaneous neurofibromas, and Figure 14.7 depicts axillary freckling. The patients depicted in questions 46 and 48 meet diagnostic criteria for NF1.

In order for a diagnosis of NF1 to be made, two or more of the following must be present:

- Six or more café au lait macules measuring more than 5 mm in diameter in prepubertal children or more than 15 mm in diameter postpuberty
- Two or more cutaneous neurofibromas or one plexiform neurofibroma (see question 54)
- Inguinal or axillary freckling (as shown in Figure 14.7)
- Optic nerve gliomas
- Two or more Lisch nodules
- NF1 diagnosed in a first-degree relative
- Sphenoid wing dysplasia, pseudoarthrosis, or cortical thinning of long bones

Café au lait spots may be seen in localized, segmental form in isolation in the setting of post-somatic mutations in the NF1 gene.

In contrast to café au lait spots, ashleaf spots are hypopigmented and are seen in tuberous sclerosis complex (TSC, discussed in questions 61 to 63). Shagreen patches are connective tissue hamartomas also seen in tuberous sclerosis. Plexiform neurofibromas are discussed in question 54.

The other disorders listed are also neurocutaneous disorders, collectively known as the phakomatoses. Unlike NF1, neurofibromatosis type 2 (NF2) is not diagnosed by the presence of specific cutaneous findings but rather by other criteria (see questions 85 and 86). Sturge-Weber syndrome is marked by the presence of hemangiomas. TSC and epidermal nevus syndrome have specific cutaneous findings that differ from NF1.

Bradley WG, Daroff RB, Fenichel GM, et al. Neurology in Clinical Practice, 5th ed. Philadelphia, PA: Elsevier; 2008.

Swaiman KF, Ashwal S, Ferriero DM. Pediatric Neurology Principles and Practice, 4th ed. Philadelphia, PA: Mosby Elsevier; 2006.

49. e

The cobblestone lissencephalies are mainly autosomal recessive in inheritance although X-linked forms have also been identified.

Cobblestone lissencephaly, or lissencephaly type II, is a neuronal migration disorder in which the cortical gray matter has reduced number of gyri and sulci that appear like cobblestones. There is reduced and abnormal white matter, and the cerebellum and brain stem are hypoplastic. Microscopically, the cortex has no recognizable layers. Hydrocephalus frequently occurs because of the presence of fibroglial bands and abnormal vascular channels disrupting the subarachnoid space. Cobblestone lissencephaly is seen in three autosomal recessive syndromes: Walker-Warburg syndrome, Fukuyama muscular dystrophy, and muscle-eye-brain disease of Santavuori. These three syndromes share similar clinical features, including microcephaly, global developmental delay, epilepsy, hypotonia, and evidence of muscular dystrophy.

Walker-Warburg is the most severe form. Several gene mutations have been identified in patients with Walker-Walburg and muscle-eye-brain disease of Santavuori. Eye abnormalities in the latter two conditions include retinal hypoplasia, optic nerve atrophy, glaucoma, and cataracts. Muscle-eye-brain disease of Santavuori is seen most commonly in Finland but also occurs in other European populations. Fukuyama muscular dystrophy, which results from a mutation in the gene fukutin, is most common in Japan and is rare in other populations. It has the least amount of cortical abnormalities, but the muscular dystrophy is severe with progressive weakness and joint contractures. An elevated level of serum creatine kinase is seen.

Bradley WG, Daroff RB, Fenichel GM, et al. Neurology in Clinical Practice, 5th ed. Philadelphia, PA: Elsevier; 2008.

Spalice A, Parisi P, Nicita F, et al. Neuronal migration disorders: clinical, neuroradiologic and genetic aspects. Acta Paediatr. 2009; 98:421–433.

Swaiman KF, Ashwal S, Ferriero DM. Pediatric Neurology Principles and Practice, 4th ed. Philadelphia, PA: Mosby Elsevier; 2006.

50. e

This patient has homocystinuria, in which methionine levels in the plasma and CSF are elevated.

Homocysteine, when condensed with serine, can be converted to cystathionine, a step catalyzed by the enzyme cystathionine-β-synthase. Cystathionine is subsequently converted to cysteine. Homocysteine can also be methylated to methionine, a step that requires vitamin B_{12}.

Homocystinuria is an autosomal recessive condition caused by a deficiency of the enzyme cystathionine-β-synthase. Deficiency of this enzyme produces an elevation of blood and urine levels of homocysteine and methionine. There are two variants of this condition, one that is pyridoxine responsive and another that is not, suggesting some residual activity of the cystathionine-β-synthase in the former type.

Patients with homocystinuria are normal at birth but will later have developmental delay and mental retardation. Some have seizures and psychiatric manifestations. Given the accumulation of homocysteine, collagen metabolism is affected, leading to involvement of other organs such as the eye, bones, and the vascular system. These patients have ectopia lentis and eventually may suffer lens dislocation. They have a marfanoid habitus and are tall and thin, with pectus carinatum, pes cavus, genu valgum, and osteoporosis. Vascular involvement is characterized by intimal thickening of the blood vessel walls and high incidence of thromboembolism, including strokes that may occur at early ages. There is elevation of plasma homocysteine levels, urine homocysteine concentration, and methionine levels in the plasma and CSF. Cystathionine-β-synthase enzyme activity is reduced.

All patients should be first treated with pyridoxine, since there is a pyridoxine-responsive variant. Even if there is no response, patients should be given pyridoxine daily. All patients require a low-protein diet, and specifically a diet low in methionine with cysteine supplementation. Betaine is a substance that lowers plasma homocysteine level by promoting its conversion to methionine. Folate and vitamin B_{12} also promote the conversion of homocysteine to methionine and decrease the levels of homocysteine.

This condition is screened for by extended newborn screening, thus allowing for presymptomatic treatment in most patients with the classic or severe form of the disease.

Fenichel GM. Clinical Pediatric Neurology: A Signs and Symptoms Approach, 6th ed. Philadelphia, PA: Saunders Elsevier; 2009.

51. c, 52. b

Figure 14.8 shows Lisch nodules, or iris melanocytic hamartomas, that are pathognomonic for neurofibromatosis type 1 (NF1). Lisch nodules do not have any clinical implications beyond their occurrence in NF1; they do not cause symptoms or progress to other ophthalmologic abnormalities. They most commonly appear after the age of 6 years and most commonly in adolescence and young adulthood, and their absence does not exclude the diagnosis of NF1. Asymptomatic retinal hamartomas less commonly occur in NF1 as well. Congenital or childhood glaucoma is another ophthalmologic manifestation of NF1. The diagnostic criteria for NF1 are discussed in questions 46 to 48.

Kayser-Fleisher rings are seen in Wilson disease. Brushfield spots are white spots in the iris seen in Down syndrome. Iris colobomas (defects in the iris) are seen in a variety of disorders, including epidermal nevus syndrome and CHARGE syndrome (coloboma, heart defects, atresia of the choanae, retardation of development, genitourinary abnormalities, ear abnormalities), but not in NF1. Iris mamillations are hyperpigmented iris lesions that can be confused with Lisch nodules.

Bradley WG, Daroff RB, Fenichel GM, et al. Neurology in Clinical Practice, 5th ed. Philadelphia, PA: Elsevier; 2008.

Neurofibromatosis Conference Statement. National Institutes of Health Consensus Development Conference. Arch Neurol. 1988; 45:575–578.

Swaiman KF, Ashwal S, Ferriero DM. Pediatric Neurology Principles and Practice, 4th ed. Philadelphia, PA: Mosby Elsevier; 2006.

53. a

A heterotopia is a cluster of abnormally located neurons that are otherwise normal in morphology. Heterotopias result from abnormal neuronal migration. The most common form of heteropia is periventricular nodular heterotopia (also known as subependymal nodular heterotopia), located, as the name implies, near the lateral ventricles, but heterotopias can be found in various regions (such as subcortical nodular heterotopias, or transmantle heterotopias, which extend from the ventricles to the cortex).

In periventricular nodular heterotopia, neurons are thought to have never begun migration but rather remained in the subventricular area (where cortical neurons originate). This disorder is most often bilateral, but it can also be unilateral. In more than half of cases, this disorder results from mutations in the FLNa gene on chromosome X. This FLNa gene encodes a protein involved in actin cytoskeleton reorganization, and abnormalities in this protein lead to disruption in cell migration by impeding the generation of forces needed for cell movement. Periventricular nodular heterotopias may be seen in isolation or as part of a syndrome associated with multiple other anomalies. Epilepsy is a common clinical manifestation, with partial seizures being most common. Intelligence may be entirely normal; males are more likely to have developmental delay.

Spalice A, Parisi P, Nicita F, et al. Neuronal migration disorders: clinical, neuroradiologic and genetic aspects. Acta Paediatr. 2009; 98:421–433.

Swaiman KF, Ashwal S, Ferriero DM. Pediatric Neurology Principles and Practice, 4th ed. Philadelphia, PA: Mosby Elsevier; 2006.

54. e

Figure 14.9 depicts a plexiform neurofibroma. Plexiform neurofibromas enlarge in approximately half of patients, particularly when they are present prior to the age of 10 years.

Neurofibromas, seen in neurofibromatosis type 1 (NF1, discussed in questions 46 to 48), occur in two types: cutaneous neurofibromas, as shown in Figure 14.6, which originate in the dermis or adjacent layers, and plexiform neurofibromas, which originate in peripheral nerves. They consist predominantly of Schwann cells and fibroblasts but also contain mast cells. Plexiform neurofibromas may occur in the face and can be disfiguring; invasion into the overlying skin causes hypertrophy, hyperpigmentation, and thickening of the skin. Neurofibromas that arise from dorsal root ganglia can grow in a dumbbell shape, invading the spinal canal and leading to nerve root and even spinal cord compression. Neurofibromas can arise also in the gastrointestinal tract, leading to intestinal obstruction or gastrointestinal hemorrhage.

As mentioned, in approximately half of patients, plexiform neurofibromas enlarge and can become disfiguring when superficial, particularly when present from an early age (before the age of 10 years). These lesions should be monitored closely, since in a minority, they can undergo malignant degeneration into a malignant peripheral nerve sheath tumor.

Bradley WG, Daroff RB, Fenichel GM, et al. Neurology in Clinical Practice, 5th ed. Philadelphia, PA: Elsevier; 2008.

Swaiman KF, Ashwal S, Ferriero DM. Pediatric Neurology Principles and Practice, 4th ed. Philadelphia, PA: Mosby Elsevier; 2006.

55. b

Urea cycle disorders are a group of conditions caused by deficiency of enzymes responsible for urea synthesis and more importantly ammonia and ammonia-containing compound removal. Ornithine transcarbamylase (OTC) deficiency is the most common and is X-linked. The other ones are inherited in an autosomal recessive fashion and include carbamyl phosphate synthetase deficiency, argininosuccinic acid synthetase deficiency, argininosuccinic acid lyase deficiency, and arginase deficiency. These enzyme defects will lead to hyperammonemia, which is the main cause of the clinical manifestations. Ammonia induces glutamine accumulation, which leads to astrocyte swelling and brain edema.

The triad of hyperammonemia, encephalopathy, and respiratory alkalosis is suggestive of this group of disorders. These patients have very high concentrations of ammonia, no evidence of organic acidemias, normal anion gaps, and normal serum glucose level. Amino acid analyses help to distinguish specific urea cycle disorders, and enzyme activity can be evaluated in liver biopsy specimens.

Clinical manifestations often begin in the newborn period with progressive lethargy, vomiting, hypotonia, and seizures. Higher levels of ammonia may be associated with coma and eventually death. Females with OTC deficiency, and some patients with partial deficiencies, may have late-onset presentations and become symptomatic after large amounts of protein ingestion or intercurrent illnesses. Arginase deficiency does not cause symptoms in the newborn, whereas newborn presentation is common in the rest of urea cycle disorders.

Treatment includes limitation of nitrogen intake in the diet and administration of essential amino acids. Calories can be supplied with carbohydrates and fat. During acute episodes, sodium benzoate and sodium phenylacetic acid are used, and sometimes dialysis may be required. Mannitol has been used for brain edema and increased intracranial pressure. Long-term treatment with low-protein diet and essential amino acids, as well as arginine supplementation (except in arginase deficiency), may stabilize the neurologic deterioration.

Fenichel GM. Clinical Pediatric Neurology: A Signs and Symptoms Approach, 6th ed. Philadelphia, PA: Saunders Elsevier; 2009.

56. d

Porencephaly is distinguished from schizencephaly in that the cleft of schizencephaly is lined uniformly with gray matter. Porencephalic cysts are not due to malformations of cortical development but are rather CSF-filled cysts that most often result from in utero infarction or other insult.

In malformations of cortical organization, neurons migrate relatively normally but formation of the cortical layers or cortical-cortical connections are abnormal. These thus occur later in gestation. Malformations of cortical organization include polymicrogyria, in which there are excessive abnormal gyri that are small and separated by shallow sulci, and schizencephaly, a deep cleft that extends from the pial surface to the ventricle and is lined with cortex. These often co-occur in the same patient.

Polymicrogyria can be unilateral or bilateral, generalized, perisylvian, predominantly frontal, or in a variety of other patterns. The perisylvian form is the most common. Polymicrogyria often occurs as part of various syndromes, either sporadically or in familial forms. Perisylvian polymicrogyria occurs particularly in the setting of peroxisomal disorders such as Zellweger syndrome. Several genetic mutations have been identified in association with polymicrogyria. Clinical manifestations depend on the location and the extent of the abnormality; epilepsy is common.

Schizencephaly, or cleft brain, most often occurs in the perisylvian region but can occur anywhere. In closed-lip schizencephaly, the cerebral cortical walls on either side of the cleft are in contact. In open-lipped schizencephaly, the two walls are separated by CSF. Schizencephaly is most often an isolated finding or is associated with polymicrogyria but can rarely be seen in patients with septo-optic dysplasia (see question 30). Mutations in homeobox genes, which encode for transcription factors expressed during different times of embryologic development and modulate neuronal proliferation and migration, may be implicated in schizencephaly.

Prayson RA, Goldblum JR. Neuropathology, 1st ed. Philadelphia, PA: Elsevier; 2005.

Spalice A, Parisi P, Nicita F, et al. Neuronal migration disorders: clinical, neuroradiologic and genetic aspects. Acta Paediatr. 2009; 98:421–433.

Swaiman KF, Ashwal S, Ferriero DM. Pediatric Neurology Principles and Practice, 4th ed. Philadelphia, PA: Mosby Elsevier; 2006.

57. c

Schwannomas and ependymomas rarely occur in neurofibromatosis type 1 (NF1); they more commonly occur in neurofibromatosis type 2 (NF2).

Thickening of the left optic nerve as seen in Figure 14.10 likely represents an optic nerve glioma. Optic nerve gliomas are the most common tumor of the CNS seen in NF1 patients and may be unilateral or bilateral. These are often low-grade lesions but may cause symptoms due to mass effect, including diplopia, pain, and proptosis (eye protrusion). Optic pathway gliomas can occur anywhere along the optic pathways, from the optic nerve to the optic radiations. Optic chiasm gliomas may present with precocious puberty when they lead to pressure on diencephalic structures. Because these lesions are often benign, serial imaging over time is often used to monitor these tumors, with chemotherapy, radiation, or surgery instituted as necessary.

Nonspecific subcortical hyperintensities (in the basal ganglia, thalamus, and other regions) are common in NF1 patients and are of unclear etiology and significance.

Figure 14.10 shows enlargement of the pons, which likely represents a low-grade glioma. As mentioned, schwannomas and ependymomas can occur in NF1, but this is rare; they more commonly occur in NF2. NF1 patients are at an increased risk of cerebral, cerebellar, and brain stem astrocytomas. NF1 patients are also at an increased risk for leukemia.

Bradley WG, Daroff RB, Fenichel GM, et al. Neurology in Clinical Practice, 5th ed. Philadelphia, PA: Elsevier; 2008.

Swaiman KF, Ashwal S, Ferriero DM. Pediatric Neurology Principles and Practice, 4th ed. Philadelphia, PA: Mosby Elsevier; 2006.

58. a

The patient's history is consistent with autism. Autistic spectrum disorder is characterized by the triad of impaired social skills, impaired communication skills, and restricted repertoire of activities and interests. Impaired communication skills entail both verbal and nonverbal skills. Social skill abnormalities include lack of eye contact or atypical eye contact, failure to develop peer relationships, and lack of emotional reciprocity. Motor stereotypies, repetitive voluntary behaviors such as those described in the case, lack of flexibility, persistent preoccupation with specific objects or part of an object, and ritualistic patterns of behavior occur. This spectrum is broad, ranging from high-functioning individuals as seen in Asperger disorder to nonverbal children with little interaction and sometimes no language skills. Cognitive delay is not a diagnostic criterion but may be an associated feature, although supranormal IQs may occur in some. Some improvements occur in adolescence, although seizures, mood disorders, or other comorbidities may also emerge.

A genetic basis has been postulated on the basis of high concordance rates among monozygotic twins and increased incidence in families with one child with autism. Neuropathology seen in patients with autism include under-development of limbic structures and reduced cerebellar Purkinje cells. Several genetic and metabolic disorders have been associated with autism, including neurofibromatosis, Down syndrome, fetal alcohol syndrome, and peroxisomal disorders. A diagnostic workup for these disorders based on the patient's history and examination is indicated.

This patient does not meet diagnostic criteria for schizophrenia (see Chapter 13), and the history is not consistent with depression, particularly given his age. Similarly, a diagnosis of personality disorder (see Chapter 13) cannot be made at this time, and although some of the personality disorders include rigid behavior, the symptom complex presented is more consistent with autism.

American Psychiatric Association. Diagnostic and Statistical Manual of Mental Disorders: DSM-IV-TR, 4th ed, text revision. Washington, DC: American Psychiatric Association; 2000.

Bradley WG, Daroff RB, Fenichel GM, et al. Neurology in Clinical Practice, 5th ed. Philadelphia, PA: Elsevier; 2008.

59. C

In Down syndrome, or trisomy 21, the frontal lobes are small and under-developed, and the superior temporal gyri are small and thin.

Developmental delay is defined by performance on standardized tests of function, that is, 2 standard deviations below the mean. Mental retardation is a diagnosis made on the basis of testing intelligence quotient (IQ) and is characterized as mild, moderate, or severe on the basis of the IQ, the degree of impairment, and the level of assistance in daily activities and other activities that are required. Mild mental retardation is defined by an IQ of 55 to 70, whereas severe mental retardation is defined by an IQ of 25 to 40. A myriad of causes for developmental delay exist, including but not limited to genetic disorders, toxin exposure, and metabolic disorders. Some causes of mental retardation due to gross chromosomal abnormalities are discussed later. Some of the other genetic causes of mental retardation are discussed in questions 64 and 65. Some of the acquired causes are discussed in question 68.

Down syndrome, or trisomy 21, results from trisomy of the 21st chromosome or, less commonly, chromosomal translocations. Diagnosis is made in the majority through karyotyping. Increased maternal age is a risk factor. The frontal lobes are small and under-developed, and the superior temporal gyri are small and thin. Clinical features include presence of medial epicanthal folds, slanting palpebral fissures, micrognathia (small mouth) leading to an apparently large tongue, the so-called simian crease (in which there is a single palmar crease), Brushfield spots (white spots of depigmentation in the iris), clinodactyly (incurving of the fingers), short stature, and other features. In addition to varying degrees of mental retardation, seizures, hematologic malignancies, and congenital heart defects occur. Early dementia with Alzheimer type pathology is seen, as the β-amyloid gene is on chromosome 21. These patients are at risk of cervical spinal cord compression due to atlantoaxial instability.

Trisomy 13 or Patau syndrome is characterized by microcephaly, microphthalmia, iris coloboma, low-set ears, cleft lip and palate, polydactyly (excess number of fingers), prominence of the heels, and cardiac abnormalities. Life expectancy is typically not beyond early childhood.

Trisomy 18 is characterized by microcephaly, ptosis, overlapping of the third finger over the second finger, rocker-bottom feet, umbilical hernia, congenital heart disease, and other findings. Life expectancy is typically not beyond early infancy.

In Klinefelter syndrome, two X chromosomes are present in a male: XXY. Clinical features include mental retardation, a wide arm span, high-pitched voice, gynecomastia (enlarged breasts), and small testes.

Ropper AH, Samuels MA. Adams and Victor's Principles of Neurology, 9th ed. New York, NY: McGraw-Hill; 2009.

60. C

The history depicted in question 60 is consistent with Rett syndrome, a syndrome of motor and cognitive regression with eventual severe disability. The presentation is one of initially normal development with subsequent regression at approximately 6 to 18 months of age. Hand wringing and other motor stereotypies are a classic feature; patients with Rett syndrome often place their hands in their mouth or may hold their hands fisted, with their fingers flexed over their thumb. Arrest of head growth with eventual microcephaly, seizures, scoliosis, dysautonomia including respiratory dysfunction with apneas, and spasticity emerge as the disease progresses. It results from various types of mutations in the gene that encodes methyl CpG binding protein 2 (MeCP2), which is involved in binding to methylated DNA, modulating gene expression. It is most often seen in females, and it is thought to be most often fatal in boys, although cases of MeCP2 mutation in male infants and children with mental retardation and other features have been identified. Another disorder of severe mental retardation in females results from a mutation in the gene CDKL5.

Chahrour M, Zoghbi Y. The story of Rett syndrome: from clinic to neurobiology. Neuron. 2007; 56(3):422–437.

Ropper AH, Samuels MA. Adams and Victor's Principles of Neurology, 9th ed. New York, NY: McGraw-Hill; 2009.

61. a, 62. c, 63. a

Given the combination of cutaneous findings shown, ashleaf spots in Figure 14.11, and facial angiofibromas in Figure 14.12, this patient's diagnosis is tuberous sclerosis complex (TSC). TSC is a neurocutaneous disorder that affects multiple organ systems including the skin, brain, heart, lungs, and kidneys among others.

The diagnosis of TSC can be made when two of the following major criteria or one major and two minor criteria are present:

Major criteria: facial angiofibroma (Figure 14.12) or forehead plaque (Figure 14.13); periungual, ungual, or subungual fibroma (Figure 14.14); shagreen patch; more than three hypomelanotic macules (including ashleaf spots, Figure 14.11); retinal hamartomas; cortical tubers; subependymal nodules (see Figure 14.17); subependymal giant cell astrocytoma (see Figure 14.15), cardiac rhabdomyoma, lymphangiomyomatosis, or renal angiomyolipoma.

Minor criteria: dental pits, rectal hamartomatous polyps, bone cysts, radial migration lines in the cerebral white matter, gingival fibromas, nonrenal hamartomas, retinal achromic patches, confetti skin lesions (hypopigmented, stippled lesions on the extremities), and multiple renal cysts.

Figure 14.11 shows three hypopigmented (hypomelanotic) patches known as ashleaf spots. These are not specific for TSC but occur in the majority of patients with TSC and are often present at birth but become more obvious with age; in newborns, examination under ultraviolet light makes them more apparent. Tinea corporis, a fungal infection, also leads to circular lesions on the trunk, but tinea has a different appearance.

Figure 14.12 shows facial angiofibromas, also known as adenoma sebaceum, which are hamartomatous lesions consisting of vascular and connective tissue. They often become apparent in early childhood as papules in the malar region and become more apparent and numerous with time: they characteristically progress to involve the nasolabial folds and sometimes the chin. Facial angiofibromas may resemble acne if not examined closely and if other historical and clinical features are not taken into consideration. Shagreen patches are cutaneous hamartomas that have irregular borders and are raised. Shagreen patches most often occur on the trunk (back or flank). These lesions may not be present in childhood but may appear later in life. Hamartomas can occur in a variety of body parts in TSC including the retina and gastrointestinal tract.

The other disorders listed in the choices are also neurocutaneous disorders but with distinct cutaneous and other clinical features and with specific diagnostic criteria. Cutaneous neurofibromas are shown in Figure 14.6 and café au lait spots in Figure 14.5; these occur in neurofibromatosis (discussed in questions 46 to 48). Hypomelanosis of Ito is associated with hypopigmented lesions that may be patchy but more often follow skin lines, in streaks (discussed in question 43). Sturge-Weber syndrome is discussed in questions 80 and 81 and epidermal nevus syndrome in question 93.

Bradley WG, Daroff RB, Fenichel GM, et al. Neurology in Clinical Practice, 5th ed. Philadelphia, PA: Elsevier; 2008.

Roach ES, Gomez MR, Northrup H. Tuberous sclerosis complex consensus conference: revised clinical diagnostic criteria. J Child Neurol. 1998; 13(12):624–628.

Swaiman KF, Ashwal S, Ferriero DM. Pediatric Neurology Principles and Practice, 4th ed. Philadelphia, PA: Mosby Elsevier; 2006.

64. e

There are a variety of causes of mental retardation. Fragile X syndrome is the most common inherited form of mental retardation. It results from expansion of the CGG repeat in the familial mental retardation 1 gene on chromosome X. The function of this gene is yet to be fully elucidated (as of 2010). Because this gene is on the X chromosome, and because random X inactivation (lyonization) occurs in females, females are less often and less severely affected. Clinical manifestations in males include an elongated face, with a high forehead and elongated jaw, and protuberant ears and enlarged testes. The degree of mental retardation ranges from mild and subtle to severe. A family history of mental retardation in males may be present. In adults with a premutation, other neurologic manifestations may occur (see Chapter 6).

Ropper AH, Samuels MA. Adams and Victor's Principles of Neurology, 9th ed. New York, NY: McGraw-Hill; 2009.

65. b

There are various causes of mental retardation. Prader-Willi syndrome is a genetic disorder characterized by infantile hypotonia, short stature, dysmorphic facies including a wide mouth, small feet, developmental delay, hypogonadism, hyperphagia, and obesity. Infants feed poorly, but then become hyperphagic when older. Another disorder associated with developmental delay and obesity is Laurence-Moon syndrome.

Angelman syndrome is a genetically related disorder characterized by mental retardation, microcephaly, intractable epilepsy, ataxia, inappropriate laughter with a wide-based stance and flailing of the arms at the sides during ambulation (hence the name "happy puppet syndrome"), prominent jaw with thin upper lip, and impaired speech development. Another genetic disorder associated with developmental delay and a happy affect is William syndrome, which is associated with congenital heart disease.

Prader-Willi and Angelman syndrome both result from a microdeletion on chromosome 15q11-q13. The same mutation leads to Prader-Willi syndrome when it is paternally inherited and to Angelman syndrome when it is maternally inherited, so-called imprinting.

Cri-du-chat syndrome is characterized by an abnormal, cat-like cry, mental retardation, presence of epicanthal folds, hypertelorism (in which the eyes are farther apart than normal), micrognathia, and other features. It is caused by a deletion on chromosome 5p.

Rett syndrome is discussed in question 60.

Ropper AH, Samuels MA. Adams and Victor's Principles of Neurology, 9th ed. New York, NY: McGraw-Hill; 2009.

66. b

In methylmalonic acidemia, propionyl-CoA accumulates, and its levels are increased.

Methylmalonic acidemia is an autosomal recessive condition caused by the deficiency of D-methylmalonyl-CoA mutase. This enzyme normally catalyzes the isomerization of L-methylmalonyl-CoA to succinyl-CoA, which then enters the Krebs cycle. Adenosylcobalamin is a required cofactor. A defect in this metabolic pathway leads to accumulation of propionyl-CoA, propionic acid, and methylmalonic acid, causing metabolic acidosis, hyperglycinemia, and hyperammonemia.

These children appear normal at birth, becoming symptomatic within the first week of life, manifesting with lethargy, failure to thrive, vomiting, dehydration, hypotonia, and respiratory distress. Hematologic abnormalities, including bleeding disorders leading to intracranial hemorrhage, may also occur. Patients who survive are left with mental retardation, developmental delay, and recurrent acidosis. The diagnosis should be suspected in newborn patients with metabolic acidosis, ketosis, hyperglycinemia, and hyperammonemia. Methylmalonic acid is elevated in plasma and urine, and the enzyme activity can be analyzed in fibroblasts.

These patients should be treated with protein restriction and supplementation of hydroxycobalamin and carnitine. Antibiotics are also helpful to reduce the production of propionic acid. In the acute setting, these patients need hydration and glucose administration with discontinuation of protein intake.

This condition is screened for by extended newborn screening, thus allowing for presymptomatic treatment in most patients with the classic or severe form of the disease.

Fenichel GM. Clinical Pediatric Neurology: A Signs and Symptoms Approach, 6th ed. Philadelphia, PA: Saunders Elsevier; 2009.

67. a

Figure 14.13 shows a forehead plaque. This is one of the cutaneous findings of tuberous sclerosis complex and is one of the major criteria for diagnosis (discussed in question 61 to 63). Neurofibromatosis type 1 is discussed in questions 46 to 48. Hypomelanosis of Ito is discussed in question 43. Sturge-Weber syndrome is discussed in questions 80 and 81 and epidermal nevus syndrome in question 93.

Bradley WG, Daroff RB, Fenichel GM, et al. Neurology in Clinical Practice, 5th ed. Philadelphia, PA: Elsevier; 2008.

Swaiman KF, Ashwal S, Ferriero DM. Pediatric Neurology Principles and Practice, 4th ed. Philadelphia, PA: Mosby Elsevier; 2006.

68. e

In utero exposure to alcohol has been associated with congenital heart disease.

There are a myriad of established or suspected exposures associated with mental retardation. Congenital infections such as cytomegalovirus and rubella lead to mental retardation with a variety of other features such as congenital blindness and periventricular calcifications. Environmental exposures including exposure to radiation during the first trimester of pregnancy have also been associated with mental retardation. Malnutrition during the first few months of life can lead to reversible cognitive delay. Maternal intake of alcohol, antiepileptics, vitamin A, and thalidomide are also linked to various nervous system and systemic malformations as well as mental retardation, as are several other agents.

Maternal alcohol intake is a common cause of acquired (nongenetic) mental retardation. Other features of fetal alcohol syndrome include behavioral problems such as hyperactivity, microcephaly, short palpebral fissure (a short distance between the inner and outer canthi of the eyes), presence of epicanthal folds, hypoplasia of the maxilla, micrognathia, and thin upper lip with flattened philtrum. Congenital heart disease is also part of fetal alcohol syndrome.

Bradley WG, Daroff RB, Fenichel GM, et al. Neurology in Clinical Practice. 5th ed. Philadelphia, PA: Elsevier; 2008.

Ropper AH, Samuels MA. Adams and Victor's Principles of Neurology, 9th ed. New York, NY: McGraw-Hill; 2009.

69. d

Figure 14.14 shows a periungual fibroma. This is one of the cutaneous findings of tuberous sclerosis complex (TSC) and is one of the major criteria for diagnosis (discussed in questions 61 to 63). This should be distinguished from traumatic periungual hematomas, which are typically darker in color and resolve with time. Subungual fibromas occur under the nail and are also one of the major criteria for TSC. Cutaneous neurofibromas are shown in Figure 14.6. Angiokeratomas are purplish lesions seen in intertriginous regions in patients with Fabry disease.

Bradley WG, Daroff RB, Fenichel GM, et al. Neurology in Clinical Practice, 5th ed. Philadelphia, PA: Elsevier; 2008.

Roach ES, Gomez MR, Northrup H. Tuberous sclerosis complex consensus conference: revised linical diagnostic criteria. J Child Neurol. 1998; 13(12):624–628.

Swaiman KF, Ashwal S, Ferriero DM. Pediatric Neurology Principles and Practice, 4th ed. Philadelphia, PA: Mosby Elsevier; 2006.

70. a

Biotin is a water soluble B-complex vitamin that is necessary in multiple metabolic reactions including gluconeogenesis, fatty acid synthesis, catabolism of amino acids, and gene expression. Its deficiency can be caused by biotinidase deficiency. This enzyme normally cleaves biocytin, thereby recycling biotin, and also participates in processing of dietary protein-bound biotin, making it available to the free biotin pool. Biotinidase deficiency has previously been known as late-onset multiple carboxylase deficiency, and it is inherited in an autosomal recessive fashion.

Children with this enzymatic defect manifest with seizures, hypotonia, ataxia, developmental delay, hearing and visual loss, spastic paraparesis, and cutaneous abnormalities, including alopecia. Laboratory studies demonstrate ketoacidosis, hyperammonemia, and organic aciduria. The enzyme activity can be analyzed in serum.

Treatment is biotin supplementation, which prevents mental retardation and reverses most of the symptoms.

This condition is screened for by extended newborn screening, thus allowing for presymptomatic treatment in most patients with the classic or severe form of the disease.

Fauci AS, Braunwald E, Kasper DL, et al. Harrison's Principles of Internal Medicine, 17th ed. New York, NY: McGraw-Hill; 2008.

Fenichel GM. Clinical Pediatric Neurology: A Signs and Symptoms Approach, 6th ed. Philadelphia, PA: Saunders Elsevier; 2009.

Wolf B. Biotinidase: its role in biotinidase deficiency and biotin metabolism. J Nutr Biochem. 2005; 16:441–445.

71. e

The molar tooth sign (discussed in question 23) is seen in various disorders associated with cerebellar hypoplasia, including Joubert syndrome, COACH syndrome (cerebellar vermis hypoplasia, oligophrenia, congenital ataxia, coloboma, and hepatic fibrocirrhosis), and Leber congenital amaurosis. However, this radiologic sign is not seen in Dandy-Walker malformation. Dandy-Walker malformation is characterized by cerebellar vermis hypoplasia, fourth ventricular cystic dilatation, and elevation of the torcula and the tentorium cerebelli. Posterior fossa enlargement and hydrocephalus are common. It is associated with various chromosomal anomalies. Neural tube defects, including encephalocele, and anomalies in other organ systems, including the heart, may occur. Another association is with facial hemangiomas.

Clinical presentation is variable and depends on the presence of hydrocephalus and associated anomalies. In severe forms, there is neonatal macrocephaly from hydrocephalus, brain stem dysfunction, and feeding and respiratory problems. Severe developmental delay and ataxia may be present. However, in other cases, no symptoms may be present and the malformation may be detected only incidentally on imaging in adulthood. Treatment involves surgical management of hydrocephalus and supportive care.

Swaiman KF, Ashwal S, Ferriero DM. Pediatric Neurology Principles and Practice, 4th ed. Philadelphia, PA: Mosby Elsevier; 2006.

72. a

Subependymal giant cell astrocytoma (SEGA) is an uncommon tumor, but it is seen almost exclusively in patients with tuberous sclerosis complex (TSC) and is a major diagnostic criterion for TSC (questions 61 to 63). This is a benign, low-grade astrocytoma but leads to symptoms due to mass effect and ventricular obstruction. Surgery is usually curative. Rapamycin may be of benefit in the treatment of SEGA. SEGA does not typically occur in the other neurocutaneous disorders described. Neurofibromatosis type 1 (NF1) is discussed in questions 46 to 48, neurofibromatosis type 2 (NF2) is discussed in questions 85 and 86, and Sturge-Weber syndrome is discussed in questions 80 and 81.

Bradley WG, Daroff RB, Fenichel GM, et al. Neurology in Clinical Practice, 5th ed. Philadelphia, PA: Elsevier; 2008.

Swaiman KF, Ashwal S, Ferriero DM. Pediatric Neurology Principles and Practice, 4th ed. Philadelphia, PA: Mosby Elsevier; 2006.

73. e

Betz cells are the upper motor neurons of the nervous system; these are large cells found in the primary motor cortex.

The majority of the cerebral cortex (>90%) consists of neocortex (also known as isocortex), a six-layered cortex (as opposed to more primitive cortex with less numbers of layers, as occurs in the paleocortex (found in olfactory and limbic cortices) and archicortex, seen in the hippocampus). The six layers of the neocortex are molecular layer (layer I, deepest), external granular cell layer (layer II), external pyramidal cell layer (layer III), internal granular cell layer (layer IV), internal pyramidal cell layer (layer V), and multiform layer (layer VI, most superficial). Corticocortical efferents (projections from one area of cortex to another) arise mainly in layer III and project predominantly to layers II and III. Layers I, IV, and VI receive the majority of thalamic efferents. Layer V gives rise to corticostriate projections (from cortex to striatum), and layer VI gives rise to corticothalamic projections (from cortex to thalamus).

Pyramidal cells constitute the largest number of cortical neurons and are found in highest numbers in cortical areas that give rise to efferents; granular (or stellate) cells function predominantly as cortical interneurons and predominate in regions involved in sensory function or integration (secondary association cortices, etc.). Betz cells are the upper motor neurons of the nervous system; these are large cells found in layer V of the primary motor cortex.

Formation of gyri and sulci normally occurs between weeks 20 and 36 of gestation. Abnormalities in this process can lead to a variety of malformations of cortical development.

Prayson RA, Goldblum JR. Neuropathology, 1st ed. Philadelphia, PA: Elsevier; 2005.

74. a

This patient has Gaucher disease, which is inherited in an autosomal recessive fashion and is caused by deficiency of the enzyme glucocerebrosidase (acid β-glucosylceramidase) leading to lysosomal accumulation of glucocerebrosides (glucosylceramide). It is caused by mutations in the gene GBA on chromosome 1q21 and is more common in Ashkenazi Jews.

There are three phenotypes:

- Type 1 is the most common and does not involve the CNS. It is characterized by hepatosplenomegaly with anemia and thrombocytopenia, skeletal involvement, and pulmonary infiltrates.
- Type 2 has its onset before the age of 2 years, with psychomotor involvement, spasticity, choreoathetosis, oculomotor abnormalities, and progresses to death by 2 to 4 years of age. These patients may also have hepatosplenomegaly, hydrops fetalis, and cutaneous changes.
- Type 3 begins after the age of 2 years and progresses slowly, with hepatosplenomegaly, psychomotor deterioration, spasticity, ataxia, and oculomotor involvement.

The diagnosis can be made with an analysis of the enzyme β-glucosylceramidase or glucocerebrosidase in leukocytes. This enzyme can also be tested for in amniocytes and through chorionic villous sampling, allowing for prenatal diagnosis.

Gaucher cells are caused by the lysosomal storage of glucocerebroside in macrophages. These cells are found in the liver, spleen, lymph nodes, and bone marrow, and have large a cytoplasm with striated appearance, what has been likened to "wrinkled tissue paper." In the CNS, the brain stem and deep nuclei are most severely affected, and neuronal degeneration is seen, likely from neurotoxic action of glucosylsphingosine.

Enzyme replacement with imiglucerase can be effective for liver and spleen involvement and for the hematologic abnormalities. Type 3 may benefit from bone marrow transplantation.

Fenichel GM. Clinical Pediatric Neurology: A Signs and Symptoms Approach, 6th ed. Philadelphia, PA: Saunders Elsevier; 2009.

Prayson RA, Goldblum JR. Neuropathology, 1st ed. Philadelphia, PA: Elsevier; 2005.

75. e

Figure 14.16 shows multiple hyperintense lesions in the cortex and gray-white junction. These are cortical tubers, also known as cortical hamartomas, findings seen in tuberous sclerosis complex (TSC). Cortical tubers contain large bizarre neurons, abnormal glia, predominantly astrocytes, and hypomyelinated axons. These lesions are not premalignant.

CNS manifestations of TSC include mental retardation, although up to half of the patients with TSC have normal intelligence. Seizures occur in the majority of TSC patients; the majority of patients with TSC and mental retardation will have seizures, but not all TSC patients with seizures will have mental retardation. A variety of seizure types may occur in patients with TSC; TSC is the most common cause of infantile spasms and, in such cases, treatment with vigabatrin is often of benefit. Other common neuropsychiatric manifestations of TSC include behavioral problems including attention-deficit/hyperactivity disorder and learning disabilities. The burden of cortical tubers correlates to some extent with cognitive function and presence, frequency, and severity of seizures.

Bradley WG, Daroff RB, Fenichel GM, et al. Neurology in Clinical Practice, 5th ed. Philadelphia, PA: Elsevier; 2008.

Swaiman KF, Ashwal S, Ferriero DM. Pediatric Neurology Principles and Practice, 4th ed. Philadelphia, PA: Mosby Elsevier; 2006.

76. b, 77. b

The patient in question 76 has a GM2 gangliosidosis, more specifically Tay-Sachs disease caused by hexosaminidase A deficiency. The patient in question 77 has another GM2 gangliosidosis, more specifically Sandhoff disease caused by deficiency of hexosaminidase A and B.

β-Galactosidase deficiency causes GM1 but not GM2 gangliosidosis. Sphingomyelinase deficiency causes Niemann-Pick types A and B.

GM2 gangliosidosis is caused by deficiency of hexosaminidase A in Tay-Sachs disease or hexosaminidase A and B in Sandhoff disease. Both are autosomal recessive.

Tay-Sachs disease or infantile GM2 gangliosidosis is more common in Ashkenazi Jews but may also occur in other populations with less frequency, and the CNS is the only affected organ. Onset is between 3 and 6 months of age, with increased startle response and subsequent motor regression, spasticity, blindness with optic atrophy, and seizures. There is a delay in reaching developmental milestones, with subsequent regression. A cherry-red spot in the macula is commonly seen, and these patients have macrocephaly. Progression to severe mental retardation occurs, and most children die by the age of 5 years. The diagnosis is suspected in patients with psychomotor retardation and a cherry-red spot and is confirmed with the detection of hexosaminidase A deficiency with normal activity of hexosaminidase B. Treatment is supportive.

Sandhoff disease occurs from combined deficiency of hexosaminidase A and B. The clinical features are similar to those seen in Tay-Sachs disease; however, as mentioned, in Tay-Sachs disease, the brain is the only organ involved, whereas in Sandhoff disease, the GM2 gangliosides accumulate in the brain and viscera, causing hepatosplenomegaly that is not seen in Tay-Sachs disease. The diagnosis is based on these clinical features and confirmed with analysis of the enzymatic activity of the enzymes involved.

Fenichel GM. Clinical Pediatric Neurology: A Signs and Symptoms Approach, 6th ed. Philadelphia, PA: Saunders Elsevier; 2009.

Prayson RA, Goldblum JR. Neuropathology, 1st ed. Philadelphia, PA: Elsevier; 2005.

78. d

Figure 14.17 shows multiple periventricular hyperdense lesions. These are known as subependymal nodules, and their presence is one of the major diagnostic criteria of tuberous sclerosis complex (TSC, see question 61 to 63). Subependymal nodules, as their name suggest, most commonly occur in the periventricular region, often at the caudo-thalamic groove. They are thought to arise from remnants of the germinal matrix. They have the potential to grow over time and, in a minority, transform into subependymal giant cell astrocytoma (see question 72). Unlike cortical tubers (discussed in question 75), the presence and number of subependymal nodules are not thought to correlate with cognitive function or seizures.

Benign hereditary calcification of the basal ganglia (Fahr disease, see Chapter 6) is on the differential diagnosis of subcortical calcifications, but the distribution of these calcifications is typically within the striatum or thalamus and they are not as nodular as these subependymal nodules are. There is no association between TSC and Fahr disease.

Bradley WG, Daroff RB, Fenichel GM, et al. Neurology in Clinical Practice, 5th ed. Philadelphia, PA: Elsevier; 2008.

Swaiman KF, Ashwal S, Ferriero DM. Pediatric Neurology Principles and Practice, 4th ed. Philadelphia, PA: Mosby Elsevier; 2006.

79. a

This patient has Canavan disease, which is an autosomal recessive disorder caused by deficiency of aspartoacylase, leading to accumulation of N-acetylaspartic acid in the brain. This condition occurs more commonly in Ashkenazi Jews, and the gene alteration is on chromosome 17p13. These patients have an onset of symptoms between 10 weeks and 4 months of life and present with poor fixation and tracking, psychomotor arrest and regression, irritability, feeding difficulties, hypotonia with poor head control and inability to sit, and subsequent spasticity. Megalencephaly (enlarged brain) is present.

Urinary N-acetylaspartic acid level is elevated, and MRI demonstrates diffuse symmetric T2 hyperintensity in the white matter, with characteristic involvement of the U fibers. MR spectroscopy shows an increased peak of N-acetylaspartic acid. CSF is normal and there is no inflammation. There is no specific treatment available.

Adrenoleukodystrophy is discussed in question 31. Alexander disease is discussed in question 88. Zellweger syndrome is discussed in question 28. Fabry disease is discussed in questions 24 and 29.

Fenichel GM. Clinical Pediatric Neurology: A Signs and Symptoms Approach, 6th ed. Philadelphia, PA: Saunders Elsevier; 2009.

Prayson RA, Goldblum JR. Neuropathology, 1st ed. Philadelphia, PA: Elsevier; 2005.

80. d, 81. e

This patient has Sturge-Weber syndrome, in which gyral calcifications result from angiomatosis of the leptomeninges and brain. Sturge-Weber syndrome is a neurocutaneous disorder characterized by the presence of cutaneous angioma of the face, also known as the port-wine nevus, which often occurs in a trigeminal distribution, as seen in Figure 14.18a, but may involve any part of the body. Associated features in some cases include angiomatosis of the ipsilateral and less commonly bilateral leptomeninges and the cortex, as seen in Figure 14.18b.

Some patients have only cutaneous findings without CNS involvement; this is most often the case if cutaneous angiomas are present only in the limbs (without facial involvement). Neurologic manifestations are variable; some patients may have no neurologic signs or symptoms, whereas others may have seizures, contralateral hemiparesis, and/or developmental delay. CNS involvement is most common in those with cutaneous angiomas involving the face. Cobb syndrome, or cutaneomeningospinal angiomatosis, is a variant of Sturge-Weber syndrome (SWS) in which cutaneous angiomas occur in a dermatome corresponding to a spinal dural angioma. Glaucoma may be a complication of Sturge-Weber syndrome but presenile cataracts are not. The pathophysiology of SWS is thought to relate to persistence of embryonal blood vessels that normally regress during gestation; it is considered a congenital malformation rather than a genetic disorder and is not hereditary.

The classic radiographic finding is one of gyral calcifications giving a tram-track appearance that may be initially best seen on a CT scan. Cerebral hemiatrophy, rather than hemimegalencephaly, is also seen, as shown in Figure 14.18b. MRA is useful in assessing the extent of intracranial involvement. Cerebral venous thrombosis may occur uncommonly.

The other options listed are also neurocutaneous syndromes but each with distinct cutaneous and other neurologic findings. Neurocutaneous melanosis and incontinentia pigmenti are discussed in question 37, Hypomelanosis of Ito in question 43, and epidermal nevus syndrome in question 93.

Bradley WG, Daroff RB, Fenichel GM, et al. Neurology in Clinical Practice, 5th ed. Philadelphia, PA: Elsevier; 2008.

Swaiman KF, Ashwal S, Ferriero DM. Pediatric Neurology Principles and Practice, 4th ed. Philadelphia, PA: Mosby Elsevier; 2006.

82. d

Neurofibromatosis type 1 (NF1) is an autosomal dominant disorder with markedly variable expression but complete penetrance. It results from a mutation in the neurofibromin gene on chromosome 17. Approximately half of cases are sporadic. Neurofibromin is a tumor suppressor protein that normally activates a GTPase that inhibits ras, a proto-oncogene involved in cell proliferation. More than 100 mutations in the NF1 gene have been identified, but no specific genotype-phenotype correlations occur.

Bradley WG, Daroff RB, Fenichel GM, et al. Neurology in Clinical Practice, 5th ed. Philadelphia, PA: Elsevier; 2008.

Swaiman KF, Ashwal S, Ferriero DM. Pediatric Neurology Principles and Practice, 4th ed. Philadelphia, PA: Mosby Elsevier; 2006.

83. c

The MRI shown in Figure 14.19 shows partial agenesis of the corpus callosum. A diagnosis of glycine encephalopathy (formerly called nonketotic hyperglycinemia) can be made on the basis of this MRI finding, along with the clinical picture and the high CSF glycine levels. Available treatment options for this condition are limited and not effective.

Glycine encephalopathy is an autosomal recessive. The onset is in newborns who, within a few hours after birth, become irritable with poor feeding and hiccups. Subsequently, they develop a progressive encephalopathy with hypotonia, myoclonic seizures, and respiratory failure requiring mechanical ventilation. Patients who survive the acute phase will have mental retardation, spasticity, and epilepsy. Brain MRI may reveal a hypoplastic or absent corpus callosum and gyral malformations and cerebellar hypoplasia. In the acute phase, the EEG shows burst suppression and hypsarrhythmia.

Nonketotic hyperglycinemia or glycine encephalopathy is caused by a defect in the P-protein (glycine decarboxylase) gene, which encodes a component of the mitochondrial glycine cleavage system, therefore affecting the degradation of glycine, with accumulation of this substance. Serum and CSF glycine levels are elevated, and the ratio of CSF to plasma glycine concentration is more than 0.6, whereas normally, it is less than 0.4.

No effective treatments are available; sodium benzoate decreases plasma glycine concentrations, but the CSF level does not normalize with this therapy, and neurologic dysfunction is not reversible. Benzodiazepines can be used for seizures.

Dextromethorphan and ketamine can be used to inhibit NMDA receptor excitation by glycine.

Bradley WG, Daroff RB, Fenichel GM, et al. Neurology in Clinical Practice, 5th ed. Philadelphia, PA: Elsevier; 2008.

Fenichel GM. Clinical Pediatric Neurology: A Signs and Symptoms Approach, 6th ed. Philadelphia, PA: Saunders Elsevier; 2009.

84. C

This patient has Krabbe disease on the basis of the history and histopathologic findings.

Krabbe disease or globoid cell leukodystrophy is a disorder with autosomal recessive inheritance, with the affected gene mapped to chromosome 14. This disorder is characterized by the accumulation of galactocerebroside in macrophages of the white matter in the CNS, leading to the formation of globoid cells and to progressive demyelination, but with sparing of the U fibers. The cause is a deficiency of the enzyme galactosylceramidase (also known as galactocerebroside β-galactosidase). It can involve the peripheral nervous system, leading to a demyelinating neuropathy, but affects predominantly the CNS.

There are three forms:

- Infantile form: the most common variant and presents between 4 and 6 months of age with irritability, hypersensitivity to stimuli, increasing hypertonicity with eventual opisthotonos, unexplained low-grade fevers, optic atrophy with blindness, psychomotor developmental arrest, and subsequent regression with loss of previously achieved milestones. These children also have a demyelinating polyneuropathy with arreflexia. They usually die by the age of 1 year.
- Juvenile form: the onset is between 3 and 10 years of age, with vision loss, spasticity, ataxia, gait disturbance, and cognitive impairment.
- Adult form: usually starts between the third and the fifth decade of life, with spastic paraparesis, weakness, vision loss, and evidence of neuropathy, but intellectual function tends to be normal.

Pathologically, there is symmetric demyelination of the cerebral white matter, with relative sparing of the subcortical arcuate or U fibers. The pathologic specimen shown in Figure 14.20 is typical of Krabbe disease, demonstrating clusters of globoid cells, which are multinucleated macrophages with cytoplasmic accumulation of galactocerebroside.

Radiologically, there is symmetric periventricular white matter signal abnormality and cerebral atrophy. NCS demonstrate slow conduction velocities and prolonged distal latencies. CSF examination shows elevated protein levels.

Fenichel GM. Clinical Pediatric Neurology: A Signs and Symptoms Approach, 6th ed. Philadelphia, PA: Saunders Elsevier; 2009.

Prayson RA, Goldblum JR. Neuropathology, 1st ed. Philadelphia, PA: Elsevier; 2005.

85. b, 86. d

The patient in question 85 likely has neurofibromatosis type 2 (NF2). Cutaneous findings seen in neurofibromatosis type 1 (NF1) are less common in NF2. NF2 is less common than NF1 and has distinct diagnostic criteria, clinical manifestations, and pathophysiology.

Diagnostic criteria for NF2 include one of the following:

- Bilateral schwannomas of cranial nerve (CN) VIII (although other CNs can be affected, most commonly CN V)
- A unilateral CN VIII schwannoma with a first-degree relative with NF2
- A family history of a first-degree relative with NF2 combined with any two of the following lesions: neurofibroma, meningioma, glioma, subcapsular (presenile) cataracts

In contrast to NF1, cutaneous lesions such as café au lait spots and neurofibromas (see Figures 14.5 and 14.6) are uncommon in NF2, but they may occur. The main cutaneous findings seen in NF2 are café au lait spots and plexiform cutaneous schwannomas. On the other hand, various CNS tumors occur more commonly in NF2, often in the same patient, including schwannomas, meningiomas, ependymomas, and astrocytomas of the brain and spine. Lisch nodules do not occur in NF2, but subcapsular cataracts and epiretinal folds may occur.

NF2 is one of the neurocutaneous syndromes that is often not diagnosed until adulthood. NF2 is autosomal dominant, with variable expression and complete penetrance. It results from a mutation in the merlin (also known as schwannomin) gene on chromosome 22. Merlin is a tumor suppressor gene, and mutations in this gene account for the various neoplasms seen in NF2. A variety of mutations in the NF2 gene have been identified, and the type of mutation correlates with clinical severity, with missense mutations leading to some functional protein production and milder clinical phenotype, and frameshift mutations leading to more severe disease.

Gorlin syndrome and Rubinstein-Taybi syndrome are rare syndromes associated with multiple meningiomas, but this patient's history of bilateral schwannomas combined with the family history is suggestive of NF2. Tuberous sclerosis complex has distinct cutaneous and CNS findings as discussed in questions 61 to 63.

Schwannomatosis is a distinct disorder characterized by the occurrence of multiple schwannomas affecting various CNs but not CN VIII. It may be segmental, and a pure spinal form also exists. It may be familial and has in some cases been associated with a mutation on chromosome 22 in a gene near, but different from, the gene mutated in NF2; less than 15% of cases of schwannomatosis are hereditary.

Bradley WG, Daroff RB, Fenichel GM, et al. Neurology in Clinical Practice, 5th ed. Philadelphia, PA: Elsevier; 2008.

MacCollin M, Chiocca EA, Evans DG, et al. Diagnostic criteria for schwannomatosis. Neurology. 2005; 64(11):1838–1845.

Swaiman KF, Ashwal S, Ferriero DM. Pediatric Neurology Principles and Practice, 4th ed. Philadelphia, PA: Mosby Elsevier; 2006.

87. b

This patient has GM1 gangliosidosis in which gangliosides accumulate in the brain and visceral organs.

GM1 gangliosidosis is an autosomal recessive disorder that occurs secondary to a deficiency in the lysosomal enzyme β-galactosidase, which is encoded on chromosome 3p21. Patients present between 6 and 18 months of age with incoordination, weakness, spasticity, seizures, psychomotor developmental arrest with subsequent regression, and a cherry-red spot. Dysmorphic, coarse facial features, and hepatosplenomegaly are also present. These patients may be confused with Hurler syndrome, except that in GM1 gangliosidosis, patients have a cherry-red spot in the macula and do not have mucopolysacchariduria.

Diagnosis is based on the detection of β-galactosidase deficiency in leukocytes or cultured fibroblasts. This enzymatic deficiency is responsible for the accumulation of GM1 gangliosides, keratan sulfate, and glycoproteins.

Macroscopically, the brain may be large initially, but as neuronal loss occurs, brain atrophy ensues. Pathologically, initially there is lipid storage in the neurons and proximal axons leading to neuronal ballooning. Subsequently, there is neuronal loss and gliosis. Treatment is supportive.

Fenichel GM. Clinical Pediatric Neurology: A Signs and Symptoms Approach, 6th ed. Philadelphia, PA: Saunders Elsevier; 2009.

Prayson RA, Goldblum JR. Neuropathology, 1st ed. Philadelphia, PA: Elsevier; 2005.

88. c

This patient has Alexander disease, which is a progressive disorder of astrocytes caused by mutations in the gene for glial fibrillary acidic protein. It has been proposed to have an autosomal dominant mode of inheritance, although this is controversial. There are infantile, juvenile, and adult forms. Patients with the infantile form have megalencephaly, developmental delay, seizures, psychomotor retardation, spasticity, and quadriparesis. The juvenile form has onset in childhood, and these patients have more significant bulbar symptoms. The adult form manifests with bulbar signs, hyperreflexia, dysautonomia, ataxia, and sleep apnea.

The brain MRI demonstrates diffuse white matter signal hyperintensity, predominantly in the frontal lobes and anterior cerebral regions, with involvement of the U fibers. In the adult-onset form, the "tadpole sign" on sagittal MRI results from dramatic thinning of the upper cervical spinal cord. The brains of these patients are large, and histopathologically, there are Rosenthal fibers. The histopathologic specimen shown in Figure 14.22 shows multiple Rosenthal fibers, which are elongated eosinophilic fibers seen on hematoxylin eosin, and they are diffusely distributed throughout the brain with clusters in the subpial, subependymal, and perivascular areas. Rosenthal fiber deposition is associated with severe myelin loss and cavitation of the white matter. They are not pathognomonic for Alexander disease and are seen in other conditions associated with gliosis. There is no specific treatment.

Canavan disease is discussed in question 79. Adrenoleukodystrophy is discussed in question 31. Zellweger syndrome is discussed in question 28. Fabry disease is discussed in questions 24 and 29.

Fenichel GM. Clinical Pediatric Neurology: A Signs and Symptoms Approach, 6th ed. Philadelphia, PA: Saunders Elsevier; 2009.

Prayson RA, Goldblum JR. Neuropathology, 1st ed. Philadelphia, PA: Elsevier; 2005.

89. a

Tuberous sclerosis complex (TSC) is an autosomal dominant disorder with variable penetrance. TSC may be either inherited or more commonly sporadic. TSC is caused either by a mutation in the TSC1 gene on chromosome 9 that encodes for the protein tuberin or by a mutation in the TSC2 gene on chromosome 16 that encodes for the protein hamartin. Tuberin and hamartin interact with each other and normally function as tumor suppressor genes, and abnormalities in these proteins lead to unregulated cell growth and proliferation. Although there are some genotype-phenotype correlations, the clinical manifestations of each mutation overlap significantly, so the two mutations cannot be distinguished between reliably on the basis of clinical features alone. TSC is also discussed in questions 61 to 63.

Bradley WG, Daroff RB, Fenichel GM, et al. Neurology in Clinical Practice, 5th ed. Philadelphia, PA: Elsevier; 2008.

Swaiman KF, Ashwal S, Ferriero DM. Pediatric Neurology Principles and Practice, 4th ed. Philadelphia, PA: Mosby Elsevier; 2006.

90. b

This patient has Pelizaeus-Merzbacher disease, which is a demyelinating disorder inherited in an X-linked recessive fashion. The gene involved is PLP1 on chromosome Xq22, and the mutation leads to abnormal synthesis of proteolipid protein 1. Mutations in this same gene also account for one form of hereditary spastic paraplegia.

The onset of clinical manifestations is in the first few months of life, with intermittent nodding movements of the head, pendular nystagmus, and other abnormal eye movements. Ataxia, chorea, athetosis, dystonia, spasticity, and laryngeal stridor also occur, and psychomotor development arrests with subsequent regression. Late manifestations include seizures and optic atrophy. Patients with later onset may have slower progression, and some patients survive into adulthood.

The MRI demonstrates diffuse demyelination. Pathologically, there is a noninflammatory demyelination sparing the U fibers and islands of white matter, giving it a "tigroid" appearance. Peripheral myelin is spared; and therefore, peripheral nerves are not involved.

Genetic testing is available for diagnosis, and there is no specific treatment.

This patient does not have Alexander disease, which is described in question 88 and which is caused by a defect in the gene for glial fibrillary acidic protein (GFAP).

Fenichel GM. Clinical Pediatric Neurology: A Signs and Symptoms Approach, 6th ed. Philadelphia, PA: Saunders Elsevier; 2009.

Prayson RA, Goldblum JR. Neuropathology, 1st ed. Philadelphia, PA: Elsevier; 2005.

91. a, 92. d

The patient in question 91 has Hunter syndrome, which is inherited in an X-linked fashion. Patients with Morquio syndrome have no mental retardation.

Mucopolysaccharidoses (MPS) are caused by impaired lysosomal degradation of glucosaminoglycans, which are long unbranched molecules of repeating disaccharides. Various enzymatic defects lead to the accumulation of glucosaminoglycans in lysosomes and the extracellular matrix.

The MPS are all autosomal recessive except for Hunter disease, which is X-linked. In general, MPS are a group of progressive multisystemic disorders that affect the cornea, cartilage, bone, connective tissue, reticuloendothelial system, and nervous system.

Hurler syndrome is MPS type I and is caused by α-L-iduronidase deficiency. The gene is localized to chromosome 4, and there is accumulation of both dermatan and heparan sulfate. These patients are normal at birth, but within the first 2 years of life, they will develop coarsening of facial features, with progressive skeletal dysplasia with dysostosis multiplex and growth impairment (dwarfism). These patients have restricted range of motion of the joints, hearing loss, corneal clouding, macroglossia, hernias, visceromegaly, valvular heart disease, and prominent mental retardation. Mild MPS type I is also known as Scheie syndrome, and the intermediate form is known as Hurler-Scheie syndrome. Most recently, MPS type I has been classified as severe MPS type I and attenuated MPS type I. The diagnosis of MPS type I is based on elevated urinary excretion of dermatan and heparan sulfate and confirmed with enzyme analysis in leukocytes and fibroblasts. Pathologically, there are cells with vacuolated appearance, expansion of perivascular spaces in the CNS, and neuronal lipidosis. Electron microscopy demonstrates reticulogranular material in epithelial and mesenchymal cells, and lamellar material in neurons, some of which adopt a layered appearance and are called zebra bodies. Enzyme replacement therapy can be used to treat noncentral nervous system manifestations of the disease. Stem cell transplantation can be potentially helpful.

Hunter syndrome or MPS type II is caused by a defect in iduronate sulfatase, with accumulation of dermatan sulfate and heparan sulfate. These patients have the Hurler phenotype but lack the corneal clouding and have characteristic nodular ivory-colored lesions on the back, shoulders, and upper arms. These children have short stature, macrocephaly, macroglossia, hoarse voice, hearing loss, visceromegaly, dysostosis multiplex, joint contractures, entrapment neuropathies such as carpal tunnel syndrome, and mental retardation. The diagnosis is based on mucopolysacchariduria and confirmed with analysis of the enzyme activity. Treatment is symptomatic.

Other MPS include types III, IV, VI, VII, and IX as follows:

- MPS type III or Sanfilippo syndrome has several subtypes (A, B, C, and D) and is associated with accumulation of heparan sulfate only. The main manifestation is mental retardation.
- MPS type IV or Morquio syndrome has two subtypes (A and B), and they manifest with corneal clouding, dysostosis multiplex, and heart disease, with normal intelligence.
- MPS type VI is also known as Maroteaux-Lamy syndrome and manifests with normal intelligence, dysostosis multiplex, corneal clouding, heart disease, and other features similar to Hurler syndrome.
- MPS type VII is also known as Sly syndrome, and these patients have hydrops fetalis, mental retardation, dysostosis multiplex, corneal clouding, and other features of Hurler syndrome.
- MPS type IX is caused by deficiency of hyaluronidase with accumulation of hyaluronan.

Fenichel GM. Clinical Pediatric Neurology: A Signs and Symptoms Approach, 6th ed. Philadelphia, PA: Saunders Elsevier; 2009.

Prayson RA, Goldblum JR. Neuropathology, 1st ed. Philadelphia, PA: Elsevier; 2005.

93. e

Lisch nodules are a feature of neurofibromatosis, not epidermal nevus syndrome (ENS). Iris colobomas are the most frequent ocular abnormality in patients with ENS.

ENS includes several disorders that are characterized by the presence of epidermal nevi and neurologic manifestations. These disorders include Proteus syndrome, which is characterized by asymmetric and often marked hypertrophy of soft tissues and bones, and other rare disorders such as sebaceous nevus syndrome and Becker nevus syndrome. Epidermal nevi are slightly raised patches of hyperpigmentation that are present at birth or appear in childhood. They enlarge over time. Not all patients have neurologic manifestations; occurrence of nevi over the face and scalp predict neurologic involvement. Neurologic manifestations may include mental retardation, seizures, and cranial neuropathies. In patients with hemimegalencephaly (which often occurs ipsilateral to a facial nevus), contralateral hemiparesis may be seen. Other brain malformations seen in patients with ENS include focal pachygyria, agenesis of the corpus callosum, Dandy-Walker syndrome, and neural tube defects. Cerebral vascular abnormalities including leptomeningeal hemangiomas and arteriovenous malformations may also occur.

Patients with ENS are at increased risk of malignancy; the nevus itself may undergo malignant transformation into basal cell carcinoma or other skin malignancies, and there is an increased risk of astrocytoma and other, systemic, malignancies. Various skeletal abnormalities may occur in ENS, including kyphoscoliosis. Ocular abnormalities include iris colobomas (most common), retinal lesions, and strabismus. Cardiac and genitourinary abnormalities also occur.

Bradley WG, Daroff RB, Fenichel GM, et al. Neurology in Clinical Practice, 5th ed. Philadelphia, PA: Elsevier; 2008.

Swaiman KF, Ashwal S, Ferriero DM. Pediatric Neurology Principles and Practice, 4th ed. Philadelphia, PA: Mosby Elsevier; 2006.

94. a

This patient has a porphyria, likely acute intermittent porphyria (AIP) given the lack of cutaneous manifestations and the absence of increased coproporphyrin III in the urine and stool, therefore making variegate porphyria (VP) and hepatic coproporphyria (HCP) less likely. The enzyme involved in AIP is porphobilinogen deaminase.

Porphyrias are a group of metabolic disorders caused by deficiency of a specific enzyme involved in the heme biosynthetic pathway. Most of the porphyrias are inherited in an autosomal dominant fashion, except 5-aminolevulinic acid dehydratase deficient porphyria, which is autosomal recessive.

AIP has primarily neurologic manifestations, HCP and VP have a combination of neurologic and cutaneous manifestations with photosensitivity, and porphyria cutanea tarda has cutaneous, with no neurologic, manifestations.

The acute porphyrias manifest with attacks of neurovisceral symptoms, with markedly elevated levels of plasma and urinary concentrations of the porphyrin precursors aminolevulinic acid (ALA) and porphobilinogen (PBG). Levels are usually elevated during attacks and may be normal in between. The attacks may be triggered by drugs such as barbiturates, sulfonamides, AEDs, and hormones among other medications. Attacks may also be triggered by a low-carbohydrate diet, infections, or other intercurrent illnesses.

AIP is the most common of the acute porphyrias with neurovisceral symptoms and is caused by deficiency of PBG deaminase, with the gene localized on chromosome 11. Onset occurs after puberty, with acute attacks of abdominal pain, sometimes associated with nausea, vomiting, diarrhea, fever, tachycardia, and leukocytosis. Commonly these patients experience limb pain and muscle weakness resulting from a peripheral neuropathy that is predominantly motor and axonal, affecting more proximal than distal segments and more the upper than the lower extremities. Deep tendon reflexes are depressed. The radial nerve has been described as being classically involved, and in severe cases, there may be bulbar, and respiratory involvement. Seizures can occur from neurologic involvement or may result from the hyponatremia that is seen in these patients. Neuropsychiatric symptoms such as anxiety, insomnia, depression, disorientation, hallucinations, and paranoia may occur.

The diagnosis is based on clinical suspicion and elevated urinary excretion of ALA and PBG during the attacks. Genetic testing and enzyme analysis are also helpful.

Management is focused on preventing attacks by avoiding precipitating factors. During attacks, these patients may need hospitalization for hydration and pain control. Carbohydrates decrease the synthesis of porphyrins, and an infusion may be required. Hematin infusions may be helpful. For seizures, clonazepam and gabapentin may be helpful. Unfortunately, many AEDs precipitate attacks, especially barbiturates, which should be avoided.

HCP is caused by coproporphyrinogen oxidase deficiency, and VP is caused by protoporphyrinogen oxidase deficiency. In both, the neurovisceral manifestations are similar to AIP, but in HCP and VP, there are cutaneous manifestations with photosensitivity, abnormal skin fragility, and bullous skin lesions on sun-exposed areas. HCP and VP cause increased urinary and fecal levels of coproporphyrin III.

Fauci AS, Braunwald E, Kasper DL, et al. Harrison's Principles of Internal Medicine, 17th ed. New York, NY: McGraw-Hill; 2008.

Fenichel GM. Clinical Pediatric Neurology: A Signs and Symptoms Approach, 6th ed. Philadelphia, PA: Saunders Elsevier; 2009.

95. d

This patient has Tangier disease, which is an autosomal recessive familial neuropathy, caused by mutation affecting the adenosine triphosphate cassette transporter protein, resulting in a deficiency of high density lipoprotein (HDL) and very low serum cholesterol and high triglyceride concentrations. Given the severely reduced HDL level, cholesteryl esters accumulate in various tissues, including tonsils, peripheral nerves, cornea, bone marrow, and other organs of the reticuloendothelial system. A typical clinical finding is the enlarged orange tonsils. Peripheral neuropathy is common and manifests with sensory loss to pain and temperature that may have a pattern in the upper extremities similar to that seen in syringomyelia and may affect the entire body. Motor involvement may manifest with weakness that affects the upper and lower extremities and particularly the hand muscles. A symmetric polyneuropathy is common; however, a mononeuropathy presentation can also be seen. Deep tendon reflexes are depressed. Cranial nerves may also be involved. Premature atherosclerosis also occurs. The diagnosis is suspected on the basis of clinical features, and a lipid profile showing HDL deficiency, with low total cholesterol and high triglyceride levels. Foamy macrophages are present in the bone marrow and other tissues. There is no specific treatment.

Fauci AS, Braunwald E, Kasper DL, et al. Harrison's Principles of Internal Medicine, 17th ed. New York, NY: McGraw-Hill; 2008.

Ropper AH, Samuels MA. Adams and Victor's Principles of Neurology, 9th ed. New York, NY: McGraw-Hill; 2009.

96. a

Menkes disease, also known as kinky hair syndrome, is a neurocutaneous disorder characterized by the presence of brittle hair (pili torti), hyperelastic skin, and thin or absent eyebrows. Abnormal fullness of the cheeks, high-arched palate, micrognathia, osteoporosis, and metaphyseal dysplasia are also seen. Neurologic manifestations include cerebral vasculopathy and progressive cerebral atrophy leading to subdural hematomas and/or hygromas. Seizures and severe developmental delay occur. Other organ systems are involved, including the skeletal, gastrointestinal, and genitourinary tract. Menkes disease is an X-linked recessive disorder resulting from a mutation in ATP7A, a copper transporter, resulting in defective copper transport across the intestines and widespread copper deficiency in the brain and other organs. Various enzymes require copper as a cofactor, including cytochrome c oxidase, dopamine β-hydroxylase, and lysyl oxidase among others.

Histopathologically, the cortex, thalamus, and subcortical nuclei demonstrate loss of neurons and gliosis. The cerebellum shows loss of granular neurons and Purkinje cells. Laboratory studies demonstrate low serum levels of ceruloplasmin and copper.

The presence of subdural hematomas in an infant may raise question of nonaccidental injury, although the cutaneous findings and other manifestations allow the distinction to be made. Menkes disease is a disorder of copper deficiency, unlike Wilson disease, a disorder of copper toxicity, which is due to a mutation in the ATP7B enzyme. Ehlers-Danlos syndrome is discussed in question 29 and Hypomelanosis of Ito in question 43.

Bradley WG, Daroff RB, Fenichel GM, et al. Neurology in Clinical Practice, 5th ed. Philadelphia, PA: Elsevier; 2008.

Prayson RA, Goldblum JR. Neuropathology, 1st ed. Philadelphia, PA: Elsevier; 2005.

Swaiman KF, Ashwal S, Ferriero DM. Pediatric Neurology Principles and Practice, 4th ed. Philadelphia, PA: Mosby Elsevier; 2006.

97. b

Mitochondrial encephalopathy, lactic acidosis and strokes (MELAS) is a mitochondrial disorder with typical maternal inheritance; however, sporadic cases may occur. The most common mutation is in the mtDNA MTTL1 gene encoding for an mtDNA tRNA. The onset is often between 2 and 10 years of age, although symptoms may begin at any age, including adulthood. Patients are normal at birth, later manifesting with seizures, migraine headaches, vomiting with anorexia, exercise intolerance, and weakness. Failure to thrive, growth retardation, and progressive deafness are common in these children. Stroke-like episodes occur, presenting with transient hemiparesis, cortical blindness, and altered consciousness, with cumulative residual effects leading to gradually progressive neurologic impairment, leading to mental deterioration and encephalopathy. The MRI shown in Figure 14.23 demonstrates multifocal infarcts that do not correlate with definite vascular territories. Initially, the infarcts occur in the posterior cerebral regions, with eventual involvement of other cerebral and cerebellar cortices, basal ganglia, and the thalamus. The infarcts are extremely epileptogenic. Lactate level is elevated in the blood and CSF. Muscle biopsy may demonstrate ragged red fibers.

There is no specific treatment. These patients may have some benefit from coenzyme Q10 and L-carnitine. L-arginine may attenuate the severity of strokes and reduce the frequency of these events.

Kearns-Sayre syndrome is discussed in question 33. Myoclonic epilepsy with ragged red fibers is discussed in Chapter 5. Leigh disease is discussed in question 32. Neuronal ceroid lipofuscinosis is discussed in question 26.

Fenichel GM. Clinical Pediatric Neurology: A Signs and Symptoms Approach, 6th ed. Philadelphia, PA: Saunders Elsevier; 2009.

Prayson RA, Goldblum JR. Neuropathology, 1st ed. Philadelphia, PA: Elsevier; 2005.

98. a

Abetalipoproteinemia, or Bassen-Kornzweig syndrome, is an autosomal recessive disorder caused by a molecular defect in the gene for the microsomal triglyceride transfer protein, which is localized to chromosome 4q22.24. This protein normally catalyzes the transport of triglyceride, cholesteryl ester, and phospholipid from phospholipid surfaces. The defect of this protein results in fat malabsorption and liposoluble vitamin deficiency, especially of vitamin E, which is the culprit of most of the clinical manifestations.

This condition manifests since birth, with failure to thrive, vomiting, and loose stool. During infancy, there is progressive psychomotor retardation with cerebellar ataxia and gait disturbance. Proprioceptive sensation is lost in the hands and feet, with less compromise of pinprick and temperature sensation. Deep tendon reflexes are depressed. This is likely from demyelination of posterior columns and peripheral nerves. Visual disturbance is the result of retinitis pigmentosa, and nystagmus is common.

Laboratory studies demonstrate acanthocytosis, absence of very low-density lipoproteins, absence of apolipoprotein B, low levels of vitamin E, and severe anemia.

Treatment involves the restriction of triglycerides in the diet, and large doses of vitamin E with supplementation of vitamins A, D, and K.

Fenichel GM. Clinical Pediatric Neurology: A Signs and Symptoms Approach, 6th ed. Philadelphia, PA: Saunders Elsevier; 2009.

Buzz Phrases	Key Points
Anterior neuropore fusion defects	Anencephaly, encephalocele
Posterior neuropore fusion defects	Spina bifida, myelomeningocele
Signals for ventral neural tube differentiation	From mesoderm of notochord: bone morphogenic proteins and sonic hedgehog
Risk factors for neural tube defect	Folate deficiency, antiepileptics, maternal diabetes, vitamin A (or vitamin A analogs) toxicity
Cell of origin of CNS	Ectoderm, derived from neural tube
Cell of origin of peripheral nervous system	Ectoderm, derived from neural crest cells
Cell of origin of vertebral bodies	Mesoderm of notochord
Balloon cells	Focal cortical dysplasia, a cortical developmental disorder of cell proliferation
Holoprosencephaly	Failure of prosencephalon to divide into cerebral hemisphere and other structures. Problem during 4 to 8 weeks of gestation
Reduced visual acuity, panhypopituitarism, absent septum pellucidum	Septo-optic dysplasia
Smooth brain, small chin, thin upper lip, intractable seizures	Lissencephaly type I, Miller-Dieker syndrome, LIS1 gene, chromosome 17, disorder of microtubules and dynein
DCX gene (doublecortin protein) abnormality: phenotype, mode of inheritance	Lissencephaly type I, DCX gene, X-linked: gene mutation leads to smooth brain in males, double cortex in females
Three disorders associated with lissencephaly type II (cobblestone lissencephaly)	Walker-Warburg syndrome, Fukuyama muscular dystrophy, and muscle-eye-brain of Santavuori. Developmental delay, seizures, muscular dystrophy, eye abnormalities
Molar tooth sign	Joubert syndrome and other disorders of cerebellar hypoplasia
Childhood obesity and mental retardation	Prader-Willi syndrome, Laurence-Moon syndrome
Inappropriate laughter, arm flapping, mental retardation, seizures, prominent jaw	Angleman syndrome
Genetic disorder in Prader-Willi and Angleman syndrome	Chromosome 15q11-q13. Prader-Willi when paternally inherited, Angleman when maternally inherited
Mental retardation, low-set ears, small testes	Fragile X, CGG trinucleotide repeat expansion

(*continued*)

Buzz Phrases	Key Points
Developmental regression at approximately 6 to 18 months of age, with hand wringing and microcephaly in female	Rett syndrome, MeCP2 gene mutation
Café au lait spots	Neurofibromatosis type 1
Shagreen patch	Tuberous sclerosis complex
Cutaneous neurofibromas	Neurofibromatosis type 1
Gene in neurofibromatosis type 2	Merlin gene, chromosome 22
Gene in neurofibromatosis type 1	Neurofibromin gene, chromosome 17
Axillary or inguinal freckling	Neurofibromatosis type 1
Bilateral vestibular schwannomas	Neurofibromatosis type 2
Lisch nodules	Iris hamartomas, Neurofibromatosis type 1
Subependymal giant cell astrocytoma	Tuberous sclerosis complex
Sphenoid wing dysplasia	Neurofibromatosis type 1
Ashleaf spots	Hypomelanotic lesions, tuberous sclerosis complex
Lymphangiomyomatosis	Tuberous sclerosis complex, females > males
Treatment that may inhibit growth of hamartomas in tuberous sclerosis complex	Rapamycin
Multiple intracranial arteriovenous malformations	Hereditary hemorrhagic telangiectasia or Osler-Weber-Rendu syndrome
Hypopigmented streaks that follow skin lines	Hypomelanosis of Ito
Dental enamel pits	Tuberous sclerosis complex
Hyperpigmented cutaneous lesions and leptomeningeal melanoma	Neurocutaneous melanosis
Hemifacial atrophy	Parry-Romberg syndrome
Multiple endochondromas and secondary hemangiomas	Mafucci syndrome
Retinal, cerebellar, and spinal hemangioblastomas; chromosome; mode of inheritance	von Hippel-Lindau disease, chromosome 3, autosomal dominant
X-linked dominant disorder with skin lesions and variable neurologic involvement; gene	Incontinentia pigmenti; NEMO gene
Freckles, multiple skin and systemic malignancies, neuropathy, ataxia, cognitive decline; pathophysiology	Xeroderma pigmentosa, due to defect in DNA repair, leading to sensitivity to ultraviolet light
Brittle hair, bilateral subdural hematomas, developmental delay; cause	Menkes disease (kinky hair syndrome); copper deficiency due to copper transporter ATP7A mutation
Epileptic encephalopathy and low CSF glucose level	Glucose transporter type 1 deficiency
Developmental delay, dysmorphic features, inverted nipples, and prominent fat pads Carbohydrate-deficient transferrin in the CSF	Congenital disorders of glycosylation
Urine with musty odor	Phenylketonuria

Buzz Phrases	Key Points
Cystathionine-β-synthase deficiency	Homocystinuria
Accumulation of branched-chain amino acids: leucine, isoleucine, and valine	Maple syrup urine disease
Mental retardation, aggressiveness, self-mutilation, hyperuricemia (gout and nephrolithiasis)	Lesch-Nyhan syndrome: Hypoxanthine guanine phosphoribosyltransferase deficiency
Gaucher cells: "wrinkled tissue paper" cells	Gaucher disease: Glucocerebrosidase deficiency
Globoid cells	Krabbe disease: Galactocerebroside β-galactosidase deficiency
β-Galactosidase deficiency	GM1 gangliosidosis
Hexosaminidase A deficiency	Tay-Sachs disease
Hexosaminidase A and B deficiency	Sandhoff disease
Acid sphingomyelinase deficiency	Niemann-Pick types A and B
Disorder of cholesterol trafficking in the intracellular domain	Niemann-Pick type C
Arylsulfatase A deficiency	Metachromatic leukodystrophy
Angiokeratomas, renal failure, hypertension, strokes, autonomic dysfunction	Fabry disease: α-Galactosidase deficiency
Symmetric white matter involvement predominantly in the posterior regions, sparing the U fibers	Adrenoleukodystrophy: Acyl coenzyme A synthetase deficiency
Megalencephaly, symmetric white matter disease involving the U fibers. N-acetylaspartic acid peak on MR spectroscopy	Canavan disease: Aspartoacylase deficiency
Megalencephaly, symmetric white matter involvement predominantly in the anterior regions Rosenthal fibers on histopathology	Alexander disease: Mutation in glial fibrillary acidic protein
White matter demyelination with "tigroid" appearance sparing the U fibers	Pelizaeus-Merzbacher disease: Gene PLP1
Enlarged orange-colored tonsils	Tangier disease
"Kinky" hair	Menkes disease
Progressive external ophthalmoplegia, onset younger than 20 years, short stature, ataxia, heart block, retinitis pigmentosa, CSF protein > 100 mg/dL	Kearns-Sayre syndrome
Get an electrocardiogram, and if there is heart block, place a pacemaker	Kearns-Sayre syndrome
Feeding difficulties, vomiting, diarrhea, jaundice, hepatosplenomegaly, failure to thrive, cataracts, and reducing substances in the urine	Galactosemia

(*continued*)

Buzz Phrases	Key Points
Triad of hyperammonemia, encephalopathy, and respiratory alkalosis No evidence of organic acidemias, normal anion gaps, and normal serum glucose level	Urea cycle disorders
Newborn babies with ketoacidosis, anion gap, elevated propionic acid level in the blood	Propionic acidemia
Alopecia, skin rash, hypotonia, seizures, optic atrophy, hearing loss, and hyperammonemia	Biotinidase deficiency
Psychomotor retardation, myoclonic seizures, and blindness. Intraneuronal deposits seen on electron microscopy (fingerprint bodies, granular osmiophilic deposits, curvilinear bodies, and rectilinear profiles)	Neuronal ceroid lipofuscinosis
Myoclonic epilepsy and cherry-red spot	Sialidosis

Chapter 15

Infectious Diseases of the Nervous System

Questions

1. A 32-year-old male intravenous drug user, whose partner was recently diagnosed with HIV, presents with headache, flu-like symptoms, fever (temperature of 39°C), and mild neck stiffness. His CSF analysis shows 0 RBCs, 15 WBCs (normal up to 5 lymphocytes/μL) with 85% lymphocytes, a protein level of 85 mg/dL (normal up to 45 mg/dL), and normal glucose level. CSF bacterial cultures are negative. Which of the following options is correct regarding this condition?

   a. A negative HIV serology (Enzyme Immunoassay and Western blot) result rules out HIV meningitis, and no further serologic tests for HIV are needed
   b. Acyclovir is the treatment of choice for HIV meningitis
   c. Positive HIV serology along with clinical manifestations would confirm the diagnosis of HIV meningitis, and no other tests are required
   d. Acute aseptic meningitis occurs only as a late manifestation of HIV
   e. Patients with acute aseptic meningitis have preserved alertness and cognition

2. A 20-year-old college student who lives in Connecticut presents with right-sided Bell's palsy and is prescribed steroids and acyclovir. One week later, he presents with left-sided facial nerve paralysis. He reports that recently he went hiking in a forest nearby, and over the past 3 weeks, he has been experiencing headaches and arthralgias and does not feel well in general. His CSF shows 98 WBCs with 78% lymphocytes (normal up to 5 lymphocytes/μL), protein level of 69 mg/dL (normal up to 45 mg/dL), and normal glucose level. Which of the following is correct regarding this condition?

   a. The causative agent is the spirochete *Treponema pallidum*
   b. Antibodies against *Borrelia burgdorferi* are present in the CSF
   c. Treatment of choice is isoniazid, pyrazinamide, ethambutol, and rifampin
   d. CSF VDRL test is very sensitive but not specific for this condition
   e. Erythema marginatum is a manifestation of this disease

3. While on a volunteer trip to Central America, you see a patient in the hospital with diabetic ketoacidosis and a destructive lesion on his face, affecting his nose, the maxillary bone, and

his right eye, with prominent proptosis. The patient rapidly deteriorates, and his condition gets complicated by cavernous sinus thrombosis. A histopathologic specimen from sinus biopsy showed nonseptated hyphae. Which among the following is not true regarding this condition?

a. The pathogenic agent is angioinvasive
b. Immunosuppressed patients are predisposed to this infection
c. Patients on long-term deferoxamine therapy are predisposed to this infection
d. Weakly acid-fast bacilli are detected
e. It is a zygomycosis

Questions 4–5

4. A 52-year-old man with a history of intravenous drug use, hepatitis C, and HIV diagnosed 10 years ago comes for evaluation of progressive cognitive decline. He has been noncompliant with his antiretroviral therapy and is presumed to have HIV-associated dementia. Which of the following is correct regarding this condition?

a. HIV-associated dementia is most commonly seen with CD4 counts between 200 and 400 cells/mm^3
b. Cognitive and psychomotor dysfunction are the main components of the HIV-associated dementia syndrome
c. More than 50% of patients have focal neurologic findings at the time of diagnosis
d. Cortical involvement with subcortical sparing is the neuropathologic hallmark
e. HIV-associated dementia is caused by an opportunistic infection

5. Which of the following is correct regarding the treatment of this patient?

a. Acyclovir is a specific treatment used along with antiretroviral therapy
b. A complex antiretroviral regimen, with multiple medications and more frequent dosing, is required to obtain better outcomes in these patients
c. Amphotericin is frequently used for the treatment of HIV-associated dementia
d. The prognosis is usually good and antiretroviral therapy can be curative
e. Antiretroviral therapy can prevent this condition and improve neuropsychological performance in patients with HIV-associated dementia

6. While you are working your 4th of July shift in the emergency department, a 62-year-old farmer with mental status changes and generalized weakness is brought by his wife. The patient has been having low-grade fevers, malaise and back pain, body aches, and headaches for the past 10 days; however, he did not want to come to the hospital. Over the past 5 days, he has developed bilateral hand tremors and difficulty walking. About 3 days ago, he became confused, and today, he was noticed to be unable to move his legs. On examination, he is lethargic and confused and noticed to be flaccid in his lower extremities, with areflexia. Which of the following is the most likely diagnosis?

a. Tuberculous meningitis and Pott's disease
b. Subacute combined degeneration of the spinal cord
c. Neurosyphilis with tabes dorsalis
d. West Nile encephalitis
e. HSV encephalitis

Questions 7–9

7. A 42-year-old woman presented with low-grade fevers of 1-month duration, headache, photophobia and neck stiffness for at least 1 week, and altered mental status on admission. A lumbar puncture was performed, and the opening pressure was 30 cm H_2O. CSF analysis showed 0 RBCs, 55 WBCs with 70% lymphocytes (normal up to 5 lymphocytes/μL), protein of 60 mg/dL (normal up to 45 mg/dL), and glucose of 50 mg/dL. India ink smear was positive in the CSF. The patient eventually died, and the brain specimen is shown in Figure 15.1. Which of the following is the most likely etiologic agent?

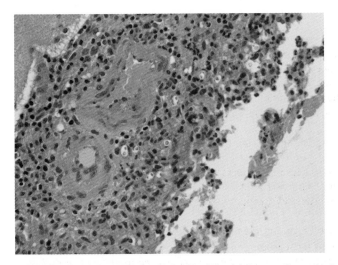

FIGURE 15.1   Brain specimen. Courtesy of Dr. Richard A. Prayson. Shown also in color plates

    a. *Mycobacterium tuberculosis*
    b. *Coccidioides immitis*
    c. *Cryptococcus neoformans*
    d. *Histoplasma capsulatum*
    e. *Streptococcus pneumoniae*

8. Which of the following is correct regarding the condition depicted in question 7?
    a. The most clinically useful diagnostic test is culture of the organism from the CSF
    b. CSF antigen detection has poor sensitivity and low specificity
    c. It commonly occurs in patients with AIDS and CD4 counts greater than 400/μL
    d. Increased intracranial pressure is a common finding and is associated with higher mortality
    e. It is frequently seen in early stages of HIV infection

9. Which of the following is correct regarding treatment of the condition depicted in question 7?
    a. Adverse effects of amphotericin, commonly used to treat this condition, include renal failure, hyperkalemia, and hypermagnesemia
    b. Fluconazole at 200 mg daily is first-line chronic maintenance therapy
    c. Vancomycin and ceftriaxone are the treatment of choice
    d. CSF drainage with frequent lumbar puncture is contraindicated in this condition
    e. Isoniazid and rifampin are first-line initial therapy

Question 10–11

10. A 50-year-old man with long-standing AIDS, noncompliant with antiretroviral therapy, presented with a seizure, mild right-sided weakness, and confusion. Brain MRI showed at least three ring enhancing lesions with surrounding edema, the most prominent one in the left subcortical white matter. A brain biopsy was obtained, and the histopathologic specimen is shown in Figure 15.2. Which of the following is correct regarding the most likely organism causing this opportunistic infection?

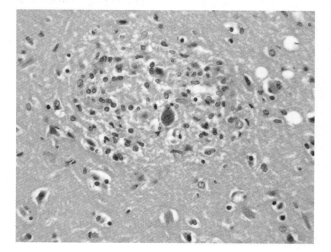

FIGURE 15.2 Brain specimen. Courtesy of Dr. Richard A. Prayson. Shown also in color plates

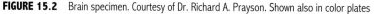

a. It is an encapsulated fungus
b. It is an intracellular protozoan
c. It belongs to the family of Herpesviridae
d. It is a mycobacterium
e. It is a spirochete

11. Which of the following is incorrect regarding the treatment of this opportunistic infection?
a. Standard therapy is sulfadiazine plus pyrimethamine
b. Trimethoprim-sulfamethoxazole is used for prophylaxis
c. Folinic acid can be used instead of sulfadiazine in sulfa-allergic patients
d. A patient with HIV, CD4 count of less than 100/μL, and immunoglobulin G (IgG) antibodies against this organism should receive prophylaxis
e. Clindamycin can be used for the treatment of this infection

12. A 49-year-old man with long-standing AIDS presents with progressive aphasia and right hemiparesis. His MRI shows a mass in the left frontal periventricular white matter, with mild contrast enhancement and surrounding edema. CSF analysis shows 20 WBCs with 90% lymphocytes (normal up to 5 lymphocytes/μL), protein of 55 mg/dL (normal up to 45 mg/dL), and normal glucose level. Epstein-Barr virus PCR in the CSF is positive. Which of the following options is correct?
a. This patient most likely has cerebral toxoplasmosis
b. CSF flow cytometry will show monoclonal B lymphocytes

c. Highly active antiretroviral therapy has not improved the prognosis of this condition
d. Cytology is 95% sensitive and specific
e. Corticosteroid therapy does not affect the results of brain biopsy

13. A 53-year-old man with AIDS and CD4 count of 30 cells/μL is seen for altered mental status. Over the prior 4 months, he had developed multiple focal neurologic findings, initially with left arm numbness, followed by right leg weakness, and eventually right hemiparesis. He later developed difficulty speaking and a deficit in his left visual field. About 1 week ago, he started to be confused. Brain MRI shows multiple coalescent nonenhancing white matter lesions in various locations. A brain biopsy was obtained and is shown in Figure 15.3. Which of the following is correct regarding this condition?

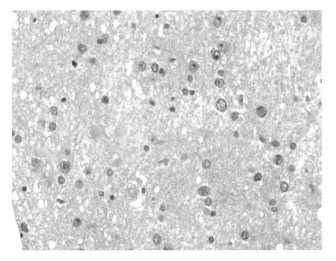

FIGURE 15.3   Brain specimen. Courtesy of Dr. Richard A. Prayson. Shown also in color plates

a. Acyclovir 10 mg/kg every 8 hours for 10 days is an effective therapy
b. Bilateral temporal periodic lateralized epileptiform discharges are useful for the diagnosis
c. The prognosis is good when specific therapy for the virus is given early
d. Presence of serum antibodies to this virus is specific to the diagnosis
e. The etiologic agent is a polyomavirus

14. A 60-year-old woman with HIV diagnosed approximately 6 years ago comes to the clinic for distal and symmetric foot pain and paresthesias that had slowly developed over the prior 12 months. She reports that she was started on new antiretroviral therapy approximately 2 months ago when her CD4 counts were found to be decreasing. Which of the following is the most likely diagnosis?

a. HIV neuropathy
b. Nucleoside analog-associated neuropathy
c. Cytomegalovirus polyradiculomyelitis
d. Acute inflammatory demyelinating polyradiculoneuropathy
e. Mononeuropathy multiplex

15. Muscle damage and wasting can be seen in patients with HIV. Which of the following mechanisms does not account for muscle problems in this patient population?
    a. Mitochondrial myopathy associated with antiretrovirals
    b. Myositis from autoimmune muscle fiber injury
    c. Muscle wasting syndrome
    d. Pyomyositis
    e. Myositis from direct HIV invasion of muscle fibers

Questions 16–18

16. Which of the following is the least common cause of bacterial meningitis in neonates?
    a. *Neisseria meningitidis*
    b. *Escherichia coli*
    c. Enteric gram-negative bacilli
    d. *Listeria monocytogenes*
    e. Group B streptococci

17. A 35-year-old man suffers an SAH with intraventricular extension and develops hydrocephalus. An external ventricular drain is placed. Over the next several days, he develops fever, and his CSF shows 210 WBCs/μL with 75% neutrophils (normal up to 5 lymphocytes/μL) and a protein level of 80 mg/dL (normal up to 45 mg/dL). Which of the following is the least likely pathogen causing this infection?
    a. *Staphylococcus aureus*
    b. *Staphylococcus epidermidis*
    c. *Pseudomonas aeruginosa*
    d. *Streptococcus pneumoniae*
    e. *Propionibacterium acnes*

18. A 79-year-old woman with diabetes, hypertension, and chronic leg ulcers develops headaches and fever. On examination, she has neck stiffness and mild confusion. Brain CT scan is unremarkable. Lumbar puncture is performed, and CSF shows 112 WBCs/μL (normal up to 5 lymphocytes/μL) with 81% neutrophils, protein level of 60 mg/dL (normal up to 45 mg/dL), and glucose of 80 mg/dL, with a blood glucose of 198 mg/dL. CSF is sent for culture. Which empiric antibiotic regimen would you start?
    a. Vancomycin and ceftriaxone
    b. Vancomycin, ceftriaxone, and ampicillin
    c. Vancomycin, ceftriaxone, and acyclovir
    d. Ampicillin and gentamicin
    e. Penicillin and gentamicin

19. *Mycobacterium tuberculosis* may invade the spinal column. Which of the following is incorrect?
    a. The mid-thoracic region is most commonly affected
    b. Back pain and muscle spasms are common symptoms
    c. Spinal disease usually starts in the spinous processes
    d. Kyphotic deformities are common
    e. Long-standing disease may produce vertebral body destruction and collapse

20. According to the Infectious Disease Society of America guidelines, which of the following patients does not need a brain CT scan prior to an lumbar puncture for evaluation of bacterial meningitis?
   a. A 62-year-old patient with a history of oligodendroglioma
   b. A 35-year-old patient with HIV
   c. A 40-year-old patient with diplopia and left pronator drift
   d. A 45-year-old obese woman with papilledema
   e. A 27-year-old man with a history of controlled epilepsy

21. The likelihood of a positive Gram stain result is lower with which of the following bacterial agents?
   a. *Haemophilus influenzae*
   b. Gram-negative bacilli
   c. *Streptococcus pneumoniae*
   d. *Neisseria meningitidis*
   e. *Listeria monocytogenes*

22. While you are on a trip to South America as a volunteer health care worker, you see a 49-year-old man who has various well-demarcated hypopigmented skin lesions with hair loss and anhidrosis. He also has a few anesthetic spots, and asymmetric peripheral nerve palsies. His ulnar nerves at the ulnar grooves are palpable and thickened. A smear from a skin lesion shows weakly positive acid-fast bacilli. Which of the following is correct?
   a. This patient has nocardiosis
   b. The most likely cause is *Mycobacterium tuberculosis*
   c. The causative organism has tropism toward nerves in warmer regions of the body
   d. This condition most commonly causes a respiratory illness from which the organisms may spread to the skin and peripheral nerves
   e. The tuberculoid variant occurs in patients with good cellular immunity

23. Which of the following antibiotics is appropriate treatment for the specified bacterium?
   a. *Streptococcus pneumoniae*—penicillin G
   b. *Neisseria meningitidis*—ceftriaxone
   c. *Listeria monocytogenes*—vancomycin
   d. *Haemophilus influenzae* β-lactamase positive—ampicillin
   e. *Pseudomonas aeruginosa*—ceftriaxone

Questions 24–25

24. A 25-year-old man was involved in a motor vehicle accident 8 months ago and suffered head trauma, requiring multiple craniofacial surgeries. He also has a history of chronic sinusitis. He now presents with fever and change in mental status. His brain MRI is shown in Figure 15.4. Which of the following is correct regarding this condition?
   a. It can be polymicrobial
   b. Highly active antiretroviral therapy is the treatment of choice
   c. CSF shows atypical lymphocytes with monoclonal B cells
   d. He should be treated with pyrimethamine and sulfadiazine
   e. It is caused by mycobacteria

25. Which of the following is not seen during the evolution of these lesions through different stages?
   a. Cerebritis
   b. Central necrosis

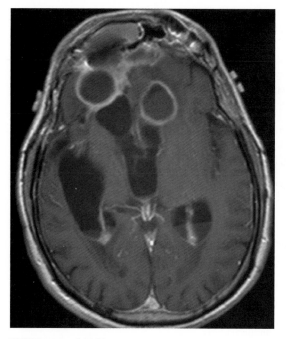

FIGURE 15.4 Axial CT scan

c. Capsule formation
d. Caseating granulomas
e. Vasogenic edema

26. A 21-year-old woman with a history of recurrent sinusitis presents with fever, diplopia and facial pain. On examination, she has proptosis of the right eye with periorbital edema, limited extraocular movements of the right eye, and reduced sensation over her right upper face and cheek. Fundoscopic examination demonstrates papilledema and retinal hemorrhages. What is the most likely diagnosis?
a. Superior sagittal sinus thrombosis
b. Meningitis
c. Brain abscess
d. Cavernous sinus thrombosis
e. Transverse sinus thrombosis

Questions 27–28

27. A 55-year-old man from South America who immigrated to the United States approximately 8 months ago presented with 2 months of low-grade fever, headaches, neck stiffness, and diplopia. On examination, he had bilateral cranial nerve VI palsies. CSF analysis showed 250 WBCs with 80% lymphocytes, (normal up to 5 lymphocytes/μL), 180 mg/dL of protein (normal up to 45 mg/dL), and 39 mg/dL of glucose. Brain MRI showed leptomeningeal enhancement, and a biopsy was obtained and is shown in Figure 15.5. Which of the following is the most likely etiology?
a. *Mycobacterium avium intracellulare complex*
b. HIV

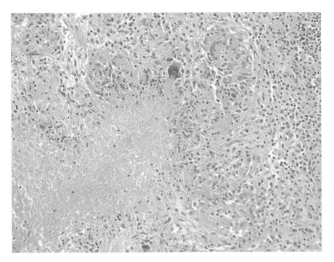

FIGURE 15.5   Leptomeningeal biopsy specimen. Courtesy of Dr. Richard A. Prayson. Shown also in color plates

    c. *Cryptococcus neoformans*
    d. *Mycobacterium tuberculosis*
    e. *Mycobacterium leprae*

28. Which of the following is correct regarding this condition?
    a. A combination of at least four drugs should be used for initial treatment
    b. CSF cultures are positive in 95% of cases
    c. Thickened nerves and mononeuritis multiplex are common manifestations
    d. Noncaseating granulomas are the pathologic hallmark
    e. The etiologic organism is anaerobic

Questions 29–30

29. A 43-year-old woman from South East Asia comes to the clinic. She has multiple hypopigmented skin lesions with sensory loss to pinprick and temperature. You notice that she also has claw-hand deformities and bilateral footdrop, and her ulnar and common peroneal nerves are enlarged on palpation. A sural nerve biopsy shows granulomas and acid-fast bacilli. Which of the following is the most likely cause of the neuropathy in this patient?
    a. Lyme disease
    b. Hansen disease (leprosy)
    c. Tuberculosis
    d. Parasitic infection
    e. Diabetes mellitus

30. Which of the following is incorrect regarding this condition?
    a. There is a tuberculoid variant
    b. There is lepromatous variant
    c. The causative organism is *Mycobacterium leprae*
    d. It tends to involve warmer regions of the body
    e. The causative organism invades Schwann cells

31. A 35-year-old woman who has a history of intravenous drug use and multiple sexual partners developed right hemiparesis and aphasia. Brain MRI showed restricted diffusion in the left hemisphere but in an unusual distribution. Rapid plasma reagin was detected as positive. CSF VDRL test was also found to be reactive. Based on the information provided, which of the following best describes this patient's disease?
    a. Primary syphilis
    b. Secondary syphilis
    c. Meningovascular syphilis
    d. Tabes dorsalis
    e. Parenchymal syphilis

32. A 54-year-old woman has a history of abdominal pain, diarrhea, weight loss, and an undetermined form of arthritis that she developed approximately 6 months earlier. She presents with a progressive dementia and abnormal eye movements associated with rhythmic chewing movements of the nose and mouth. A duodenal biopsy is performed and shows periodic acid Schiff-positive material. Which of the following is correct?
    a. The causative agent is *Tropheryma whippelii*
    b. A positive 14–3-3 protein in the CSF makes the diagnosis
    c. Avoiding gluten is the treatment of choice
    d. Vitamin B$_{12}$ deficiency is the major cause of these neurologic manifestations
    e. Angiotensin-converting enzyme levels in the CSF are usually elevated in this condition

33. A 57-year-old aerospace engineer is brought to the clinic by his wife because of cognitive decline and various neurologic symptoms. Approximately 6 months ago, he stopped worrying about his job and began exhibiting odd behavior, leaving the house without showering or brushing his teeth. He progressively became apathetic and paranoid. He could not solve simple mathematical problems and was having trouble paying his bills. Over the past month, he has developed unsteady gait, ataxia and frequent falls. His wife also reports that he "jerks all over." An MRI is obtained and is shown in Figure 15.6. Which of the following is the most likely cause?

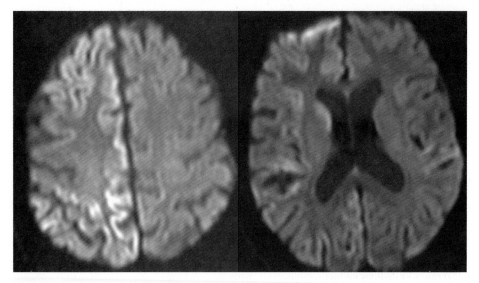

FIGURE 15.6 Axial diffusion-weighted MRI

a. Progressive multifocal leukoencephalopathy
b. CJD
c. Alzheimer disease
d. AIDS dementia
e. FTD

34. Primary CNS lymphoma occurs more frequently in patients with AIDS but may also be diagnosed in immunocompetent patients. Regarding CNS lymphoma, which of the following differs between these two patient populations?
a. Association with Epstein Barr virus
b. Findings on cytology
c. Response to steroids
d. B-cell origin
e. MRI findings

35. A 64-year-old man who has not seen a physician in many years is brought to the hospital because he has been unsteady on his feet for the past 6 months. On examination, he has asymmetric pupils, which are poorly reactive to light. His lower extremity strength is preserved; however, his sensory examination is abnormal to vibration and proprioception, and he has gait ataxia with a broad-based gait. When he closes his eyes, he falls to the floor. Serum rapid plasma reagin (RPR) is reactive. Which of the following is correct?
a. This patient has secondary syphilis
b. RPR is very specific but not sensitive for the diagnosis of syphilis
c. Treatment with penicillin will cure the disease and reverse the neurologic deficits
d. Treatment requires intravenous penicillin G, up to 4 million units every 4 hours for 14 days
e. Neurologic manifestations will occur in 99% of the patients who are initially infected and left untreated

36. Regarding CJD, which of the following is correct?
a. Granulovacuolar degeneration and neurofibrillary tangles are seen on histopathologic specimens
b. The familial form is autosomal recessive caused by a mutation in the prion protein gene
c. It is caused by scrapie prion protein (PrP^{Sc}), which has decreased β-sheet content as compared with cellular prion protein (PrP^{C})
d. The EEG finding shows a repetitive periodic pattern
e. It is associated with very low CD4 counts

37. A 26-year-old woman is brought to the emergency department after having a seizure. As per her roommate, the patient had been behaving oddly over the past week. Approximately 3 days ago, she developed fever, and for the past 2 days, she has been confused, talking strangely, and very lethargic. Today she had a generalized tonic-clonic seizure. Her CSF was reported as "reddish" in color, with 59 WBCs (normal up to 5 lymphocytes/μL), 3500 RBCs, protein of 58 mg/dL (normal up to 45 mg/dL), and normal glucose levels. An MRI is obtained and is shown in Figure 15.7. Which is the most likely diagnosis?
a. West Nile encephalitis
b. Bacterial meningitis
c. HSV encephalitis
d. Enterovirus meningitis
e. Tuberculous meningitis

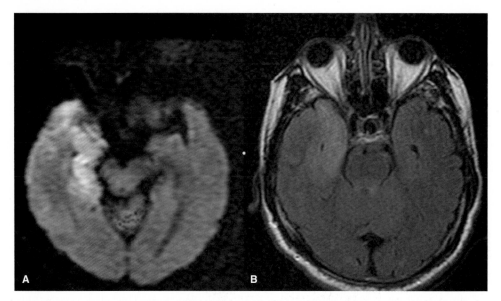

FIGURE 15.7 (**A**) Axial diffusion-weighted MRI; (**B**) Axial FLAIR MRI

38. A 40-year-old Italian man with progressive cognitive decline, ataxia, and tremors is brought to the emergency department because his family cannot take care of him anymore. He seems to be agitated at night and more confused than usual, and his wife reports that for the past month, he has not been able to sleep at all. His wife, who is a nurse, has also noticed that he becomes tachycardic, hypertensive, and diaphoretic, sometimes with mild fever. On the basis of supportive diagnostic information, he is thought to have a prion disease. Which of the following is the most likely diagnosis?
    a. Fatal familial insomnia
    b. Gerstmann-Straussler-Scheinker disease
    c. Familial CJD
    d. Sporadic CJD
    e. Iatrogenic CJD

39. In HSV encephalitis, which of the following is a characteristic EEG finding?
    a. Occipital seizures
    b. Triphasic waves
    c. Periodic lateralized epileptiform discharges
    d. 14- and 6-Hz spikes
    e. 3-Hz spike and wave complexes

40. An MRI is performed on a patient with HSV encephalitis. Which of the following is suggestive of this condition?
    a. Hemorrhagic changes in the temporal lobes
    b. T2 hyperintensity and restricted diffusion in the posterior cortical regions
    c. Hockey-stick and pulvinar signs
    d. Leptomeningeal enhancement in the basal regions
    e. Diffuse white matter hyperintensity on T2 sequences

41. Which of the following is not caused by an arbovirus?
a. Saint Louis virus encephalitis
b. West Nile encephalitis
c. La Crosse (California) encephalitis
d. Japanese encephalitis
e. Subacute sclerosing panencephalitis

42. A 49-year-old woman with a history of liver transplantation 5 years ago presents with altered mental status. MRI of the brain shows multiple areas of restricted diffusion bilaterally, with no clear vascular distribution. A histopathologic specimen is obtained and is shown in Figure 15.8. Which of the following is the most likely diagnosis?

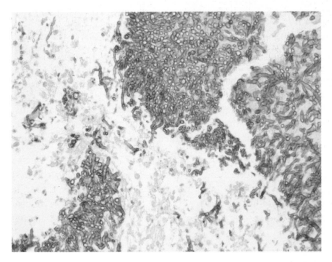

FIGURE 15.8   Pathologic specimen. Courtesy of Dr. Richard A. Prayson. Shown also in color plates

a. Cryptococcosis
b. Aspergillosis
c. Histoplasmosis
d. Candidiasis
e. HSV encephalitis

43. A 36-year-old man from South America comes to the epilepsy clinic for evaluation of new-onset partial seizures. His CT scan shows multiple cystic lesions in different locations and some small calcified masses. A biopsy was obtained and is shown in Figure 15.9. Which of the following is correct regarding this condition?
a. It is caused by *Taenia saginata*
b. India ink will be positive on CSF examination
c. Human ingestion of cooked pork meat containing the adult tapeworm leads directly to this clinical presentation
d. Albendazole is the treatment of choice
e. It is transmitted by the tsetse fly

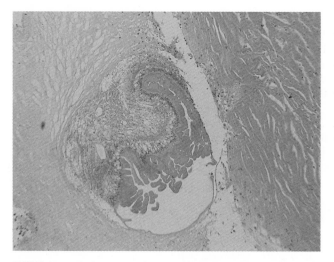

FIGURE 15.9   Brain specimen. Courtesy of Dr. Richard A. Prayson. Shown also in color plates

44. A 20-year-old man is admitted for evaluation of fever, neck stiffness, and altered mental status. Approximately 5 days prior, he had gone swimming with his friends in a pond nearby his house. During hospitalization, he rapidly worsened and eventually died. On autopsy, a brain specimen was obtained and is shown in Figure 15.10. Which of the following is the most likely diagnosis?

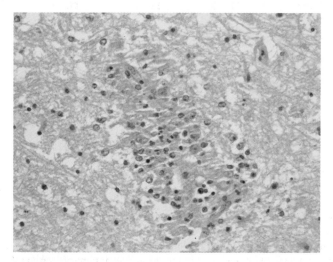

FIGURE 15.10   Brain specimen. Courtesy of Dr. Richard A. Prayson. Shown also in color plates

   a. Amebic meningoencephalitis
   b. Viral encephalitis
   c. Bacterial meningitis
   d. Tuberculous meningitis
   e. Fungal infection

Questions 45–46

45. A 24-year-old man goes camping in Connecticut and presents 5 weeks later with headache and severe pain radiating down his low back to the left leg. He also has paresthesias in his right hand and left foot. The patient recalls having a rash that started 2 weeks ago, which seems to be migrating and looks round and erythematous with a paler center. Which of the following is incorrect regarding this condition?

a. Ceftriaxone is used for the treatment of this condition
b. Doxycycline can be used for the treatment in the setting of normal CSF
c. Bacterial meningitis with predominance of neutrophils is a common manifestation
d. There are early and late neurologic manifestations of the disease
e. Approximately 10% of asymptomatic people in endemic areas may be seropositive for this organism

46. Which of the following neurologic presentations is not typical with this condition?

a. Cranial neuropathy
b. Mononeuritis multiplex
c. Aseptic meningitis
d. Subdural empyema
e. Polyradiculitis

Answer key

1. e	9. b	17. d	25. d	33. b	41. e
2. b	10. b	18. b	26. d	34. a	42. b
3. d	11. c	19. c	27. d	35. d	43. d
4. b	12. b	20. e	28. a	36. d	44. a
5. e	13. e	21. e	29. b	37. c	45. c
6. d	14. a	22. e	30. d	38. a	46. d
7. c	15. e	23. b	31. c	39. c	
8. d	16. a	24. a	32. a	40. a	

Answers

1. e

By definition, in meningitis, alertness and cognition are preserved, distinguishing it from encephalitis and meningoencephalitis.

Acute HIV meningitis is a syndrome that occurs in patients with progressive HIV disease and as CD4 count declines. It is occasionally present during the initial stages of HIV infection as part of the seroconversion syndrome and/or may be precipitated by a concomitant infection. Patients with acute HIV meningitis present with a febrile illness, headache, and symptoms of meningeal irritation. By definition, alertness and cognition are preserved. The CSF of these patients usually shows a lymphocytic pleocytosis (but usually less than 25 cells/μL) and mildly increased protein level (less than 100 mg/dL), with normal glucose levels.

In a patient with HIV, meningitis due to HIV itself is a diagnosis of exclusion; an extensive evaluation to rule out other etiologies is mandatory, including other viruses, tuberculosis, fungi, bacteria, lymphoma or meningeal carcinomatosis, and other inflammatory conditions. The diagnosis is made once other etiologies have been ruled out in a patient with signs of meningeal irritation and confirmed HIV infection. However, this syndrome may occur at early stages of infection during which HIV antibodies may not be detected. In these cases, subsequent serologic testing for HIV is required later.

Acute HIV meningitis requires no specific therapy and will eventually subside, although early initiation of treatment of antiretroviral therapy for the HIV infection itself is important.

Bradley WG, Daroff RB, Fenichel GM, et al. Neurology in Clinical Practice, 5th ed. Philadelphia, PA: Elsevier; 2008.

2. b

This patient has bilateral Bell's palsy and lymphocytic meningitis, most likely associated with Lyme disease, which is caused by *Borrelia burgdorferi*. This spirochete is transmitted by the deer tick *Ixodes* and is frequently seen in the northeast United States. Clinically, the disease manifests in three stages:

- Primary stage (within first 4 weeks of the tick bite): erythema chronicum migrans, which is a "bull's eye rash" (not erythema marginatum, which is seen in rheumatic fever). Patients usually have constitutional symptoms during this stage.
- Secondary stage (weeks after the rash): systemic manifestations, including cardiac involvement (cardiac conduction blocks), arthralgias and arthritis, lymphocytic meningitis, and neuropathies
- Tertiary stage (months after the secondary stage): neuropathy, encephalomyelitis, encephalopathy, and dementia

The diagnosis of Lyme disease is based on epidemiologic data, clinical information, and CSF and serologic studies. The presence of anti–*B. burgdorferi* antibodies in the serum and intrathecal production of these antibodies is helpful in making the diagnosis. PCR is also available. MRI studies may show leptomeningeal enhancement in some cases.

Patients with CNS abnormalities should be treated with intravenous antibiotics such as ceftriaxone or penicillin G for up to 2 to 4 weeks. If CSF findings are unremarkable and there are no neurologic manifestations, oral doxycycline may be sufficient. Option c provides a list of medications used in tuberculosis, which is not the diagnosis in this patient. This patient does not have syphilis; therefore, CSF VDRL test is not helpful.

Bradley WG, Daroff RB, Fenichel GM, et al. Neurology in Clinical Practice, 5th ed. Philadelphia, PA: Elsevier; 2008.

3. d

This patient has mucormycosis, which is a zygomycosis. This fungus tends to enter through the respiratory tract, producing nasal and sinus disease and pulmonary infections. In the presence of predisposing factors and trauma, it may invade blood vessels and gain entry into the CNS, where it can produce an acute necrotizing reaction and vascular thrombosis, including sinus venous thrombosis, especially affecting the cavernous sinus. Externally, patients have a destructive inflammatory and necrotizing lesion affecting the face, especially in the nasal and maxillary areas. Diabetes mellitus and diabetic ketoacidosis are major and frequent risk factors for this condition. Other predisposing conditions include malignancies, high-dose steroids, organ transplantation, immunosuppression, and iron chelation therapy (with deferoxamine). The organisms causing this infection are mucor, rhizopus, and rhizomucor, which are fungi and not acid-fast bacilli. These fungi are seen as infrequently septated or nonseptated hyphae on histopathologic specimens.

Bradley WG, Daroff RB, Fenichel GM, et al. Neurology in Clinical Practice, 5th ed. Philadelphia, PA: Elsevier; 2008.

Fauci AS, Braunwald E, Kasper DL, et al. Harrison's Principles of Internal Medicine, 17th ed. New York, NY: McGraw-Hill; 2008.

4. b, 5. e

HIV-associated dementia is a complication of HIV occurring at late stages of the disease, in patients with CD4 counts below 200 cells/mm^3, meeting the diagnostic criteria for AIDS. HIV-associated dementia is also called AIDS-dementia complex. The etiology of this condition is the retrovirus itself rather than an opportunistic infection. Progressive cognitive decline and prominent psychomotor dysfunction are the main clinical manifestations. These patients have significant difficulties with attention and concentration, along with fine motor dysfunction, gait incoordination, and tremors. However, focal neurologic findings are not common.

CSF analysis is nonspecific, frequently revealing mild lymphocytic pleocytosis and slightly elevated protein levels. Neuropathological studies show diffuse white matter pallor, activated macrophages, multinucleated giant cells, and vacuolar changes in the brain. The main findings are in the subcortical region, and the cerebral cortex is relatively spared.

Neuropsychologic testing is useful in the diagnosis and follow-up of these patients, as well as to monitor these patients while on therapy.

HIV-associated dementia can be prevented by adequate early treatment of HIV with highly active antiretroviral therapy (HAART), with the goals of attaining higher CD4 counts and suppressing the virus. Treatment of patients with HIV-associated dementia leads to improvements in neuropsychological performance.

Given the cognitive impairment of these patients, successful treatment requires the use of simpler HAART regimens, with the least number of drugs and simple dosing intervals, and using a regimen that minimizes side effects. Complex regimens are associated with poor compliance. Family or friend support is very important, and directly observed therapy may be required. Besides HAART, there are no other specific therapies for HIV-associated dementia.

Bradley WG, Daroff RB, Fenichel GM, et al. Neurology in Clinical Practice, 5th ed. Philadelphia, PA: Elsevier; 2008.

6. d

This patient has West Nile virus (WNV) encephalitis, which is an arboviral infection that spreads in the summer months, can occur in epidemics, and is transmitted by mosquitoes of the genus *Culex*. Most infected patients are asymptomatic, up to 20% may show signs of a febrile viral illness, and less than 1% develop a severe neurologic presentation; elderly patients are particularly at risk for neurologic disease and death. Patients with this neurologic presentation will have manifestations of encephalitis; however, WNV can also invade the anterior horn cells leading to flaccid weakness with areflexia, similar to poliomyelitis. WNV infection may also manifest with cranial neuropathies and tremors.

WNV encephalitis is diagnosed by serology and detection of immunoglobulin M (IgM) antibodies in the CSF. CSF PCR is less sensitive, but is diagnostic when positive. MRI is nondiagnostic. Treatment is supportive.

This patient does not have findings to support the other conditions listed.

Bradley WG, Daroff RB, Fenichel GM, et al. Neurology in Clinical Practice, 5th ed. Philadelphia, PA: Elsevier; 2008.

7. c, **8.** d, **9.** b

On the basis of the clinical history, presentation, elevated CSF opening pressure, and the presence of a positive India ink smear, this patient has cryptococcal meningitis, which is caused by the encapsulated yeast *Cryptococcus neoformans*. Furthermore, the histopathologic specimen demonstrates budding yeasts near blood vessels and surrounded by an inflammatory infiltrate, which is consistent with infection by this organism.

Cryptococcal meningitis usually occurs in immunocompromised patients and is an opportunistic infection seen in advanced HIV infection, usually when CD4 counts fall below 200 cells/μL. However, it may rarely be seen in otherwise immunocompetent patients; in such cases, a history of exposure to bird droppings, as occurs with roofers, may be elicited.

Patients usually present with fever, headache, neck stiffness, personality and behavioral changes, and altered mental status. Brain CT scan and MRI are performed to rule out other conditions and may demonstrate hydrocephalus, gelatinous pseudocysts, infarcts, or cryptococcomas. Lumbar puncture demonstrates an increased opening pressure, and CSF analysis shows mononuclear lymphocytosis with increased protein and low glucose levels. India ink smear is not very sensitive; however, it is useful when it is positive. Cryptococcal antigen detection in the CSF is rapid, sensitive and specific, and clinically useful, since fungal culture may take several days to weeks for a positive result to be obtained.

The initial treatment regimen is amphotericin plus flucytosine for 2 to 3 weeks. These patients should be monitored closely, since amphotericin is associated with renal failure, hypokalemia, and hypomagnesemia; and flucytosine may cause hematologic abnormalities. If the patient is doing well on amphotericin and flucytosine, or the meningitis is mild, the treatment can be switched to fluconazole 200 mg twice daily for 8 to 10 weeks. Afterward, the patient should be kept on long-term maintenance therapy with fluconazole 200 mg daily to prevent recurrences. Highly active antiretroviral therapy, by promoting immune reconstitution, plays a major role in the long-term treatment of HIV patients with cryptococcal meningitis, after the acute infection has cleared.

Mortality rate in the acute setting may be related to elevated intracranial pressure, which should be treated. Patients with increased intracranial pressure may need frequent CSF drainage by repeated lumbar punctures or even ventriculostomy.

Since this patient does not have a bacterial or tuberculous meningitis, there is no role for vancomycin, ceftriaxone, isoniazid, or rifampin.

Bradley WG, Daroff RB, Fenichel GM, et al. Neurology in Clinical Practice, 5th ed. Philadelphia, PA: Elsevier; 2008.

10. b, **11.** c

This patient has toxoplasmosis of the CNS, which is caused by *Toxoplasma gondii*, an intracellular protozoan. The diagnosis in this case can be suspected based on the history and clinical findings and confirmed with the histopathologic findings showing a microglial nodule, in which an encysted bradyzoite can be seen surrounded by an inflammatory infiltrate.

Cerebral toxoplasmosis is the most frequent opportunistic infection in patients with AIDS. The organism is usually acquired earlier in life and remains dormant until the immune system declines and *T. gondii* becomes active. This occurs in advanced stages of immunodeficiency in the setting of CD4 counts of less than 100/μL.

Patients present with headaches, focal neurologic deficits, seizures, and altered mental status that can progress to coma. Brain MRI typically demonstrates multiple ring enhancing lesions with surrounding edema. Since these cases present with a mass lesion in the brain, the differential diagnoses include primary CNS lymphoma, tuberculomas, fungal masses, or bacterial abscesses.

Definitive diagnosis is made with brain biopsy; however, this is not commonly performed, and patients are typically treated empirically.

Standard therapy is sulfadiazine plus pyrimethamine. Since both agents affect the folate metabolism pathways, folinic acid should be provided to avoid hematologic complications. An alternative therapy is clindamycin, especially in patients who are allergic to the sulfa components and cannot take sulfadiazine. Long-term suppressive therapy is needed to prevent relapses. Highly active antiretroviral therapy promotes immune reconstitution, and patients whose CD4 counts rise above 200/μL may not need further suppressive therapy. Trimethoprim-sulfamethoxazole is used for prophylaxis. Patients with HIV and CD4 counts of less than 200/μL with positive immunoglobulin G (IgG) antibodies to toxoplasma should be given prophylaxis.

Bradley WG, Daroff RB, Fenichel GM, et al. Neurology in Clinical Practice, 5th ed. Philadelphia, PA: Elsevier; 2008.

12. b

This patient has primary CNS lymphoma (PCNSL) in the setting of AIDS. These patients usually present with focal neurologic manifestations, which progress slowly over weeks to months. Since PCNSL in AIDS patients is frequently associated with Epstein-Barr virus, positive CSF PCR for this virus helps to make the diagnosis. CSF findings usually demonstrate a lymphocytic pleocytosis, elevated protein, and low to normal glucose levels. Cytology may detect atypical cells; however, this test has low sensitivity. Flow cytometry is helpful in making the diagnosis when it shows monoclonal B lymphocytes. CT scan has poor sensitivity, and MRI is a better tool, showing one or more lesions usually in the periventricular and deep regions of the brain. These lesions may have contrast enhancement, surrounding edema, and produce mass effect. Definitive diagnosis is done with brain biopsy.

Corticosteroids are helpful in the treatment of edema and mass effect, and the lesion itself tends to shrink with this treatment. However, the use of steroids should be reserved until after the brain biopsy has been obtained, since the results may be altered and the sensitivity of the biopsy reduced with corticosteroid exposure. Chemotherapy has been used, especially methotrexate; however, this therapy may be toxic and not optimal in patients with a baseline poor performance status related to the underlying disease. Radiation therapy is used as palliative treatment. The use of highly active antiretroviral therapy has improved the overall prognosis in patients with AIDS and PCNSL.

Bradley WG, Daroff RB, Fenichel GM, et al. Neurology in Clinical Practice, 5th ed. Philadelphia, PA: Elsevier; 2008.

13. e

This patient has progressive multifocal leukoencephalopathy (PML), caused by JC virus, which is a polyomavirus. PML occurs in patients with end-stage AIDS and is the only known manifestation of JC virus. A large percentage of the general population has antibodies against this virus, certainly without clinical manifestations; and therefore, the presence of serum antibodies is not helpful for the diagnosis. Only those patients with severe immunosuppression and CD4 counts less than 200 cells/μL develop clinical manifestations; PML in immunocompetent individuals is exceedingly rare but can occur.

PML presents with a gradually progressive course of multiple focal neurologic manifestations, with visual field deficits and visual agnosias being common, given the predominant involvement of parieto-occipital regions. Seizures also occur.

The diagnosis can be suspected with the history and clinical manifestations, supported with MRI findings and CSF JC virus DNA PCR and confirmed with brain biopsy (though brain biopsy is not necessary in the setting of typical clinical, imaging, and CSF findings).

MRI shows multiple white matter nonenhancing lesions that tend to coalesce and predominate in the parieto-occipital regions. Brain biopsy is the gold standard diagnostic test; neuropathologic findings include myelin loss, giant astrocytes, and altered oligodendrocytes, with enlarged nuclei and viral inclusions. On electronic microscopy, the viral particles give a "spaghetti and meatballs" appearance. The specimen shown in Figure 15.3 demonstrates enlarged oligodendrocytes with intranuclear inclusions consistent with PML. CSF JC virus DNA PCR is specific for the diagnosis, and because of the wide availability of this test, brain biopsy is rarely necessary.

Patients with PML have poor prognosis, as it denotes the presence of an already severely altered immune system. There is no specific therapy for this condition; however, some patients may improve with antiretroviral therapy and immune reconstitution. There are no specific EEG findings in PML, and acyclovir does not treat this condition.

Bradley WG, Daroff RB, Fenichel GM, et al. Neurology in Clinical Practice, 5th ed. Philadelphia, PA: Elsevier; 2008.

14. a

This patient has HIV neuropathy, which is a distal sensory neuropathy seen in patients with HIV, more frequently as the CD4 count drops. This condition is a predominantly sensory, axonal length-dependent symmetric polyneuropathy. It is thought to be related to direct effects of the virus and cytokine upregulation. These patients should continue antiretroviral therapy for virus suppression, and the treatment is symptomatic for the neuropathic pain.

Options b to e mention other types of neuropathy that can be seen in patients with HIV. Nucleoside analog-associated neuropathy occurs over weeks following the initiation of therapy, and the treatment is to discontinue the offending drug. In this patient, the symptoms of neuropathy had evolved over months and not in direct relationship with initiation of the antiretrovirals; therefore, it is most likely that she has HIV neuropathy. Acute inflammatory demyelinating polyradiculoneuropathy can occur secondary to dysregulation of the immune system and is seen most frequently at the time of seroconversion. Cytomegalovirus polyradiculomyelitis is an uncommon syndrome seen in patients with very low CD4 counts, presenting with leg pain, sensory symptoms, and weakness, along with areflexia and sphincteric dysfunction evolving over days. Mononeuropathy multiplex can occur with HIV disease, more frequently late in the course of the illness, and may be associated with superimposed infection, lymphomatous infiltration, or vasculitis. However, clinically, this case does not represent a mononeuropathy multiplex, but rather a distal symmetric polyneuropathy.

Bradley WG, Daroff RB, Fenichel GM, et al. Neurology in Clinical Practice, 5th ed. Philadelphia, PA: Elsevier; 2008.

15. e

HIV does not seem to invade muscle fibers directly, but rather it induces major histocompatibility complex I expression with autoimmune muscle fiber injury. This myositis can occur at any time during HIV infection. Patients on zidovudine can develop a mitochondrial myopathy. Pyomyositis is rare, but since the HIV epidemic, it has been more frequently seen. Patients with end-stage AIDS may develop a muscle wasting syndrome known as AIDS cachexia.

Bradley WG, Daroff RB, Fenichel GM, et al. Neurology in Clinical Practice, 5th ed. Philadelphia, PA: Elsevier; 2008.

16. a, 17. d, 18. b

Bacterial meningitis can be caused by different groups of bacteria, depending on the age group, risk factors, and associated circumstances. *Escherichia coli*, other enteric gram-negative bacilli, *Listeria monocytogenes*, and group B streptococci are the most common pathogens of bacterial meningitis in neonates. In patients from 1 to 23 months of age, the most common agents are

Streptococcus pneumoniae, Neisseria meningitidis, Streptococcus agalactiae, Haemophilus influenzae, and *Escherichia coli.* In patients in the 2 to 50 years age group, the most common agents are *Streptococcus pneumoniae* and *Neisseria meningitidis.* In older adults, such as the patient depicted in question 18, *Listeria monocytogenes* should be considered, as well as aerobic gram-negative bacilli, *Streptococcus pneumoniae* and *Neisseria meningitidis.* Neurosurgical patients are predisposed to meningitis with aerobic gram-negative bacilli (including *Pseudomonas aeruginosa*), *Staphylococcus aureus,* and *Staphylococcus* coagulase negative (such as epidermidis). In the setting of CNS instrumentation, these same agents and *Propionibacterium acnes* should be considered. Unlike in community-acquired meningitis, *Streptococcus pneumoniae* is not a common cause of hospital-acquired meningitis.

Empiric antibiotic therapy should be started before specific agents are identified from CSF cultures. Usually, vancomycin and a third-generation cephalosporin (such as ceftriaxone) are initiated in adult patients with suspicion for bacterial meningitis caused by *Streptococcus pneumoniae, Neisseria meningitidis,* and/or *Haemophilus influenzae.* In the extremes of life (younger and older patients) and in immunocompromised patients, *Listeria monocytogenes* should be considered and, therefore, ampicillin should be added to the empiric therapy.

Allan RT, Hartman BJ, Kaplan SL, et al. Practice guidelines for the management of bacterial meningitis. Clin Infect Dis. 2004; 39:1267–1284.

Bradley WG, Daroff RB, Fenichel GM, et al. Neurology in Clinical Practice, 5th ed. Philadelphia, PA: Elsevier; 2008.

19. c

Tuberculosis can affect the spine, more specifically the vertebral column (Pott's disease). The most commonly affected region is the midthoracic spine. Patients frequently present with constitutional symptoms, back pain, and muscle spasms, sometimes with findings of compressive radiculopathy or myelopathy.

Mycobacterium tuberculosis invades the body of the vertebral column, usually starting in the anterior region of the vertebral bodies, not at the spinous processes. The infectious process tends to disrupt the bone and the intervertebral spaces, leading to vertebral body destruction and collapse, as well as vertebral column deformities with kyphosis and scoliosis.

Bradley WG, Daroff RB, Fenichel GM, et al. Neurology in Clinical Practice, 5th ed. Philadelphia, PA: Elsevier; 2008.

20. e

In patients with increased intracranial pressure, or an intracranial mass, lumbar puncture may precipitate a herniation syndrome. Therefore, in most cases, a brain CT scan is recommended before performing an lumbar puncture, in order to rule out an intracranial process. Various studies have been performed in the past to evaluate which clinical features are associated with abnormalities detected on CT scan, and based on these findings, specific guidelines have been recommended for adults undergoing CT scan before lumbar puncture.

The following are the recommended criteria for adult patients with suspected bacterial meningitis who should have a brain CT scan prior to lumbar puncture:

– Immunocompromised patients (HIV patients, AIDS patients, patients on immunosuppressive therapy, transplant patients)
– History of CNS disease (mass, stroke, focal infection)
– New-onset seizure (especially within 1 week)
– Papilledema
– Abnormal level of consciousness
– Focal neurologic deficit.

In this case, a known history of epilepsy does not fit the recommended criteria, and a brain CT scan does not necessarily need to be done prior to the lumbar puncture.

Tunkel AR, Hartman BJ, Kaplan SL, et al. Practice guidelines for the management of bacterial meningitis. Clin Infect Dis. 2004; 39:1267–1284.

21. e

Gram stain results depend on multiple factors, such as the CSF concentration of bacteria and the specific bacterial agent. Approximately 90% of meningitis cases caused by *Streptococcus pneumoniae*, 86% of those caused by *Haemophilus influenzae*, 75% of those caused by *Neisseria meningitidis*, 50% of those caused by gram-negative bacilli, and 33% of cases caused by *Listeria monocytogenes* have positive Gram stain results.

Even though the yield of CSF Gram stain can be as low as 20% in patients who have received antibiotics, this test is easy to do, is rapid and inexpensive, and is recommended for all patients with suspected bacterial meningitis.

Tunkel AR, Hartman BJ, Kaplan SL, et al. Practice guidelines for the management of bacterial meningitis. Clin Infect Dis. 2004; 39:1267–1284.

22. e

This patient has Hansen disease, or leprosy. This disease has a long incubation period (from months to decades) and is caused by *Mycobacterium leprae*, which is thought to spread through the respiratory tract but does not typically produce a respiratory illness. This mycobacterium has tropism toward peripheral nerves, especially in cooler areas of the body.

Leprosy has two major variants, a lepromatous variant and a tuberculoid variant, in addition to forms intermediate between the two. The lepromatous variant occurs in patients with impaired cell-mediated immunity, making it possible for the organism to spread to the skin and peripheral nerves, causing a maculopapular rash, nodules, and poorly demarcated skin lesions. The manifestations can be systemic, and patients will present with thickened nerves and multiple neuropathies. The tuberculoid form occurs in patients with good cellular immunity, in which the disease is less disseminated, the skin lesions are better localized, and the patient will also have asymmetric peripheral neuropathies with thickened nerves. The ulnar nerve is commonly affected, and the syndrome may resemble mononeuritis multiplex.

The diagnosis is supported by skin smears showing weakly positive acid-fast bacilli. Skin and/or nerve biopsies are sometimes needed. The lepromin test is an intradermal test similar to the purified protein derivative test. Chronic therapy is usually needed, using rifampin, dapsone, and clofazimine.

As opposed to tuberculosis, there is no pulmonary illness in Hansen disease. *Nocardia asteroides* stains partially acid-fast; however, it is associated with respiratory infections, cutaneous abscesses and fistulas, and sometimes cerebral abscesses, but not peripheral neuropathies.

Bradley WG, Daroff RB, Fenichel GM, et al. Neurology in Clinical Practice, 5th ed. Philadelphia, PA: Elsevier; 2008.

23. b

Neisseria meningitidis should be treated with a third-generation cephalosporin, either ceftriaxone or cefotaxime, and the recommended duration of treatment is 7 days.

Streptococcus pneumoniae should be treated initially with vancomycin and ceftriaxone, and the duration of treatment is between 10 and 14 days.

Listeria monocytogenes, which is a potential cause of meningitis particularly at the extremes of age (younger and older) and in immunocompromised patients, should be treated with ampicillin for more than 21 days, or for 2 weeks after the CSF culture is sterile. *Haemophilus influenzae* can be treated with ampicillin if the organism is β-lactamase negative; however, if it is β-lactamase positive, a third-generation cephalosporin should be used. *Pseudomonas aeruginosa* is usually a hospital-acquired infection and is typically resistant to ceftriaxone. Ceftazidime and cefepime have been used to treat this infection with a duration of treatment of at least 21 days.

Tunkel AR, Hartman BJ, Kaplan SL, et al. Practice guidelines for the management of bacterial meningitis. Clin Infect Dis. 2004; 39:1267–1284.

24. a, 25. d

This patient has multiple ring enhancing lesions, with a history and clinical findings consistent with brain abscesses. These lesions originate from invasion of brain parenchyma by bacterial organisms, commonly polymicrobial, with a combination of streptococci, staphylococci, enterobacteria, and anaerobes. The bacterial agents spread via hematogenous routes or from a contiguous infected site, such as the sinuses, ears, or teeth. They also can be encountered after open trauma or neurosurgical interventions.

Patients may present with fever, headaches, neck stiffness, focal neurologic findings, and altered mental status. The diagnosis is made on the basis of clinical suspicion and the presence of risk factors, along with clinical and radiologic findings, with the MRI showing ring enhancing lesions with surrounding edema.

Lumbar puncture may be contraindicated in the presence of mass effect; however, if a CSF sample is obtained, there may be increased WBC and protein levels, with normal to decreased glucose level. Atypical lymphocytes and monoclonal B cells are seen in lymphoproliferative disorders and not in brain abscesses.

Brain abscesses evolve through different stages, with initial cerebritis in the first few days, then the formation of central necrosis with surrounding vasogenic edema, and the subsequent formation of a capsule. The abscess eventually matures, with the development of collagenous tissue in the capsule and regression of the vasogenic edema. Caseating granulomas are not seen in cerebral bacterial abscesses.

Given that these lesions are polymicrobial, the treatment of choice is a combination of antibiotics, usually a third-generation cephalosporin (for streptococci and gram-negative bacilli), metronidazole (for anaerobes), and vancomycin (for staphylococci). The IV antibiotic regimen is continued for 6 to 8 weeks, and subsequent continuous oral antibiotics may be required for 2 to 3 months. Some cases may require surgical intervention, with stereotactic aspiration or excision. Vasogenic edema is treated with steroids and sometimes hyperosmolar agents are required.

Pyrimethamine and sulfadiazine are used for cerebral toxoplasmosis, which is not the diagnosis in this patient. Antiretroviral therapy plays no role in the treatment of cerebral abscesses. These lesions are not typically caused by mycobacteria.

Bradley WG, Daroff RB, Fenichel GM, et al. Neurology in Clinical Practice, 5th ed. Philadelphia, PA: Elsevier; 2008.

26. d

This patient has septic cavernous sinus thrombosis, which can be a complication of bacterial sinus infections, and manifests with proptosis, compromise of the cranial nerves (CNs) traveling within the sinus (CNs V1 and V2, III, IV, and VI), retinal vein engorgement with retinal hemorrhages, and papilledema.

Patients with intracranial infections may also develop thrombosis of other sinuses such as the superior sagittal or the transverse sinuses. Diagnosis is based on clinical suspicion and radiologic studies. MRV or angiographies with venous phases are very useful. Treatment involves antibiotic therapy, covering gram-positive agents, staphylococci, gram-negative organisms, and anaerobes.

    This patient's proptosis and cranial nerve abnormalities suggest involvement of the cavernous sinus rather than the superior sagittal or the transverse sinus. Basilar meningitis can cause cranial neuropathies; however, basilar meningitis and brain abscess would not produce the constellation of neurologic manifestations that this patient has.

Bradley WG, Daroff RB, Fenichel GM, et al. Neurology in Clinical Practice, 5th ed. Philadelphia, PA: Elsevier; 2008.

27. d, 28. a

This patient has tuberculous (TB) meningitis. This diagnosis is suspected on the basis of his epidemiologic factors, clinical findings, and CSF findings and confirmed with the leptomeningeal biopsy, which demonstrates a granulomatous inflammatory response with multinucleated giant cells and caseating necrosis, as seen in Figure 15.5.

    TB meningitis is caused by *Mycobacterium tuberculosis*, which is an aerobic mycobacterium that spreads via respiratory droplets leading to a primary infection (usually pulmonary) and subsequent reactivation (usually in the setting of immunosuppression). TB meningitis tends to affect the base of the brain and commonly presents with fever, headache, neck stiffness, multiple cranial neuropathies (due to involvement of the basilar aspect of the brain) and altered mental status. Focal neurologic manifestations and seizures may also occur.

    CSF demonstrates elevated protein level (80 to 400 mg/dL), low glucose level (less than 40 mg/dL), and lymphocytic pleocytosis (200 to 400 cells/μL). Opening pressure is usually elevated but may be normal. Acid fast bacillus (AFB) smear is diagnostic in 10% to 30% of the cases, and CSF cultures may be positive in 45% to 70%; however, the results may take between 6 and 8 weeks to become positive. PCR has higher sensitivity and may be helpful for a faster diagnosis. Brain MRI may be normal or may demonstrate meningeal enhancement, especially on the basal surface. Pathologic specimens show caseating granulomas, mononuclear inflammatory infiltrates, and multinucleated giant cells as described in this case.

    Combinations of multiple anti-TB agents are used to kill the organisms and avoid inducing resistance. Commonly used medications are isoniazid, rifampin, pyrazinamide, streptomycin, and ethambutol. Usually, four drugs are initially administered for 2 months, after which the regimen can be reduced to two drugs that can be continued for several months.

    Mycobacterium tuberculosis can affect the spinal cord and the brain parenchyma, where it can lead to the formation of tuberculomas. These lesions behave like space-occupying lesions, and the treatment is with anti-TB medications.

    Peripheral nerves are more commonly affected by *Mycobacterium leprae* rather than *Mycobacterium tuberculosis*; in leprosy, nerve thickening occurs, and mononeuritis multiplex is a common manifestation (discussed in questions 29–30).

Bradley WG, Daroff RB, Fenichel GM, et al. Neurology in Clinical Practice, 5th ed. Philadelphia, PA: Elsevier; 2008.

29. b, 30. d

This patient has Hansen disease, which is the cause of her neuropathy. Hansen disease, or leprosy, is caused by *Mycobacterium leprae* and is an important cause of neuropathy and skin disease worldwide. Most cases in the United States occur in immigrants, especially from Asia, the South Pacific, India, South America, and certain parts of Africa. *Mycobacterium leprae* is transmitted after prolonged and close contact with a patient with the disease, with an incubation period that is very long, lasting for years. The organism is thought to spread through the respiratory tract, from where it disseminates to other regions, especially the skin and superficial nerves, and mainly to cooler regions of the body. When invading the peripheral nerves, the mycobacterium tends to involve the Schwann cells preferentially.

There are two main variants determined by the immune reaction against this mycobacterium, and these variants are the tuberculoid and lepromatous forms. In between these, there are three borderline variants: borderline tuberculoid, borderline intermediate, and borderline lepromatous forms. The tuberculoid variant presents in patients with strong cell-mediated immunity and an intense delayed hypersensitivity reaction, causing destruction of peripheral nerves and inflammatory lesions in the skin. These patients typically have demarcated hypopigmented lesions and areas of sensory loss, especially to temperature and pinprick. Peripheral nerves are involved, indurated, hypertrophic, and palpable, and sensory loss may be prominent, leading to trauma. Nerves predominantly involved are the ulnar, radial, common peroneal, sural, and greater auricular. Claw-hand from ulnar involvement and footdrop from common peroneal involvement may be present.

The lepromatous form is present in patients with poor cell-mediated immunity with proliferation of the mycobacteria as they invade the tissues. It is characterized by skin infiltration by the mycobacteria, leading to diffuse cutaneous involvement in the coolest regions such as the pinna of the ear, tip of the nose, and dorsum of the hands and feet. Nerves may also be involved but usually at later stages.

The treatment of Hansen disease is prolonged, usually with a combination of dapsone and rifampin, sometimes with the addition of clofazimine.

Bradley WG, Daroff RB, Fenichel GM, et al. Neurology in Clinical Practice, 5th ed. Philadelphia, PA: Elsevier; 2008.

Ropper AH, Samuels MA. Adams and Victor's Principles of Neurology, 9th ed. New York, NY: McGraw-Hill; 2009.

31. C

This patient has manifestations of neurosyphilis, more specifically meningovascular syphilis. Syphilis is caused by the spirochete *Treponema pallidum*, which transmits vertically from mother to child or via sexual contact. In infected adults, three phases with a latent period and various neurologic complications are described:

- Primary syphilis is characterized by the development of a painless chancre at the site of entry (genital region). There is asymptomatic systemic spread of the organism, and the chancre eventually disappears
- Secondary syphilis develops approximately 2 to 12 weeks after the contact, with manifestations of systemic dissemination, including constitutional symptoms, lymphadenopathy, and rash (classically palms and soles). Syphilitic meningitis and cranial neuropathies may occur in this second stage
- Latent period is an asymptomatic phase with serologic evidence of the disease, which may last for years
- Tertiary syphilis is characterized by cardiovascular complications (such as aortitis), gummatous complications, and neurologic complications

Major neurologic complications include pure meningeal syphilis, meningovascular syphilis, tabes dorsalis and parenchymatous neurosyphilis. Meningeal invasion of the treponemes can lead to meningitis and meningovascular syphilis, in which there is endarteritis obliterans and vasculitis, which can lead to strokes in different arterial distributions; this can occur at any stage but often occurs within the first 4–7 years of infection with syphilis. Tabes dorsalis is the classical myelopathy with areflexia, lightning pains, sensory ataxia, loss of pain and temperature sensation, and relatively preserved strength, leading to gait instability and the development of Charcot joints. Parenchymatous syphilis (general paresis) is the encephalitic form in which patients develop progressive dementia, neuropsychiatric manifestations, speech disturbance, and pupillary abnormalities. Argyll-Robertson pupils, which accommodate but do not react to light, may be seen in patients with neurosyphilis. Manifestations of neurosyphilis may overlap in the same patient, usually presenting with a combination of findings.

Bradley WG, Daroff RB, Fenichel GM, et al. Neurology in Clinical Practice, 5th ed. Philadelphia, PA: Elsevier; 2008.

32. a

This patient has Whipple disease, caused by *Tropheryma whippelii*. Whipple disease is a multisystemic disease, initially affecting the gastrointestinal tract, producing abdominal pain, diarrhea, and weight loss. It can also produce arthritis, cutaneous hypopigmentation, adrenal insufficiency, and various neurologic manifestations, including dementia, supranuclear ophthalmoplegia, ataxia, oculomasticatory myorrhythmia (such as described in this case), meningitis, neuropathy, and myopathy. Some patients with Whipple disease may present only with CNS manifestations, without the characteristic diarrhea and joint symptoms.

The diagnosis is made on the basis of gastrointestinal biopsy demonstrating periodic acid Schiff-positive macrophage inclusions. CSF-PCR for *Tropheryma whippelii* can also be helpful. A prolonged course of trimethoprim-sulfamethoxazole is the treatment of choice.

Angiotensin-converting enzyme is utilized for the evaluation of sarcoidosis, and the 14–3-3 protein is used in the diagnostic workup for CJD, neither of which are the diagnosis in this patient. This patient does not have vitamin B_{12} deficiency. She does not have celiac sprue and, therefore, avoiding gluten is not recommended.

Bradley WG, Daroff RB, Fenichel GM, et al. Neurology in Clinical Practice, 5th ed. Philadelphia, PA: Elsevier; 2008.

33. b

This patient has CJD, which is a transmissible spongiform encephalopathy. The MRI shown in Figure 15.6 demonstrates restricted diffusion of the cortex (cortical ribboning) and the head of the caudate, which are findings not seen in the diagnoses provided in the other options. Other MRI findings seen in some CJD variants include bilateral signal hyperintensity in both thalami (especially in the pulvinar region, known as the pulvinar sign) and in the anterior portions of the putamen. The combination of anterior putamen and caudate head hyperintensity is known as the "hockey-stick" sign.

Patients with CJD present clinically with a rapidly progressive dementia, neuropsychiatric symptoms, cerebellar ataxia, and myoclonus. These patients deteriorate rapidly and inexorably die within months. The diagnosis is suspected on the basis of clinical features and supported by ancillary tests such as MRI, EEG, and CSF studies. EEG shows a typical periodic pattern. CSF 14-3-3 protein can be seen in many other causes of neuronal destruction, but for sporadic CJD, it can be up to 94% sensitive and 93% specific. CSF tau is also used in the diagnosis. Neuropathologic evaluation may be required in some cases and demonstrates significant spongiform degeneration with neuronal loss, vacuolar changes, and astrocytosis (discussed in chapter 12).

Bradley WG, Daroff RB, Fenichel GM, et al. Neurology in Clinical Practice, 5th ed. Philadelphia, PA: Elsevier; 2008.

34. a

Primary CNS lymphoma (PCNSL) is more frequently diagnosed in immunocompromised patients, especially in patients with AIDS. Almost all of these cases are associated with Epstein-Barr virus (EBV), and CSF EBV PCR is helpful in the diagnosis. In contrast, PCNSL in immunocompetent patients is not commonly associated with EBV.

In general, PCNSL in immunocompromised patients occurs at earlier ages than in those who are immunocompetent. It is not possible to differentiate PCNSL in immunocompromised patients versus immunocompetent patients only on the basis of imaging, CSF findings, or cytology. There is no clear evidence of differences in response to steroids in either group.

Bradley WG, Daroff RB, Fenichel GM, et al. Neurology in Clinical Practice, 5th ed. Philadelphia, PA: Elsevier; 2008.

35. d

This patient has tabes dorsalis, which is caused by syphilis in its tertiary phase, and occurs if syphilis in its primary stages is untreated and the spirochete invades the CNS, in this case the spinal cord. However, not all cases of untreated syphilis progress to the subsequent stages, and only less than 10% of patients with untreated syphilis will develop symptomatic neurosyphilis.

The diagnosis of syphilis is based on clinical manifestations along with supportive laboratory evidence. There are treponemal and nontreponemal tests. Nontreponemal tests are the Venereal Disease Research Laboratory (VDRL) test and the Rapid Plasma Reagin test. These tests are more sensitive but less specific than treponemal tests and become negative some time after treatment. Treponemal antibodies remain positive for life and include the fluorescent treponemal antibody, syphilis immunoglobulin G, and microhemagglutination assay among others. For the diagnosis of neurosyphilis, CSF should be analyzed, usually showing mononuclear pleocytosis with elevated protein levels. CSF VDRL is very specific for neurosyphilis but may be negative in as many as 25% of cases. Intrathecal antibody production against *Treponema pallidum*, oligoclonal bands, and PCR are also helpful for the diagnosis.

Treatment of neurosyphilis involves intravenous antibiotics, and the first choice is penicillin G 4 million units every 4 hours for 14 days. Antibiotic therapy may clear the infection; however, it will not reverse already established neurologic manifestations of tertiary syphilis. Follow-up CSF analysis is recommended to assess the response to therapy.

Bradley WG, Daroff RB, Fenichel GM, et al. Neurology in Clinical Practice, 5th ed. Philadelphia, PA: Elsevier; 2008.

36. d

CJD is a prion disease, caused by conformational changes of the prion protein from cellular prion protein (PrP^C) to scrapie prion protein (PrP^{Sc}), which has an increased β-sheet content. This leads to physico-chemical changes in the protein, making it resistant to proteinases, poorly soluble in water, and with a tendency to polymerize, which leads to neuronal death. PrP^{Sc} has the ability to bind to PrP^C and induce its conformational change, therefore making this agent infective.

CJD can be sporadic or familial, caused by mutations in the prion protein gene. The familial form can be inherited in an autosomal dominant fashion. EEG is helpful in making the diagnosis, showing a repetitive periodic pattern. CJD is not necessarily associated with compromised immunity, and therefore does not depend on CD4 counts. Granulovacuolar degeneration and neurofibrillary tangles are seen in Alzheimer disease and not in CJD.

Bradley WG, Daroff RB, Fenichel GM, et al. Neurology in Clinical Practice, 5th ed. Philadelphia, PA: Elsevier; 2008.

37. c

This patient has HSV encephalitis, likely from HSV type 1, which is the most common cause of fatal sporadic viral encephalitis in the United States. This virus is transmitted via respiratory or salivary secretions, spreading to the CNS, where it tends to affect the orbitofrontal and temporal regions. Patients present with fever, headaches, behavioral changes, altered mental status, focal neurologic findings, and seizures. CSF analysis is the most important diagnostic test, demonstrating a lymphocytic pleocytosis (10 to 1000 WBCs/μL), moderately elevated protein and normal glucose levels. Increased RBC count in the CSF or xanthochromia is seen frequently; however, this finding is neither sensitive nor specific. CSF HSV PCR is 95% sensitive and almost 99% specific for this condition; however, there may be false-negative results if the CSF is sampled in the first 24 hours of the illness. The MRI, as shown in Figure 15.7 demonstrates FLAIR T2 hyperintensities and restricted diffusion in the temporal regions—in this case, on the right side. Treatment with intravenous acyclovir 10 mg/kg every 8 hours should be started as soon as possible and continued for a minimum of 14 days.

This patient does not have West Nile virus (WNV) encephalitis, which is an arthropod-borne viral encephalitis that occurs in the summer months. WNV encephalitis is discussed in question 6. The CSF findings are not consistent with bacterial meningitis, which typically causes neutrophilic pleocytosis. Since this patient has findings of parenchymal involvement, this is an encephalitis rather than a meningitis; therefore, this is not consistent with enteroviral meningitis. Tuberculous meningitis is discussed in questions 27 and 28.

Bradley WG, Daroff RB, Fenichel GM, et al. Neurology in Clinical Practice, 5th ed. Philadelphia, PA: Elsevier; 2008.

38. a

This patient has features suggestive of fatal familial insomnia, which is a prion disorder characterized by progressive intractable insomnia and symptoms of sympathetic hyperactivity such as hypertension, tachycardia, hyperthermia, and hyperhidrosis. Patients may also have cognitive impairment, tremor, ataxia, hyperreflexia, and myoclonus.

CJD exists in different variants, including sporadic, familial, iatrogenic, and new variant forms. The sporadic form is the typical form that was described in question 33. The familial variant is similar; however, it may present earlier, and the course is more protracted and insidious. The iatrogenic form is very rare and has been described in the past in patients who received cadaver-derived human growth hormone, and after neurosurgical procedures or corneal transplants. Gerstmann-Straussler-Scheinker is an inherited prion disease that progresses slowly over years. It is characterized by cerebellar ataxia and dysarthria, sometimes extrapyramidal features followed by dementia. These patients may also have gaze palsies, deafness, cortical blindness, extensor plantar response, and hyporeflexia in the lower extremities. The new variant CJD was first described in 1996 and is believed to occur from infection through consumption of cattle products contaminated with the agent of bovine spongiform encephalopathy. In contrast to traditional forms of CJD, new variant CJD affects younger patients (third to fourth decade of life), and the duration is more protracted.

Bradley WG, Daroff RB, Fenichel GM, et al. Neurology in Clinical Practice, 5th ed. Philadelphia, PA: Elsevier; 2008.

39. c

Abnormal EEG findings are common in patients with HSV encephalitis. Periodic lateralized epileptiform discharges (PLEDs) in the temporal regions are characteristic and support the diagnosis. Diffuse slowing, which is nonspecific, can also be seen.

Occipital seizures can be seen in various conditions, including occipital lobe epilepsies, and in posterior reversible encephalopathy syndrome.

Triphasic waves are seen typically in hepatic encephalopathy, but they are seen also in other metabolic encephalopathies, including uremic encephalopathy. While 14- and 6-Hz spikes are normal and benign findings, 3-Hz spike and wave complexes are seen in absence epilepsy.

Bradley WG, Daroff RB, Fenichel GM, et al. Neurology in Clinical Practice, 5th ed. Philadelphia, PA: Elsevier; 2008.

40. a

MRI is helpful in the evaluation of HSV encephalitis, demonstrating the structural lesions that occur, typically focal abnormalities in the temporal lobes with increased signal intensity on T2-weighted images (see Figure 15.7). The presence of hemorrhagic changes in the temporal regions is suggestive of HSV encephalitis, correlating with the pathologic findings of foci of hemorrhages and necrosis.

T2 hyperintensity and restricted diffusion in the posterior head regions are not typically seen in HSV encephalitis and are more consistent with posterior reversible encephalopathy syndrome. The hockey-stick and pulvinar signs are seen in CJD (see question 33). Leptomeningeal enhancement in the basal regions is nonspecific and may be seen in conditions such as tuberculous meningitis or neurosarcoidosis. Diffuse white matter hyperintensities on T2-weighted images is also nonspecific but may be seen in acute disseminated encephalomyelitis or in leukodystrophies.

Bradley WG, Daroff RB, Fenichel GM, et al. Neurology in Clinical Practice, 5th ed. Philadelphia, PA: Elsevier; 2008.

41. e

Subacute sclerosing panencephalitis (SSPE) is a rare and late complication of measles, which is not an arbovirus. Measles can cause four major neurologic syndromes:

- Acute encephalitis
- Postviral encephalomyelitis
- Measles inclusion body encephalitis, which is a rapidly progressive dementing illness with seizures, myoclonus, and coma, occurring 1 to 6 months after measles infection in patients with cell-mediated immunodeficiency
- SSPE, which is caused by defective measles virus maturation in neural cells

Children infected in the first two years of life are the ones at the greatest risk for SSPE, which may develop 2 to 12 years after the infection. It begins with behavioral and personality changes, later causing seizures, myoclonus, spasticity, choreoathetoid and ballistic movements, ataxia, optic atrophy, quadriparesis, autonomic instability, akinetic mutism, and eventually coma. Neurons contain nuclear and cytoplasmic viral inclusion bodies, and levels of CSF and serum antibodies are elevated. MRI demonstrates T2 hyperintensity in the gray and subcortical white matter more in the posterior regions. EEG shows periodic slow-wave complexes at regular intervals and a background of depressed activity.

Regarding the arboviruses, these are arthropod-borne viruses, transmitted by mosquitoes, and more than 500 arbovirus-transmitted RNA viruses exist, including Saint Louis encephalitis virus, West Nile virus, La Crosse encephalitis virus, Japanese encephalitis virus, and Eastern and Western Equine encephalitis viruses.

Bradley WG, Daroff RB, Fenichel GM, et al. Neurology in Clinical Practice, 5th ed. Philadelphia, PA: Elsevier; 2008.

42. b

This patient has aspergillosis, which is caused by the aspergillus fungus. This organism is capable of causing various manifestations, such as allergic syndromes, respiratory tract infections, and sinusitis. However, it may also cause an invasive syndrome that can spread to the CNS, especially in neutropenic patients, immunocompromised patients, or those on chronic steroids. *Aspergillus fumigatus* is the organism that causes most of the invasive syndromes, invading blood vessels, causing stroke-like syndromes, infarcts, and hemorrhagic transformation. A vasculitis-like phenomenon occurs as the fungus invades the vessel walls and may eventually progress to parenchymal disease, forming granulomas and abscesses. This fungus may invade multiple other organs and cause systemic disease.

Histopathologically, invading hyphae are detected in blood vessels, with the findings of necrosis, hemorrhage, and inflammation. The specimen shown in Figure 15.8 is a Gomori methenamine silver stain demonstrating septate hyphae that branch at acute angles, which is consistent with aspergillus infection. Aspergillosis does not typically present with meningitis.

Cryptococcus causes meningitis and not typically a vasculitis-type syndrome. Histoplasmosis causes pulmonary disease more frequently, but when it invades the CNS, it can produce a form of basilar meningitis, focal cerebritis, or granulomas. Candidiasis can also cause systemic disease, with histopathological findings of budding yeasts and pseudohyphae. This patient does not have clinical features or pathologic findings of HSV encephalitis (discussed in question 37).

Bradley WG, Daroff RB, Fenichel GM, et al. Neurology in Clinical Practice, 5th ed. Philadelphia, PA: Elsevier; 2008.

Fauci AS, Braunwald E, Kasper DL, et al. Harrison's Principles of Internal Medicine, 17th ed. New York, NY: McGraw-Hill; 2008.

43. d

The specimen in Figure 15.9 shows a parasite consistent with cysticercosis. Neurocysticercosis is caused by the pork tapeworm *Taenia solium* and has a worldwide distribution, being endemic in Latin America, Africa, the Indian subcontinent, and parts of Asia.

Human ingestion of undercooked pork meat containing cysticerci may lead to infection with the intestinal tapeworms but does not cause the manifestations of neurocysticercosis, which occurs only with infection at a specific stage of the tapeworm life cycle. When the adult tapeworm resides in the small bowel of either the pig or the human, proglottids are released and excreted in to the feces. The eggs in these proglottids are infective to humans and animals. After humans ingest these eggs, larvae are released that penetrate the intestinal wall and migrate to various tissues, causing cysticercosis and neurocysticercosis. Clinical manifestations may occur years later, including seizures, focal neurologic symptoms, a vasculitic-type syndrome with strokes, increased intracranial pressure, headaches, hydrocephalus, and rarely coma.

Neuroimaging is helpful in the diagnosis of neurocysticercosis, showing cystic lesions that may have contrast enhancement and calcifications. The treatment of choice is albendazole.

Praziquantel is an alternative. Since patients commonly have seizures, antiepileptic agents are used and may be required for life.

Taenia saginata is the beef tapeworm but does not cause neurocysticercosis.

India ink is used to detect *Cryptococcus* but is not useful in cysticercosis.

Cysticercosis is not transmitted by flies. The tsetse fly transmits *Trypanosoma brucei*, which causes African trypanosomiasis, or sleeping sickness.

Bradley WG, Daroff RB, Fenichel GM, et al. Neurology in Clinical Practice, 5th ed. Philadelphia, PA: Elsevier; 2008.

Fauci AS, Braunwald E, Kasper DL, et al. Harrison's Principles of Internal Medicine, 17th ed. New York, NY: McGraw-Hill; 2008.

44. a

This patient has amebic meningoencephalitis. The diagnosis is based on clinical history and epidemiological factors and is confirmed by the histopathologic specimen, which shows an inflammatory infiltrate and trophozoites, consistent with an amebic infection.

Amebic meningoencephalitis is caused by free-living amebae, such as *Naegleria fowleri*, *Acanthamoeba*, and *Balamuthia mandrillaris*. Patients acquire the amebae by swimming in contaminated ponds or lakes. The parasites enter the brain by passing through the cribriform plate and along the olfactory nerve to enter the frontal lobes and cause a necrotizing inflammation with destruction. Acanthamoeba can also enter the CNS through hematogenous dissemination and from a primary corneal infection acquired by using contact lenses stored in contaminated solution.

Patients with amebic encephalitis present with rapid progression of headaches, fever, neck stiffness, nausea, and vomiting and eventually develop focal neurologic findings, seizures, and altered mental status. The progression is rapid, and the disease is usually fatal.

CSF opening pressure is increased, and CSF analysis shows a neutrophilic pleocytosis, increased protein, and decreased glucose levels. Gram stain will not show the organism, but trophozoites may be seen on a wet preparation of unspun spinal fluid. Pathologically, there are findings consistent with a purulent meningitis, with microabscesses in the parenchyma, and an extensive necrotizing destruction of the parenchyma. A polymorphonuclear inflammatory infiltrate and trophozoites can be seen, such as in the histopathologic specimen shown in Figure 15.10.

Bradley WG, Daroff RB, Fenichel GM, et al. Neurology in Clinical Practice, 5th ed. Philadelphia, PA: Elsevier; 2008.

Ropper AH, Samuels MA. Adams and Victor's Principles of Neurology, 9th ed. New York, NY: McGraw-Hill; 2009.

45. c, 46. d

This patient has Lyme disease, which has a broad variety of neurologic presentations; however, bacterial meningitis with neutrophilic predominance is unlikely to occur. Subdural empyema is not seen in Lyme disease.

Lyme disease is caused by *Borrelia burgdorferi*. It is more commonly acquired in the Northeastern United States and is transmitted by a tick bite, more specifically the *Ixodes* tick. Lyme disease has an early phase and a late phase, and neurologic complications occur in both. In the early phase, patients may have a rash called erythema migrans, which is characteristic and has a "bull's eye" appearance. Other nonneurologic manifestations include carditis, arthralgias, lymphadenopathy, and fever. Neurologic manifestations in the early phase include the following:

– Aseptic meningitis: these patients have a mononuclear pleocytosis and mild elevation of protein levels in the CSF, as well as intrathecal production of antibodies against *Borrelia burgdorferi*
– Encephalitis
– Cranial neuropathy: commonly cranial nerve VII, and this can be uni- or bilateral
– Peripheral nervous system: including mononeuritis multiplex, peripheral neuropathy, polyradiculopathy, or even a Guillain-Barre type presentation (which is not common).

Neurologic presentations in the late phase are encephalopathy, encephalomyelitis, and peripheral neuropathy.

The diagnosis of CNS Lyme disease is based on clinical and epidemiological suspicion, supported by the presence of positive serology, CSF abnormalities, and intrathecal production of antibodies. Serology is positive in 10% of people living in endemic areas, and this should be taken into account. The treatment is antibiotic therapy with intravenous ceftriaxone, up to 2 g daily for 2 to 4 weeks. For late presentations, a longer course may be required. Oral antibiotic therapy with doxycycline can be used in patients without CSF abnormalities.

Bradley WG, Daroff RB, Fenichel GM, et al. Neurology in Clinical Practice, 5th ed. Philadelphia, PA: Elsevier; 2008.

Ropper AH, Samuels MA. Adams and Victor's Principles of Neurology, 9th ed. New York, NY: McGraw-Hill; 2009.

Buzz Phrases	Key Points
Erythema migrans	Lyme disease
Nasal and maxillary necrotizing lesion and diabetic ketoacidosis	Mucormycosis
Meningitis, positive India ink ± budding yeasts	Cryptococcus
AIDS and MRI showing ring enhancing masses with edema	Consider toxoplasmosis and CNS lymphoma
AIDS with mass lesion and positive Epstein-Barr virus PCR	Primary CNS lymphoma
AIDS and multiple nonenhancing lesions in the parieto-occipital regions. Pathology showing myelin loss, giant astrocytes, and altered oligodendrocytes, with enlarged nuclei and viral inclusions	JC virus, progressive multifocal leukoencephalopathy
Meningitis in the very young or very elderly	Consider *Listeria monocytogenes*
Hypopigmented lesions and enlarged peripheral nerves	*Mycobacterium leprae*
Oculomasticatory myorrhythmia	Whipple disease
Progressive dementia, 14–3-3 protein, EEG with periodic pattern, MRI with hyperintensity in the cortex, bilateral thalami, pulvinar, and head of the caudate	CJD
Encephalitis and bilateral temporal hemorrhages	HSV encephalitis

Chapter 16

Neurologic Complications of Systemic Diseases and Pregnancy

Questions

1. A 52-year-old woman with a prosthetic aortic valve presents to the emergency department with complaints of fever, chills, and generalized malaise of 3 weeks' duration. She is found to have *Staphylococcus epidermidis* bacteremia, and a transesophageal echocardiogram shows an echodensity on her aortic valve. Two days after admission, she develops left hemiparesis. MRI of the brain shows multiple bilateral cortical foci of restricted diffusion, the largest being in the right MCA territory. Which of the following is incorrect regarding this patient's condition?
   a. Ischemic strokes due to septic emboli are the most common neurologic complication of infective endocarditis
   b. Cerebral septic emboli lead to arteritis of the involved vessel with subsequent development of mycotic aneurysms in some cases
   c. Hemorrhagic conversion of an ischemic infarct is the most common cause of intracerebral hemorrhage in patients with infective endocarditis
   d. Patients with ischemic stroke due to infective endocarditis should be immediately anticoagulated to prevent further strokes
   e. Neurologic complications are more common in patients with native valve endocarditis than in those with prosthetic valve endocarditis

2. A 16-year-old boy with sickle cell anemia (Hemoglobin [Hb] SS disease) presents with sudden onset of left hemiparesis. He has had a fever with productive cough for 4 days. Chest radiograph shows pneumonia. CT scan of the brain shows a hypodensity in the right MCA territory. Which of the following statements is incorrect regarding this patient's condition?
   a. Patients with sickle cell anemia (Hb SS disease) are more likely to suffer from neurologic complications as compared to those with hemoglobin SC (Hb SC) disease

677

b. Intracerebral hemorrhage is more common than ischemic stroke in patients with Hb SS disease

c. Patients with Hb SS disease are at risk of developing intracerebral aneurysms with subsequent subarachnoid hemorrhage

d. Myelopathy and radiculopathy may be complications of vertebral body infarction in patients with Hb SS disease

e. In children found to have elevated cerebral blood flow velocities on transcranial Doppler ultrasonography, blood transfusion reduces the risk of ischemic stroke

Questions 3–4

3. Which of the following statements is incorrect regarding neurologic involvement in patients with plasma cell dyscrasias and other hematological disorders?

a. Infiltration of vertebral bones from myeloma cells can be complicated by spinal cord and nerve root compression

b. POEMS syndrome (plasma cell dyscrasia with polyneuropathy, organomegaly, endocrinopathy, monoclonal gammopathy, and skin changes) is a constellation of abnormalities seen in some patients with plasma cell dyscrasias, particularly plasmacytoma

c. Plasma cell dyscrasias are associated with both paraneoplastic and infiltrative neuropathies

d. Causes of encephalopathy in patients with plasma cell dyscrasias include hypercalcemia, hyperviscosity syndrome, and CNS infections due to their immunocompromised state

e. Presence of neuropathy in a patient with monoclonal gammopathy invariably indicates that the patient has multiple myeloma

4. A 62-year-old woman presented with a 4-month history of paresthesias that began in her toes and later extended up to her shins and began involving her fingertips. Over the prior few weeks, she had noticed herself to be tripping more frequently than usual. Examination showed bilateral foot dorsiflexion and plantar flexion to be Modified Research Council grade 4/5. Wrist extension was 4/5 on the left. Otherwise, motor examination was normal. Sensory examination revealed reduced sensation to all modalities in the feet, including reduced vibratory sense and impaired proprioception. Deep tendon reflexes could not be elicited in any extremity. She had no family history of neuropathy, and there was no evidence of hammer toes or high-arched feet. EMG/NCS showed a demyelinating neuropathy with mild axon loss. Serum monoclonal protein immunofixation showed an immunoglobulin M monoclonal band. Which of the following tests would be indicated in this patient?

a. Genetic panel for Charcot-Marie-Tooth disease

b. A technetium bone scan

c. Antibodies against myelin-associated glycoprotein

d. Superoxide dismutase gene mutation

e. Anti-GQ1b antibodies

5. A 62-year-old woman has been feeling tired and sluggish and had appeared pale to her husband for several days. She complained of headache and felt feverish. While at the grocery store, she is witnessed to have a generalized tonic-clonic seizure and is brought to the emergency department. Her temperature is 39.1°C. Laboratory evaluation reveals a hemoglobin level of 6.6 g/dL (normal 13 to 17 g/dL), platelet count of 30,000/μL (normal 150 to 400/μL), and creatinine level of 1.8 mg/dL (normal 0.7 to 1.4 mg/dL). Review of a peripheral smear shows evidence of red blood cell fragmentation. Coagulation tests are normal. Lactate dehydrogenase level is elevated, and serum haptoglobin level is low. What is the most likely diagnosis in this patient?

a. Hemolytic-uremic syndrome

b. Idiopathic thrombocytopenic purpura

c. Thrombotic thrombocytopenic purpura

    d. Disseminated intravascular coagulation

    e. Anti-phospholipid antibody syndrome

6. A 42-year-old man with nonalcoholic steatohepatitis cirrhosis of the liver was brought to the emergency department by his wife, with confusion. One week earlier, he had started to show some signs of confusion, and over the prior few days, he had been sleeping most of the day, and at night, he would wake up distinctly confused and agitated. On examination, he appears restless and agitated and is mumbling incomprehensibly. Asterixis is noted on examination. An EEG shows moderate generalized slowing and triphasic waves. On reexamination a few hours later, he is somnolent but arousable to noxious stimuli. Which of the following is correct regarding the most likely cause of this patient's encephalopathy?

    a. A serum ammonia level can be used to assess for the severity of his condition and serially checked as a means of assessing response to therapy

    b. Given the extent of his encephalopathy, he must also have a history of alcoholism

    c. This patient should undergo a transjugular intrahepatic portosystemic shunt procedure to help treat his encephalopathy

    d. Treatment for this type of encephalopathy includes reducing absorption of ammonia in the colon and may include lactulose or neomycin

    e. A high-protein diet should be instituted in this patient

7. A 32-year-old woman presents with unsteadiness of walking. She reports that over the prior year, her gait has become progressively more unsteady. On review of systems, she reports chronic diarrhea, significant weight loss, and multiple food intolerances, including pasta, bread, and pastries. On examination, she has bilateral dysmetria and a wide-based, lurching gait. Examination also shows reduced sensation to pinprick and light touch on her extremities distally. MRI of the brain shows cerebellar atrophy. Upper gastrointestinal endoscopy with small bowel biopsy is obtained, and pathological examination of the biopsy specimens shows atrophy of the villi. Periodic acid-Schiff (PAS) staining of the biopsies does not show PAS-positive macrophage inclusions. Which of the following statements is incorrect regarding this patient's condition?

    a. Other neurologic complications that could be seen include inflammatory myopathy, cognitive dysfunction, and myoclonus

    b. There is an increased risk of seizures in patients with this condition

    c. Her neurologic symptoms are expected to improve with a gluten-free diet

    d. In some patients with this disorder, neurologic symptoms may be the presenting feature, without diarrhea or other gastrointestinal manifestations

    e. This patient should be treated with a prolonged course of a sulfonamide

8. A 24-year-old woman with ulcerative colitis is admitted to the hospital with increasing frequency of bowel movements and hematochezia. While being treated for her exacerbation, she experiences severe diffuse headache. MRV shows superior sagittal sinus thrombosis. Which of the following statements is incorrect regarding the neurologic complications of inflammatory bowel disease (IBD)?

    a. Neurologic complications are most common during acute exacerbations of IBD but can occur at any time

    b. Both demyelinating and axonal neuropathies can occur

    c. Patients are at increased risk of neurologic complications from vitamin deficiencies resulting from chronic malabsorption

    d. Patients with IBD are at increased risk of cerebral venous thrombosis, but there is not an increased risk of arterial thrombosis in these patients

    e. Patients with recurrent facial nerve palsies, angioedema, and tongue fissuring (Melkersson-Rosenthal syndrome) should be evaluated for IBD

9. Which of the following statements regarding the neurologic complications of renal failure are incorrect?
   a. Uremic encephalopathy often presents with impaired concentration and attention, apathy, and, in severe cases, obtundation
   b. Mononeuritis multiplex is the most common neuropathy seen in patients with chronic renal failure
   c. Seizures may occur in patients with acute or chronic renal failure
   d. Asterixis and multifocal myoclonus are often seen in uremic encephalopathy
   e. Dialysis disequilibrium syndrome may present with a range of neurologic manifestations ranging from mild encephalopathy to fatal cerebral edema

10. Various electrolyte abnormalities can lead to a spectrum of neurologic manifestations ranging from mild encephalopathy to seizures, coma, and even cerebral edema with death. Which of the following electrolyte abnormalities is not commonly associated with CNS complications?
    a. Hyponatremia
    b. Hypokalemia
    c. Hypocalcemia
    d. Hypercalcemia
    e. Hypomagnesemia

11. A 73-year-old woman is brought to the clinic by her daughter who is concerned about her mother's memory. Over the prior few months, she had become more forgetful, disinterested in social activities she used to enjoy, and slept most of the day. Her gait had also become somewhat more unsteady, and her daughter had noticed that her mother was having more difficulty climbing stairs. She has also noticed weight gain, constipation, and dry skin. Which of the following laboratory tests should be ordered on this patient?
    a. Serum growth hormone
    b. Anti-neuronal antibody
    c. Thyroid stimulating hormone
    d. Vitamin D
    e. Anti-microsomal antibodies

12. Which of the following statements is incorrect regarding the neurologic manifestations of thyroid disorders?
    a. The most common cause of treatable mental retardation is congenital hypothyroidism; it most commonly results from dysgenesis of the thyroid gland
    b. Pseudomyotonia (a delay in muscle relaxation following elicitation of deep tendon reflex) is a feature of hyperthyroidism
    c. Myopathy can result from both hypothyroidism and hyperthyroidism
    d. Tremor is present in the majority of patients with untreated hyperthyroidism
    e. Restricted upward gaze is the most common eye movement abnormality seen in patients with thyroid eye disease

13. A 73-year-old man with non–insulin-dependent diabetes since the age of 32 presents with non-healing, painless ulcers on his feet. On examination, he has absent vibratory sense from the toes to the knees bilaterally, reduced sensation to pinprick with a gradient up to the mid-thigh bilaterally, and impaired proprioception in the toes. Which of the following statements is correct regarding the peripheral nervous system complications of diabetes?

a. Sensory loss associated with significant motor weakness is the most common manifestation of diabetic polyneuropathy
b. A proximal predominantly motor neuropathy is the most common manifestation of diabetic polyneuropathy
c. Neuropathy can result from impaired glucose tolerance alone in patients not otherwise meeting laboratory criteria for diabetes
d. Diabetes rarely affects the autonomic nervous system
e. Diabetic neuropathy is reversible with adequate glycemic control

14. A 52-year-old man with recently diagnosed diabetes presents to the clinic with multiple complaints including headache, difficulty climbing stairs, and impotence. His wife reports that he is very moody and has become verbally and even physically aggressive, which is highly unusual for him. On examination, he has central obesity with abdominal striae and has multiple ecchymoses all over his body. On confrontation testing, he is found to have a bitemporal hemianopia. Hip flexors are Medical Research Council grade 4/5 bilaterally. What is the most likely diagnosis in this patient?
a. Hypothyroidism
b. Graves disease
c. Cushing disease
d. Addison disease
e. Hyperparathyroidism

15. Consultation is requested for a 22-year-old woman who was admitted to the orthopedic service for pathologic fracture of the right femur. She has a history of bilateral hearing loss of unclear etiology. On examination, she was noted to have reduced visual acuity, weakness of the right upper and lower facial muscles, and reduced sensation in the distribution of all three branches of the trigeminal nerve. Serum alkaline phosphatase level is elevated. What is the most likely diagnosis in this patient?
a. Achondroplasia
b. Osteopetrosis
c. Ankylosing spondylitis
d. Osteomalacia
e. Relapsing polychondritis

16. A 32-year-old woman is brought to the emergency department by her mother. Over the prior 2 weeks, the patient had been suffering from fever, headache, and facial rash that she had attributed to a viral illness and had not sought medical attention for. However, in the prior 2 days, the patient had become confused, with significant delusions and hallucinations. General examination revealed a rash on both her cheeks and a systolic murmur. Neurologic examination showed her to be severely encephalopathic, restless, and agitated. Otherwise, there were no focal neurologic abnormalities on examination. Laboratory evaluation showed elevated creatinine level, anemia, leucopenia, thrombocytopenia, and elevated antinuclear antibody. CSF analysis showed pleocytosis with elevated protein and normal glucose levels; CSF cultures and other testing for microorganisms were negative. What is the most likely diagnosis in this patient?
a. Systemic lupus erythematosus
b. Systemic sclerosus
c. Sarcoidosis
d. Behçet syndrome
e. Sjögren syndrome

Questions 17–18

17. A 52-year-old woman presents with gait instability. She began to experience left lower extremity painful paresthesias 2 years earlier, which were attributed to an L5-S1 radiculopathy and not further evaluated. Subsequently, her right leg became involved. Over the following 2 years, she experienced slowly progressive sensory loss in both of her extremities and began having frequent falls a few months prior to presentation. She reported falling even when she was just leaning over the sink to wash her face. Examination showed normal cranial nerve and motor examination, reduced sensation to pinprick over the upper and lower extremities, face, and trunk, and impaired proprioception, temperature discrimination, and vibratory sense in the fingers and toes. Deep tendon reflexes were hypoactive throughout. On review of systems, she endorsed multiple complaints including dry eyes, dry mouth, and orthostatic light-headedness. NCS showed reduced amplitude of the SNAPs in the arms and legs, but motor NCS is normal. What is the most likely diagnosis in this patient?

a. Small fiber neuropathy due to systemic lupus erythematosis
b. Subacute combined degeneration due to vitamin B_{12} deficiency
c. Sensory neuronopathy due to Sjögren syndrome
d. Generalized sensorimotor polyneuropathy due to Sjögren syndrome
e. Small fiber neuropathy due to Churg-Strauss syndrome

18. Which of the following diagnostic studies would not be helpful in making the diagnosis?

a. Schirmer test
b. Anti-Ro (SSA) antibody
c. Anti-La (SSB) antibody
d. Lip biopsy
e. Rectal biopsy

19. Which of the following disorders is most commonly associated with atlanto-axial dislocation?

a. Rheumatoid arthritis
b. Systemic sclerosis
c. Sarcoidosis
d. Behçet syndrome
e. Sjögren syndrome

Questions 20–21

20. A 44-year-old man with a history of hepatitis B infection due to blood transfusion presents to the clinic with complaints of pain in the right forearm with inability to extend his wrist or fingers and an inability to dorsiflex his left foot. He also complains of recent onset of severe abdominal pain. He is later admitted to the hospital with worsening abdominal pain and elevated serum lactate level. Because of concerns for bowel ischemia, he undergoes a mesenteric angiogram, which shows multiple mesenteric aneurysms. He later undergoes nerve biopsy, shown in Figure 16.1. Serum perinuclear anti-neutrophil cytoplasmic (P-ANCA) antibody is positive. Which of the following diagnoses is the most likely in this patient?

a. Churg-Strauss syndrome
b. Polyarteritis nodosa
c. Wegener granulomatosis
d. Kawasaki disease
e. Behçet syndrome

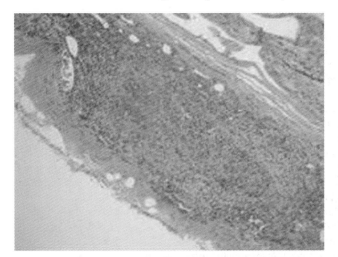

FIGURE 16.1   Nerve biopsy specimen. Courtesy of Dr. Richard Prayson. Shown also in color plates.

21. Which of the following systemic necrotizing vasculitides is not associated with the listed manifestations?
    a. Churg-Strauss syndrome—asthma, nasal polyps, peripheral eosinophilia, peripheral neuropathy
    b. Wegener granulomatosis—glomerulonephritis, inflammatory sinusitis, peripheral and cranial neuropathy
    c. Hepatitis C—vasculitis with type 2 cryoglobulinemia
    d. Kawasaki disease—aseptic meningitis
    e. Polyarteritis nodosa—recurrent oral and genital ulcers

22. A 19-year-old woman from Thailand had reported to family members feeling unwell for weeks, with fevers and malaise. She had a history of erythema nodosum and mild anemia that was under investigation. Other symptoms she had previously reported included pain in the calves whenever she walked more than approximately 50 meters without rest. One morning, she is found collapsed on the floor of her apartment, unresponsive. She is taken to an emergency department where a CT scan of the brain showed an acute infarct involving the entire territory of the left MCA. MRI of the brain also shows an extensive right lateral medullary infarct. Angiogram shows significant disease of the aortic arch, bilateral severe narrowing of the subclavian arteries and left carotid, and right vertebral occlusion. What is the most likely diagnosis in this patient?
    a. Primary angiitis of the CNS
    b. Polyarteritis nodosa
    c. Takayasu arteritis
    d. Temporal arteritis
    e. Microscopic polyangiitis

23. A 32-year-old woman from Turkey presents to the ophthalmologist, complaining of painful vision loss. Examination reveals uveitis. On review of systems, the patient endorses multiple recurrent oral and genital ulcers of several years duration. Which of the following is incorrect regarding this patient's disorder?

   a. The skin pathergy test is typically positive in this disorder
   b. Headaches are the most common neurologic manifestation
   c. Focal inflammation affecting the basal ganglia or brain stem is one pattern of CNS involvement that may occur
   d. Increased intracranial pressure with dural venous sinus thrombosis occurs
   e. A symmetric sensorimotor axonal polyneuropathy is a frequent occurrence in this disorder

24. Which of the following has not been associated with increased risk of venous thrombosis that may involve the CNS?
   a. Anti-phospholipid antibody syndrome
   b. Acquired factor VIII deficiency
   c. G20210 A prothrombin polymorphism
   d. Antithrombin III deficiency
   e. Factor V Leiden

Questions 25–26

25. A 32-year-old African American woman presented to the clinic, complaining of a moderate holocephalic headache of 3 weeks' duration. She denied a prior history of headaches. On review of systems, she endorsed a dry cough of several months' duration, which she had not sought medical evaluation for. On examination, the patient had normal cranial nerve, motor, and sensory examination. MRI of the brain is shown in Figure 16.2. CSF analysis showed 21 WBCs/μL (normal 0 to 5 WBCs/μL), protein level of 86 mg/dL (normal 50 to 75 mg/dL), and glucose level of 86 mg/dL (normal 15 to 45 mg/dL). CT scan of the chest revealed bilateral hilar adenopathy. Bronchoscopy was performed, and pathological review of the specimens obtained showed multiple noncaseating granulomas. What is the most likely diagnosis in this patient?

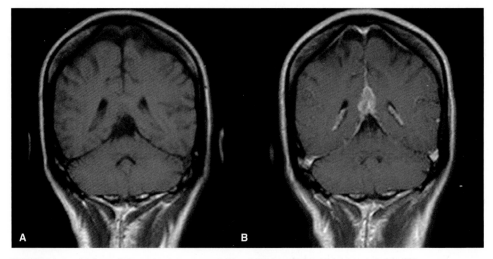

FIGURE 16.2   **(A)** Coronal T1-weighted precontrast MRI and **(B)** Coronal T1-weighted postcontrast MRI

   a. Wegener granulomatosis
   b. Primary CNS lymphoma

c. Disseminated tuberculosis
d. Metastatic breast cancer
e. Sarcoidosis

26. Regarding the disorder depicted in question 25, which of the following is incorrect?
a. Myelopathy is the most common presentation
b. Corticosteroids are the mainstay of therapy
c. Both large and small fiber neuropathy as well as myopathy may occur
d. Cranial nerve (CN) VII is the most commonly involved CN
e. Serum angiotensin-converting enzyme levels are neither sensitive nor specific for diagnosis

27. A 52-year-old woman presents to the emergency department with episodes of severe headaches, palpitations, and diaphoresis that have been occurring daily for the past several weeks. She had seen two other physicians, one of which had ordered an MRI of the brain and an MRA of the Circle of Willis, which were normal. Her attacks had been attributed to panic disorder. While being evaluated in the ED, she experiences a similar attack. Blood pressure during the attack is 190/110 mm Hg. Which of the following statements is correct?
a. These symptoms are likely hot flashes due to menopause, and she should be treated with hormone replacement therapy
b. She is likely suffering from panic attacks and should be referred to a psychiatrist
c. She may be suffering from pheochromocytoma and should under go exploratory laparotomy to find the tumor
d. She may be suffering from pheochromocytoma and plasma free metanephrine level should be checked
e. She may be suffering from pheochromocytoma and should undergo 24-hour urine collection for 5-hydroxyindoleacetic acid

28. Which of the following statements is incorrect regarding the pituitary?
a. The anterior pituitary is derived embryologically from Rathke's pouch, which evaginates from the oropharyngeal membrane during fetal development
b. The pituitary derives its blood supply from perforating branches of the basilar artery
c. Secretion of hormones from the anterior pituitary is controlled by the hypothalamus; the hypophyseal-portal system serves for regulation of hormone release controlled by the hypothalamus
d. Antidiuretic hormone and oxytocin are synthesized in the supraoptic and paraventricular nucleus of the hypothalamus and are secreted from the posterior pituitary
e. The classic visual field deficit occurring due to sellar lesions is a bitemporal hemianopia due to pressure on the optic chiasm

29. A 63-year-old woman undergoes transsphenoidal resection of a pituitary mass. Following surgery, she reports feeling markedly thirsty and reports urinating excessively. Her serum sodium level is noted to be 161 mmol/L (normal 135 to 146 mmol/L). Which of the following statements is correct regarding the likely cause of this patient's hypernatremia?
a. Her urine osmolality is likely high
b. If this patient is administered desmopressin, her urine osmolality will increase
c. Water deprivation is the treatment of choice in this patient
d. Hypertonic saline is the treatment of choice for this patient
e. This patient's serum sodium level is elevated because of an excess of antidiuretic hormone

30. A 62-year-old man with aneurysmal subarachnoid hemorrhage (SAH) is admitted to the ICU. Seven days into the hospitalization, he is noted to have a serum sodium concentration of 129 mmol/L (normal 135 to 146 mmol/L). Further testing reveals elevated urinary sodium and urinary osmolarity. He is noted to be hypotensive and tachycardic. Central venous pressure is low. Which of the following statements is correct?

 a. His hyponatremia is likely due to syndrome of inappropriate antidiuretic hormone secretion (SIADH), and he should be treated with fluid restriction
 b. His hyponatremia is likely due to cerebral salt wasting, and he should be treated with fluid restriction
 c. His hyponatremia is likely due to SIADH, and he should be treated with intravenous fluids
 d. His hyponatremia is likely due to cerebral salt wasting, and he should be treated with intravenous fluids
 e. He should be treated with a loop diuretic such as furosemide

31. A 22-year-old woman delivers a healthy baby. A few hours after delivery, the woman complains of a severe headache. Shortly afterward, she becomes sleepy but is still arousable to minor stimuli. Her blood pressure is not elevated. Urine protein level is not elevated. She develops right arm and leg paresthesias. MRI of the brain does not show any abnormalities; MRA shows multifocal stenoses involving bilateral MCAs, PCAs, and left ACA. What is the most likely diagnosis in this patient?

 a. Eclampsia
 b. Cerebral venous sinus thrombosis
 c. Postpartum cerebral angiopathy
 d. Meningitis
 e. Amniotic fluid embolism to the brain through a patent foramen ovale

32. A 32-year-old woman is 2 weeks postpartum from an uneventful pregnancy and delivery. She presents to the emergency department with a severe holocephalic headache, nausea, and two episodes of vomiting. Examination shows bilateral papilledema but is otherwise normal. She is otherwise healthy. Family history is remarkable for a history of spontaneous lower extremity deep venous thrombosis in her mother and recurrent miscarriages in her sister. Noncontrast CT scan of the brain is normal. Which of the following tests should be ordered in this patient?

 a. CT scan of the brain with contrast
 b. MRV
 c. Cerebral angiogram
 d. Transcranial Doppler ultrasonography
 e. LP

Questions 33–34

33. A 28-year-old woman in her last trimester of pregnancy is witnessed to have a generalized tonic-clonic seizure of 2 minutes duration. She is brought to the emergency department (ED). On arrival, she is somnolent but arousable and follows simple commands. Blood pressure when is 180/100 mm Hg. Urine analysis shows 3+ proteinuria. In the ED, she has another generalized seizure of 1 minute duration. What is the most likely diagnosis in this patient?

 a. Preeclampsia
 b. Eclampsia
 c. Gestational hypertension
 d. Venous sinus thrombosis
 e. Meningitis

34. Regarding the patient depicted in question 33, which of the following management strategies is appropriate?
   a. Intravenous phenobarbital
   b. Intravenous pentobarbital
   c. Oral angiotensin-converting enzyme inhibitor for long-term blood pressure control
   d. Oral diazepam
   e. Intravenous magnesium sulfate

35. Which of the following statements is correct regarding the activity of neurologic disorders in pregnancy?
   a. Pregnant women with epilepsy invariably have a worsening of seizures during pregnancy
   b. Multiple sclerosis commonly improves during pregnancy
   c. Multiple sclerosis relapse rates accelerate during pregnancy and then slow down after pregnancy
   d. The majority of women with a history of migraines have increased migraine frequency during pregnancy
   e. Myasthenia gravis typically goes into complete remission during pregnancy

36. In which of the following cases is the specified test not indicated given the patient's presentation?
   a. A 32-year-woman in the second trimester of pregnancy who complains of creepy-crawly feelings in her legs in the evening and at night—ferritin
   b. A 21-year-old woman in the first trimester of pregnancy who presents to the emergency department with involuntary dancing-like movements of her right arm—anti-phospholipid antibodies
   c. A 23-year-old woman who is planning a pregnancy but wishes to be tested for Huntington disease, given a strong family history—genetic counseling and genetic testing for Huntington disease
   d. A 36-year-old woman in the second trimester of pregnancy who presents with a high-frequency postural tremor and palpitations—thyroid stimulating hormone
   e. A 21-year-old woman with bipolar disorder started on risperidone after becoming manic during pregnancy presents with fever and muscle rigidity—serum copper

Answer key

1. d	**7.** e	**13.** c	**19.** a	**25.** e	**31.** c
2. b	**8.** d	**14.** c	**20.** b	**26.** a	**32.** b
3. e	**9.** b	**15.** b	**21.** e	**27.** d	**33.** b
4. c	**10.** b	**16.** a	**22.** c	**28.** b	**34.** e
5. c	**11.** c	**17.** c	**23.** e	**29.** b	**35.** b
6. d	**12.** b	**18.** e	**24.** b	**30.** d	**36.** e

Answers

1. d

Because of increased risk of hemorrhagic conversion, anticoagulation in patients with ischemic stroke due to infective endocarditis is warranted only in specific cases such as in patients with mechanical valves.

Infective endocarditis can lead to a variety of neurologic complications due to septic cerebral embolization, including but not limited to ischemic stroke (most common), intracranial hemorrhage (most often due to hemorrhagic conversion of an ischemic infarct), subarachnoid hemorrhage, cerebral abscess, meningoencephalitis, and seizures. Headaches and encephalopathy also occur, often as a symptom of the latter complications. Neurologic complications occur in both patients with native and prosthetic valve endocarditis, although they are more common with native valve endocarditis.

Septic cerebral emboli can lead to mycotic aneurysms by causing intraluminal arterial wall necrosis and destruction of the adventitia and muscularis with subsequent dilatation. Mycotic aneurysms are usually located at distal arterial bifurcations and are best detected by conventional cerebral angiography.

The mainstay of therapy for the neurologic complications of infective endocarditis is antibiotic therapy and acute symptomatic management (such as AEDs in patients with seizures).

Aminoff MJ. Neurology and General Medicine, 4th ed. Philadelphia, PA: Elsevier; 2008.

2. b

Intracranial hemorrhage is less common than ischemic stroke in patients with sickle cell anemia (Hemoglobin [Hb] SS disease).

Neurologic complications of Hb SS disease include ischemic stroke, intracranial hemorrhage, cranial neuropathies, spinal cord infarction (although rare), intracranial aneurysm formation with subarachnoid hemorrhage, ischemic optic neuropathy, optic atrophy, seizures, and headaches. Ischemic stroke is more common in children with Hb SS disease than in adults. In children, transcranial Doppler ultrasonography should be periodically performed, and when elevated velocities are detected, blood transfusions have been shown to reduce the risk of ischemic stroke. Patients with Hb SS disease are more likely than those with hemoglobin SC (Hb SC) disease to suffer from neurologic complications.

Adams R, McKie V, Hsu L, et al. Prevention of a first stroke by transfusion in children with abnormal results on transcranial Doppler ultrasonography. N Engl J Med. 1998; 339:5–11.

Aminoff MJ. Neurology and General Medicine, 4th ed. Philadelphia, PA: Elsevier; 2008.

3. e, 4. c

Monoclonal gammopathy of undetermined significance (MGUS) alone can lead to neuropathy, and the presence of neuropathy in a patient with a monoclonal paraproteinemia does not necessarily indicate that the patient has multiple myeloma.

The plasma cell dyscrasias include Waldenström macroglobulinemia, MGUS, multiple myeloma, plasmacytomas, and others. Neurologic complications of the plasma cell dyscrasias may result from infiltration of the peripheral nervous system by abnormal plasma cells. Infiltration of vertebral bodies can lead to spinal cord or nerve root compression, and infiltration of peripheral nerves leads to a sensorimotor predominantly axonal neuropathy. Neuropathy in patients with plasma cell dyscrasias can also be due to amyloidosis or a paraneoplastic syndrome. Patients with plasma cell dyscrasias may develop encephalopathy due to hypercalcemia, hyperviscosity syndrome (due to hypergammaglobulinemia), and CNS infections, which such patients are prone to due to their immunocompromised state. CNS involvement in the plasma cell dyscrasias can occur but is relatively rare. POEMS syndrome (plasma cell dyscrasia with polyneuropathy, organomegaly, endocrinopathy, monoclonal gammopathy, and skin changes) is a constellation of abnormalities seen in some patients with plasma cell dyscrasias.

A patient with immunoglobulin M (IgM) monoclonal gammopathy associated with antibodies against myelin-associated glycoprotein (MAG) is depicted in question 4. Patients with MGUS (which is characterized by the presence of a monoclonal protein in the absence of significant bone marrow involvement, anemia, renal failure, lytic lesions, or hypercalcemia) are at risk of developing symptomatic multiple myeloma. However, MGUS without evidence of other hematologic disorders can be associated with neuropathy. The neuropathy is often primarily demyelinating, and in some cases, particularly in patients with IgM MGUS, antibodies against MAG are detected in the serum.

Neuropathy in patients with monoclonal proteinemias can also occur because of the presence of cryoglobulins. Cryoglobulins are serum protein complexes that precipitate at specific temperatures. They occur in a variety of conditions as follows: Type I cryoglobulins are monoclonal proteins seen in the monoclonal paraproteinemias such as multiple myeloma and Waldenström macroglobulinemia. Type II cryoglobulins are seen in lymphoproliferative and autoimmune disorders, and infectious hepatitis. Type III cryoglobulins are seen with underlying infectious and autoimmune disorders. The most common neuropathic complication of cryoglobulinemia is generalized neuropathy, although mononeuritis or mononeuritis multiplex and cerebral vasculitis with ischemic stroke can also occur.

While Charcot-Marie-Tooth disease can present in adulthood, in the absence of family history or other evidence of a hereditary neuropathy on examination (discussed in Chapter 9), a costly genetic panel would not be of high yield. A technetium bone scan is not useful in investigating for the presence of bone lesions due to multiple myeloma (rather, plane film radiographs are used). Anti-GQ1b antibodies are typically seen in the Miller-Fisher variant of Guillain-Barré syndrome (discussed in Chapter 9). Genetic abnormalities of superoxide dismutase are detected in some patients with familial amyotrophic lateral sclerosis (discussed in Chapter 11), which is not the diagnosis in this case.

Aminoff MJ. Neurology and General Medicine, 4th ed. Philadelphia, PA: Elsevier; 2008.

5. **C**

This patient's laboratory studies point to the presence of hemolytic anemia, renal failure, and thrombocytopenia. Given her presentation with a seizure, her history is consistent with thrombotic thrombocytopenic purpura (TTP). The diagnostic pentad of TTP includes a microangiopathic hemolytic anemia, low platelet counts, renal dysfunction, neurologic signs or symptoms, and fever, although not all five features may necessarily be present. TTP results from a deficiency of von Willebrand factor–cleaving protease, leading to abnormal platelet aggregation. Neurologic manifestations include seizures, headaches, encephalopathy, and in severe cases coma, cranial neuropathies, and focal neurologic deficits. Treatment includes emergency plasma exchange.

Hemolytic-uremic syndrome (HUS) shares several features with TTP but HUS is associated with more severe renal dysfunction. It is predominantly a disorder of childhood, often associated with an infection with Shiga toxin–producing bacteria such as certain strains of *Escherichia coli* and *Shigella*. The syndrome is typically preceded by abdominal pain and diarrhea, not present in the case depicted in question 5. Seizures, encephalopathy, cranial nerve palsies, and neuropathy may occur.

Idiopathic thrombocytopenic purpura does not typically have primary neurologic manifestations (unless intracranial bleeding occurs, which is rare even with markedly low platelet levels), and it is not associated with a hemolytic anemia. Disseminated intravascular coagulation (DIC) results in a coagulopathy; in this patient, the coagulation tests were normal. Because DIC typically occurs in the setting of a severe illness, there is often associated encephalopathy, and seizures and other neurologic manifestations may complicate the underlying illness.

Anti-phospholipid antibody syndrome is discussed in question 24.

Aminoff MJ. Neurology and General Medicine, 4th ed. Philadelphia, PA: Elsevier; 2008.

Bradley WG, Daroff RB, Fenichel GM, et al. Neurology in Clinical Practice, 5th ed. Philadelphia, PA: Elsevier; 2008.

6. d

This patient's history is consistent with hepatic encephalopathy, or portosystemic encephalopathy. Hepatic encephalopathy is seen in patients with liver cirrhosis of any cause (not only in those with alcoholic cirrhosis), and the extent of liver dysfunction, rather than the cause of cirrhosis, correlates with the degree of encephalopathy. Clinical manifestations are variable, ranging from mildly decreased attention, disorientation, and personality changes to somnolence and in severe cases coma. Asterixis, or negative myoclonus, is seen in hepatic encephalopathy and other metabolic encephalopathies. EEG findings include generalized slowing and triphasic waves (discussed also in Chapter 5).

Although hyperammonemia has been largely implicated in the pathophysiology of hepatic encephalopathy, other abnormalities of neurotransmission, including abnormal GABA and glutamate neurotransmission, and abnormalities in fatty acids are also implicated. Ammonia is normally produced in the colon and is taken to the liver through the hepatic portal vein, where it is converted to urea and excreted in the urine. With liver dysfunction, ammonia and other toxic substances are shunted to the systemic circulation (so-called portosystemic shunting). Transjugular intrahepatic portosystemic shunt, used to treat certain complications of portal hypertension such as recurrent esophageal variceal hemorrhage, increases the risk of hepatic encephalopathy, as it enhances shunting of ammonia from the liver to the systemic circulation.

Serum ammonia levels may be elevated, but hepatic encephalopathy may occur even at relatively low serum ammonia levels, due to the impaired cerebral ammonia uptake and metabolism seen in patients with cirrhosis. Clinical improvement in mental status is the best indicator of response to therapy, and serum ammonia concentrations are not reliable for this purpose. Treatment of hepatic encephalopathy includes correction of precipitating factors (hypovolemia, gastrointestinal bleed, infection, and others) and reduction of ammonia absorption from the colon by using the disaccharide lactulose, sometimes in combination with the antibiotics rifaximin or neomycin.

The pathological hallmark of hepatic encephalopathy is the Alzheimer type II astrocyte, which is seen in various areas of the cortex and subcortical regions, including the basal ganglia, thalamus, dentate of the cerebellum, and red nuclei.

Aminoff MJ. Neurology and General Medicine, 4th ed. Philadelphia, PA: Elsevier; 2008.

Romero-Gomez M. Pharmacotherapy of hepatic encephalopathy in cirrhosis. Expert Opin Pharmacother. 2010; 11:1317–1327.

7. e

This patient's history, examination, and biopsy findings are consistent with celiac disease. Sulfonamides are used for the treatment of Whipple disease rather than celiac disease; absence of periodic acid Schiff -positive macrophage inclusions on bowel biopsy makes Whipple disease less likely (see Chapter 15).

Celiac disease, also known as gluten-sensitive enteropathy, results from an immune-mediated insensitivity to gluten, a protein found in foods containing cereal grains. Chronic diarrhea with malabsorption is common, and small bowel biopsy shows atrophy of intestinal villi. Celiac disease can have a variety of neurologic manifestations; in fact, neurologic manifestations may be the only clinical features in a minority of patients. These include a predominantly axonal peripheral neuropathy, inflammatory myopathy, cerebral calcifications, and seizures. Prominent cerebellar involvement is often seen because of loss of Purkinje cells in the cerebellum. The mainstay of treatment is a gluten-free diet, although some of the neurologic manifestations, such as cerebellar atrophy, may not be reversible. Patients with celiac disease can also have neurologic complications resulting from vitamin E deficiency (discussed in Chapter 17) due to chronic malabsorption.

Aminoff MJ. Neurology and General Medicine, 4th ed. Philadelphia, PA: Elsevier; 2008.

8. d

Patients with inflammatory bowel diseases are at increased risk of both venous and arterial thrombosis, including ischemic stroke.

Crohn's disease and ulcerative colitis are inflammatory bowel diseases (IBD). Neurologic complications of these disorders are most common during exacerbations (manifested by worsening diarrhea, abdominal pain, and other gastrointestinal symptoms) but can occur at any time. Patients with IBD are at an increased risk of both venous and arterial thrombosis, which may be due to activation of the coagulation cascade, impaired fibrinolysis, platelet activation, and systemic activation. Cerebral venous thrombosis and ischemic strokes may occur. Other neurologic complications include demyelinating and axonal neuropathies, myopathies, and cranial neuropathies, particularly cranial nerve VII palsy as is seen in Melkersson-Rosenthal syndrome, which also includes tongue fissuring and angioedema. White matter abnormalities resembling the demyelinating lesions of multiple sclerosis are seen in some patients with IBD; the significance of these findings is unclear. Patients with IBD can also have neurologic complications resulting from malabsorption of vitamin E, vitamin B_{12}, or other nutrients (discussed in Chapter 17).

Aminoff MJ. Neurology and General Medicine, 4th ed. Philadelphia, PA: Elsevier; 2008.

Pfeiffer RF. Neurologic presentations of gastrointestinal disease. Neurol Clin. 2010; 28:75–87.

9. b

A generalized sensorimotor polyneuropathy is the most common type of neuropathy in patients with chronic renal failure. Patients with renal failure can have a variety of neurologic signs and symptoms. Alteration in awareness from renal failure, or uremic encephalopathy, may manifest as reduced alertness, poor attention and concentration, perceptual errors, and hallucinations. In more severe cases, the patient may be obtunded. Patients with uremic encephalopathy, as with other metabolic encephalopathies, may exhibit multiple motor symptoms including asterixis, myoclonus (so-called uremic twitching, attributed to alterations in cerebral phosphate metabolism), and gait ataxia. Seizures can occur in both acute and chronic renal failure. When treating seizures in patients with renal failure, attention must be given to the pharmacokinetic changes that occur in such patients. Uremic neuropathy is typically a distal, symmetric sensorimotor axonal polyneuropathy; mononeuritis multiplex is typically not associated with renal failure itself, unless there is an underlying connective tissue disorder leading to both the renal failure and the mononeuropathies. Mononeuropathies can occur as a complication of arteriovenous shunt placement.

Dialysis disequilibrium syndrome is a spectrum of neurologic signs and symptoms occurring during or after dialysis. It is most common during initiation of urgent dialysis but may occur at any time. It is thought to result at least in part from shifts of water into the brain due to changes in the osmotic gradient. Clinical manifestations can range from mild encephalopathy to fatal cerebral edema. Other neurologic manifestations in patients with renal failure include dementia and restless legs syndrome.

Aminoff MJ. Neurology and General Medicine, 4th ed. Philadelphia, PA: Elsevier; 2008.

10. b

Hypokalemia typically manifests with peripheral nervous system abnormalities such as muscle cramps or tetany; CNS manifestations rarely, if ever, occur.

Various electrolyte abnormalities can lead to neurologic manifestations. Hyponatremia typically causes more severe neurologic symptoms when it develops rapidly, but they can occur also in chronic hyponatremia. A nonspecific encephalopathy is the most frequent manifestation. Seizures can occur with acute hyponatremia, usually with serum sodium levels of 115 mEq/L or less. Correction of serum sodium levels is the mainstay of treatment of hyponatremia-associated seizures, but care must be taken not to correct serum sodium levels too rapidly, given the risk of central pontine myelinolysis (discussed in Chapter 3). CNS manifestations of hypernatremia typically occur with serum sodium concentrations higher than 160 mEq/L and include encephalopathy, seizures, and in severe cases coma.

Both hypokalemia and hyperkalemia are associated with peripheral rather than CNS manifestations. Hypokalemia can lead to myalgias and proximal limb weakness (with sparing of bulbar muscles). Rhabdomyolysis can occur with severe hypokalemia. Tetany may be a manifestation of hypokalemia (or hypocalcemia). Hyperkalemia is associated with muscle weakness in the context of hyperkalemic periodic paralysis (discussed in Chapter 10) or Addison disease, but rarely otherwise.

Neurologic manifestations of hypercalcemia include encephalopathy and in severe cases coma. Other manifestations include headache and rarely seizures. Hyperparathyroidism can lead to depression, encephalopathy, and myopathy. Seizures are a much more common complication of hypocalcemia. Hypocalcemia also leads to tetany, which is due to spontaneous repetitive nerve action potentials. Initial symptoms of hypocalcemia include tingling in the perioral area and the digits. In more severe later stages, tonic muscle spasms occur, beginning in the fingers and toes (carpopedal spasm) but in some cases involving more proximal musculature; when the tetany involves truncal musculature, opisthotonos is present.

Hypomagnesemia can lead to encephalopathy, tremor, myoclonus, and in severe cases seizures. Hypermagnesemia is rare, usually occurring in the setting of renal failure. Neurologic manifestations of severe hypermagnesemia include muscle weakness that when severe may progress to respiratory failure.

Aminoff MJ. Neurology and General Medicine, 4th ed. Philadelphia, PA: Elsevier; 2008.

11. c

In a patient presenting with cognitive dysfunction, apathy, and hypersomnolence, hypothyroidism is a diagnostic possibility, and serum thyroid stimulating hormone (TSH) level should be tested. Thyroid function should be assessed in all patients presenting with cognitive dysfunction, but particularly older adults (see discussion of question 12 for other neurologic manifestations of thyroid disease). Growth hormone deficiency is unlikely to lead to the mentioned presentation; vitamin D deficiency should be checked for in older adults, but symptoms (if any) include myalgias and other pains. There is no suggestion of an autoimmune condition in this case, and a TSH would be more important to order than an anti-neuronal antibody. Anti-microsomal antibodies may be checked in the evaluation of a patient with thyroid dysfunction but would not be the first test to order. Anti-microsomal antibodies are also checked in patients with a relapsing-remitting encephalopathy or with other neurologic manifestations that raise concern for steroid-responsive encephalopathy with autoimmune thyroiditis (SREAT, or Hashimoto encephalopathy).

Aminoff MJ. Neurology and General Medicine, 4th ed. Philadelphia, PA: Elsevier; 2008.

12. b

Pseudomyotonia, or a delay in muscle relaxation following elicitation of deep tendon reflex, is a feature of hypothyroidism.

Congenital hypothyroidism is the most treatable cause of mental retardation. Untreated, it leads to cretinism, which is manifested by cognitive dysfunction, gait dysfunction, and hearing loss. The most common cause is dysgenesis of the thyroid, but severe maternal iodine deficiency also can lead to it.

Both hypothyroidism and hyperthyroidism can lead to myopathy. Serum creatine kinase level is typically elevated. Gait dysfunction in patients with thyroid disorders could be due to cerebellar ataxia, myopathy, neuropathy, or a combination of these.

Tremor is almost universally present in patients with untreated hyperthyroidism. It is typically a postural, high-frequency tremor that is thought to result from increased β-adrenergic activity. Other abnormal movements seen in patients with hyperthyroidism include parkinsonism, dyskinesias, chorea, and myoclonus.

Thyroid eye disease in patients with Graves disease results from an immune-mediated increase in connective tissue of the orbit. Manifestations include proptosis, extraocular muscle enlargement with restricted movement, optic nerve compression, and ocular neuromyotonia. Restricted upward gaze is the most common extraocular abnormality seen in patients with thyroid eye disease, but impaired abduction, adduction, and downward gaze also occur. Eyelid retraction in patients with Graves disease may be due to overactivation of Muller muscle (a sympathetically innervated muscle) or eyelid fibrosis.

Myxedema coma, due to severe untreated hypothyroidism, typically occurs in older adults and is often precipitated by intercurrent illnesses. Clinical features include hypothermia and encephalopathy. Seizures occur in some patients.

Patients with hypothyroidism may develop diffuse peripheral neuropathy with both axonal and/or demyelinating features and entrapment neuropathy, most commonly carpal tunnel syndrome (discussed in Chapter 9), resulting from deposition of mucopolysaccharides.

Other neurologic manifestations of thyroid disease include both obstructive and central sleep apnea, headache, and hearing impairment with tinnitus.

Aminoff MJ. Neurology and General Medicine, 4th ed. Philadelphia, PA: Elsevier; 2008.

13. c

Peripheral nervous system complications of diabetes include both small and large fiber neuropathy, autonomic neuropathy, radiculopathy (including thoracic radiculopathy), cranial neuropathies (most commonly, cranial nerves III and VI), and diabetic amyotrophy (discussed in Chapter 9). Diabetic polyneuropathy occurs in more than half of patients with diabetes. It is pathophysiologically complex but is in part related to increased activity of the aldose reductase pathway, which leads to accumulation of intraneuronal sorbitol and fructose with subsequent impairment in intracellular signaling, impaired auto-oxidation of glucose, accumulation of advanced glycation end products, oxidative stress, and impaired neuronal microvascular function.

Early in diabetes, small nerve fibers are predominantly affected, leading to positive sensory symptoms such as tingling and pain. Large-fiber involvement may also lead to positive sensory symptoms, although later in the disease, sensory loss predominates. Diabetic polyneuropathy is most commonly a distal, symmetric, sensorimotor polyneuropathy. Sensory loss is the most common clinical manifestation of diabetic polyneuropathy; motor weakness typically occurs only in advanced cases or from other complications of diabetes (discussed in Chapter 9). With involvement of nociceptive fibers, injuries may be painless, with the development of painless ulcers that often heal poorly, as in the case depicted in question 13. Charcot joints, or relatively painless progressive deformities of the foot and ankle, also occur.

Autonomic neuropathy is common in diabetics and can result in a variety of abnormalities including impotence, bladder dysfunction, abnormal pupillary reaction, orthostatic hypotension, and gastroparesis.

Neuropathy can result from impaired glucose tolerance alone in patients not otherwise meeting laboratory criteria for diabetes. In fact, impaired glucose tolerance is often found in patients with otherwise idiopathic neuropathy, and treatment including diet and exercise may halt progression of the neuropathy. Diabetic polyneuropathy is irreversible, but slowing the progression is accomplished by adequate glycemic control. Painful neuropathy is treated with medications including nonsteroidal anti-inflammatory agents, antidepressants (tricyclic antidepressants, selective serotonin reuptake inhibitors, norepinephrine serotonin reuptake inhibitors), anticonvulsants (gabapentin and pregabalin), and topical agents such as capsaicin.

Diabetic oculomotor palsy may present acutely and be associated with ipsilateral forehead pain. It results from ischemia to the third nerve; pupillomotor fibers are spared, given their more circumferential location, distinguishing it from other causes of acute oculomotor palsy such as cerebral aneurysms (see also Chapter 1). Cranial nerve VI palsy is another manifestation of diabetes.

CNS complications of diabetes may result from diabetic ketoacidosis and hyperosmolar hyperglycemic state, both of which can lead to encephalopathy and in severe cases stupor and coma. Cerebrovascular disease due to atherosclerosis and arteriosclerosis due to frequently comorbid hypertension can lead to various CNS manifestations resulting from ischemic stroke. Acute and sometimes permanent chorea can occur in patients with nonketotic hyperglycemia.

Aminoff MJ. Neurology and General Medicine, 4th ed. Philadelphia, PA: Elsevier; 2008.

Smith AG, Singleton R. Impaired glucose tolerance and neuropathy. Neurologist. 2008; 14:23–29.

14. c

This man's history and examination are consistent with Cushing disease, which results from hypercortisolism in the setting of an ACTH-secreting pituitary adenoma. Neurologic manifestations of Cushing disease include headache, proximal myopathy, cognitive dysfunction, and behavioral changes, with psychosis in severe cases.

In this patient, the bitemporal hemianopia is a clue to a compressive lesion of the optic chiasm, distinguishing Cushing disease from Cushing syndrome, which can result from cortisol-secreting tumors or from ectopic ACTH production as can occur with paraneoplastic syndromes or other causes.

Hypothyroidism (discussed in question 12) can lead to weight gain, cognitive dysfunction, and proximal myopathy but not typically the skin changes and aggressive behavior depicted in question 14. Hyperthyroidism (discussed in question 12) leads to weight loss and lacks the skin findings depicted. Hypocortisolism, as occurs in primary adrenal insufficiency or Addison disease, can lead to fatigue, cognitive dysfunction, myopathic weakness, and psychiatric symptoms, but typically not weight gain. Skin manifestations in Addison disease include hyperpigmentation. Hyperparathyroidism can lead to depression, encephalopathy, and myopathy, but not the other features depicted in the case.

Aminoff MJ. Neurology and General Medicine, 4th ed. Philadelphia, PA: Elsevier; 2008.

15. b

This patient's history is consistent with osteopetrosis, a sclerosing bone disorder characterized by pathologically increased bone mass due to impaired bone resorption by osteoclasts. It is caused by a mutation in an ATPase or a chloride channel. Autosomal dominant and recessive forms exist, each differing in their age at presentation and clinical manifestations. Some of the younger-onset forms are severe. The majority of patients are asymptomatic, but symptoms may include bone pain, joint deformities, secondary osteoarthritis, and fractures. Many adults with osteopetrosis are asymptomatic, but cranial neuropathies may occur because of skull thickening with subsequent narrowing of cranial nerve (CN) foramina in the base of the skull. The most commonly involved CNs are CNs II (in some cases leading to optic atrophy with blindness), VII, and VIII, leading to irreversible hearing loss, as in this patient. Elevated serum alkaline phosphatase level is a clue to this diagnosis. The olfactory nerve is also commonly involved.

A bone disorder with similar neurologic complications to osteopetrosis is Paget disease. Paget disease results from excessive bone turnover and abnormal compensatory bone formation. It is often asymptomatic and diagnosed incidentally, but it may also result in cranial neuropathies (most commonly CN VIII, but also CN II), spinal stenosis with resulting myelopathy, radiculopathy, or a combination of these. Serum alkaline phosphatase level is also elevated in Paget disease.

Achondroplasia is an autosomal dominant bone dysplasia characterized by short stature. Cognition often develops normally, but in some, developmental delay may be present. Other neurologic complications include cervical myelopathy due to craniocervical junction abnormalities, radiculopathy, and hydrocephalus.

Ankylosing spondylitis is a chronic polyarticular inflammatory disorder that involves the spine and sacroiliac joints. Uveitis and aortic insufficiency may occur. Neurologic complications include vertebral fracture with secondary spinal cord injury and spinal stenosis, leading to radiculopathy and/or myelopathy. Cauda equina syndrome due to arachnoiditis may occur.

Relapsing polychondritis results from recurrent episodes of inflammation and destruction of cartilage. Episodes commonly involve not only the ears but also the upper airway. Neurologic manifestations include vertigo and hearing loss due to involvement of the vestibulocochlear system. Ocular motor palsies and optic neuritis may rarely occur. Other neurologic manifestations of relapsing polychondritis include cerebral vasculitis, peripheral neuropathy, and aseptic meningitis.

Aminoff MJ. Neurology and General Medicine, 4th ed. Philadelphia, PA: Elsevier; 2008.

Ruiz-Garcia M, Tovar-Baudin A, Del Castillo-Ruiz V, et al. Early detection of neurological manifestations in achondroplasia. Childs Nerv Syst. 1997; 13:208–213.

Steward CG. Neurological aspects of osteopetrosis. Neuropathol Appl Neurobiol. 2003; 29:87–97.

16. a

This patient's history and examination are consistent with systemic lupus erythematosis (SLE). This is an autoimmune disorder characterized by multiorgan involvement and presence of various antibodies including anti–double-stranded DNA and anti-Smith antigen. There are specific diagnostic criteria based on hematologic, dermatologic, neurologic, renal, cardiac, and serologic features.

SLE may involve both the CNS and the peripheral nervous system. Neuropsychiatric manifestations of SLE include cognitive dysfunction, depression, anxiety, and psychosis. Headaches and seizures are among the most common neurologic manifestations; others include aseptic meningitis (as is likely the case in this patient), chorea, and myelopathy. There is an increased risk of ischemic strokes due to a variety of mechanisms including cardioembolism, antiphospholipid antibody–associated thrombosis, premature intracranial atherosclerosis, and rarely secondary cerebral vasculitis. Intracerebral hemorrhage may also occur. Peripheral nervous system manifestations include cranial neuropathies, peripheral mononeuropathy or mononeuritis multiplex, demyelinating or axonal polyneuropathy, and plexopathy.

Systemic sclerosis is a multiorgan disorder that leads to fibrosis. Scleroderma is the term used to describe the skin thickening that is seen in this disorder. Subcutaneous calcinosis, Raynaud phenomenon, esophageal dysfunction, sclerodactyly, and telangiectasia (CREST) syndrome is seen in some patients with systemic sclerosis. The diagnosis is made on the basis of the presence of clinical features and antibodies against centromeres and topoisomerases. Intracerebral vasculopathy leading to TIAs, ischemic stroke, or intracranial hemorrhage may occur. Peripheral nervous system manifestations include carpal tunnel syndrome, trigeminal neuropathy, peripheral polyneuropathy, and mononeuritis multiplex.

Sarcoidosis is discussed in questions 25 and 26, Behçet syndrome in question 23, and Sjögren syndrome in questions 17 and 18.

Aminoff MJ. Neurology and General Medicine, 4th ed. Philadelphia, PA: Elsevier; 2008.

17. c, 18. e

This patient's history and examination are consistent with a sensory neuronopathy due to Sjögren syndrome. Rectal biopsy is used to diagnose amyloidosis and is not helpful in the diagnosis of Sjögren syndrome.

Sjögren syndrome is an inflammatory multiorgan disorder primarily affecting exocrine glands (such as the salivary and lacrimal glands), leading to xerostomia and xerophthalmia (which when severe can lead to keratoconjunctivitis sicca). Sjögren syndrome often co-occurs with other autoimmune disorders. Constitutional symptoms are often present.

Peripheral nervous system involvement in Sjögren syndrome manifests most commonly as a distal predominantly sensory or mixed sensorimotor axonal polyneuropathy. A sensory neuronopathy, or dorsal root ganglionopathy, as depicted question 17, may occur, and results from involvement of the dorsal root ganglia. With sensory neuronopathy, the sensory loss may not follow a length-dependent pattern but rather can affect the face or trunk before distal segments of the limbs (discussed further in Chapter 9). Sensory ataxia is often prominent in such cases. Other manifestations of Sjögren syndrome include isolated small fiber neuropathy (without large fiber involvement), autonomic neuropathy, and cranial neuropathy. CNS manifestations of Sjögren syndrome are uncommon but include cognitive dysfunction, focal brain lesions most often affecting subcortical white matter, aseptic meningitis, optic neuritis, and myelopathy.

Diagnosis is made on the basis of the presence of symptoms of xerostomia and xerophthalmia, objective documentation of xerophthalmia with Schirmer test, serologic testing for the autoantibodies anti-Ro (SSA) or anti-La (SSB), and/or minor salivary gland biopsy. Treatment is a combination of symptomatic therapies and immunosuppressants in some cases.

This patient's examination and nerve conduction findings are not consistent with an isolated small fiber neuropathy, in which NCS are normal. Normal motor NCS would not be seen in a sensorimotor polyneuropathy. Churg-Strauss syndrome is discussed in questions 20 and 21. Small fiber neuropathy due to systemic lupus erythematosus would not be associated with abnormal NCS, and other systemic features would be present. Vitamin B_{12} deficiency can lead to a variety of neurologic manifestations (discussed in Chapter 17) but would not be associated with the dry eyes and mouth that this patient describes.

Aminoff MJ. Neurology and General Medicine, 4th ed. Philadelphia, PA: Elsevier; 2008.

Segal B, Carpenter A, Walk D. Involvement of nervous system pathways in primary Sjögren's syndrome. Rheum Dis Clin N Am. 2008; 34:885–906.

19. a

Atlanto-axial dislocation is most common in patients with rheumatoid arthritis, a polyarticular symmetric inflammatory disorder. In addition to an inflammatory arthritis, other features include subcutaneous nodules, hypersplenism, amyloidosis, scleritis, cardiac, and pulmonary involvement. Diagnosis is made on the basis of the presence of clinical features, rheumatoid factor, and cyclic citrullinated peptide. Atlanto-axial dislocation in rheumatoid arthritis results from inflammation and resulting laxity of the ligaments, with pannus formation. Myelopathy may also occur. The most common neurologic manifestation of rheumatoid arthritis is carpal tunnel syndrome. Other neurologic manifestations of rheumatoid arthritis include headaches, compressive mononeuropathies, distal sensorimotor polyneuropathy, mononeuritis multiplex, and rarely ischemic stroke.

Systemic sclerosis is discussed in question 16, sarcoidosis in questions 25 and 26, Behçet syndrome in question 23, and Sjögren syndrome in questions 17 and 18.

Aminoff MJ. Neurology and General Medicine, 4th ed. Philadelphia, PA: Elsevier; 2008.

20. b, 21. e

The patient mentioned in question 20 has a history consistent with polyarteritis nodosa. Recurrent oral and genital ulcers are seen in Behçet disease (see discussion to question 23), not in polyarteritis nodosa.

Polyarteritis nodosa, Wegener granulomatosis, Kawasaki disease, and Churg-Strauss syndrome are systemic necrotizing vasculitides involving medium and small vessels. These diseases typically involve multiple organs with often prominent constitutional symptoms. Neurologic manifestations of the systemic vasculitides of medium and small vessels include seizures, mononeuritis multiplex, cranial neuropathies (with the most frequently involved being cranial nerve VIII), and peripheral polyneuropathies. The neuropathy seen in these vasculitides is a necrotizing vasculitic ischemic neuropathy due to involvement of vasa vasorum. Figure 16.1 shows a nerve biopsy specimen demonstrating perivascular neutrophilic inflammatory infiltrate with necrosis. Arteritis of cerebral blood vessels may also lead to ischemic stroke.

Although overlap occurs in these different disorders, certain features help distinguish them. Diagnostic criteria for Churg-Strauss syndrome include asthma, eosinophilia, and sinus and pulmonary involvement. Features of Wegener granulomatosis include glomerulonephritis, paranasal sinusitis, and pulmonary involvement. The presence of granulomas on biopsy and the presence of cytoplasmic anti-neutrophil cytoplasmic (C-ANCA) antibody and antibodies to proteinase-3 allow for the diagnosis. Polyarteritis nodosa leads to a vasculopathy in multiple organ systems. It leads to prominent constitutional symptoms, renal, cardiac, and gastrointestinal involvement, and is associated with chronic hepatitis B infection. Skin manifestations include livedo reticularis, skin ulcerations, and subcutaneous nodules. Kawasaki disease is a disorder of childhood and is characterized by acute onset of fever, conjunctivitis, mucositis, polymorphous rash, lymphadenopathy, and other findings, including increased risk coronary artery aneurysms; neurologic involvement includes the occurrence of aseptic meningitis. Cryoglobulinemia is discussed in question 4. The systemic necrotizing vasculitides are treated with immunosuppression, often including corticosteroids and cyclophosphamide.

Aminoff MJ. Neurology and General Medicine, 4th ed. Philadelphia, PA: Elsevier; 2008.

22. c

This patient's history and angiographic findings are consistent with Takayasu arteritis, or pulseless disease, a large-vessel vasculitis most common in females of Asian descent. Commonly involved vessels include the subclavian arteries, but the aorta and cerebral vessels can also be involved, leading to ischemic stroke as in the case depicted in question 22. Takayasu arteritis manifests with constitutional symptoms and symptoms related to organ ischemia such as peripheral claudication. Treatment is with immunosuppression and in some cases surgical or endovascular treatment of vessel stenosis or occlusion.

Polyarteritis nodosa, microscopic polyangiitis, and temporal arteritis affect medium or small vessels as opposed to large ones. Temporal arteritis, or giant cell arteritis (discussed in Chapter 4), most commonly leads to headaches, but ischemic strokes or transient ischemic attacks can also occur in a minority due to involvement of the carotid and vertebral arteries.

Aminoff MJ. Neurology and General Medicine, 4th ed. Philadelphia, PA: Elsevier; 2008.

23. e

Peripheral nervous system involvement with Behçet syndrome is rare. Behçet syndrome is a systemic inflammatory disorder that typically affects multiple organs, including the eyes, skin, gastrointestinal tract, joints, and vascular system. Uveitis and orogenital ulcers are characteristic manifestations. Diagnostic criteria include recurrent oral ulceration, plus two of the following: recurrent genital ulceration, eye lesions including uveitis, skin lesions (such as papulopustular lesions), or a positive pathergy skin test. Patients may also have arthritis, subcutaneous thrombophlebitis, deep venous thrombosis, and gastrointestinal lesions.

Behçet syndrome is most common in younger woman of Mediterranean or east Asian descent. Diagnosis is based on clinical features; in many patients with Behçet syndrome, the skin pathergy test is positive but is nonspecific. The most common CNS manifestation is headache. CNS involvement may also include focal inflammatory brain lesions most commonly affecting the basal ganglia and/or brain stem. Progressive personality change, psychiatric disorders, and dementia may develop. Increased intracranial pressure associated with venous sinus thrombosis is another potential pattern of CNS involvement. Unlike other systemic vasculitides, peripheral nervous system involvement with Behçet syndrome is rare, although peripheral neuropathy or myopathy may occur.

Al-Araji A, Kidd DP. Neuro-Behçet's disease: epidemiology, clinical characteristics, and management. Lancet Neurol. 2009; 9:192–204.

Aminoff MJ. Neurology and General Medicine, 4th ed. Philadelphia, PA: Elsevier; 2008.

24. b

Acquired factor VIII deficiency, or acquired hemophilia, leads to increased risk of hemorrhage rather than thrombosis.

Anti-phospholipid antibody syndrome (APLS) and most of the so-called hereditary thrombophilias, including G20210 A prothrombin polymorphism, mutation in the methylene tetrahydrofolate reductase gene (leading to hyperhomocysteinemia), and factor V Leiden, as well as others including antithrombin III, protein C, and protein S deficiency, lead to venous thrombosis. Therefore, venous sinus thrombosis is the most common neurologic manifestation of these disorders. However, arterial ischemia in the form of venous infarction is seen, as are paradoxical emboli to the cerebral vasculature from the venous system through an intracardiac right-to-left shunt. Other causes of both venous and arterial thrombosis include malignancy, heparin-induced thrombocytopenia, systemic vasculitides (discussed in questions 20 and 21) and myeloproliferative diseases (such as essential thrombocythemia, polycythemia rubra vera, and others).

APLS is a disorder of thrombosis resulting from the presence of circulating antibodies against phospholipid-bound proteins such as anticardiolipin antibodies and lupus anticoagulant antibodies. In addition to venous and less commonly arterial thrombosis, other neurologic manifestations seen in APLS include chorea, headaches, and seizures.

Aminoff MJ. Neurology and General Medicine, 4th ed. Philadelphia, PA: Elsevier; 2008.

Landolfi R, Di Gennaro L, Falanga A. Thrombosis in myeloproliferative disorders: pathogenetic facts and speculation. Leukemia. 2008; 22:2020–2028.

Levy JH, Hursting MJ. Heparin-induced thrombocytopenia, a prothrombotic disease. Hematol Oncol Clin North Am. 2007; 21:65–88.

25. e, 26. a

The patient depicted in question 25 has sarcoidosis. The most commonly involved organs in sarcoidosis are the lungs. Myelopathy can occur but is relatively uncommon.

Sarcoidosis is a granulomatous, immune-mediated disorder that may involve multiple organ systems including (but not limited to) the lungs (most commonly), skin, heart, and central and peripheral nervous system. In the United States, it is more common in African American females. Neurologic signs or symptoms as the primary presentation are rare; less than 10% of sarcoidosis cases present with extrapulmonary involvement leading to diagnosis. The most common presentation of neurosarcoidosis is cranial neuropathy, with cranial nerve VII being the most frequently affected. Multiple cranial neuropathies may occur in some patients. Other neurologic manifestations include aseptic meningitis (as in the case presented in question 25), hydrocephalus, parenchymal disease/mass lesion, myelopathy, small and large fiber peripheral neuropathy, and myopathy. Hypothalamic or pituitary involvement may lead to endocrinopathy.

The diagnosis of sarcoidosis is established on the basis of the history, examination, and demonstration of noncaseating granulomas on biopsy. Serum angiotensin-converting enzyme (ACE) is neither sensitive nor specific, but increased serum ACE levels are a marker of disease activity. In patients with known systemic sarcoidosis, neurosarcoidosis is diagnosed in the setting of neurologic signs or symptoms and/or findings of LP or MRI of the brain or spine (although alternative causes, such as in CNS infections in sarcoidosis patients being treated with immunosuppressive therapy must also be considered and excluded). Diffuse leptomeningeal enhancement, often with a predominance at the base of the brain, is the classic finding, although focal parenchymal enhancing brain lesions can also occur (as shown in Figure 16.2 in the splenium of the corpus callosum) as can intramedullary or extramedullary enhancing spine lesions. Treatment is with immunosuppressive therapy including corticosteroids and, in some cases, steroid-sparing agents such as methotrexate.

Lymphoma and breast cancer are not associated with the presence of granulomas on biopsy. Wegener granulomatosis is associated with granulomas and can also lead to multiple cranial neuropathies, but a history of recurrent sinusitis and other serologic findings help distinguish Wegener granulomatosis (discussed in questions 20 and 21) from neurosarcoidosis. Biopsy specimens in tuberculosis show caseating as opposed to noncaseating granulomas.

Aminoff MJ. Neurology and General Medicine, 4th ed. Philadelphia, PA: Elsevier; 2008.

27. d

This patient's history is concerning for pheochromocytoma, which may present with episodes of headache, diaphoresis, and palpitations in the setting of elevated blood pressure. Pheochromocytomas are neuroendocrine tumors derived from amine precursor uptake decarboxylation (APUD) cells. Included in the group of APUD cell tumors are carcinoid tumor, paraganglioneuromas, neuroblastoma, and others. Pheochromocytomas arise from chromaffin cells and secrete catecholamines. The majority arise from the adrenal medulla, although in a minority, they arise from the sympathetic ganglia, in which case they are termed catecholamine-secreting paragangliomas. Pheochromocytomas are most commonly sporadic, although in a minority, they occur as part of other syndromes such as neurofibromatosis, von Hippel-Lindau disease, tuberous sclerosis, and Sturge-Weber syndrome (discussed in Chapter 14). They are most commonly benign but are malignant in a minority of patients. Diagnosis of pheochromocytomas may be aided by measurement of catecholamines, metanephrines, and vanillylmandelic acid in a 24-hour urine collection; measurement of plasma free metanephrines is the most sensitive test.

The differential diagnosis for patients with the presentation depicted in the case is broad, but elevated blood pressure in the setting of these symptoms warrants exclusion of pheochromocytoma before a diagnosis of anxiety or hot flashes due to menopause is made. Carcinoid syndrome can present with episodic flushing and headache associated with other symptoms; diagnosis is made by measurement of urinary 5-hydroxyindoleacetic acid.

Aminoff MJ. Neurology and General Medicine, 4th ed. Philadelphia, PA: Elsevier; 2008.

28. b

The pituitary derives its blood supply from the superior and inferior hypophyseal arteries, which arise from the ICA.

The anterior pituitary, or adenohypophysis, is derived embryologically from Rathke's pouch, which evaginates from the oropharyngeal membrane during fetal development. The hypothalamus modulates pituitary function, and pituitary hormones in turn modulate hypothalamic function. The pituitary derives its blood supply from the superior and inferior hypophyseal arteries, which arise from the ICA. The superior hypophyseal artery forms a capillary plexus in the hypothalamic median eminence. Blood carrying regulatory hypothalamic hormones flows from there in the hypophyseal portal vein, through the infundibulum (or pituitary stalk) to the anterior pituitary. Secretion of prolactin by the anterior pituitary is modulated by dopamine. Growth hormone–releasing hormone secreted by the hypothalamus regulates growth hormone release by the anterior pituitary. Thyrotropin-releasing hormone secreted by the hypothalamus modulates thyroid stimulating hormone release, and gonadotropic-releasing hormone secreted by the hypothalamus modulates release of follicle-stimulating hormone and luteinizing hormone from the anterior pituitary. ACTH release by the anterior pituitary is modulated by corticotrophin-releasing hormone from the hypothalamus.

Magnocellular neurons in the supraoptic and paraventricular nuclei of the hypothalamus synthesize antidiuretic hormone and oxytocin. These are then moved via axonal transport, where they are stored and released by the posterior pituitary, also called the neurohypophysis.

Bradley WG, Daroff RB, Fenichel GM, et al. Neurology in Clinical Practice, 5th ed. Philadelphia, PA: Elsevier; 2008.

Ropper AH, Samuels MA. Adams and Victor's Principles of Neurology, 9th ed. New York, NY: McGraw-Hill; 2009.

29. b

Given this patient's recent history of a neurosurgical procedure in the pituitary region, she most likely has central diabetes insipidus (DI), due to deficiency of antidiuretic hormone (ADH).

ADH is synthesized by the magnocellular and supraoptic nuclei of the hypothalamus and secreted by the posterior pituitary. Synthesis and secretion of ADH is modulated by serum osmolality; increases in serum osmolality normally lead to release of ADH, which stimulates renal tubular resorption of water.

Central DI manifests clinically with thirst, polydipsia, and polyuria. It is not uncommon following neurosurgery and may be transient. Other causes of central DI include trauma, hypoxic-ischemic insult, compressive lesions in the sellar or suprasellar region, and infiltration of the hypothalamus due to granulomatous diseases such as sarcoidosis (discussed in questions 25 and 26). In some cases, the disorder is idiopathic. In patients with DI, urine osmolality is low: the urine is dilute due to inadequate resorption of water and hence excessive excretion of water in the urine.

Central DI is distinguished from nephrogenic DI, which results from inadequate renal response to ADH. In patients with central DI, administration of desmopressin, an ADH analog, will lead to urinary concentration and therefore an increase in urine osmolality and a reduction in serum sodium concentration. In nephrogenic DI, urine osmolality does not decrease in response to desmopressin. One of the causes of nephrogenic DI is lithium carbonate.

The treatment of central DI includes allowing free access to water (allowing patients to maintain adequate intake of water) and administration of vasopressin; water restriction will worsen hypernatremia, as will hypertonic saline.

Aminoff MJ. Neurology and General Medicine, 4th ed. Philadelphia, PA: Elsevier; 2008.

Bradley WG, Daroff RB, Fenichel GM, et al. Neurology in Clinical Practice, 5th ed. Philadelphia, PA: Elsevier; 2008.

30. d

In the setting of subarachnoid hemorrhage, and given evidence of hypovolemia, this patient's hyponatremia is most likely due to cerebral salt wasting. This results from excessive renal losses of sodium and is seen in patients with severe CNS dysfunction. Unlike patients with syndrome of inappropriate antidiuretic hormone secretion (SIADH) who are typically euvolemic, in cerebral salt wasting syndrome, the patient is hypovolemic, and the treatment is with salt supplementation and intravenous isotonic fluid administration. The pathophysiology of cerebral salt wasting syndrome is not clear, but it may in part relate to increased levels of atrial natriuretic peptide released from the cardiac atria.

SIADH may occur following head trauma, neurosurgery SAH and with paraneoplastic ectopic antidiuretic hormone production. Several medications may also cause SIADH. Treatment of SIADH is with fluid restriction and correction of underlying causes; in severe cases, furosemide may be used. Vasopressin receptor antagonists are being investigated in the neuro-critical care setting.

Aminoff MJ. Neurology and General Medicine, 4th ed. Philadelphia, PA: Elsevier; 2008.

Ropper AH, Samuels MA. Adams and Victor's Principles of Neurology, 9th ed. New York, NY: McGraw-Hill; 2009.

Wright WL, Asbury WH, Gilmore JL, et al. Conivaptan for hyponatremia in the neurocritical care unit. Neurocrit Care. 2009; 11:6–13.

31. c

This patient's history and imaging findings are consistent with postpartum cerebral angiopathy, a disorder along the spectrum of reversible cerebral vasoconstriction syndrome. The pathophysiology of this disorder is unclear but is related to the occurrence of multifocal vasospasm. Clinically, patients present most commonly with headache, although seizure and/or focal neurologic deficit may occur. This disorder is typically benign, responsive to calcium channel blockers and/or corticosteroids. Rarely, ischemic strokes occur.

Normal blood pressure and urine protein level distinguish postpartum cerebral angiopathy from preeclampsia (discussed in questions 33 and 34). Absence of infarcts on MRI make amniotic fluid emboli unlikely; the presence of arterial vasospasm and absence of abnormalities on MRI of the brain make cerebral venous sinus thrombosis less likely. The history is not consistent with meningitis, and the presence of vasospasm further points to the diagnosis of postpartum angiopathy.

Calabrese LH, Dodick DW, Schwedt TJ, et al. Narrative review: reversible cerebral vasoconstriction syndrome. Ann Intern Med. 2007; 146(1):34–44.

Turan TN, Stern BJ. Stroke in pregnancy. Neurol Clin. 2004; 22:821–840.

32. b

Given this patient's presentation, cerebral venous sinus thrombosis should be excluded, and MRV would be the most appropriate test to order. Pregnancy and the postpartum period are hypercoagulable states, predisposing to venous sinus thrombosis. In pregnancy, levels of several of the procoagulant factors are elevated, including fibrinogen and factors VII, VIII, IX, and X. These elevations, associated with a reduction in protein S levels, increase susceptibility to venous thrombosis. Given this patient's family history, a hereditary thrombophilia or anti-phospholipid antibody syndrome may also have contributed to her risk of thrombosis (see discussion to question 24).

Venous sinus thrombosis can occur during pregnancy or in the postpartum period. In addition to headache and other signs and symptoms of increased intracranial pressure, seizures can occur.

A CT scan with contrast would be of little utility in this case; it may show a triangular area of central hypodensity surrounded by a rim of hyperintensity in the superior sagittal sinus (the so-called empty delta sign), but absence of this sign would not exclude the diagnosis. Cerebral angiogram is not indicated, although if this patient's condition deteriorates significantly, angiogram with venous thrombolysis may be necessary.

Transcranial Doppler ultrasonography could be used to exclude vasospasm as occurs in postpartum angiopathy (discussed in question 31), but the presence of papilledema in this case makes the diagnosis of venous sinus thrombosis more likely. Similarly, while subarachnoid hemorrhage, meningitis, and other indications for LP in the postpartum period can occur, the presence of papilledema makes an MRV of higher priority.

Aminoff MJ. Neurology and General Medicine, 4th ed. Philadelphia, PA: Elsevier; 2008.

Karnad DR, Guntupalli KK. Neurologic disorders in pregnancy. Crit Care Med. 2005; 33(10)(suppl):S362–S371.

33. b, 34. e

This patient's history, laboratory findings, and elevated blood pressure are consistent with eclampsia. Preeclampsia is characterized by gestational hypertension and proteinuria, often associated with edema in the face and hands. Eclampsia is the occurrence of seizures in association with hypertension and edema during pregnancy or in the postpartum period. The pathophysiology may relate to impaired trophoblast invasion of the endometrium and immune-mediated and endocrinologic mechanisms. Associated symptoms may include headache, visual disturbance, and epigastric abdominal pain. Postpartum eclampsia is more commonly associated with complications including disseminated intravascular coagulation and respiratory distress. In more severe cases, ischemic stroke, intracerebral hemorrhage, and/or posterior reversible encephalopathy syndrome (discussed in Chapter 3) can occur.

Management of eclampsia includes delivery (which should be the priority if the pregnancy is at or close to term) and intravenous medications such as hydralazine or labetalol for blood pressure reduction (although excessive reductions should be avoided to maintain fetal blood flow). Angiotensin-converting enzyme inhibitors should be avoided given potential effects on the fetal kidney. Intravenous magnesium sulfate should be administered; it reduces vasospasm and improves cerebral perfusion. Close monitoring is necessary as magnesium toxicity may lead to maternal respiratory distress. The use of AEDs is controversial, but medications that depress the fetus, such as pentobarbital or phenobarbital, should be avoided; oral diazepam is likely to be of little utility in seizure control and may depress the fetus.

Gestational hypertension is the presence of hypertension without associated proteinuria occurring beyond 20 weeks of gestation. Venous sinus thrombosis can lead to seizures and should be on the differential diagnosis of a patient in the peripartum period presenting with seizures, but the presence of proteinuria and hypertension point to eclampsia. Similarly, the history and laboratory features make meningitis less likely.

Kaplan PW. Neurologic aspects of eclampsia. Neurol Clin. 2004; 22:841–861.

35. b

Multiple sclerosis typically improves during pregnancy. The rate of multiple sclerosis relapses decline during pregnancy but may rebound afterward. Seizure frequency in pregnant patients with epilepsy is variable and unpredictable; approximately one-third have increased seizure frequency in pregnancy, whereas the rest have a reduction or no change in seizure frequency. The majority of women with a history of migraine have a reduction in migraines during their pregnancy, although some women may have a worsening, and migraines can occur for the first time in pregnant women without pre-existing migraines. In the latter patients, exclusion of other causes of headache such as venous sinus thrombosis (discussed in question 32) is important. The effects of pregnancy on myasthenia gravis are variable. Approximately one-third of women have significant worsening; improvement in the second and third trimesters occurs in others, and this is thought to be related to the relative immunosuppression that occurs during this period. Sudden worsening in the postpartum period may occur.

Ciafaloni E, Massey JM. Myasthenia gravis and pregnancy. Neurol Clin. 2004; 22:771–782.

Hughes M. Multiple sclerosis and pregnancy. Neurol Clin. 2004; 22:757–769.

Pennel PB. Pregnancy in women who have epilepsy. Neurol Clin. 2004; 22:799–820.

Silberstein S. Headaches in pregnancy. Neurol Clin. 2004; 22:727–756.

36. e

In question 36, the first case depicts a pregnant woman with restless legs syndrome (RLS). RLS may first present during pregnancy, and preexisting RLS often worsens during this state. RLS is associated with iron deficiency, which is not uncommon during pregnancy. Testing serum ferritin level is indicated, and iron supplementation should be initiated if the ferritin level is less than 50 ng/mL.

The second case in question 36 depicts a pregnant woman with chorea gravidarum. Previously associated most often with rheumatic fever, with the decline in incidence of rheumatic fever in recent decades, other causes such as anti-phospholipid antibody syndrome have emerged as being more common and should be checked for.

In the third case depicted in question 36, a young woman with a family history of Huntington disease wishes to be tested prior to pregnancy. Referral to a genetic counselor and genetic testing is appropriate.

In the fourth case, assessment for hyperthyroidism is indicated in the setting of new-onset tremor during pregnancy.

The fifth case depicts a patient with fever and rigidity following initiation of an antipsychotic, a story that may be consistent with neuroleptic malignant syndrome (discussed in Chapter 3). The diagnosis is a clinical one, although measurement of serum creatine kinase level is indicated as it is often elevated. Checking serum copper and ceruloplasmin levels, tests for Wilson disease (discussed in chapter 6), may be indicated as part of the initial workup of this patient's underlying neuropsychiatric illness but would not be the first line of testing for this acute presentation.

Russel CS, Lang C, McCambridge M, et al. Neuroleptic malignant syndrome in pregnancy. Obstest Gynecol. 2001; 98:906–908.

Smith M, Evatt M. Movement disorders in pregnancy. Neurol Clin. 2004; 22:783–798.

Buzz Phrases	Key Points
Dry eyes, dry mouth, painful dysesthesias with sensory loss	Sjögren syndrome, sensory neuronopathy
Headache, oral and genital ulcers in a woman of Mediterranean descent	Behçet disease
Recurrent sinusitis, renal disease, multiple cranial neuropathies	Wegener granulomatosis, check cytoplasmic antineutrophil cytoplasmic antibody
Fever, abdominal pain, headache, mononeuritis multiplex in patient with hepatitis B	Polyarteritis nodosa, check perinuclear antineutrophil cytoplasmic antibody
Multiple cranial neuropathies, thick skull, elevated alkaline phosphatase level	Osteopetrosis
Pentad of thrombotic thrombocytopenic purpura	Microangiopathic hemolytic anemia, low platelet counts, renal dysfunction, neurologic signs or symptoms, and fever
Facial palsy involving both upper and lower face, hilar adenopathy	Sarcoidosis
Test to check when there is demyelinating neuropathy with immunoglobulin M monoclonal gammopathy	Antibodies against myelin-associated glycoprotein

Chapter 17

Nutritional and Toxic Disorders of the Nervous System

Questions

1. Which of the following drugs is not associated with withdrawal symptoms?
   a. Cocaine
   b. Lysergic acid diethylamide
   c. Amphetamine
   d. Alcohol
   e. Opiates

Questions 2–6

2. A 32-year-old man with a history of opiate abuse presents to the emergency department in suspected opiate overdose. Which of the following is not a typical finding in someone with opiate intoxication?
   a. Hypotension
   b. Decreased respirations
   c. Bradycardia
   d. Mydriasis
   e. Decreased cough reflex

3. What would be the most appropriate treatment for symptom reversal in this patient with suspected opiate overdose?
   a. Intravenous naltrexone
   b. Intravenous thiamine
   c. Intravenous glucose
   d. Intravenous flumazenil
   e. Intravenous naloxone

4. The following day when you are examining the patient on morning rounds, you suspect that he is having opiate withdrawal. Which of the following findings would not be expected in opiate withdrawal?
    a. Nausea and vomiting
    b. Diarrhea
    c. Dry eyes
    d. Myalgias
    e. Diaphoresis

5. What are the two main structures in the reward circuit that are thought to mediate drug addiction?
    a. Amygdala and locus coeruleus
    b. Ventral tegmental area and nucleus accumbens
    c. Periaqueductal gray matter and arcuate nucleus
    d. Nucleus accumbens and periaqueductal gray matter
    e. Ventral tegmental area and periaqueductal gray matter

6. Which opiate receptor class is involved with spinal analgesia?
    a. Kappa (κ)
    b. Beta (β)
    c. Mu (μ)
    d. Delta (δ)
    e. Nociceptin (ORL$_1$)

Questions 7–9

7. A 41-year-old man presents with suspected amphetamine intoxication. What is the most complete answer regarding the mechanism of action of this substance?
    a. Blocks reuptake of dopamine and norepinephrine
    b. Causes direct release of dopamine and norepinephrine but does not block their reuptake
    c. Causes direct release of dopamine
    d. Causes direct release of dopamine and norepinephrine and blocks their reuptake
    e. Causes direct release of norepinephrine

8. Which of the following would be an unexpected finding in the patient depicted in question 7?
    a. Tachycardia
    b. Miosis
    c. Hypertension
    d. Cardiac arrhythmia
    e. Dyskinesia

9. Cocaine intoxication can present similarly to amphetamine intoxication. What is the primary mechanism of action of cocaine?
    a. Causes direct release of dopamine and norepinephrine and inhibits their reuptake
    b. Inhibits reuptake of dopamine and norepinephrine
    c. Causes direct release of norepinephrine
    d. Causes direct release of dopamine and norepinephrine but does not inhibit their reuptake
    e. Causes direct release of dopamine

Questions 10–15

10. A 52-year-old man presents to the emergency department with altered mental status and somnolence. He smells strongly of alcohol and his blood alcohol level confirms your suspicion of intoxication. What would be the best next step in treatment of this patient?

   a. Intravenous folate
   b. Intravenous glucose
   c. Intravenous thiamine
   d. Intravenous flumazenil
   e. Intravenous naloxone

11. On closer examination, you find that besides the confusion, he also has nystagmus, ophthalmoplegia, and ataxia. You suspect Wernicke's encephalopathy. Which of the following structures would you not expect to find abnormalities in on an MRI of the brain?

   a. Hypothalamus
   b. Mammillary bodies
   c. Caudate nucleus
   d. Periaqueductal gray matter
   e. Medial thalami

12. Two days after admitting the patient depicted in question 10, you begin to notice new-onset tremors, tachycardia, and hypertension. There is no history of epilepsy. What is the next most important medication to add for this patient, assuming initial standard therapy has been started?

   a. Propranolol
   b. Nimodipine
   c. Lorazepam
   d. Phenytoin
   e. Zolpidem

13. The effect of alcohol on the CNS is mediated primarily by what mechanism of action?

   a. $GABA_B$ receptor stimulation
   b. $GABA_A$ receptor stimulation
   c. $GABA_B$ and $GABA_A$ receptor stimulation
   d. $GABA_B$ receptor inhibition
   e. $GABA_A$ receptor inhibition

14. How long after the last drink does delirium tremens typically begin in an alcoholic patient?

   a. 6 to 12 hours
   b. 12 to 24 hours
   c. 24 to 36 hours
   d. 36 to 48 hours
   e. 48 to 96 hours

15. When seizures occur in an alcoholic patient, which of the following would be the least likely time frame for them to occur after the last drink?

   a. 6 to 12 hours
   b. 12 to 24 hours
   c. 24 to 36 hours
   d. 36 to 48 hours
   e. 72 to 96 hours

16. What is the primary mechanism of action of nicotine?
   a. Nicotinic acetylcholine receptor inhibition
   b. Acetylcholine reuptake inhibition
   c. Norepinephrine receptor activation
   d. Nicotinic acetylcholine receptor activation
   e. Dopamine reuptake inhibition

17. What is the primary mechanism of action that explains the stimulant effects of caffeine?
   a. Adenosine agonist
   b. Nicotinic acetylcholine antagonist
   c. Nicotinic acetylcholine agonist
   d. Adenosine antagonist
   e. Adenosine diphosphate antagonist

Questions 18–21

18. A 38-year-old man was brought to the emergency department in handcuffs. He had broken out of the first set of handcuffs. He was found running down the street naked and throwing concrete blocks through windows because he thought he was invisible and was fighting "clear, flat aliens." On examination, after being wrestled in place by six police officers, he is found to be hypertensive, tachycardic, and hyperthermic and have rotatory nystagmus. What intoxicating substance do you suspect?
   a. Lysergic acid diethylamide
   b. 3, 4-Methylenedioxymethamphetamine
   c. Phencyclidine
   d. Psilocybin (4-phosphoryloxy-N,N-dimethyltryptamine)
   e. Mescaline (peyote)

19. What is the primary mechanism of action of the suspected substance ingested by the patient in question 18?
   a. Serotonin receptor agonist
   b. Dopamine receptor agonist
   c. NMDA receptor agonist
   d. Serotonin receptor antagonist
   e. NMDA receptor antagonist

20. The hallucinogenic drugs, such as lysergic acid diethylamide, are all theorized to act predominantly at what neurotransmitter receptor system?
   a. Dopamine
   b. Serotonin
   c. Norepinephrine
   d. Acetylcholine
   e. NMDA

21. Which of the following would be an uncommon finding with hallucinogen intoxication?
   a. Tachycardia
   b. Anxiety
   c. Diaphoresis
   d. Miosis
   e. Synesthesias

Questions 22–23

22. A 29-year-old woman presents with a slowly progressive spastic paraparesis of her legs over 2 years. In addition to this finding on examination, you also see that she has absent vibratory sense and proprioception in her feet. She also mentions that she takes zinc supplementation twice daily for the last several years to prevent "colds." Which of the following is the most likely etiology of these findings?

a. Vitamin E deficiency
b. Vitamin B_{12} deficiency
c. Copper excess
d. Zinc deficiency
e. Copper deficiency

23. Which of the following would be one of your primary treatment recommendations for the patient depicted in question 22?

a. Vitamin B_{12} replacement therapy
b. Chelation therapy
c. Copper supplementation
d. Increase zinc supplementation
e. Vitamin E supplementation

Questions 24–25

24. A 38-year-old woman with Crohn's disease, chronic diarrhea, and steatorrhea is referred to your office for evaluation of gait instability and ataxia. On examination, you find that she has some dysmetria, mild dysarthria, and absent reflexes. What is the likely cause of these neurologic findings?

a. Vitamin A deficiency
b. Vitamin D deficiency
c. Vitamin B_{12} deficiency
d. Copper deficiency
e. Vitamin E deficiency

25. Which of the following would be one of your primary treatment recommendations for the patient depicted in question 24?

a. Vitamin E supplementation
b. Vitamin A supplementation
c. Copper replacement
d. Increased sunlight and vitamin D supplementation
e. Vitamin B_{12} replacement

26. Which of the following would be the least likely finding related to thiamine (vitamin B_1) deficiency?

a. Neuropathy
b. Arrhythmia
c. Extensor plantar responses
d. Congestive heart failure
e. Wernicke-Korsakoff syndrome

27. A defect in production of which of the following underlies the pathophysiology of the neurologic findings in vitamin B$_{12}$ deficiency?
 a. Threonine
 b. Serotonin
 c. Homocysteine
 d. Methionine
 e. Serine

Questions 28–29

28. A 49-year-old woman and her very anxious husband present to your office with progressively worsening sensory loss and weakness, which began distally in her legs and moved proximally beginning approximately a week ago. You notice she has a diffuse macular rash that is pruritic and scaling on her palms and soles. Records indicate that she had presented to the emergency department 3 weeks prior with complaints of severe nausea, vomiting, and diarrhea, and the physician had noted that her breath smelled strongly of garlic. What do you suspect is the cause for these symptoms?
 a. Guillain-Barré syndrome
 b. Cyanide poisoning
 c. Thallium poisoning
 d. Arsenic poisoning
 e. Mercury poisoning

29. For the patient depicted in question 28, what test finding would have confirmed your suspicion if it had been completed during her emergency department visit 3 weeks prior?
 a. LP revealing albumino-cytologic dissociation
 b. Elevated urinary arsenic level
 c. Elevated urinary thallium level
 d. Elevated urinary mercury level
 e. Elevated urinary cyanide level

30. A 34-year-old man who works at an industrial electroplating plant presents to the emergency department with complaints of nausea, vomiting, headache, anxiety, eye and mucous membrane irritation, cough, and dyspnea. His skin is also flushed with a cherry-red color. He mentions that he just started this job and forgot to wear protective work gear. He mentions that he smelled a bitter, almond odor while working all day. What do you suspect as the cause of these symptoms?
 a. Arsenic poisoning
 b. Carbon monoxide poisoning
 c. Thallium poisoning
 d. Mercury poisoning
 e. Cyanide poisoning

31. A 45-year-old mine worker is brought to your office by his wife. She says he has been exhibiting progressive personality changes and has become very anxious. On examination, you find a prominent intention tremor and notice that his gums appear very inflamed and tender to touch. What do you suspect may be the cause of these symptoms?
 a. Lead toxicity
 b. FTD
 c. Mercury toxicity

d. Thallium toxicity
e. Manganese toxicity

32. A 19-year-old girl with a history of migraine presents to the emergency department with her parents during the first cold week in the fall months. She complains of a generalized headache, nausea, dizziness, and malaise. You notice her skin is quite flushed and, interestingly, her parents both exhibit similar symptoms. What should be the first-line treatment at this time?
a. Symptomatic management
b. An antibiotic for possible early bacterial infection
c. An antiviral for possible early influenza
d. High-flow oxygen
e. High-rate IV fluids

33. A 5-year-old boy is brought to your office with his parents. They had recently moved into a house built in the 1920s. They are concerned because their son has been having behavioral changes, psychomotor slowing, clumsiness, lethargy, frequent abdominal pain, and suffered an unprovoked seizure 4 days ago. In addition, you notice that he has more weakness with extension of his hands compared with flexion. What is the most likely explanation?
a. Carbon monoxide toxicity
b. Autistic spectrum disorder
c. Lead toxicity
d. Mercury toxicity
e. HSV encephalitis

34. While on hospital neurology consult service, you are asked to see a 46-year-old man with chronic liver disease on long-standing total parenteral nutrition who has become confused and uncoordinated with a new tremor, bradykinesia, and other parkinsonian features. What do you suspect to be the cause of these symptoms?
a. Parkinson disease
b. Manganese toxicity
c. Lead toxicity
d. Severe malnutrition
e. Copper deficiency

35. A 56-year-old man who is an alcoholic presents to the emergency department with headache, reduced visual acuity of new onset, and nausea. He tells you he has been drinking "anything he can get his hands on containing alcohol, even that stuff you put in a car." What toxicity to you suspect?
a. Hexacarbon toxicity
b. Lead toxicity
c. Gasoline ingestion
d. Acrylamide toxicity
e. Methanol toxicity

36. A 49-year-old farmer presents to the emergency department after finishing spraying his crop for the year against insect damage. He thinks he accidentally sprayed some in his mouth approximately 20 minutes ago, and his wife reports he had a brief seizure before arriving. He is salivating and having difficulty breathing with excess secretions. On examination, you notice frequent fasciculations. On the basis of your suspicion, which of the following would not be a recommended treatment at this time?

a. Activated charcoal
b. Benzodiazepines
c. Pralidoxime
d. Gastric lavage
e. Atropine

37. A 67-year-old man who lives on a farm with his wife presents with complaints of blurred and double vision, difficulty swallowing, and neck and shoulder weakness. There is no diurnal variation. These symptoms have been progressively worsening over the last 2 days. He reports being very healthy otherwise and attributes his good health to growing his own food and storing all excess by canning. On examination, you find multiple cranial nerve abnormalities and fixed pupillary dilation, and he is unable to contract his deltoids against resistance. What diagnosis would you first suspect?

a. Myasthenia gravis
b. Lambert-Eaton myasthenic syndrome
c. Botulism
d. Guillain-Barré syndrome
e. Leptomeningeal carcinomatosis

Answer key

1. b	**8.** b	**15.** e	**22.** e	**29.** b	**36.** d
2. d	**9.** b	**16.** d	**23.** c	**30.** e	**37.** c
3. e	**10.** c	**17.** d	**24.** e	**31.** c	
4. c	**11.** c	**18.** c	**25.** a	**32.** d	
5. b	**12.** c	**19.** e	**26.** c	**33.** c	
6. a	**13.** b	**20.** b	**27.** d	**34.** b	
7. d	**14.** e	**21.** d	**28.** d	**35.** e	

Answers

1. b

Lysergic acid diethylamide does not produce a withdrawal syndrome. Lysergic acid is one of the ergot fungus' diverse alkaloid components, and it is a potent mood-changing and hallucinogenic drug. It is discussed further in question 18. Cocaine, amphetamine, alcohol, and opiates all have well-defined withdrawal syndromes and are discussed in further questions.

A marijuana (Cannabis) withdrawal syndrome has been debated. The DSM-IV-TR criteria for cannabis dependence include physiologic tolerance but do not include a withdrawal syndrome. The World Health Organization's International Classification of Diseases-10th Revision does recognize a cannabis withdrawal syndrome, which is not life threatening. The most common symptoms of a possible cannabis withdrawal syndrome include fatigue, discomfort, yawning, anxiety, depression, hypersomnia, anxiety, and psychomotor slowing. Marijuana is typically smoked, although it is also ingested orally when added to other foods or drinks. The active ingredient in cannabis is δ-9-tetrahydrocannabinol (THC). Common side effects include increased appetite (THC is sometimes used for anorexia and as an anti-emetic in cancer and AIDS patients), tachycardia, dry mouth, conjunctival injection, excessive laughter, memory impairment, poor attention span, sedation, paranoia, anxiety, delusions, impaired coordination, and poor insight and judgment. Chronic use frequently causes flat affect, apathy, and lack of motivation. THC is active in the ventral tegmental area, nucleus accumbens, hippocampus, caudate nucleus, and cerebellum. THC's effects on the hippocampus may help explain the memory problems that can develop with the use of cannabis, and those on the cerebellum may help explain the loss of coordination and imbalance sometimes seen.

Bradley WG, Daroff RB, Fenichel GM, et al. Neurology in Clinical Practice, 5th ed. Philadelphia, PA: Elsevier; 2008.

Hasin DS. Cannabis withdrawal in the United States: results from NESARC. J Clin Psychiatry. 2008; 69:1354–1363.

Ropper AH, Samuels MA. Adams and Victor's Principles of Neurology, 9th ed. New York, NY: McGraw-Hill; 2009.

2. d, 3. e, 4. c, 5. b, 6. a

Opiate use and intoxication classically are associated with miosis, or pinpoint pupils, not mydriasis. Of note, this must be differentiated from pontine lesions, which can also cause pinpoint pupils. All of the other options can be seen with opiate intoxication, including decreased body temperature and coma. In addition to these findings, common side effects include euphoria, drowsiness, analgesia, and constipation (hence the use of opiates and opiate derivatives as antidiarrheals). Opiate toxicity/overdose creates a "silent gut", which can help in the diagnosis. Because of its cough suppressant effects, codeine is sometimes used in cough medicines.

Treatment of suspected opiate overdose includes the opioid antagonist naloxone at 0.4 to 2 mg intravenously every 2 to 3 minutes. The diagnosis should be questioned if there is no response even after administration of 10 mg. Naltrexone is also an opioid antagonist used in longer-term treatment opioid and alcohol dependence as opposed to naloxone, which is used in emergency settings. Thiamine is classically given before glucose in suspected Wernicke encephalopathy. Flumazenil is given for benzodiazepine overdose. The dose of flumazenil is 0.2 to 0.5 mg intravenously every minute to a maximum total dose of 5 mg.

Opiate withdrawal occurs within hours to several days of cessation. Withdrawal symptoms are often quite severe and cause significant functional impairment. They include dysphoria, myalgias, nausea, vomiting, rhinorrhea, lacrimation, piloerection, diaphoresis, diarrhea, mydriasis, fever, and insomnia. Difficulty often exists in differentiating opiate from sedative (e.g., alcohol, benzodiazepines) withdrawal. Hyperactive deep tendon reflexes (DTRs) can help in this differentiation because increased DTRs are typical in alcohol or sedative withdrawal but not opioid withdrawal. Therefore, if you see increased DTRs and give more opioids for suspected opioid withdrawal in the setting of actual sedative withdrawal, benzodiazepine or alcohol withdrawal seizures will be a likely complication.

Opiates are one of multiple euphoria-producing drugs. All euphoria-producing drugs cause release of dopamine from the midbrain to the forebrain in the reward circuit (ventral tegmental area and the nucleus accumbens). The caudate nucleus is included in this pathway. These areas contain especially high concentrations of dopaminergic synapses. The opiates also interact with other structures modulated by endorphins, including the amygdala, locus coeruleus, arcuate nucleus, thalamus, and the periaqueductal gray matter, which influence dopaminergic pathways indirectly. There are natural and synthetic forms of opiates. Opioid receptors are a group of G-protein coupled receptors, with opioids acting as ligands. The endogenous opioids are dynorphins, enkephalins, endorphins, endomorphins, and ORL_1. There are four major subtypes of opioid receptors. The first is δ, including subtypes δ_1 and δ_2. They are involved with analgesia, antidepressant effects, and physical dependence. The second is κ and includes κ_1, κ_2, and κ_3. These are involved in spinal analgesia, sedation, miosis, and inhibition of antidiuretic hormone release. The third is μ and includes μ_1, μ_2, and μ_3. The subtype μ_1 is involved in supraspinal analgesia and physical dependence; μ_2 is involved in respiratory depression, miosis, euphoria, reduced gastrointestinal motility, and physical dependence. The actions of μ_3 are not clear. The fourth is ORL_1/orphanin, which is involved in anxiety, depression, appetite, and development of tolerance to μ agonists.

Bonci A, Bernardi G, Grillner P, et al. The dopamine-containing neuron: maestro or simple musician in the orchestra of addiction? Trends Pharmacol Sci. 2003; 24:172–177.

Bradley WG, Daroff RB, Fenichel GM, et al. Neurology in Clinical Practice, 5th ed. Philadelphia, PA: Elsevier; 2008.

Corbett AD, Henderson G, McKnight AT, et al. 75 years of opioid research: the exciting but vain quest for the Holy Grail. Br J Pharmacol. 2006; 147(suppl 1):S153-S162.

Gussow L. Myths of toxicology: thiamine before dextrose. Emerg Med News. 2007; 29(4):3–11.

Ropper AH, Samuels MA. Adams and Victor's Principles of Neurology, 9th ed. New York, NY: McGraw-Hill; 2009.

7. d, 8. b, 9. b

Amphetamines work by causing direct release of dopamine and norepinephrine and inhibiting their reuptake. Cocaine works by primarily inhibiting presynaptic reuptake of dopamine (as well as serotonin and norepinephrine). Amphetamine and cocaine use present with similar findings, which include mydriasis (as opposed to opiates, which cause miosis), euphoria, tachycardia, cardiac arrhythmias, hypertension, nausea/vomiting, weight loss, diaphoresis, agitation, anxiety, respiratory depression, seizures, psychosis, formication (sensation of crawling bugs on skin), dyskinesias, and dystonia. Stroke and myocardial infarctions can occur.

Similar to all of the euphoria-producing drugs, the effects of amphetamines and cocaine are predominantly on the reward circuit (the ventral tegmental area and nucleus accumbens). Withdrawal symptoms are also similar with amphetamines and cocaine and include dysphoria, vivid/unpleasant dreams, increased appetite, insomnia or hypersomnia, agitation, or psychomotor retardation. The routes of amphetamine use are oral, nasal (snorting), inhalational (smoking), or intravenous. The routes of cocaine use are nasal (snorting), inhalational (smoking; crack cocaine), intravenous, or oral (chewing coca leaves).

Bradley WG, Daroff RB, Fenichel GM, et al. Neurology in Clinical Practice, 5th ed. Philadelphia, PA: Elsevier; 2008.

Derlet RW, Rice P, Horowitz BZ, et al. Amphetamine toxicity: experience with 127 cases. J Emerg Med. 1989; 7:157–161.

Ritz MC, Lamb RJ, Goldberg SR, et al. Cocaine receptors on dopamine transporters are related to self-administration of cocaine. Science. 1987; 237:1219–1223.

Ropper AH, Samuels MA. Adams and Victor's Principles of Neurology, 9th ed. New York, NY: McGraw-Hill; 2009.

10. c, 11. c, 12. c, 13. b, 14. e, 15. e

This patient has suspected alcohol intoxication. Symptoms include confusion, somnolence, ataxia, dysarthria, hypotension (later hypertension), impaired judgment, and tachycardia. When this is suspected, intravenous thiamine has been classically recommended to precede intravenous glucose administration to avoid precipitation of Wernicke encephalopathy due to acute thiamine deficiency. However, more recent literature raises questions regarding the validity of this practice. Thiamine is converted to thiamine pyrophosphate, which acts as a cofactor in several metabolic pathways necessary in energy metabolism. When there is a high metabolic demand (such as after a glucose load) in the setting of thiamine deficiency, cellular damage occurs and Wernicke encephalopathy may result. Wernicke encephalopathy is characterized by confusion/mental status changes, ataxia, ophthalmoplegia, and nystagmus. The chronic phase of Wernicke encephalopathy is known as Korsakoff syndrome and is associated with anterograde amnesia, although there are components also of retrograde amnesia. MRI findings in Wernicke encephalopathy may include petechial hemorrhages classically in the mammillary bodies, but also in hypothalamus, medial thalami, and periaqueductal gray matter, sometimes even extending into the medulla, with atrophy in chronic stages. Acute thiamine deficiency does not typically lead to changes in the caudate nucleus.

Alcohol and other sedative-hypnotic drugs affect not only the basic structures of the reward circuit but also several other structures that use GABA as a neurotransmitter. GABA is one of the most widespread neurotransmitters in several parts of the brain, including the cortex, the cerebellum, hippocampus, amygdala, and superior and inferior colliculi. Alcohol exerts its effects by stimulation of the GABA$_A$ receptor, similar to the mechanism of action of benzodiazepines. This is why benzodiazepines are used to prevent withdrawal symptoms. Alcohol also inhibits glutamate-induced excitation, which leads to additive CNS-depressant effects.

Chronic alcohol use has detrimental multi-systemic effects. Alcohol withdrawal can be quite severe and can even lead to death if not treated appropriately. Minor withdrawal symptoms begin within 6 to 36 hours from the last drink and include headache, tremors, diaphoresis, palpitations, insomnia, gastrointestinal upset, diarrhea, anorexia, agitation, and anxiety. Mentation is preserved during this period. Seizures can occur generally 6 to 48 hours after the last drink. Alcoholic hallucinosis begins at 12 to 48 hours and includes hallucinations (mostly visual but can also be auditory and tactile), intact orientation, and stable vital signs. Delirium tremens occurs at 48 to 96 hours if adequate prophylaxis is not initiated and is characterized by delirium, hallucinations, disorientation, agitation, encephalopathy, hypertension, tachycardia, arrhythmias, low-grade fever, and diaphoresis. In severe cases, delirium tremens can be fatal. β-Blockers and calcium channel blockers can be used for hypertension and tachycardia, although these will merely mask symptoms. Use of phenytoin or other anticonvulsants is appropriate in those with seizures and pre-existing epilepsy. This history is not present in the patient described, so it is not indicated here. Benzodiazepines such as lorazepam should be given as scheduled doses to prevent withdrawal symptoms (including seizures), and these are the most important medications to add in this setting. Alcohol withdrawal symptoms often occur in unrecognized alcoholic patients who are admitted for surgeries or other reasons. Zolpidem is a nonbenzodiazepine hypnotic used to treat insomnia, and not indicated in this setting.

Bradley WG, Daroff RB, Fenichel GM, et al. Neurology in Clinical Practice, 5th ed. Philadelphia, PA: Elsevier; 2008.

Ropper AH, Samuels MA. Adams and Victor's Principles of Neurology, 9th ed. New York, NY: McGraw-Hill; 2009.

Turner RC, Lichstein PR, Peden JG Jr, et al. Alcohol withdrawal syndromes: a review of pathophysiology, clinical presentation, and treatment. J Gen Intern Med. 1989; 4:432–444.

16. d

Nicotine is an agonist at nicotinic acetylcholine receptors. Nicotine leads to increased levels of several neurotransmitters, especially dopamine, in the reward circuits of the brain. This leads to euphoria, relaxation, and addiction. Nicotine in tobacco stimulates several areas in the reward circuit and its connections, such as the noradrenergic neurons of the locus coeruleus. Several other areas in the brain that secrete acetylcholine, such as the hippocampus and cortex, also appear to be affected by nicotine, and this may explain the increased attentiveness that smokers often describe after nicotine ingestion.

Katzung, Bertram G. Basic and Clinical Pharmacology. New York, NY: McGraw-Hill; 2006.

17. d

Adenosine is a purine nucleotide that is released in the brain, primarily from astrocytes. Adenosine normally inhibits release of excitatory neurotransmitters, leading to reduced neuronal firing rate and decreased cortical excitability. Caffeine competitively antagonizes the adenosine A1 and A2A G-protein–coupled receptor subtypes. The resulting decreased activity of adenosine by caffeine leads to increased release of excitatory neurotransmitters, and thus the stimulating effects noted with caffeine.

Shapiro RE. Caffeine and Headaches. Curr Pain Headache Rep. 2008; 12:311–315.

18. c, 19. e, 20. b, 21. d

This patient exhibits symptoms of intoxication with phenylcyclohexyl piperidine, more commonly known as phencyclidine (PCP). This was a drug developed initially as a dissociative anesthetic, primarily used in animals. It is structurally similar to ketamine, which is used for medical anesthesia. Hypertension, tachycardia, nystagmus (vertical, lateral, horizontal, or rotatory), decreased pain sensation (often causing superhuman appearance of strength), rage, muscle rigidity, seizures, bizarre behaviors, hallucinations, delusions, impaired judgment, confusion, dysarthria, ataxia, and myoclonic jerks are all characteristic findings in PCP intoxication. Its use can also lead to hyperthermia, autonomic instability, and multiorgan failure.

PCP is used by oral, intravenous, or intranasal routes. It acts as a noncompetitive antagonist at the glutamate NMDA receptor. PCP has been shown to affect biogenic amine (dopamine, norepinephrine, serotonin) release and reuptake. These actions probably account for the sympathomimetic effects of PCP.

PCP is structurally similar to ketamine, but it differs from ketamine in that it is longer acting, is more likely to cause seizures, and tends to cause more emergent confusion and delirium. Ketamine also acts as a noncompetitive antagonist of the NMDA receptor. It also has interactions with muscarinic, nicotinic, and cholinergic receptors and inhibits reuptake of norepinephrine, dopamine, and serotonin.

The other choices listed are of the psychedelic, or hallucinogenic, category. Although some symptoms can overlap with PCP intoxication, the symptoms described in this case are characteristic of PCP. Psilocybin (4-phosphoryloxy-N,N-dimethyltryptamine) comes from specific types of mushrooms, and mescaline comes from the peyote cactus. Lysergic acid is one of the ergot fungus' diverse alkaloid components, and lysergic acid diethylamide was popularized as a potent mood-changing and hallucinogenic drug. Use of the different hallucinogens leads to many similar symptoms including sensory distortions (such as synesthesias; "feeling" colors, "seeing" sound), illusions, hallucinations, euphoria, anxiety, tachycardia, palpitations, pupillary dilation (as opposed to opiates, which cause miosis), and diaphoresis. The hallucinogens primarily work at various serotonergic receptors. Different receptor subtypes are modulated by these various drugs, some of which may do so through agonism, whereas others through antagonism. The serotonin $5HT_2$ receptor is particularly thought to be involved in the action of these drugs. Some of these drugs may have some effects at dopamine and norepinephrine receptors. In addition, 3, 4-methylenedioxymethamphetamine (MDMA), or ecstasy, blocks reuptake of serotonin, and prolonged use of MDMA results in destruction of serotonergic neurons in the brain.

Fantegrossi WE, Murnane KS, Reissig CJ. The behavioral pharmacology of hallucinogens. Biochem Pharmacol. 2008; 75(1):17–33.

Romanelli F. Club drugs: methylenedioxymethamphetamine, flunitrazepam, ketamine hydrochloride, and gamma-hydroxybutyrate. Am J Health Syst Pharm. 2002; 59(11):1067–1076.

Ropper AH, Samuels MA. Adams and Victor's Principles of Neurology, 9th ed. New York, NY: McGraw-Hill; 2009.

Smith KM, Larive LL, Fischer C, et al. Reorganization of ascending 5-HT axon projections in animals previously exposed to recreational drug 3,4-methelenedioxymetham-phetamine (MDMA, "Ecstasy"). J Neurosci. 1995; 15(8):5476–5485.

22. e, 23. c

This patient has copper deficiency related to excess zinc intake. This can be related to excess dietary intake (as in this case), overuse of denture cream, parenteral feeding deficiency, and gastrointestinal surgery. This syndrome occurs because zinc increases enterocyte metallothionein synthesis. These excess enterocyte metallothioneins easily bind copper. The resultant excessively bound copper within the enterocytes is then excreted when the enterocytes are sloughed off, resulting in impaired absorption. Copper deficiency myelopathy syndrome resembles the subacute combined degeneration seen with vitamin B_{12} deficiency. Copper deficiency causes a sensorimotor peripheral neuropathy with axonal loss features on electrodiagnostic studies combined with myelopathy in the form of spastic paraparesis and posterior column dysfunction. Pancytopenia is also frequently associated. Copper deficiency is discussed also in Chapter 11. The history of excess zinc makes this more likely than vitamin B_{12} deficiency in this particular patient. Vitamin E deficiency can mimic symptoms of spinocerebellar ataxia, which is not present in this patient.

Goodman BP, Bosch EP, Ross MA, et al. Clinical and electrodiagnostic findings in copper deficiency myeloneuropathy. J Neurol Neurosurg Psychiatry. 2009; 80:524–547.

Kumar N, Gross JB Jr, Ahlskog JE. Copper deficiency myelopathy produces a clinical picture like subacute combined degeneration. Neurology. 2004; 63:33–39.

24. e, 25. a

This patient's neurologic findings are likely the result of vitamin E deficiency related to chronic diarrhea and subsequent malabsorption of fat-soluble vitamins, that is, vitamins D, A, K, and E. These vitamins need to be supplemented, especially vitamin E as in this case. Symptoms resemble a spinocerebellar ataxia syndrome such as Friedrich ataxia and may include ataxia, dysarthria, areflexia, extensor plantar responses, and large fiber sensory loss. Presentation can occur at any age in the setting of chronic diarrhea and malabsorption diseases. Vitamin E deficiency is more likely to occur in childhood when a genetic etiology is present, such as α-tocopherol-transfer protein mutation or abetalipoproteinemia (Bassen-Kornzweig syndrome). Abetalipoproteinemia is caused by a mutation of a microsomal triglyceride transfer protein resulting in absence of apolipoprotein B–containing proteins. Laboratory findings show low vitamin E levels. Acanthocytosis may also be seen on peripheral smear. See discussion to question 22 for copper deficiency, and that to question 27 for vitamin B_{12} deficiency.

Bradley WG, Daroff RB, Fenichel GM, et al. Neurology in Clinical Practice, 5th ed. Philadelphia, PA: Elsevier; 2008.

Ropper AH, Samuels MA. Adams and Victor's Principles of Neurology, 9th ed. New York, NY: McGraw-Hill; 2009.

Satya-Murti S, Howard L, Krohel G, et al. The spectrum of neurologic disorder from vitamin E deficiency. Neurology. 1986; 36:917–921.

26. c

Extensor plantar responses would not be seen in thiamine (vitamin B_1) deficiency. This deficiency would be more likely to cause peripheral neuropathy and flexor plantar responses. Thiamine deficiency in Wernicke-Korsakoff syndrome is discussed in question 10. Thiamine deficiency causes an axonal, sensorimotor peripheral neuropathy with weakness and distal sensory loss. This is termed "dry beriberi." When it is associated with cardiac involvement in the form of cardiomegaly, cardiomyopathy, congestive heart failure, arrhythmia and tachycardia, and peripheral edema, it is called "wet beriberi." Thiamine deficiency has also been reported to cause Leigh syndrome (Leigh subacute necrotizing encephalomyelopathy). Laboratory findings may include decreased serum thiamine, erythrocyte transketolase activity and urinary thiamine, with increased pyruvate and lactate levels, in addition to characteristic electrodiagnostic findings.

Bradley WG, Daroff RB, Fenichel GM, et al. Neurology in Clinical Practice, 5th ed. Philadelphia, PA: Elsevier; 2008.

Pincus JH. Subacute necrotizing encephalomyelopathy (Leigh's disease): a consideration of clinical features and etiology. Dev Med Child Neurol. 1972; 14:87–101.

Tanphaichitr V. In: Shils M (Ed), Modern Nutrition in Health and Medicine, 9th ed. Philadelphia, PA: Lippincott Williams & Wilkins; 2000.

27. d

The neurologic deficits in vitamin B_{12} (cobalamin) deficiency are ultimately related to a defect in methionine production. Vitamin B_{12} is a cofactor for methionine synthase, which is involved in conversion of homocysteine to methionine and production of succinyl-CoA from methylmalonyl-CoA. Methionine is subsequently a precursor for S-adenosyl-L-methionine, which helps with methylation of myelin basic protein. Without this process, abnormal myelin structure results in neurologic deficit. The syndrome resulting from vitamin B_{12} deficiency is called subacute combined degeneration because of sensorimotor peripheral neuropathy combined with myelopathy, spastic paraparesis and posterior column dysfunction. Complete blood cell count may reveal a macrocytic anemia. Occasionally, vitamin B_{12} levels may be in the low normal or even normal range despite true deficiency. If clinical suspicion is present for deficiency, the levels of metabolic intermediaries homocysteine and methylmalonic acid should be checked, both of which would be elevated in vitamin B_{12} deficiency. Animal products (meat and dairy) provide the primary dietary source of vitamin B_{12} for humans. This puts older adults, alcoholics, patients with malnutrition, and strict vegans at high risk for development of deficiency.

Bradley WG, Daroff RB, Fenichel GM, et al. Neurology in Clinical Practice, 5th ed. Philadelphia, PA: Elsevier; 2008.

Green R, Kinsella LJ. Current concepts in the diagnosis of cobalamin deficiency. Neurology. 1995; 45(8):1435–1440.

Hemmer B, Glocker FX, Schumacher M, et al. Subacute combined degeneration: clinical, electrophysiological, and magnetic resonance imaging findings. J Neurol Neurosurg Psychiatry. 1998; 65:822–827.

Lindenbaum J, Savage DG, Stabler SP, et al. Diagnosis of cobalamin deficiency, II: relative sensitivities of serum cobalamin, methylmalonic acid, and total homocysteine concentrations. Am J Hematol. 1990; 34:99–107.

28. d, 29. b

This patient exhibits symptoms consistent with arsenic poisoning. Arsenic is a naturally occurring element most commonly incorporated into organic or inorganic compounds, both of which are very toxic. It can also occur in gas form. With acute exposure, symptoms may develop within minutes to hours and usually begin with gastrointestinal symptoms such as abdominal pain, nausea, vomiting, and diarrhea. A garlic odor on the breath is characteristic. These symptoms can be followed by hypotension, dehydration, and cardiac and respiratory instability. Delirium, encephalopathy, coma, and seizures may occur. Other acute manifestations include proteinuria, hematuria, and acute tubular necrosis. If patients survive, within 1 to 3 weeks, they can develop hepatitis, pancytopenia, and a symmetric sensorimotor peripheral neuropathy, which typically begins with distal paresthesias, followed rapidly by an ascending sensory loss and weakness, which mimics Guillain-Barré syndrome. The neuropathy can progress to intense burning pain, especially in the soles. In addition, dermatologic lesions can occur and may include alopecia, oral mucosal ulcerations, diffuse pruritic macular rash, and scaly rash on the palms and soles. A dry hacking cough and Mees lines (horizontal 1- to 2-mm white lines on the nails) may also occur. In chronic poisoning, the peripheral neuropathy and dermatologic symptoms are usually more prominent than the gastrointestinal symptoms. Cancers of the liver, bladder, kidney, skin, lung, nasal mucosa, and prostate have been reported with chronic exposure.

After a suspected acute ingestion of arsenic, abdominal radiographs may reveal gastrointestinal radiopaque material. Urine arsenic levels are preferable to blood arsenic levels, but both can be used. Fish or shellfish intake within the previous 48–72 hours can cause falsely elevated levels of arsenic. For chronic exposure, hair and nail samples can be analyzed for the presence of arsenic, and 24-hour urine arsenic or spot urine arsenic and creatinine levels can be checked. Additional evaluations should include renal and liver function tests, complete blood cell count, urinalysis, and electrodiagnostic testing if there are symptoms of peripheral neuropathy. A distal sensorimotor axonopathy is the typical finding.

Acute treatment includes fluid and electrolyte replacement, cardiac monitoring, activated charcoal, and chelation therapy. Chelation agents typically used include dimercaprol (British Anti-Lewisite) and meso-2,3-dimercaptosuccinic acid (succimer).

Although symptoms can mimic Guillain-Barré syndrome, the constellation of clinical symptoms and signs described and adequate evaluation should have ruled this out. Cyanide and mercury poisoning are discussed in questions 30 and 31 respectively. Thallium causes acute gastrointestinal symptoms, confusion, painful (mostly sensory) neuropathy with autonomic features, and alopecia, which classically occurs about 2 to 4 weeks after ingestion.

Danan M, Dally S, Conso F. Arsenic-induced encephalopathy. Neurology. 1984; 34:1524.

Flomenbaum N, Goldfrank L, Hoffman R, et al. Goldfrank's Toxicologic Emergencies, 8th ed. New York, NY: McGraw-Hill; 2006.

Windebank AJ. Arsenic. In: Spencer PS, Schaumburg HH (Eds), Experimental and Clinical Neurotoxicology. New York, NY: Oxford University Press; 2000.

Yip L, Dart RC. Arsenic. In: Sullivan JB, Krieger GR (Eds), Clinical Environmental Health and Toxic Exposures. Philadelphia, PA: Lippincott Williams & Wilkins; 2001.

30. e

This patient exhibits symptoms of cyanide poisoning. In industrialized countries, the most common cause of cyanide poisoning are domestic fires due to combustion of products containing carbon and nitrogen, such as wool, silk, polyurethane (insulation/upholstery), and plastics. There are many industrial causes, such as electroplating in this case. There are also dietary causes, especially from ingestion of plant products from the family Rosaceae, including the seeds and pits of the plum, peach, pear, bitter almond, cherry laurel, apricot, and apple.

Cyanide is a rapidly lethal mitochondrial toxin that can cause death within minutes to hours of exposure. Cyanide competes with oxygen and binds to the ferric ion (Fe^{3+}) of cytochrome oxidase a_3, which inhibits this final enzyme in the mitochondrial cytochrome complex, resulting in cessation of oxidative phosphorylation. As a result, cells cannot use oxygen in their electron transport chain and must switch to anaerobic metabolism. Because of the decreased utilization of oxygen by tissues, venous oxyhemoglobin concentration will be high, making venous blood appear bright red and thus, the bright red coloration of skin, similar to the effects of carbon monoxide. Cyanide also causes toxic oxygen free radicals, release of glutamate, and inhibition of glutamic acid decarboxylase (the enzyme that helps form the inhibitory neurotransmitter GABA).

CNS symptoms include headache, anxiety, abnormal taste, encephalopathy, vertigo, and seizures. Cardiovascular symptoms include chest pain, initial tachycardia, and hypertension, then bradycardia and hypotension, atrioventricular block, and arrhythmias. Respiratory symptoms include initial tachypnea, then bradypnea and pulmonary edema. Gastrointestinal symptoms include nausea, vomiting, and abdominal pain. Skin symptoms include flushing, cherry-red color. Cyanosis may occur late. Renal and hepatic failure may also occur.

Laboratory evaluation reveals severe metabolic acidosis with increased anion gap, elevated lactate level, and elevated blood cyanide level. Levels of more than 3.0 mg/L correlate with death. Treatment must be initiated quickly, and includes removal of the cyanide source (such as from the skin) and activated charcoal. The Taylor Cyanide Antidote Package may be used. This includes amyl nitrite, sodium nitrite, and sodium thiosulfate. Hydroxocobalamin is also used to directly bind and neutralize cyanide and is often combined with sodium thiosulfate. See discussion to question 32 for carbon monoxide poisoning, question 31 for mercury poisoning, and question 28 and 29 for arsenic and thallium poisoning.

Greenberg MI, Hamilton RJ, Phillips SD. Occupational, Industrial, and Environmental Toxicology. St Louis, MO: Mosby; 1997.

Morocco AP. Cyanides. Crit Care Clin. 2005; 21:691–705.

Sauer SW, Keim ME. Hydroxocobalamin: improved public health readiness for cyanide disasters. Ann Emerg Med. 2001; 37:635–641.

Vogel S, Sultan T, Ten Eyck R. Cyanide poisoning. Clin Toxicol. 1981; 18:367–383.

31. c

This man exhibits symptoms consistent with mercury toxicity, likely from years of exposure in a mercury mine. The organic forms of mercury are the most toxic, such as dimethylmercury and methylmercury. Some fish and shellfish concentrate mercury in the form of methylmercury. However, inorganic forms of mercury, such as cinnabar, are also highly toxic by ingestion or inhalation of the dust. Besides mining, other occupational exposures to mercury include dentistry, chloralkali industries, and thermometer factories. It was called "mad hatter's disease" in the past because hat makers frequently worked with mercury to set and shape hats. If inhaled, a fatal interstitial pneumonitis may occur. It can be absorbed through the skin and orally ingested. Other symptoms include severe intention tremor, cerebellar ataxia, paresthesias, tender and inflamed gums, excessive salivation, swollen salivary glands, change in personality, and psychiatric symptoms such as anxiety, irritability, fearfulness, memory loss, depression, and fatigue. Treatment includes chelation therapy with British Anti-Lewisite, penicillamine, 2,3 dimercaptopropane-1-sulfonate, and dimercaptosuccinic acid. See discussion to question 33 for lead poisoning, question 34 for manganese toxicity, Chapter 12 for FTD, and questions 28 and 29 for thallium toxicity.

Berlin M. Mercury. In: Friberg L, Nordberg GF, Vouk VB (Eds), Handbook on the Toxicology of Metals, Vol. II. Amsterdam, The Netherlands: Elsevier; 1986.

Schutte NP, Knight AL, Jahn O. Mercury and its compounds. In: Zenz C, Dickerson OB, Horovath EP (Eds), Occupational Medicine, 3rd ed. St Louis, MO: Mosby; 1994.

32. d

This woman has carbon monoxide (CO) poisoning. It commonly occurs at the change of seasons as winter months approach and people turn on their furnaces. Other family members in the same household may have similar symptoms, which gives a clue to diagnosis. CO is an odorless, tasteless, colorless gas. It binds to the iron moiety of heme in hemoglobin with much higher affinity than does oxygen, forming carboxyhemoglobin, which results in impaired oxygen transport and utilization. It competes with oxygen in binding hemoglobin. This binding leads to a structural change, which limits the ability of the other three oxygen binding sites to release oxygen to peripheral tissues and hence the cherry-red flushed coloration. It can also lead to CNS lipid peroxidation and delayed neurologic sequelae. Some sources include poorly functioning heating systems and improperly vented fuel-burning devices such as kerosene heaters, charcoal grills, camping stoves, gasoline-powered generators, and motor vehicles. Symptoms most commonly include headache, nausea, malaise, dizziness, and cherry-red skin coloration. Severe toxicity can cause seizures, encephalopathy, coma, and cardiovascular instability. Diagnosis is based on clinical history and elevated carboxyhemoglobin levels (which may be normally elevated to an extent in smokers). Treatment should include high-flow 100% oxygen via a nonrebreather mask. In severe cases, histopathology in chronic stages reveals necrosis in the globus pallidus and confluent areas of necrosis in subcortical white matter.

Ernst A, Zibrak JD. Carbon monoxide poisoning. N Engl J Med. 1998; 339:1603–1608.

Harper A, Croft-Baker J. Carbon monoxide poisoning: undetected by both patients and their doctors. Age Ageing. 2004; 33:105–109.

Kao LW, Nanagas KA. Carbon monoxide poisoning. Emerg Med Clin North Am. 2004; 22(4):985–1018.

33. c

This boy most likely has lead intoxication, especially given the timing of symptoms in relation to moving into a very old house. Given this scenario, one must be concerned about the possibility of lead intoxication as lead-based paint in old houses has been a frequent etiology, especially in children. Many other occupational exposures are possible but would be seen more in adults. Lead inhibits the sulfhydryl-dependent enzymes such as γ-aminolevulinic acid dehydratase and ferrochelatase in heme synthesis, which causes disruption of hemoglobin synthesis and leads to the production of free erythrocyte protoporphyrins. Lead also competes with calcium in several biologic systems and processes, such as mitochondrial respiration and nerve functions, and has been implicated as contributing mechanisms in neurotoxicity. Common symptoms of lead toxicity include abdominal pain (lead colic), constipation, myalgias, arthralgias, seizures, psychomotor slowing, headache, and anorexia. Basophilic stippling of red blood cells and microcytic hypochromic anemia are often seen. In addition, a bluish pigmentation at the gum-tooth line is sometimes seen. A peripheral neuropathy classically with extensor weakness or "wrist/ankle drop" is associated with lead toxicity and is due to an axonal degeneration that primarily affects motor nerves. Generally, removal from the lead source is the only treatment needed, although chelation therapy with 2,3-dimercaptosuccinic acid succimer, and calcium disodium ethylenediaminetetraacetate are also available.

Cullen MR, Robins JM, Eskenazi B. Adult inorganic lead intoxication: presentation of 31 new cases and a review of recent advances in the literature. Medicine (Baltimore). 1983; 62:221–247.

Fischbein A, Hu H. Occupational and environmental exposure to lead. In: Environmental and Occupational Medicine, Rom WN, Markowitz SB (Eds), Philadelphia, PA: Wolters Kluwer/Lippincott Williams & Wilkins; 2007.

Thomson RM, Parry GJ. Neuropathies associated with excessive exposure to lead. Muscle Nerve. 2006; 33:732–741.

34. b

This patient most likely has manganese toxicity. It is most commonly seen in those with chronic liver disease (impaired biliary excretion), those receiving total parenteral nutrition containing manganese, and those in the welding and steel industries. Symptoms include parkinsonian features, tremors, incoordination, confusion, personality changes, hallucinations, agitation, psychosis (manganese madness), memory disturbances, headache, and aggression. Brain MRI may show high T1 signal predominantly in the globus pallidus. Chelation therapy with ethylenediaminetetraacetate has been used as treatment. Parkinson's disease is discussed in Chapter 6, lead toxicity in question 33, and copper deficiency in question 22. Although this patient could certainly be malnourished, parkinsonian features do not result from malnutrition.

Fell JM, Reynolds AP, Meadows N, et al. Manganese toxicity in children receiving long-term parenteral nutrition. Lancet. 1996; 347:1218–1221.

McMillan DE. A brief history of the neurobehavioral toxicity of manganese: some unanswered questions. Neurotoxicology. 1999; 20:499–507.

Wedler FC. Biochemical and nutritional role of manganese: an overview. In: Klimis-Tavantzis DJ (Ed), Manganese in Health and Disease. Boca Raton, FL: CRC Press; 1994.

35. e

This man likely has methanol poisoning from ingestion of a household product in an attempt to ingest alcohol. Methanol and ethylene glycol are found in automotive antifreeze, de-icing solutions, antifreeze, and windshield wiper fluid and solvents, among others. Symptoms include nausea, headache, visual complaints, blindness, dizziness and encephalopathy, inebriation, and sedation. Findings classically include necrosis of optic nerves and the putamen on neuroimaging. Toxicity occurs when methanol is oxidized by alcohol dehydrogenase and aldehyde dehydrogenase, forming the metabolite formate. Formate causes retinal injury and permanent blindness and injury to the basal ganglia (especially putamen). Fomepizole can also be used as treatment, which acts as an alcohol dehydrogenase inhibitor. Ethanol can also be used to competitively bind to alcohol dehydrogenase, preventing breakdown of methanol into its toxic metabolites. Treatment also consists of correction of systemic acidosis.

Acrylamide can cause seizures, encephalopathy, and peripheral neuropathy. Hexacarbon solvents are found in paints, glues (glue sniffing), and solvents, and they also cause peripheral neuropathy, euphoria, hallucinations, and headache. These symptoms do not fit with this patient's clinical presentation, especially blindness.

Kerns W, Tomaszewski C, McMartin K, et al. Formate kinetics in methanol poisoning. J Toxicol Clin Toxicol. 2002; 40:137–143.

Liesivuori J, Savolainen H. Methanol and formic acid toxicity: biochemical mechanisms. Pharmacol Toxicol. 1991; 69:157–163.

Sivilotti ML, Burns MJ, Aaron CK, et al. Reversal of severe methanol-induced visual impairment: no evidence of retinal toxicity due to fomepizole. J Toxicol Clin Toxicol. 2001; 39:627–631.

36. d

This patient likely has organophosphate/carbamate poisoning related to the use of insecticide/pesticide. The only listed item that is not recommended in this clinical situation is gastric lavage because of a substantial risk of aspiration, given the increased secretions and decreased mental status in many patients. Organophosphates and carbamates are potent cholinesterase inhibitors leading to severe cholinergic toxicity. Toxicity can result from ingestion, cutaneous exposure, or inhalation. Some organophosphates are also used as terrorist nerve agents and include tabun, sarin, and soman.

Two common mnemonics used to remember the cholinergic/muscarinic crisis signs are as follows:

SLUDGE: Salivation, Lacrimation, Urination, Defecation, Gastric Emesis

DUMBELS: Defecation, Urination, Miosis, Bronchorrhea/Bronchospasm/Bradycardia, Emesis, Lacrimation, Salivation

Often these patients will develop the "intermediate syndrome," approximately 12 to 96 hours after exposure that consists of weakness, fasciculations, tachycardia, hypertension, decreased deep tendon reflexes, cranial nerve abnormalities, proximal muscle weakness, and respiratory insufficiency. In addition, some organophosphates can cause organophosphorus-induced delayed neuropathy, occurring 2 to 3 weeks after exposure. Symptoms include painful but transient "stocking-glove" paresthesias followed by a symmetrical motor polyneuropathy with flaccid weakness of the lower extremities, which ascends to the upper extremities. Neurobehavioral symptoms may also occur as chronic sequelae.

Atropine competes with acetylcholine at muscarinic receptors to help prevent cholinergic activation. Since atropine does not bind to nicotinic receptors, it is ineffective in treating neuromuscular dysfunction, so the cholinesterase-reactivating agent pralidoxime is typically given concurrently with atropine and is effective in treating manifestations resulting from activation of both muscarinic and nicotinic receptors. Benzodiazepines are used for organophosphate-related seizures and sometimes for seizure prophylaxis. Activated charcoal is recommended if presentation is within 1 hour of ingestion. Gastric lavage is not recommended as mentioned earlier.

Eddleston M, Roberts D, Buckley N. Management of severe organophosphorus pesticide poisoning. Crit Care. 2001; 5(4):211–215.

Moretto A, Lotti M. Poisoning by organophosphorus insecticides and sensory neuropathy. J Neurol Neurosurg Psychiatry. 1998; 64:463–468.

Roberts DM, Aaron CK. Managing acute organophosphorus pesticide poisoning. Br Med J. 2007; 334:629–634.

Rusyniak DE, Nañagas KA. Organophosphate poisoning. Semin Neurol. 2004; 24(2): 197–204.

Sevim S, Aktekin M, Dogu O, et al. Late onset polyneuropathy due to organophosphate (DDVP) intoxication. Can J Neurol Sci. 2003; 30:75–78.

37. c

This patient describes symptoms most consistent with botulism, likely related to foodborne source from home canning. Botulism is a potentially life-threatening neuroparalytic syndrome resulting from exposure to botulinum toxin, produced by *Clostridium botulinum*. There are at least eight distinct types of botulinum toxin, although the most commonly involved is botulinum toxin A. There are multiple forms of botulism including foodborne botulism (ingestion of food contaminated by botulinum toxin), wound botulism (infection of a wound by *C. botulinum*, with subsequent production of neurotoxin), infantile botulism (ingestion of clostridial spores that then colonize the gastrointestinal tract and release toxin), adult enteric infectious botulism (toxin produced in the gastrointestinal tract), and inhalational botulism (aerosolized toxin related to acts of bioterrorism).

Botulinum toxin binds to the synaptotagmin II receptor on presynaptic cholinergic synapses and neuromuscular junctions. After the heavy chain of the toxin binds to the receptors, the light chain translocates into the nerve cell via endocytosis. Upon entering the cytoplasm, the toxin irreversibly inhibits acetylcholine release by cleaving various proteins involved in neuroexocytosis of acetylcholine. Botulinum toxin A and E cleave SNAP-25; botulinum toxin C cleaves SNAP-25 and syntaxin; and botulinum B, D, F, and G cleave synaptobrevin. Reversal of this inhibition requires sprouting of a new presynaptic terminal and formation of a new synapse. This generally takes 3 to 6 months. Although the toxin can be quite harmful, these effects are used for therapeutic purposes, such as for the treatment of dystonia, spasticity, and other neurologic disorders.

Symptoms related to foodborne botulism may begin within 12 to 36 hours after ingestion of the toxin but may be delayed for several days. Symptoms include acute onset of multiple cranial neuropathies, blurred vision (due to fixed pupillary dilation), symmetric descending weakness, urinary retention, and constipation. Gastrointestinal symptoms such as diarrhea, abdominal pain, nausea, and vomiting often precede neurologic symptoms in foodborne botulism.

Symptoms are not consistent with myasthenia gravis (there is no diurnal variation or other historical points to suggest fatigability; discussed in Chapter 10), Lambert-Eaton myasthenic syndrome (discussed in Chapter 10), or Guillain-Barré syndrome (which presents with ascending, not descending, weakness and without pupillary involvement; discussed in Chapter 9). He has no history of cancer and is otherwise healthy, making leptomeningeal carcinomatosis unlikely, especially with the abrupt onset of symptoms.

Abrutyn E. Botulism. In: Fauci AS, Isselbacher KJ, Braunwald E, et al. (Eds), Principles of Internal Medicine, 14th ed. New York, NY: McGraw-Hill; 1998.

Hughes JM, Blumenthal JR, Merson MH, et al. Clinical features of types A and B food-borne botulism. Ann Intern Med. 1981; 95:442–445.

Jin R, Rummel A, Binz T, et al. Botulinum neurotoxin B recognizes its protein receptor with high affinity and specificity. Nature. 2006; 444(7122):1019–1020.

Buzz Phrases	Key Points
Pinpoint pupils	Opiate overdose (also pontine lesions)
Wernicke encephalopathy	Thiamine deficiency
Confusion, ataxia, ophthalmoplegia, nystagmus	Wernicke encephalopathy tetrad
Wernicke treatment	Thiamine before glucose (vitamins before dessert)
Hemorrhagic mammillary bodies	Wernicke encephalopathy
Wet beriberi (thiamine deficiency)	Peripheral edema, cardiomegaly, cardiomyopathy, congestive heart failure, arrhythmia, and tachycardia
Dry beriberi (thiamine deficiency)	Sensorimotor peripheral neuropathy with weakness and distal sensory loss
Vitamin B_{12} deficiency	Subacute combined degeneration
Garlic breath	Arsenic poisoning
Almond odor	Cyanide
Alopecia and painful neuropathy	Thallium
Cherry-red skin	Carbon monoxide and cyanide poisoning
Wrist and foot drop in a patient with encephalopathy	Lead poisoning
Optic nerve necrosis	Methanol poisoning
Globus pallidus necrosis	Carbon monoxide
Putamen necrosis	Methanol

Index

Note: Page numbers followed by *f* and *t* indicate figures and tables respectively

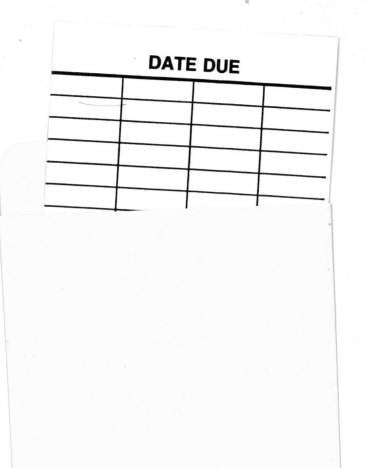

DATE DUE